## SIXTH EDITION

# Adult-Gerontology Nurse Practitioner CERTIFICATION REVIEW GUIDE

*Edited by*

**Sally K. Miller, PhD, AGPCNP-BC, AGACNP-BC, FAANP**

*Clinical Professor*
Drexel University College of Nursing and Health Professions
Philadelphia, Pennsylvania

*Nurse Practitioner*
Nevada Health Centers
Carson City, Nevada

JONES & BARTLETT
LEARNING

**World Headquarters**
Jones & Bartlett Learning
5 Wall Street
Burlington, MA 01803
978-443-5000
info@jblearning.com
www.jblearning.com

Jones & Bartlett Learning books and products are available through most bookstores and online booksellers. To contact Jones & Bartlett Learning directly, call 800-832-0034, fax 978-443-8000, or visit our website, www.jblearning.com.

Substantial discounts on bulk quantities of Jones & Bartlett Learning publications are available to corporations, professional associations, and other qualified organizations. For details and specific discount information, contact the special sales department at Jones & Bartlett Learning via the above contact information or send an email to specialsales@jblearning.com.

Copyright © 2016 by Jones & Bartlett Learning, LLC, an Ascend Learning Company

All rights reserved. No part of the material protected by this copyright may be reproduced or utilized in any form, electronic or mechanical, including photocopying, recording, or by any information storage and retrieval system, without written permission from the copyright owner.

The content, statements, views, and opinions herein are the sole expression of the respective authors and not that of Jones & Bartlett Learning, LLC. Reference herein to any specific commercial product, process, or service by trade name, trademark, manufacturer, or otherwise does not constitute or imply its endorsement or recommendation by Jones & Bartlett Learning, LLC and such reference shall not be used for advertising or product endorsement purposes. All trademarks displayed are the trademarks of the parties noted herein. *Adult-Gerontology Nurse Practitioner Certification Review Guide, Sixth Edition* is an independent publication and has not been authorized, sponsored, or otherwise approved by the owners of the trademarks or service marks referenced in this product.

There may be images in this book that feature models; these models do not necessarily endorse, represent, or participate in the activities represented in the images. Any screenshots in this product are for educational and instructive purposes only. Any individuals and scenarios featured in the case studies throughout this product may be real or fictitious, but are used for instructional purposes only.

The authors, editor, and publisher have made every effort to provide accurate information. However, they are not responsible for errors, omissions, or for any outcomes related to the use of the contents of this book and take no responsibility for the use of the products and procedures described. Treatments and side effects described in this book may not be applicable to all people; likewise, some people may require a dose or experience a side effect that is not described herein. Drugs and medical devices are discussed that may have limited availability controlled by the Food and Drug Administration (FDA) for use only in a research study or clinical trial. Research, clinical practice, and government regulations often change the accepted standard in this field. When consideration is being given to use of any drug in the clinical setting, the health care provider or reader is responsible for determining FDA status of the drug, reading the package insert, and reviewing prescribing information for the most up-to-date recommendations on dose, precautions, and contraindications, and determining the appropriate usage for the product. This is especially important in the case of drugs that are new or seldom used.

**Production Credits**
VP, Executive Publisher: Dave Cella
Executive Editor: Amanda Martin
Acquisitions Editor: Teresa Reilly
Associate Acquisitions Editor: Rebecca Myrick
Production Editor: Sarah Bayle
Marketing Communications Manager: Katie Hennessy
Art Development Editor: Joanna Lundeen
Art Development Assistant: Shannon Sheehan
VP, Manufacturing and Inventory Control: Therese Connell
Composition: diacriTech
Cover Design: Scott Moden
Manager of Photo Research, Rights & Permissions: Lauren Miller
Cover Image: © Libi Ostrovsky/ShutterStock, Inc.
Printing and Binding: Edwards Brothers Malloy
Cover Printing: Edwards Brothers Malloy

To order this product, use ISBN: 978-1-284-04967-1

**Library of Congress Cataloging-in-Publication Data**
Adult nurse practitioner certification review guide
Adult-gerontology nurse practitioner certification review guide / [edited by] Sally Miller. — Sixth edition.
  p. ; cm.
Preceded by Adult nurse practitioner certification review guide. 5th ed. / [edited by] Sally K. Miller. c2013.
 Includes bibliographical references and index.
 ISBN 978-1-284-06552-7
 I. Miller, Sally K., editor. II. Title.
 [DNLM: 1. Nurse Practitioners—Examination Questions. 2. Nurse Practitioners—Outlines. 3. Geriatric Nursing—Examination Questions. 4. Geriatric Nursing—Outlines. 5. Nursing Process—Examination Questions. 6. Nursing Process—Outlines. 7. Primary Nursing—Examination Questions. 8. Primary Nursing—Outlines. WY 18.2]
 RT82.8
 610.7306'92–dc23
                2014025423

6048

Printed in the United States of America
18 17 16 15 14  10 9 8 7 6 5 4 3 2 1

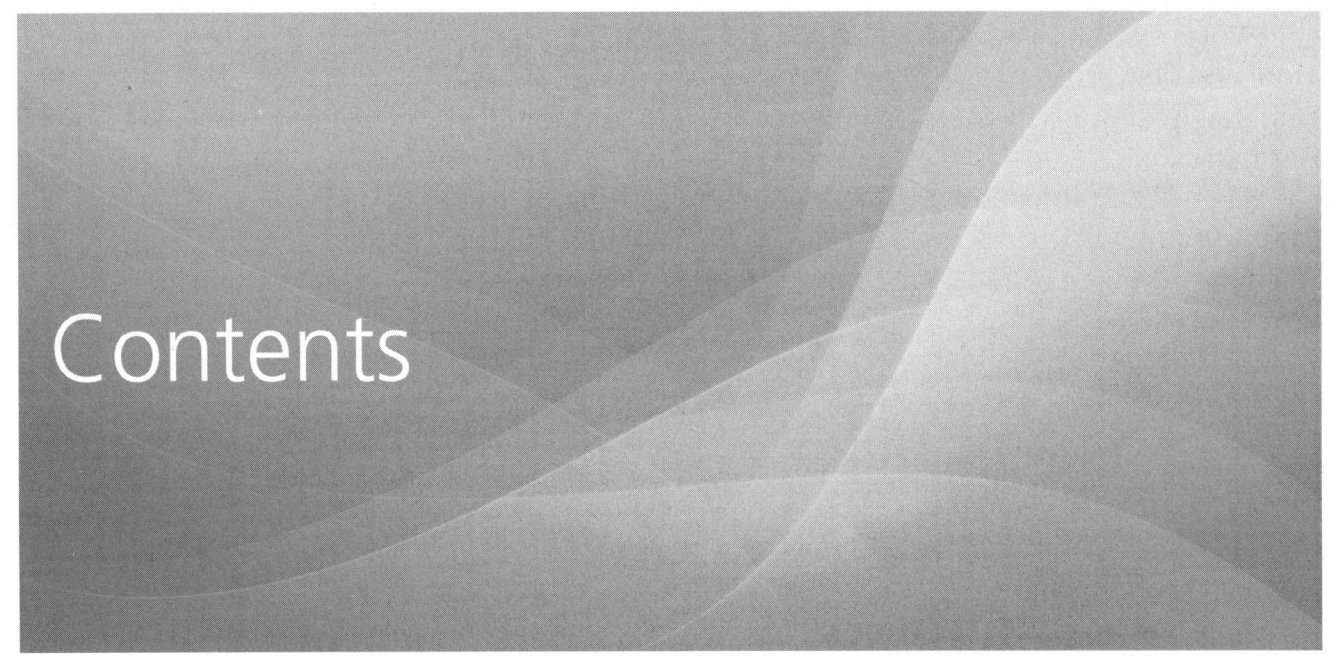

# Contents

Preface vii
Acknowledgments ix
Contributing Authors xi

## Section I
## Core Curriculum   1

### Chapter 1
### Test-Taking Strategies and Techniques   3

*Nancy A. Dickenson-Hazard*
*Virginia L. Millonig*

Strategy 1: Know Yourself   3
Strategy 2: Develop Your Thinking Skills   4
Strategy 3: Know the Content   6
Strategy 4: Become Test-Wise   9
Strategy 5: Psych Yourself Up: Taking Tests Is Stressful   11
Bibliography   12

### Chapter 2
### Health Promotion and Evaluation   15

*Rosanne H. Pruitt*

Theoretical Aspects: Health Promotion Theories and Models   15
Related Concepts   16
Lifestyle/Health Behaviors   17
Health Evaluation Across the Life Span   22
Questions   28
Answers   29
Bibliography   29

### Chapter 3
### Special Considerations in the Gerontological Patient   31

*Debbie Gilbert Kramer*

Demographics of Older Adults   31
Theories of Biological Aging   32
Theories of Psychosocial Aging   33
Interview and Health History   34
Living Situations and Income Status   36
Functional Assessment   36
Physical Assessment   37
Pharmacotherapy and the Elderly   40
Questions   42
Answers   44
Bibliography   45

### Chapter 4
### Dermatological Disorders   47

*Sylvia Torres Fletcher*
*Susan E. Chaney*

Acne Vulgaris 47
Alopecia 48
Bacterial Infections/Pyodermas 49
Dermatitis 51
Fungal and Yeast Infections 53
Papulosquamous Disorders 54
Scabies 56
Skin Cancer 56
Viral Dermatoses 58
Questions 61
Answers 63
Bibliography 64

## Chapter 5
**Eye, Ear, Nose, and Throat Disorders 65**

*Margaret Hadro Venzke*

Conjunctivitis 65
Blepharitis 67
Foreign Body in Eye 67
Corneal Abrasion 68
Glaucoma 68
Cataracts 70
Acute Otitis Media (AOM) 70
Serous Otitis Media (SOM) 71
Otitis Externa 71
Hearing Loss 72
Vertigo 73
Epistaxis 74
Nasopharyngitis 75
Influenza 75
Pharyngitis 76
Infectious Mononucleosis 77
Allergic Rhinitis 78
Sinusitis 79
Questions 81
Answers 84
Bibliography 84

## Chapter 6
**Respiratory Disorders 85**

*Margaret Hadro Venzke*

Pulmonary Function Tests 85
Acute Bronchitis 86
Pneumonia 87
Asthma 88
Chronic Obstructive Pulmonary Disease (COPD) 90
Tuberculosis (TB) 91
Lung Cancer 93
Questions 97
Answers 100
Bibliography 100

## Chapter 7
**Cardiovascular Disorders 101**

*Sally K. Miller*

Hypertension (HTN) 101
Coronary Artery Disease (CAD) 103
Dyslipidemia 106
Congestive Heart Failure (CHF) 107
Peripheral Arterial Disease (PAD) 108
Thrombophlebitis 109
Chronic Venous Insufficiency 109
Pericarditis 110
Endocarditis 110
Questions 113
Answers 115
Bibliography 115

## Chapter 8
**Hematological and Oncological Disorders 117**

*Sister Maria Salerno*

Common Anemias 117
Microcytic Anemias (MCV < 80 m$^3$) 117
Iron-Deficiency Anemia 117
Thalassemia 120
Macrocytic Anemias (MCV > 100 m$^3$) 121
Pernicious Anemia 121
Folic Acid–Deficiency Anemia 122
Normocytic Anemias (MCV 80–100 m$^3$) 124
Anemia of Chronic Disease (ACD) 124
Sickle Cell Anemia 124
Leukemia 125
Non-Hodgkin's Lymphoma 126

Hodgkin's Disease 127
Questions 130
Answers 132
Bibliography 132

## Chapter 9
**Gastrointestinal Disorders 135**

*Sister Maria Salerno*

Peptic Ulcer Disease (PUD) 135
Gastroesophageal Reflux Disease 138
Cholecystitis 139
Appendicitis 140
Diverticulitis 141
Viral Hepatitis 142
Acute Gastroenteritis 145
Irritable Bowel Syndrome (IBS) (Functional Bowel Syndrome) 148
Inflammatory Bowel Disease 149
Colorectal Cancer 150
Questions 153
Answers 156
Bibliography 156

## Chapter 10
**Endocrine Disorders 159**

*Sister Maria Salerno*

Diabetes Mellitus (DM) 159
Thyrotoxicosis 166
Adult Hypothyroidism 168
Thyroid Nodule 170
Cushing's Syndrome (Hypercortisolism) 170
Addison's Disease (Primary Adrenocortical Insufficiency) 171
Questions 176
Answers 179
Bibliography 179

## Chapter 11
**Genitourinary and Gynecological Disorders 181**

*Pamela A. Shuler*
*Mary D. Knudtson*

Acquired Immunodeficiency Syndrome (AIDS) 181
Gonorrhea (Uncomplicated Gonococcal Infections) 184
Genital Chlamydial Infection 185
Syphilis 186
Herpes Genitalis 188
Genital Warts (Condylomata Acuminata) 189
Pelvic Inflammatory Disease (PID) 191
Vulvovaginitis 192
Lower Urinary Tract Infection (LUTI; Cystitis: Acute, Uncomplicated) 194
Acute Pyelonephritis (Upper UTI) 195
Acute Bacterial Prostatitis 196
Chronic Bacterial Prostatitis 196
Epididymitis 197
Benign Prostatic Hyperplasia (BPH) 198
Prostate Cancer 199
Fibrocystic Breast Changes 200
Breast Cancer 200
Dysfunctional Uterine Bleeding (DUB) 201
Dysplasia: Abnormal Papanicolaou (Pap) Smear Management 203
Amenorrhea 205
Dysmenorrhea 206
Premenstrual Syndrome (PMS) 206
Questions 208
Answers 212
Bibliography 212

## Chapter 12
**Musculoskeletal and Associated Immunological Disorders 213**

*Madeline Turkeltaub*

Osteoarthritis (OA) 213
Rheumatoid Arthritis (RA) 214
Systemic Lupus Erythematosus (SLE) 216
Giant Cell Arteritis 217
Gout 217
Osteoporosis 218
Low Back Pain (LBP) 220
Bursitis 221

Epicondylitis (Tennis Elbow) 222
Carpal Tunnel Syndrome 222
Knee Pain 223
Ankle Sprain 224
Muscle Strain 224
Questions 225
Answers 227
Bibliography 228

## Chapter 13
## Neurological Disorders 229

*Sally K. Miller*

Headache 229
Tension Headaches 230
Migraine Headache 230
Cluster Headaches 232
Transient Ischemic Attack (TIA) 232
Seizure Disorder 234
Parkinson's Disease 236
Multiple Sclerosis (MS) 237
Dementia 238
Questions 242
Answers 245
Bibliography 245

## Chapter 14
## Psychosocial Disorders 247

*Sister Maria Salerno*

Depression (Major) 247
Suicide 251
Anxiety 253
Alcoholism 255
Psychoactive Substance Abuse 257
Delirium (Acute Confusion) 259
Questions 261
Answers 264
Bibliography 264

## Chapter 15
## Advanced Practice, Role Development, Current Trends, and Health Policy 267

*Leanne C. Busby*
*Mary A. Baroni*

Introduction 267
Advanced Practice Nursing 267
Role Development 268
Advanced Practice Trends and Issues 269
Health Policy 276
Health Insurance Portability and Accountability Act of 1996 (HIPAA): Public Law 104-191 279
Evidence-Based Practice 280
Questions 281
Answers 284
Bibliography 284

## Appendix A
## Supplement for the Primary Care Provider 287

*Beth M. Kelsey*
*Susan B. Moskosky*

Pregnancy 289
Fertility Control 301
Intrauterine Devices/Systems 307
Menopause 315
Questions 319
Answers 324
Bibliography 324

## Appendix B
## Supplement for the Acute Care Provider 325

*Sally K. Miller*

Management of the Preoperative Patient 327
Management of the Postoperative Patient 330
Common Problems in Acute Care 334
The Transplant Patient 348
Shock States 349
Questions 351
Answers 356
Bibliography 356

Index 357

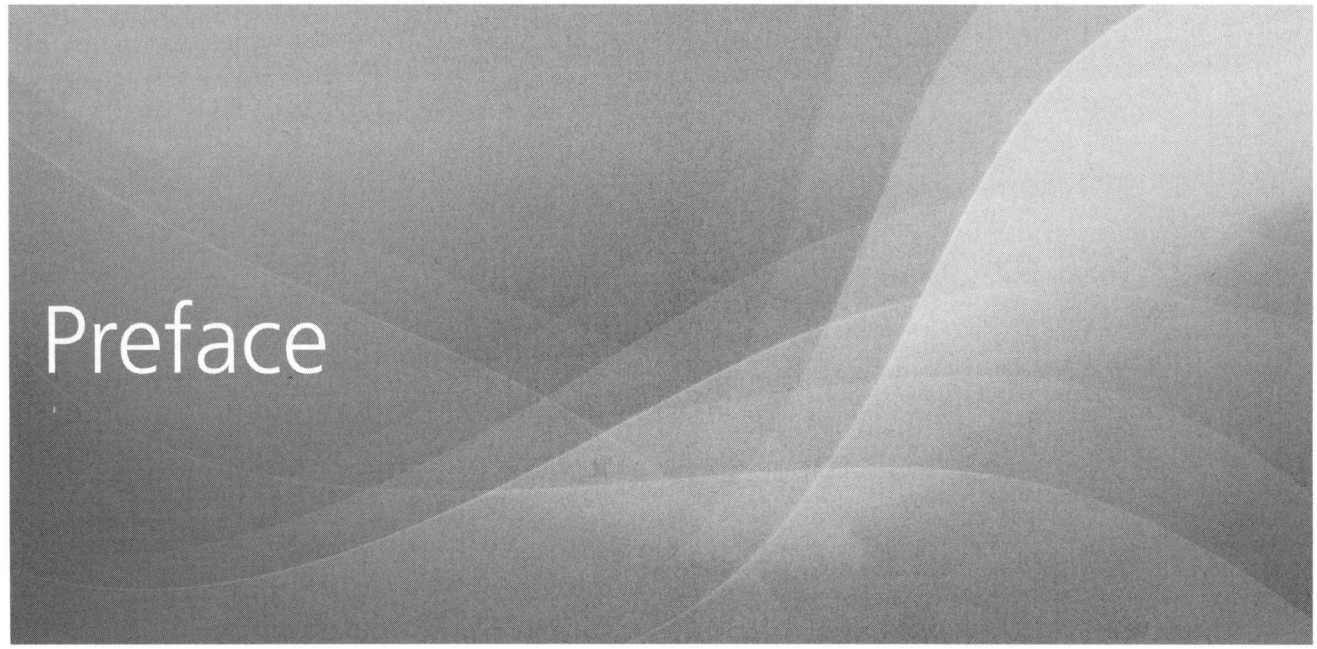

# Preface

The sixth edition of this text has been developed especially for adult–gerontology nurse practitioners preparing to take a national board certification examination in both the primary care and acute care specialties. This revised edition is developed with the understanding that the majority of clinical content in adult gerontology is relevant to both primary and acute care certification examinations, but that each specialty examination is also characterized by content specific to its setting. Therefore, core chapters are presented, along with two new appendices, each containing focused content for primary care and acute care providers, respectively. This text is also an excellent tool for use in the clinical area for those who need an abbreviated but comprehensive current clinical practice reference. All sections have been extensively revised and updated for primary and acute care providers. The practice questions have also been revised as appropriate and the chapter bibliographies updated and enhanced.

The purpose of the text is threefold. It can be used by student nurse practitioners as they progress through their academic programs, it will assist new graduates and returning clinicians engaged in self-study preparation for certification examinations, and finally, the text can be used as a reference guide in the practice setting.

The text has been organized to provide the reader with test-taking strategies first. This introductory chapter is followed by a chapter on health promotion. The next 12 chapters address common disorders and provide succinct summaries of definitions, etiology, signs and symptoms, physical findings, differential diagnoses, diagnostic evaluation, and clinical management. The final chapter addresses health policy, role, trends, and professional issues for the nurse practitioner in the healthcare industry at large.

At the end of each chapter are test questions, which are intended to help the reader assess recall and application of content and serve as an introduction to the testing arena. In addition, a bibliography is included for those who need a more in-depth discussion of the subject matter in each chapter. These references can serve as additional instructional material for the reader.

Many nurses preparing for certification examinations find that reviewing an extensive body of scientific knowledge requires a very difficult search of many sources that must be synthesized to provide a review base for the examination. This publication provides a succinct yet comprehensive review of the core material.

The editor is certified both as an adult-gerontology primary care nurse practitioner and adult-gerontology acute care nurse practitioner. All contributing authors are certified nurse practitioners. They have designed this text to help potential examinees prepare for success in the certification examination process, as well as enhance their clinical practice.

Certification is a process that is gaining recognition both within and outside of the professional community. Most states, insurers, and employers require certification for licensure, hire, and reimbursement. For the professional, it is a means of gaining special recognition as a certified nurse practitioner, which not only demonstrates a level of competency, but may also enhance professional opportunities and advancement. For the consumer, it means that a certified practitioner has met certain predetermined standards set by the profession.

# Acknowledgments

This newest edition of the *Adult-Gerontology Nurse Practitioner Certification Review Guide* has been a labor of love and learning, and so many people in my life have contributed to the effort with their love, support, and tolerance. As always, hugs to my son Michael, now the 31-year-old version of the little boy to whom I dedicated my first book, to the teachers and mentors who brought me into the profession that I love, and to the students who keep me on my toes and force me to be a life-long learner. Finally, big hugs to my Dad, who taught me to always follow through on a commitment with my very best effort. I miss you every day.

# Contributing Authors

**Mary A. Baroni, PhD, RN, CPNP**
Professor
Nursing Program Director
University of Washington, Bothell
Bothell, Washington

**Leanne C. Busby, DSN, RNC, FAANP**
Dean and Professor
Jeanette Rudy School of Nursing
Cumberland University
Lebanon, Tennessee

**Susan E. Chaney, EdD, APRN, BC, FNP-C**
Professor
College of Nursing
Graduate Program Coordinator
Texas Woman's University
Family Nurse Practitioner
Homeless Outreach Medical Services
Parkland Health and Hospital System
Dallas, Texas

**Sylvia Torres Fletcher, MS, RN, CS, FNP**
Family Nurse Practitioner
Community Oriented Primary Care—Homeless Outreach Program
Parkland Health and Hospital System
Dallas, Texas

**Nancy A. Dickenson-Hazard, MSN, CPNP, FAAN**
Executive Officer
Sigma Theta Tau International
Indianapolis, Indiana

**Beth M. Kelsey, MS, EdD(c), RNC, WHNP**
Assistant Professor
Women's Health Nurse Practitioner
School of Nursing
Ball State University
Muncie, Indiana

**Mary D. Knudtson, DNSc, NP-BC**
Professor
Family Medicine
University of California, Irvine
Irvine, California

**Debbie Gilbert Kramer, MS, RN, CS, CRNP**
Gerontological/Adult Nurse Practitioner
Risk Management Department
Johns Hopkins Bayview Medical Center
Nurse Consultant
EHA Consulting Group, Inc.
Baltimore, Maryland

**Sally K. Miller, AGPCNP-BC, AGACNP-BC, FAANP**
Clinical Professor
Drexel University College of Nursing and Health Professions
Philadelphia, Pennsylvania
Nurse Practitioner
Nevada Health Centers
Carson City, Nevada

**Virginia L. Millonig, PhD, RN, CPNP**
President
Health Leadership Associates, Inc.

**Susan B. Moskosky, MS, RNC, WHCNP**
Director, Office of Family Planning
Office of Population Affairs
U.S. Department of Health and Human Services
Washington, D.C.

**Rosanne H. Pruitt, PhD, APRN-BC**
Professor
School of Nursing
Clemson University
Clemson, South Carolina

**Sister Maria Salerno, OSF, DNSc, APRN-BC**
Associate Professor
Director Primary Care/Adult and Gerontological Nurse
    Practitioner Programs
Adult Nurse Practitioner, Gerontological Nurse
    Practitioner
Family Nurse Practitioner
Coordinator Adult CNS/Educator Program
School of Nursing
The Catholic University of America
Washington, D.C.

**Pamela A. Shuler, DNSc, RN, CFNP**
Family Nurse Practitioner
Great Smokies Medical Center
Asheville, North Carolina

**Madeline Turkeltaub, PhD, CRNP**
Nurse Practitioner
Greenbelt, Maryland

**Margaret Hadro Venzke, MS, RN, CS, FNP**
Instructor Nurse Practitioner Program
College of Nursing and Health Science
George Mason University
Fairfax, Virginia
Family Nurse Practitioner
Student Health Center
Georgetown University
Washington, D.C.

# CORE CURRICULUM

# Test-Taking Strategies and Techniques

Nancy A. Dickenson-Hazard

Virginia L. Millonig

We all respond to testing situations in different ways. What separates the successful test taker from the unsuccessful one is knowing how to prepare for and take a test. Preparing yourself to be a successful test taker is as important as studying for the test. Each person needs to assess and develop individual test-taking strategies and skills. The primary goal of this chapter is to provide potential examinees with strategies that will help them develop studying and test-taking skills. Of equal importance to this test preparation is a basic understanding of how certification examinations are developed. They are based on a universal knowledge foundation. Test items are selected from generally recognized resources available to the examinee and specific to the specialty area.

With respect to adult gerontological primary and acute care nurse practitioner certifications, the examinations are an assembly of questions derived from practice domains that are clearly identified by the relevant certifying bodies: the American Nurses Credentialing Center (ANCC) certifies both acute and primary care adult gerontological nurse practitioners, the American Academy of Nurse Practitioners (AANP) certifies adult gerontological primary care nurse practitioners, and the American Association of Critical-Care Nurses (AACN) certifies adult gerontological acute care nurse practitioners. Eligibility to take these nurse practitioner certification examinations requires successful completion of a nurse practitioner program offered by an accredited nursing program. Accredited programs have successfully demonstrated compliance with the National Organization of Nurse Practitioner Faculties' nurse practitioner core competencies. Therefore, exam candidates may refer to the core competencies and test domains of any of these organizations to understand the foundation from which their exam questions are derived.

## STRATEGY 1: KNOW YOURSELF

When faced with an examination, do you feel threatened, experience butterflies or sweaty palms, or have trouble keeping your mind focused on studying or on test questions? These common symptoms of test anxiety plague many of us but can be used advantageously if understood and handled correctly. Over the years, each of us has developed certain test-taking behaviors, some of which are beneficial, and others of which present obstacles to successful test taking. You can take control of the test-taking situation by identifying undesirable behaviors, maintaining desirable ones, and developing skills to improve test performance.

### ■ Technique 1

Find your personality type. Write down those characteristics that describe you even if they are from different personality types. Carefully review the pitfalls associated with your test-taking personality characteristics. Write down the problems that are most troublesome. Then, make a list of how you can remedy these problems from the improvement strategies list. Be sure to use these strategies as you prepare for and take examinations.

# STRATEGY 2: DEVELOP YOUR THINKING SKILLS

## ■ Understanding the Thought Process

To improve your thinking skills and subsequent test performance, you must understand the types of thinking as well as techniques to enhance the thought process.

Everyone has a personal learning style, but we all must proceed through the same process to think. Thinking occurs on six levels—from the basic levels of knowledge and comprehension to the more complex levels of application, analysis, synthesis, and evaluation (Bloom & Krathwohl, 1956). Knowledge is the ability to recall facts. Without adequate retrieval of facts, progression through the higher levels of thinking cannot occur easily. Comprehension is the ability to understand memorized facts. To be effective, comprehension skills must allow the person to translate recalled information from one context to another. Application, or the process of using information to know why something occurs, is a higher form of learning. Effective application relies on the use of understood, memorized facts to verify intended action. Analysis is the ability to use abstract or logical forms of thought to show relationships and to distinguish between the cause and effect variables in a situation.

As related to testing situations, the thought process from memory to analysis occurs quite quickly. Some examination items are designed to test memory and comprehension, whereas others test application and analysis. An example of a memory question is as follows:

Type 1 diabetes results from dysfunction of the:

a. Liver
b. *Pancreas*
c. Adrenal glands
d. Kidneys

To answer this question correctly, the individual has to retrieve a memorized fact. Understanding the fact, knowing why it is important, or analyzing what should be done in this situation is not needed. The following example is a question that tests comprehension:

You are taking a history on a 47-year-old white female during a routine health assessment visit. She reports that in the past month she has experienced increased thirst and needs to urinate frequently. She reports recurrent episodes of vaginitis and is concerned about an abrasion on her leg that will not heal. You note that her blood pressure is recorded at 150/90 mm Hg and that she is overweight at 5'9" and 195 lbs. Which of the following is the most likely cause of her symptoms?

a. Urinary tract infection
b. Hyperthyroidism
c. Type 1 diabetes mellitus
d. *Type 2 diabetes mellitus*

To answer this question correctly, an individual must retrieve facts about the physiology of diabetes mellitus and the differences between type 1 and type 2 in order to understand and differentiate the presenting symptoms.

In answering an examination question that requires a higher level of thought, an individual must be able to recall a fact, understand that fact in the context of the question, and apply this understanding to determine why one answer is correct after analyzing possible answer choices as they relate to the situation (Sides & Korchek, 1994). The following example is an application analysis question:

A 48-year-old diabetic woman wants to enroll in a low-impact aerobics class. Her diabetes is well managed with twice-daily insulin injections. Your best advice is to suggest that she:

a. Increase daily doses of insulin
b. *Have an extra snack before exercise class*
c. Administer a dose of regular insulin after exercise is completed
d. Consider an activity that does not require physical exertion

To answer this question correctly, the individual must recall physiological facts of exogenous insulin administration and action, understand what is happening in this situation, consider each option and how it applies to the patient's condition, and analyze why each advice option works or does not work for this patient. Application/analysis questions require the examinee to use a logical rationale based on a well-defined principle or fact. Problem-solving ability becomes important because the examinee must think through each question option and determine its relevance and importance to the situation in the question.

## ■ Building Your Thinking Skills

Effective memorization is the cornerstone to learning and building thinking skills (Olney, 1989). We have all experienced "memory power outages" at some time, due in part to trying to memorize too much, too fast. Developing skills to improve memorization is important for increasing the effectiveness of your thinking and subsequent test performance.

### Technique 1

Quantity is *not* quality, so concentrate on learning important content. For example, it is important to know the various pharmacological agents appropriate for the management of chronic obstructive pulmonary disease (COPD), not the specific dosages for each medication.

### Technique 2

Memory from repetition, or saying something over and over again to remember it, usually fades. Developing memory skills that trigger retrieval of needed facts is more useful. Such skills include the following:

**Acronyms:** These are mental crutches that facilitate recall. Some are already established, such as PERRLA (pupils equal, round, react to light, and accommodation), CHF (congestive heart failure), and TIA (transient ischemic attack). Developing your own acronyms can be particularly useful because they are your own word association arrangements in a singular word. Nonsense words or funny, unusual ones are often more useful because they attract your attention.

**Acrostics:** This mental tool arranges words into catchy phrases. The first letter of each word stands for something that is recalled as the phrase is spoken. Your own acrostics are most valuable in triggering recall of learned information because they are your individual situation associations. An example of an acrostic is as follows:

**S**am **E**xercises **B**y **W**eight-lifting and **R**unning stands for the aspects of nondrug therapy/management for hypertension: **S**alt restriction, **E**xercise, **B**iofeedback, **W**eight reduction, and **R**elaxation techniques.

**ABCs:** This technique facilitates information retrieval by using the alphabet as a crutch. Each letter stands for a symptom, which when put together creates a picture of the clinical presentation of the disease. For example, the characteristics of peptic ulcer disease using the ABC technique are as follows:

Antacids relieve pain
Burning epigastric pain
Cycle of pain 2 hours after eating
Discomfort awakens at night
Experiences weight loss
Food sometimes aggravates pain

**Imaging:** This technique can be used in two ways. The first is to develop a nickname for a clinical problem that, when spoken, produces a mental picture. For example, "thin, barrel-chested, pink puffer" might be used to visualize a patient with emphysema who has a muscle-wasted body appearance, absent central cyanosis, hypertrophy of respiratory accessory muscles, and an AP (anterior posterior) chest diameter (width) greater than the transverse chest (depth). A second form of imaging is to visualize a specific patient while you are trying to understand or solve a clinical problem when studying or answering a question. For example, imagine a young woman who is experiencing an acute asthma attack. You are trying to analyze the situation and place her in a position that maximizes respiratory effort. In your mind you visualize her in various positions of sidelying, angular, and forward, imagining what will happen to the woman and her respiratory effort in each position.

**Rhymes, music, and links:** The absurd is easier to remember than the common. Rhymes, music, and links can add absurdity and humor to learning and remembering (Olney, 1989). These retrieval tools are developed by the individual for specific content. For example, making up a rhyme about diabetes may be helpful in remembering the predominant female incidence, origin of disease, primary symptoms, and management, as illustrated by the following:

There once was a woman
whose beta cells failed
She grew quite thirsty
and her glucose levels sailed
Her lack of insulin caused her to
increase her intake
And her increased urinary output
was certainly not fake
So she learned to watch her diet
and administer injections
That kept her healthy, growing,
and free of complications.

Setting content to music is sometimes useful to remembering. Melodies that are repetitious jog the memory by the ups and downs of the notes and the rhythm of the music. Links connect key words from the content by using them in a story. An example given by Olney (1989) for remembering the parts of an eye is IRIS watched a PUPIL through the LENS of a RED TIN telescope while eating CORN-EA on the cob.

Additional memory aids may also include the use of color or drawing for improving recall. Use different colored pens or paper to accentuate the material being learned. For example, highlight or make notes in blue for content about respiratory problems and in red for cardiovascular content. Drawing assists with visualizing content as well. This is particularly helpful for remembering the pathophysiology of the specific health problem.

**The important thing to remember about remembering is to use good recall techniques.**

## Technique 3

Improving higher-level thinking skills involves exercising the application and analysis of memorized facts. Small-group review is particularly useful for enhancing these high-level skills. Small-group interaction allows verbalization of thought processes and receipt of input about content and thought process from others (Sides & Korchek, 1994). Individuals hear not only how they think but also how others think as well. This interaction allows individuals to identify flaws in their thought processes as well as strengthen their positive points.

Taking practice tests is also helpful in developing application/analysis thinking skills. Practice tests permit the individual to analyze thinking patterns as well as the cause-and-effect relationships between the question and its options. The problem-solving skills needed to answer application/analysis questions are tested, giving the individual more experience through practice (Dickenson-Hazard, 1990b).

## STRATEGY 3: KNOW THE CONTENT

Your ability to study is directly influenced by organization and concentration (Dickenson-Hazard, 1990d). If effort is spent on both of these aspects of exam preparation, examination success can be increased.

### ■ Preparation for Studying: Getting Organized

Study habits are developed early in our education experiences. Some of our habits enhance learning, while others do not. To increase study effectiveness, organization of study materials and time is essential. Organization decreases frustration, allows for easy resumption of study, and increases concentrated study time.

### Technique 1

Create your own study space. Select a study area that is yours alone, free from distractions, comfortable, and well lighted. The ventilation and room temperature should be comfortable because a cold room makes it difficult to concentrate and a warm room may make you sleepy (Burkle & Marshak, 1989). All study materials should be left in a specific study space. The basic premise of a study space is that it facilitates a mindset that you are there to study. When study is interrupted, it is best to leave study materials just as they are. Don't close books or put away notes because you will then have to relocate them, which wastes valuable time when study is resumed.

### Technique 2

Define and organize the content. Secure an outline or the content parameters that are to be examined from the examining body. If the outline is sketchy, develop a more detailed one for yourself using the recommended texts as guidelines. Next, identify available study resources: class notes, old exams, handouts, textbooks, review courses and books, home study programs, or study groups. For national standardized exams, such as initial licensing or certification, it is best to identify a few resources that cover the content being tested and stick to them. Attempting to review all available resources not only is mind boggling but increases anxiety and frustration as well. Make your selections and stay with them.

### Technique 3

Conduct a content assessment. Use a simple rating scale of

1 = requires no review
2 = requires minimal review
3 = requires intensive review
4 = start from the beginning

Read through the content outline and rate each content area (Dickenson-Hazard, 1990a). **Table 1-1** provides a sample exam content assessment. Be honest in your assessment. It is far better to recognize your content weaknesses when you can study and remedy them than to wish during the exam that you had studied more. Likewise with content strengths: if you know the material, your time is better used on other content. As an added value, the simple act of organizing and constructing a content assessment is a method of "studying." Simply reviewing all of the material in an effort to organize it reacquaints you with the content.

**TABLE 1-1** Sample Content Assessment

**Exam Content: Gastrointestinal Health Problems of the Adult**

| Category: Provided by Examining Body | Rating: Provided by Examinee |
|---|---|
| I. Peptic Ulcer Disease | |
| A. Etiology | 4 |
| B. Pathophysiology | 3 |
| C. Symptomatology | 3 |
| D. Differential Diagnosis | 4 |
| E. Diagnostic Tests | 3 |
| F. Management/Treatment | 4 |
| II. Esophagitis | |
| A. Etiology | 3 |
| B. Pathophysiology | 3 |
| C. Symptomatology | 2 |
| D. Differential Diagnosis | 3 |
| E. Diagnostic Tests | 2 |
| F. Management/Treatment | 4 |

| Exam Content: Gastrointestinal Health Problems of the Adult | |
|---|---|
| **Category: Provided by Examining Body** | **Rating: Provided by Examinee** |
| III. Cholecystitis | |
| A. Etiology | 2 |
| B. Pathophysiology | 2 |
| C. Symptomatology | 1 |
| D. Differential Diagnosis | 2 |
| E. Diagnostic Tests | 4 |
| F. Management/Treatment | 4 |
| IV. Appendicitis | |
| A. Etiology | 3 |
| B. Pathophysiology | 4 |
| C. Symptomatology | 3 |
| D. Differential Diagnosis | 2 |
| E. Diagnostic Tests | 3 |
| F. Management/Treatment | 4 |
| V. Diverticulitis | |
| A. Etiology | 3 |
| B. Pathophysiology | 4 |
| C. Symptomatology | 3 |
| D. Differential Diagnosis | 3 |
| E. Diagnostic Tests | 2 |
| F. Management/Treatment | 4 |
| VI. Hepatitis | |
| A. Etiology | 3 |
| B. Pathophysiology | 4 |
| C. Symptomatology | 4 |
| D. Differential Diagnosis | 4 |
| E. Diagnostic Tests | 2 |
| F. Management/Treatment | 4 |
| VII. Acute Gastroenteritis | |
| A. Etiology | 2 |
| B. Pathophysiology | 3 |
| C. Symptomatology | 2 |
| D. Differential Diagnosis | 3 |
| E. Diagnostic Tests | 4 |
| F. Management/Treatment | 3 |
| VIII. Irritable Bowel Syndrome | |
| A. Etiology | 3 |
| B. Pathophysiology | 3 |
| C. Symptomatology | 3 |
| D. Differential Diagnosis | 4 |
| E. Diagnostic Tests | 4 |
| F. Management/Treatment | 3 |

## Technique 4

Develop a study plan. Coordinate the content that needs to be studied with the time available (Sides & Korchek, 1994). Prioritize your study needs, starting with weak areas first. Allow for a general review at the end of the study plan. Finally, establish an overall goal for yourself, something that will motivate you when brought to mind.

**Table 1-2** illustrates a study plan developed on the basis of the exam content assessment in Table 1-1. Conducting an assessment and developing a study plan should require no more than 50 minutes. It is a wise investment of time with potential payoffs of reduced study stress and exam success.

## Technique 5

Begin now and use your time wisely. The smart test taker begins the study process early (Olney, 1989). Sit down, conduct the content assessment, and develop a study plan as soon as you know about the exam. *Don't procrastinate!*

## ■ Getting Down to Business: The Actual Studying

There is no better way to prepare for an examination than individual study (Dickenson-Hazard, 1989b). The responsibility to achieve the goal you set for this exam lies with you alone. The means that you employ to achieve this goal will vary and should begin with identifying your peak study times and using techniques to maximize them.

## Technique 1

Study in short bursts. Each of us has our own biological clock that dictates when we are at our peak during the day. If you are a morning person, you are generally active and alert early in the day, slowing down and becoming drowsy by evening. If you are an evening person, you don't completely wake up until late morning and hit your peak in the afternoon and evening. Each person generally has several peaks during the day. It is best to study during those times when your alertness is at its peak (Dickenson-Hazard, 1990c).

During our concentration peaks, there are mini peaks or bursts of alertness (Olney, 1989). These alertness (mini) peaks occur during a concentration peak because levels of concentration are at their highest during the first part and last part of a study period. These bursts can vary from 10 minutes to 1 hour depending on the extent of concentration. If studying is sustained for 1 hour, there are only two mini peaks: one at the beginning and one at the end. There are eight mini peaks if that same hour is divided into four 15-minute intervals. Hence, it is more helpful to study in short bursts (Olney, 1989). More can be learned in less time.

**TABLE 1-2　Sample Study Plan**

**Goal: Master Content on the Gastrointestinal Problems of the Adult Patient. Test Time Available: 2 Weeks**

| Objective | Activity | Date Accomplished |
|---|---|---|
| Master content on diverticulitis. | Read Chapter 26. Take notes on chapter content according to outline. Review class notes combined with chapter notes. Review sample test questions. | Feb. 5 & 6, 1 hour Feb. 6, 1 hour Feb. 6, 1 hour |
| Understand content on peptic ulcer disease. | Read Chapter 25. Take notes on chapter content according to content outline. Review class notes combined with chapter notes. | Feb. 7, 2 hours Feb. 8, 1½ hours |
| Master content on cholecystitis. | Read Chapter 24. Take notes on chapter content according to content outline. Review class notes combined with chapter notes. Review sample test questions. | Feb. 10, 2 hours Feb. 11, ½ hour Feb. 12, 1½ hours |
| Know material on irritable bowel syndrome. | Scan Chapter 27. Review class notes, supplementing with text notes. | Feb. 14, 2 hours |
| Know material on esophagitis. | Scan Chapter 23. Review class notes, supplementing with text notes. | Feb. 15, 2 hours |
| Know material on hepatitis. | Scan Chapter 28. Review highlights and important concepts. | Feb. 16, 2 hours |
| Know material on appendicitis and acute gastroenteritis. | Scan Chapter 29. Review highlights and important concepts. | Feb. 17, 2 hours |
| Demonstrate understanding of all material. | Review with another person. Review all notes. Take sample test questions. | Feb. 18, 2 hours Feb. 19, 1½ hours Feb. 19, 1½ hours |
| Think positively. | SMILE. Take frequent breaks. Reward myself after each study session. Keep my goal in mind. | ONGOING |

## Technique 2

"Cramming" can be useful when properly recognized and managed. Because concentration ability is highly variable, some individuals can sustain their mini peaks for 15, 20, or even 30 minutes at a time. Pushing your concentration beyond its peak is fruitless and verges on cramming, which in general is a poor study technique. There are, as mentioned, times when cramming, a short-term memory tool, is useful. Short-term memory generally is at its best in the morning. A quick review or cram of content in the morning can be useful the day of the exam (Olney, 1989). Most studying, however, is best accomplished in the afternoon or evening when long-term memory functions at its peak.

## Technique 3

Give your brain breaks. Regular times during study to rest and absorb the content are needed by the brain. The best approach to breaks is to plan them and take a conscious break (Dickenson-Hazard, 1990d). This approach eliminates the "day dreaming" or "wandering thought" approach to breaks that many of us use. It is better to get up, leave the study area, and do something unrelated to studying for longer breaks. For shorter breaks of 5 minutes or so, leave your desk, gaze out the window, or do some stretching exercises. When your brain says to give it a rest, accommodate it! You'll learn more in time that is less stressful.

## Technique 4

Study the correct content. It is easy for all of us to become bogged down in the detail of the content we are studying. However, it is best to focus on the major concepts or the "state of the art" content. Leave the details, the suppositions, and the experience at the door of your study area. Concentrate on the major textbook facts and concepts that revolve around the subject matter being tested. Remember, the foundation of these exams is evidence-based practice. Know the evidence and the national and professional guidelines that drive practice. In the day-to-day of clinical practice we may deviate from guidelines for a variety of reasons. On certification examinations, evidence-based practice guides the way. Also keep in mind that these are generalist exams—not specialty exams. Many assessment and management techniques employed in specialty practice may go beyond the evidence-based recommendations used in the general setting.

## Technique 5

Fit your studying to the test type. The best way to prepare for an objective test is to study facts, particularly anything printed in italics. Memory-enhancing techniques are particularly useful when preparing for an objective test. If preparing for an essay test, study generalities, examples, and concepts. Application techniques are helpful when studying for this type of an exam (Burkle & Marshak, 1989).

## Technique 6

Use your study plan wisely. Your study plan is meant to be a guide, not a rigid schedule. You should take your time with studying. Don't rush through the content just to remain on schedule. Occasionally, study plans need revision. If you take more or less time than planned, readjust the plan for the time gained or lost. The plan can guide you, but you must go at your own pace.

## Technique 7

Actively study. Being an active participant in study rather than trying to absorb the printed word is also helpful. Ways to be active include taking notes on the content as you study, constructing questions and answering them, and taking practice tests and discussing the content with yourself. Also, using your individual study quirks is encouraged. Some people stand, others walk around, and some play background music. You should use whatever helps you to concentrate and study better.

## Technique 8

Use study aids. While there is no substitute for individual studying, several resources, if available, are useful in facilitating learning. Review courses are an excellent means for organizing or summarizing your individual study. They generally provide the content parameters and the major concepts of the content that you need to know. Review courses also provide an opportunity to clarify less-well-understood content as well as to review known material (Dickenson-Hazard, 1990a). Study guides, certification review books, and home study programs are useful for organizing study. They provide detail on the content that is important to the exam. Study groups are an excellent resource for summarizing and refining content. They provide an opportunity for thinking through your knowledge base, with the advantage of hearing another person's point of view. Each of these study aids increases understanding of content and, when used correctly, increases effectiveness of knowledge application.

## Technique 9

Know when to quit. It is best to stop studying when your concentration ebbs. It is unproductive and frustrating to force yourself to study. It is far better to rest or unwind, and then resume at a later point in the day. Avoid studying outside your a.m. or p.m. concentration peaks and focus your study energy on your best time of day or evening.

## STRATEGY 4: BECOME TEST-WISE

The majority of nurse practitioner certification examinations are composed of multiple choice questions (MCQs). This type of question requires the examinee to select the best response for a specific circumstance or condition. Successful test taking is dependent not only on content knowledge but on test-taking skill as well. If you are unable to impart your knowledge through the vehicle used for its conveyance—for example, the MCQ—your test-taking success is in jeopardy.

### ■ Technique 1

Recognize the purpose of a test question. Most test questions are developed to examine knowledge at separate levels: memory, comprehension, or application and analysis. A memory question requires examinees to recall facts from their knowledge base, whereas an application question requires examinees to use and apply the knowledge. Memory questions test recall of facts. Comprehension questions test ability to draw reasonable inferences from facts. Analysis and application questions test the ability to analyze given facts and apply that analysis to a clinical scenario. When taking a test, you need to understand what the question is asking of you.

### ■ Technique 2

Recognize the components of a test question. Multiple choice questions may include the basic components of a background statement, a stem, and a list of options. The background statement presents information that facilitates answering the question. The stem asks or states the intent of the question. The options typically include four possible responses to the question. The correct option is called the keyed response, and all other options are called distracters (American Board of Pediatrics, 1989). Knowing the components of a test question helps you sift through the information presented and focus on the question's intent (see **Table 1-3**).

### ■ Technique 3

Identify the key word or words in a test question. Don't jump to conclusions when you read the stem. Key words are generally included in the stem of a test question, whereas key concepts or conditions appear in

| TABLE 1-3 | Anatomy of a Test Question |
|---|---|
| Background statement | A 32-year-old female is being seen for a complaint of sores in the vaginal area. She has been experiencing a low-grade fever, headache, and malaise over the past 5 days. Physical examination reveals inguinal lymphadenopathy, vaginal erythema, and multiple labial and vaginal vesicular lesions. |
| Stem | Which of the following causative organisms would you suspect? |
| Options | a. *Herpes simplex virus 2*<br>b. *Condylomata lata*<br>c. *Herpes simplex virus 1*<br>d. *Treponema pallidum* |

the background statement. You should pay particular attention to the key words in the stem and their impact on the intent of the question. Never "read between the lines" of a question or make assumptions about the information given. Answer what the question is asking of you. This is a critically important point for successful test taking. If the question asks "What is the next step in the assessment of this patient?" then the correct answer will be an assessment. Do not be distracted by a choice that seems to match the background scenario but that does not answer the question. Consider the following question:

> Ms. Stevenson is a 43-year-old female with no significant medical history. She presents with a complaint of significant pain and edema of her left lower extremity. She flew back to the United States from Hong Kong the day before yesterday and reports that she spent more than 20 hours on airplanes. She denies any history of a similar event even though she makes this trip every year. Her vital signs are within normal limits, but her left leg is clearly edematous as compared to the right. There is no discoloration. Initial management of her pain may include:
> 
> a. Venipuncture for D-dimer analysis
> b. Left lower extremity arterial and venous ultrasound
> c. A weak opioid analgesic
> d. Cardiovascular evaluation

The best answer to this question is c because the question asks very specifically about what initial pain management would include. Consistent with World Health Organization pain management guidelines, moderate pain may be appropriately managed with an opioid analgesic. Some of you may have wanted to choose option a because this would be appropriate to rule out the deep vein thrombosis that is suggested by her history; others may have preferred option b in order to examine both arterial and venous vasculature, and some may choose option d given the risk inherent in the history and the "significant pain." None of those options would be inappropriate or "wrong" in this scenario—but the answer to the *question that is asked* is option c.

### ■ Technique 4

Recognize the item types. Basically, two styles of MCQs are used for examinations. The more common type requires the examinee to select the one best answer; occasionally, an exam will require selection of multiple correct answers. When selecting an answer from the "one best answer" type, it is important to remember that several choices may be acceptable, but one will be best as compared to the others. When the test taker is stumped by the answer choices, he should re-read the question with particular attention to precisely what the question is asking. When selecting answer choices from the "choose all that apply" type (multiple correct answers), consider each answer choice on its own merits and select it if it is an appropriate response to the question.

### ■ Technique 5

Read the directions to the questions carefully. Questions are sometimes answered incorrectly because the test taker did not carefully read the directions. Similarly, be sure to read all answer choices before choosing "the best option of those provided." Many times, several answer choices will sound good, but one is better than the others. It is important always to read the entire question and all answer choices before answering the question.

### ■ Technique 6

Apply the basic rules of test taking. Examination candidates can avoid many problems associated with test taking if they give thought to the mechanics of sitting down, reading the question, and noting their answers. Timing yourself to avoid spending too much time on a question and not changing your answers are two techniques that can improve performance. Review these and apply them to the testing situation.

### ■ Technique 7

Make educated guesses. An educated guess is the selection of an option (answer) when you are unsure of the correct answer. Elimination of all options except for two, followed by a reevaluation of these two options based on your knowledge base, allows you to make an educated guess.

The more common advanced practice nursing certification examinations give credit when correct answers are selected and give no credit for incorrect answers. Directions for this type of examination may state that credit will be given for correct answers; therefore, all questions should be answered, and you will not be penalized for guessing. Consequently, an unanswered question always gets no credit. An answered question always has a chance—so do not leave anything unanswered.

### ■ Technique 8

Practice, practice, practice. Taking practice tests can improve performance. Whereas they can assist in evaluation of your knowledge, *their primary benefit is to assist you with test-taking skills.* You should use them to evaluate your thinking process; your ability to read, understand, and interpret questions; and your skills in completing the mechanics of the test. Practice tests are not typically the best way to study content—if you need help with the content, you should study the content appropriately as already described. However, if you feel confident with the content, practice tests are an excellent way to develop your test-taking technique.

### ■ Technique 9

Be prepared for exam day. It is important to familiarize yourself with the test site, the building, the parking, and the travel route prior to the exam day. The night before the exam, go to bed at a reasonable hour and avoid excessive drinking or eating (Sides & Korchek, 1994). If you must travel, allow time for this familiarization. It is helpful to make a list of things you need on the exam day: picture identification, admission card, watch, and a few pieces of hard candy as a quick energy source. On exam day allow yourself plenty of time to arrive at the site. Wear comfortable clothes and have a good breakfast that morning. The idea is to arrive on time at the test site as prepared and as rested as possible.

## STRATEGY 5: PSYCH YOURSELF UP: TAKING TESTS IS STRESSFUL

Whereas a little stress can be productive, too much can incapacitate you in your studying and test taking (Divine & Kylen, 1979). Your attitude and approach to test taking and studying can influence your outcomes. Psyching yourself up can have a positive effect and help keep examinations from becoming anxiety-laden experiences (Dickenson-Hazard, 1990b). The following techniques are based on the principles of successful test taking as presented by Sides and Cailles (1989). Incorporation of these techniques can improve response and performance in examination situations.

### ■ Technique 1

Adopt an "I can" attitude. Believing you can succeed is the key to success. Self-belief inspires and gives you the power to achieve your goals. Without a success attitude, the road to your goal is much harder. We all stand an equal chance of success in this world. Those who believe they can achieve it. This "I can" attitude must permeate all your efforts in test taking, from studying to improving your skills to actually writing the test.

### ■ Technique 2

Take control. By identifying your goal, deciding how to accomplish it, and developing a plan for achieving it, you take control. Do not leave your success or failure to chance; control it through action and attitude.

### ■ Technique 3

Think positively. Examinations are generally based on a standard that is the same for all individuals. Everyone can potentially pass. Performance is influenced not only by knowledge and skill but also by attitude. Those individuals who regard an exam as an opportunity or challenge will be more successful.

### ■ Technique 4

Project a positive self-fulfilling prophecy. While preparing for an examination, project thoughts of the positive outcomes you will experience when you succeed. Self-talk is self-fulfilling. Expect success, not failure, of yourself.

### ■ Technique 5

Feel good about yourself. Without feeling a sense of positive self-worth, passing an examination is difficult. Recognize your professional contributions and give yourself credit for your accomplishments. Think "I will pass," not "I suppose I can."

### ■ Technique 6

Know yourself. Focus exam preparation and test taking on your strengths. Try to alter your weaknesses instead of becoming hung up on them. If you tend to overanalyze, study and read test questions at face value. If you're a speed demon when taking a test, slow down and read more carefully.

### ■ Technique 7

Failure is a possibility. We all have failed at something at some point in our lives. Rather than dwelling on the failure, making excuses, and believing you will fail again, recognize your mistakes and remedy them. Failure is a time to begin again; use it as a motivator to do better. It is not the end of the world unless you allow it to be. It is best to deal with the failure and move on; otherwise, it interferes with your success.

### ■ Technique 8

Persevere, persevere, persevere! Endurance must underlie all your efforts. Call forth those reserve energies when you have had all you think you can take. Rely on yourself and your support systems to help you maintain a sense of direction and keep your goal in the forefront.

### ■ Technique 9

Motivation is muscle. Most individuals are motivated by fear or desire. The fear in an exam situation may be one of failure, the unknown, or discovery of imperfection. Put your fear into perspective; realize you are not the only one with fear and that all have an equal opportunity for success. Develop strategies to reduce fear, and use fear to your advantage by improving the imperfections. Desire is a powerful motivator, and you should keep the rewards of your desire foremost in your mind. Whatever motivates you, use it to be successful. Reward yourself during your exam preparation and after the exam has been completed. You alone hold the key to success; use what you have wisely.

### ■ Technique 10

Overprepare. One of the best ways to reduce test anxiety is to overprepare. The more prepared you are, the more confident you will be. Overpreparation requires you to study the same information over again even when you know the information. This activity reinforces your learning and builds confidence and reduces anxiety when it comes time to take the examination.

Overpreparation cannot occur unless adequate time is allowed for this process. A last-minute cramming approach will not lead to an overprepared test taker. Being overprepared definitely places an individual in control and in a position of power and confidence (Nugent & Vitale, 1997).

This chapter provides concepts, strategies, and techniques for improving study and test-taking skills. Your first task in improvement is to know yourself, how you study, and how you take a test. You should use your strengths and remedy the weaknesses. Next, you need to develop your thinking skills. Work on techniques to improve memory and reasoning. Then, you need to organize your study and concentrate on using these new skills to be successful. Create a study space, develop a plan of action, and then implement that plan during your periods of peak concentration. Before taking the exam, be sure you understand the components of a test question, can identify key words and phrases, and have practiced. Apply the test-taking rules during the exam process. Finally, believe in yourself, your knowledge, and your talent. Believing you can accomplish your goal makes it more likely that you will.

## BIBLIOGRAPHY

American Academy of Nurse Practitioners Certification Program. (2013). *AANPCP candidate and renewal certification handbook 2013.* Retrieved from http://www.aanpcert.org/ptistore/resource/documents/2013%20CandidateRenewalHandbook%20-Rev%2011%2025%202013%20forNCCA(FINAL).pdf

American Association of Critical-Care Nurses & AACN Certification Corporation. (2012). *Curriculum map illustrating integration of competency and practice standards for the adult-gerontology acute care nurse practitioner role.* Retrieved from http://www.aacn.org/wd/certifications/docs/aprn-curriculum-map-acnpc-ag.pdf

American Board of Pediatrics. (1989). *Developing questions and critiques.* Unpublished manuscript.

American Nurses Credentialing Center. (2013a). *Adult-gerontology acute care nurse practitioner board certification examination test content outline.* Retrieved from http://www.nursecredentialing.org/Documents/Certification/TestContentOutlines/AdultGeroAcuteCareNP-TCO.aspx

American Nurses Credentialing Center. (2013b). *Adult-gerontology primary care nurse practitioner board certification examination test content outline.* Retrieved from http://www.nursecredentialing.org/Documents/Certification/TestContentOutlines/AdultGeroPCNP-TCO.aspx

Bloom, B. S., & Krathwohl, D. R. (1956). *Taxonomy of educational objectives: The classification of educational goals, by a committee of college and university examiners. Handbook 1: Cognitive domain.* New York, NY: Longman.

Burkle, C. A., & Marshak, D. (1989). *Study program: Level 1.* Reston, VA: National Association of Secondary School Principals.

Dickenson-Hazard, N. (1989a). Anatomy of a test question. *Pediatric Nursing, 15,* 395–399.

Dickenson-Hazard, N. (1989b). Making the grade as a test taker. *Pediatric Nursing, 15,* 302–304.

Dickenson-Hazard, N. (1990a). Develop your thinking skills for improved test taking. *Pediatric Nursing, 16,* 480–481.

Dickenson-Hazard, N. (1990b). The psychology of successful test taking. *Pediatric Nursing, 16,* 66–67.

Dickenson-Hazard, N. (1990c). Study effectiveness: Are you a 10 a.m. or p.m. scholar? *Pediatric Nursing, 16,* 419–420.

Dickenson-Hazard, N. (1990d). Study smart. *Pediatric Nursing, 16,* 314–316.

Divine, J. H., & Kylen, D. W. (1979). *How to beat test anxiety.* New York, NY: Barrons Educational Series.

Millman, J., & Pauk, W. (1969). *How to take tests.* New York, NY: McGraw-Hill.

National Organization of Nurse Practitioner Faculties. (2012). *Nurse practitioner core competencies.* Retrieved from http://c.ymcdn.com/sites/www.nonpf.org/resource/resmgr/competencies/npcorecompetenciesfinal2012.pdf

Nugent, P. M., & Vitale, B. A. (1997). *Test success* (2nd ed.). Philadelphia, PA: F. A. Davis.

Olney, C. W. (1989). *Where there's a will, there's an A*. Chesterbrook, PA: Chesterbrook Educational Publishers.

Sides, M., & Cailles, N. B. (1989). *Nurse's guide to successful test taking.* Philadelphia, PA: Lippincott.

Sides, M., & Korchek, N. (1994). *Nurse's guide to successful test taking* (2nd ed.). Philadelphia, PA: Lippincott.

# Health Promotion and Evaluation

*Rosanne H. Pruitt*

## THEORETICAL ASPECTS: HEALTH PROMOTION THEORIES AND MODELS

- High-Level Wellness—a *continuum* that demonstrates dynamic interaction of health and environment as one moves toward high-level wellness; health is dynamic with a continuing need for health-promoting activity to maintain and improve one's health

- Maslow's Hierarchy of Needs (Maslow, 1954)
  1. Survival needs—food, water, sleep
  2. Safety and security—protection from physical hazards
  3. Love and belonging—affection, companionship
  4. Self-esteem—sense of self-worth, recognition
  5. Self-actualization—achievement of personal potential

- Health Belief Model (Becker, 1972)—health is influenced by age, sex, race, ethnicity, and income
  1. Threats to health
     a. Perceived susceptibility
     b. Perceived seriousness of condition
  2. Outcome expectation of health action
     a. Perceived benefits of action
     b. Perceived barriers to taking action
     c. Efficacy expectations

- Self-Efficacy Theory (Bandura, 1986)—explains human behavior in terms of a dynamic, reciprocal interaction between behavior, personal factors, and environmental influences; key concepts include
  1. Personal factors, including the ability to symbolize behavior meaning, to foresee outcomes of given behavior, to learn by observing others, to self-determine and self regulate, and to reflect and analyze experience
  2. Reciprocal determinism refers to behavior as dynamic and dependent on environmental and personal constructs that influence each other simultaneously

- Health Promotion Model (Pender, 2002)—health-promoting behaviors are motivated by multiple cognitive-perceptual factors such as the importance of health and perceived benefits, and the perceived control of health and self-efficacy, and are modified by factors such as demographics and interpersonal influences

- Erikson's Stages of Psychosocial Development (Erikson, 1963)—degree of success in accomplishing developmental tasks influences the accomplishment of tasks of older adults
  1. Trust versus mistrust—trust of self and others
  2. Autonomy versus shame and doubt—self-expression and cooperation with others
  3. Initiative versus guilt—focus on purposeful behavior
  4. Industry versus inferiority—belief in one's ability
  5. Identity versus role confusion—clear sense of self
  6. Intimacy versus role confusion—capacity for reciprocal love relationships
  7. Generativity versus stagnation—creativity and productivity
  8. Ego identity versus despair—acceptance of one's life as worthwhile and unique

- Health Behavior Change Models
  1. PRECEDE Model (Green & Kreuter, 1991)—involves identifying and assessing the learner's quality of life; identifying health problems and risk factors; the acronym PRECEDE stands for Predisposing, Reinforcing, and Enabling Causes in Educational Diagnosis and Evaluation: Predisposing factors (perception, knowledge, and attitudes), Reinforcing factors (significant others), and Enabling factors (environmental factors of accessibility and costs) are used to develop educational interventions for change and policies to support change
  2. Change Theory (Lewin, 1951)—advanced practice environments are dynamic; planned change involves unfreezing of current approach, implementing change, refreezing or creating, and acceptance and regular use of new approach
  3. Transtheoretical Model (Prochaska & Velicer, 1997)—temporal model of behavioral change; model emerged from comparative analysis of more than 300 theories
     a. Precontemplation—no intention to take action within next 6 months; not ready and often resistant to health promotion change efforts; appropriate to use consciousness-raising education
     b. Contemplation—intention to take action within next 6 months; not ready and ambivalent toward change; appropriate to use consciousness-raising education
     c. Preparation—intends to take action within 30 days and has taken some behavioral steps in this direction; individuals at this stage should be recruited for action toward behavior change
     d. Action—individual has changed behavior for less than 6 months
     e. Maintenance—individual has changed overt behavior for more than 6 months; support and encouragement of continued behavior change

- Systems Theories
  1. General Systems Theory (von Bertalanffy, 1968)—views world in terms of sets of integrated reactions in an effort to see parts in relation to the whole; key concepts include
     a. System—goal-directed unit with interdependent, interacting parts that also interact with environment
     b. Boundaries regulate exchange of energy, information, and matter between systems; may be open or closed depending on interaction with surrounding environment
     c. Input, output, and feedback loop provide for an exchange of energy, information, and matter
  2. Neuman's Systems Model (Neuman & Fawcett, 2002)—uses a systems format and includes levels of prevention as well as multiple dimensions of health promotion (physical, psychological, spiritual, and social); health promotion efforts are used to strengthen line barriers of defense

## RELATED CONCEPTS

- Levels of prevention from public health science are used by most authorities when differentiating health promotion activities from other interventions. *Healthy People 2020* and other federal documents use a broader interpretation, including health protection with specific screenings and safety factors, which are also included in this chapter
  1. Primary prevention includes measures to promote optimum health prior to the onset of any problems—health promotion and care intended to minimize risk factors and subsequent disease (e.g., promoting a healthy diet, exercise, stress management, safety, avoiding harmful substances)
  2. Secondary prevention focuses on early identification and treatment of existing health problems (e.g., screening for disease, Pap smear, mammogram, digital rectal exam)
  3. Tertiary prevention is care intended to improve the course of a disease, maximize function, and minimize deterioration; the rehabilitation and restoration to health (e.g., cardiac rehabilitation)

- Cultural influence must be considered with any healthcare encounter. Cultural beliefs of disease causation influence health practices (e.g., magic or evil spirits—Latino; violation of a natural law—American Indian; imbalance between "hot" and "cold" forces—Asian, Latino). Varied beliefs affect the acceptance of practices such as hand washing and immunizations. There are differences between and among cultural groups. Certain beliefs are common among cultural groups
  1. Native Americans—harmony with nature and supernatural forces are important factors in health beliefs; social networking is also important; note taking is often considered taboo; silence is a sign of respect
  2. Hispanic Americans—extended family is important in decision making; illness may be related to imbalance of hot and cold; sustaining eye contact is considered rude (*mal ojo*); higher risk of vitamin A, iron, and calcium deficiency resulting from dietary habits

3. Asian Americans—naturalistic beliefs are common; saying no is considered rude and is avoided; eye contact may be avoided out of respect; a need to balance hot and cold through food and medication is prevalent; use of acupuncture therapy is widespread
4. African Americans—diverse group with beliefs that include "health is harmony with nature" and "life is a process, not a state"; maternal grandmother is often important in decision making

## LIFESTYLE/HEALTH BEHAVIORS

- Stress management—stress is an imbalance between environmental demands and one's individual and social resources required to cope with those demands
    1. Types of stressors
        a. Major life events—discrete events that disrupt normal functioning (e.g., marriage, divorce, death of family member)
        b. Daily hassles—minor daily events perceived as frustrating
        c. Chronic strains—challenges, hardships, and problems
        d. Cataclysmic events—sudden disasters that require major adaptive responses (e.g., natural disasters)
        e. Ambient stressors—continuous and often unchanging conditions in physical environment, such as chronic pollution or noise
    2. Theoretical basis of stress
        a. General Adaptation Syndrome—Selye's (1974) continuum demonstrates how small amounts of stress are motivating and improve the quality of life (eustress or good stress); however, beyond a certain point the stress becomes psychologically and physically debilitating (distress)
        b. Physical indicators of stress
            (1) Gastrointestinal symptoms—upset stomach, change of appetite
            (2) Headache, muscle tension, elevated blood pressure (BP), tachycardia
            (3) Restlessness, tremor
            (4) Cold, sweaty palms
        c. Emotional indicators of stress
            (1) Irritability, emotional outbursts, crying
            (2) Depression, withdrawal
            (3) Hostility, tendency to blame others
            (4) Anxiety, suspiciousness
        d. Behavioral indicators of stress
            (1) Lethargy, loss of interest
            (2) Poor concentration, forgetfulness
            (3) Decreased productivity, absenteeism
            (4) Sleep disturbance
        e. Related terminology—*Karoshi* (Japanese), which means death by overwork; associated with long hours and stressful working conditions
    3. Stress management intervention techniques
        a. Stress reduction techniques
            (1) Time management—determine goals and priorities, set time priorities, and learn to say no to non-goal-related activities
            (2) Time blocking—set aside time to adapt to change and incorporate it into daily routine
            (3) Change avoidance—during periods of high life change, avoid unnecessary change to prevent need to make multiple adjustments simultaneously
            (4) Habituation—incorporate routine into daily activities during stressful situation (e.g., park in same place to avoid having to look for car upon return)
            (5) Environmental modification—identify experiences and/or personalities that are abrasive or stress producing and minimize contact as much as possible
            (6) Involvement with activities of interest—doing something for others and helping with activities of interest to decrease focus on self
        b. Behavioral aspects to build stress resistance
            (1) Increase self-esteem—focus on own strengths and attributes
            (2) Increase assertiveness—substitute positive assertive behavior for negative passive actions
            (3) Meditation/prayer (includes Zen and yoga)
        c. Counter-conditioning to lower stress response
            (1) Autogenic training—repetition of autogenic suggestions such as "my hands are warm"
            (2) Imagery—image visualization used to relax or assist with past frightening experiences
            (3) Tension–relaxation exercises—tense muscles for 8–10 seconds, then relax; longer training sessions are usually required initially to enhance benefits (may be contraindicated in individuals with severe heart disease or hypertension)
            (4) Biofeedback—awareness and control to influence response that is not ordinarily under voluntary control
                (a) Electromyography—measures the amount of electrical discharge in

muscle fibers (usually forearm and forehead)
- (b) Skin temperature feedback—peripheral temperature measurement by vasomotor control found in bio-dots, mood rings, etc.
- (5) Exercise—produces physiological changes that counteract effects of stress
- d. Contraindications for stress management
  - (1) Severe depression
  - (2) Hallucinations or delusions
  - (3) Temporary hypotensive or hypoglycemic states
  - (4) Severe pain

- Social Support—strong relationship between social support and health (Bomar, 2004)
  1. Four types of supporting behaviors
     a. Emotional support—provision of empathy, love, trust, and caring (strongest, most consistent relationship to positive health status)
     b. Instrumental support, such as direct assistance or services, including money and time
     c. Informational support, such as advice, suggestions, and information
     d. Appraisal support or provision of information useful for self-evaluation purposes (feedback, affirmation)
  2. Related research
     a. Research evidence suggests that quality of supportive relationships, rather than quantity, is a better predictor of health—relationships are thought to provide buffering effects to protect people from the negative consequences of stressful situations
     b. The importance of social support has been demonstrated in multiple studies related to recovery from illness, disaster, success with weight loss, and other positive life changes; support groups can provide encouragement for those without a strong positive social network (Pender, 2002)

- Nutrition
  1. Healthy diet guidelines
     a. Eat a variety of foods, with more fruit, vegetables, whole grains, poultry, and fish (herbs/spices can enhance diminished taste associated with normal aging)
     b. Calorie breakdown—55–60% carbohydrates, < 30% fat, with remainder protein (0.8–1 g/kg)
     c. Limit total fat to less than 30% of total calories and saturated fat to less than 10% of total calories (low in saturated fat and cholesterol, moderate in total fat)
     d. Limit cholesterol intake to 300 mg/day
     e. Use sugar, salt, and sodium in moderation; choose and prepare foods with less salt and moderate sugar content
     f. The food guide pyramid (U.S. Department of Agriculture, 2011) includes the following daily recommendations
        (1) Bread, cereal, rice—6–11 servings; variety daily, especially whole grain
        (2) Vegetables—4–5 servings; fruits—3–4 servings
        (3) Milk, yogurt, and cheese—2–3 servings
        (4) Meat, poultry, fish, dry beans, eggs, and nuts—2–3 servings for a total of 6–7 oz
        (5) Oils, sweets, and fats used sparingly
     g. Multivitamins with folic acid (0.4 mg/day) are recommended for all women of childbearing age
     h. Vitamin D is needed for proper calcium absorption—the U.S. Department of Agriculture (USDA) recommends an intake of 600 IU/day up to age 70 years; older than age 70, 800 IU/day
     i. Calcium (see **Table 2-1**)
  2. Assessment for weight loss
     a. Symptoms indicative of underlying pathology (associated with and/or aggravated by excessive weight)
        (1) Polyuria/polyphagia/polydipsia (diabetes)
        (2) Joint pain or marked swelling (osteoarthritis or gout)
        (3) Angina/palpitations/dyspnea (cardiovascular disease)
        (4) Edema/cold intolerance (hypothyroidism)
        (5) Recent weight gain with edema, pruritus (renal disease)

**TABLE 2-1  Recommended Calcium Intakes**

| Age Group | Amount (mg/day) |
|---|---|
| Adolescents (13–18 years); Pregnant/lactating women | 1,300 |
| Men, women, pregnant women (19–50 years) | 1,000 |
| Men 51–70 years | 1,000 |
| Women 51–70 years | 1,200 |
| Men and women 71+ years | 1,200 |

Food sources of calcium: yogurt, milk, cheese, calcium-fortified juices and cereal, turnip and mustard greens, collards, kale, broccoli, sardines and salmon with bones

b. Contraindications for weight loss
   (1) Pregnancy
   (2) Chemotherapy because of already compromised nutritional status and potential impact on therapy
3. Body mass determinations—useful in determining both under- and overnutrition or weight-for-frame size; body mass index (BMI) is calculated by dividing weight in kilograms by height in meters squared. National Heart, Lung, and Blood Institute (NHLBI) categories of weight assessment are as follows:
   a. Underweight = < 18.5
   b. Normal weight = 18.5–24.9
   c. Overweight = 25–29.9
   d. Obese (class 1) = 30–34.9
   e. Obese (class 2) = 35–39.9
   f. Extreme obesity (class 3) = ≥ 40
4. Guidelines for healthy weight loss should include
   a. A diet characterized by a reduction in calories, not nutrients, with a focus on diet composition/preparation methods
      (1) 1,000–1,200 calories per day recommended for most women
      (2) 1,200–1,600 calories per day recommended for most men
      (3) A reduction of 500 calories per day will result in 1 lb weight loss per week
   b. A balanced diet (MyPlate); should not depend on vitamins, weight loss pills, prepared liquids, "fad diets"
   c. A diet that supplies all essential vitamins and minerals
   d. Adequate fiber for proper GI functioning
   e. Adequate fluid for renal functioning
   f. Enough fat to supply essential fatty acid linoleic acid
   g. Consumption of a variety of highly nutritious foods
   h. A goal of up to 3 lbs/week (gradual) weight loss
   i. A focus on eating regular meals, avoiding snacks, and modifying bad eating habits
   j. Follow tips on healthy behavior changes that consider cultural needs
   k. A plan to keep weight off after loss
5. Weight control strategies
   a. Regular physical activity increases caloric use, aids and sustains weight loss, preserves lean body mass and metabolism
   b. Social support by family, friends, colleagues, and support groups
   c. Focus on internal motivation for loss (e.g., control, personal goals, self-monitoring) and positive health benefits
   d. Smaller, more frequent meals to maintain blood sugar levels and avoid feeling hungry
   e. Control home environment (e.g., limit eating to one room, sit down at table without watching television)
   f. Control eating environment (e.g., avoid serving bowls at the table, use smaller plates and glasses, and eat slowly)
   g. Limit snacks (e.g., keep ready-to-eat, low-calorie snacks available)
   h. Control work environment (e.g., eat away from your desk, store food away from work area, and take exercise breaks)
   i. Use a shopping list; do not shop when hungry
   j. Keep a food diary (thoughts and feelings regarding eating patterns for 2 weeks) to guide intervention strategies
6. Health effects of severe dieting (metabolic response to starvation)
   a. Lower metabolic rate
   b. Hypertension as a result of norepinephrine release
   c. Overcompensation, gain beyond pre-diet weight
   d. Loss of fat and protein; regain fat
   e. Fat cells multiply as protective response against starvation
7. Weight loss prognostic factors
   a. Stability of present weight—number of years at present weight
   b. Motivation to change; conditions making weight loss a high priority
   c. Realistic expectations
8. Nutritional risk factors for older adults—three or more factors indicate a moderate nutritional risk (Hudgens & Langkamp-Henken, 2004)
   a. Illness or condition with potential impact on appetite, ability to eat, alertness, and memory
   b. Tooth loss or mouth pain
   c. Eating poorly, low variety, skipping meals, or more than two alcoholic beverages daily
   d. Inadequate finances for food (economic hardship)
   e. Physically unable to shop, cook, or feed self (needs assistance in self-care)
   f. Multiple medications related to influence on appetite and GI response
   g. Unintentional loss or gain of 10 lbs in past 6 months
   h. Elder beyond 80 years
   i. Three or more different medications taken daily
   j. Reduced social contact

- Physical Activity for Health—any physical activity performed regularly is beneficial; current

guidelines emphasize benefits of an exercise plan with optimal health benefits derived when that activity is in accordance with certain minimums. Health-derived benefits include
1. Physical fitness
    a. Psychological benefits
        (1) Increased alertness
        (2) Improved self-esteem, feeling better
        (3) Decreased depression
        (4) Lower stress
    b. Physical benefits
        (1) Heart—increases efficiency, lowers heart rate, lowers BP, increases oxygen capacity
        (2) Decreases low-density lipoprotein (LDL) cholesterol, increases high-density lipoprotein (HDL) cholesterol
        (3) Muscles—improves strength and endurance
        (4) Improves flexibility
        (5) Increases basal metabolic rate (BMR) during and after exercise
        (6) Weight loss of fat, not muscle
        (7) Body composition—lowers fat percentage
        (8) Antiaging effect
    c. Components of effective exercise
        (1) Moderate-intensity aerobic activity (brisk walking or equivalent) for 30 minutes 5 days weekly or
        (2) Vigorous activity (jogging or equivalent) for 20 minutes 2 days weekly
        (3) Approaches may be combined
        (4) All adults should also perform resistance training 2 days weekly
        (5) Enjoyable for participant
        (6) Rhythmic movement with alternating relaxation and contraction of large muscle groups
    d. Components of an exercise plan
        (1) Warm up (increases blood flow, loosens and strengthens muscles), e.g., brisk walk and deep breathing
        (2) Stretch (maintains and increases flexibility), e.g., stretch slowly and hold position several seconds to point of tightness, not pain; do not bounce
        (3) Endurance—select a variety of activities to work different muscle groups; start slow and build up gradually
        (4) Cool-down period allows body temperature and heart rate to decrease slowly, prevents pooling of blood in extremities and decreases muscle soreness, e.g., walk, deep breathe, and loosely shake extremities
    e. Exercise counseling
        (1) Exercises to avoid
            (a) Bouncing with stretch (strains involved joints)
            (b) Sit-ups with legs straight or double-leg lifts (strains lower back)
            (c) Duck or bent knee walk (stresses knees)
            (d) Toe touching (stresses hamstrings)
            (e) Leg splits and leg thrusts in kneeling position (stresses legs and groin area, also creates potential hip strain)
        (2) Exercise self-care
            (a) Appropriate clothing with layers in winter
            (b) Caps for cold weather and summer heat
            (c) Appropriate footwear, snug socks
            (d) Plenty of fluids before, during, and after exercise
            (e) Alternate exercise program during weather extremes, e.g., stationary bike, treadmills, steppers
        (3) Tolerance barometer—refers to potentially dangerous physical symptoms or early signs of injury
            (a) Breathlessness (inability to talk while exercising)
            (b) Excessive fatigue—fatigue for more than 1 hour after exercise
            (c) Chest discomfort, dizziness, faintness, exertional dyspnea, nausea, or vomiting
            (d) Stiffness in joints with slight loss of motion
            (e) Swelling and localized pain
    f. Exercise prescription components
        (1) Specify duration, intensity, and frequency
        (2) Progression of physical activity—gradual onset, increasing in intensity/duration, e.g., begin walking, then gradually replace with jogging
        (3) Individualized to patient capabilities
        (4) Patient motivation, goals, and interest (motivators)—adolescent females—weight control, improved appearance; adolescent males—increased skills, strength, competition; women—weight control, appearance, stress reduction; men—pleasure, fun, and challenge abilities
        (5) Based on available time, equipment, and facilities
        (6) Refer individuals with abnormal exercise stress tests (bicycle ergometer or

treadmill), chronic/recent heart or lung pathology, or any positive cardiac risk factors to the appropriate healthcare provider
    g. Physical fitness evaluation
        (1) Baseline—resting heart rate, blood pressure, and weight (calculate BMI)
        (2) Skinfold test or other determination of body fat composition
        (3) Back flexibility is tested with sit and reach test; joints should be evaluated with range of motion
        (4) Muscle strength—tested by determining maximum amount of weight that can be lifted comfortably, a single time, by four different muscle groups; test is usually conducted following completion of approximately 6 weeks of training
        (5) Aerobic capacity with bicycle ergometer or treadmill, heart is stressed to level of steady state
    h. Nutrition for athletic performance
        (1) Drink 17 ounces of fluid approximately 2 hours prior to exercise to promote hydration; allow time for excretion of excess ingested fluid; drink approximately 2 cups of fluid for every pound of weight loss during extended athletic activities
        (2) Maintain well-balanced diet—adequate carbohydrates to optimize respiratory metabolism, adequate protein to preserve lean body mass, adequate minerals to maximize oxygen delivery, and calcium to develop high-density bones (American College of Sports Medicine, 2003).

- Safety and Environment
  1. General
     a. Fire safety (smoke alarms, fire extinguishers)
     b. Home safety (secure locks on doors and windows, secure firearms)
     c. Automobile (use of safety belts, harnesses, defensive driving)
     d. Helmets and safety pads (bikes, motorcycles, inline skates); mouth guards appropriate for sport
     e. Personal safety (avoid risk-taking behaviors; always be alert to danger)
  2. Safety for aging adult
     a. Home safety
        (1) Adequate lighting especially around stairs; light switches near doorways and accessible from bed
        (2) Home should be surveyed for risk factors that may create walking hazards (loose rugs, furniture placement, electrical cords); maintain traffic lanes in each room free of hazards
        (3) Nightlight or flashlight by bed is recommended to avoid falls or disorientation in the dark
        (4) Avoid housekeeping hazards by cleaning up spills as they occur and avoiding clutter on floors/stairways
        (5) Bathroom—nonslip mat in tub/shower, secure "grab bar"
        (6) Stairwell—secure handrail, steps in good repair with contrasting color/surface at edge of steps
     b. Personal safety
        (1) Avoid dangers of hypothermia with adequate heat and caloric intake
        (2) Set up daily surveillance system with others
        (3) Assess ability to take medications correctly
     c. Physical deficit concerns
        (1) Gait and balance problems
            (a) Slippery or irregular surfaces
            (b) Clutter or obstructions
            (c) Stairs steep or without rails
            (d) Lack of space to maneuver assistive device (e.g., walker)
            (e) Bathtub without secure rail or slip guards
        (2) Decreased vision
            (a) Inadequate lighting
            (b) Poorly marked stairs
        (3) Decreased sensitivity to pain/heat
            (a) Hot water bottle/heating pad
            (b) Hot bath water
        (4) Potential driving/traffic hazards
            (a) Decreased visual acuity and hearing
            (b) Decreased reaction time
            (c) Difficulty moving head due to arthritis or disc problems
            (d) Ambulation too slow for traffic signals
  3. Four categories of environmental hazards
     a. Biological (e.g., viruses, microorganisms)
     b. Chemical (e.g., lead, asbestos)
     c. Physical (e.g., natural disasters)
     d. Sociological and psychological hazards (e.g., overcrowding, lack of resources)
  4. Components of an environmental assessment
     a. Home hazards—fire safety, pest control, inadequate heat or toilet facilities
     b. Work site hazards and protection—noise, inhalants, lifting, hazardous materials; related exposures
     c. Neighborhood hazards—noise, air/water pollution, inadequate police protection, overcrowding or isolation from neighbors

d. Community hazards—lack of availability of grocery stores, drugstores, public transportation

## HEALTH EVALUATION ACROSS THE LIFE SPAN

- Health History—important in identifying risk behaviors and need for health education
  1. Demographics and biographical data
  2. Chief complaint and history of present illness
     a. Reason for seeking health care or chief complaint—signs/symptoms and duration; preferably in patient's own words
     b. Symptom analysis (OPQRST) and any other relevant information to elucidate the chief complaint
        O—Onset
        P—Provocative/Palliative (better or worse)
        Q—Quality/Quantity
        R—Region/Radiation
        S—Setting
        T—Timing
  3. Past medical history
     a. General state of health (patient's perception)
     b. Past illnesses and hospitalizations
     c. Past injuries, surgery (dates, treatment, and follow-up)
     d. Emotional health (past problems including assistance, history of domestic violence)
     e. Sexual health (obstetric and contraceptive history, number of partners, sexual preference, sexual problems, disease prevention efforts)
     f. Food or drug allergies (specify reaction and treatment, if any)
     g. Medications (prescription, over the counter, herbal, folk remedies)
     h. Immunizations (type and date)
     i. Sleep patterns (approximate hours, difficulties, e.g., difficulty falling asleep [DFA], early morning awakening [EMA], nightmares)
     j. Last examinations (physical, dental, vision, hearing, radiography, electrocardiogram [ECG], cancer screenings)
  4. Personal habits
     a. Tobacco use—cigarettes, pipe, cigars, smokeless; record number of cigarettes per day, number of years used, if stopped, how long ago; approach adolescents with declarative statements related to drugs at school, drugs in common use at school, drugs used by friends, and by individuals; inquire about tobacco use in terms of number of packs smoked daily
     b. Alcohol and drug use (type, amount)
     c. Use of caffeine (coffee, colas, etc.)
     d. Diet (24-hour intake, including nutritional supplements)
     e. Exercise (type, frequency)
     f. Leisure activities (type, frequency)
     g. Sexual practices and activities (disease prevention, contraception, number of partners, and sexual preferences)
     h. Sports (type, frequency)
     i. Information required regarding sports participation, especially contact sports includes (Armado & Thomas, 2002)
        (1) Family history of heart disease, high blood pressure, or Marfan's syndrome
        (2) Prior limitation from sports
        (3) Exertional dyspnea or chest pain
        (4) Seizure, concussion, or history of unconsciousness
        (5) Ability to run ½ mile or more
        (6) Missing kidney
        (7) Recent history of mononucleosis
  5. Psychosocial history
     a. Living situation at present
     b. Education—for adolescents ask, if in school, grades, positive or negative attitudes toward school
     c. Religious beliefs in relation to health and treatment
     d. Positive or negative perspective of the future
     e. Perception of "typical day"
     f. Stress, stress management
     g. Depression or anxiety, suicide ideation (adolescents and young adults require direct questioning, e.g., have you ever thought of killing yourself)
     h. Support systems
  6. Family history—include age, health status, or cause of death of parents, siblings, children in a genogram (diabetes, heart disease, cancer, hypertension, lung disease, alcoholism, blood disorders, birth defects, and any other illnesses that seem to run in the family)
  7. Occupational and environmental history
     a. Type of work, former occupation(s)
     b. Hazardous exposures at home or work
     c. Military service, wartime employment, if any
     d. Location of home, length of time
     e. Home location adjacent to factories, shipyards, or other potentially hazardous facilities
     f. Hobbies, potential exposures
  8. Adolescent interviewing guidelines
     a. Adolescent is primary historian, interviewed alone
     b. Explain ground rules—unless serious problem emerges threatening life or health, interview is confidential

c. Home, Education, Activities, Drugs, Sex, Suicide (HEADSS) interview format is widely suggested—see age-related anticipatory guidance
9. Older adult interviewing guidelines
   a. Ensure that the patient is the primary historian; utilize caregivers and family members as additional sources of information
   b. Ensure that the patient can hear you
   c. Allow adequate time for information processing and response

- Risk Factor Identification—virtually every disease and condition has risk factors; select conditions are presented related to prevalence, in addition to protective factor
   1. Research over the past 20 years has identified factors associated with physical health and longer, healthier life (Pender, 2002)
      a. Exercise—regular (see exercise, this chapter)
      b. Nonsmoker, recently extended to smoke-free environment
      c. Seven to eight hours of sleep
      d. Moderate or no alcohol
      e. Regular and moderate eating (including breakfast)
      f. Weight control
   2. Cardiac risk factors
      a. Age—male 45+, female 55+ or premature menopause
      b. Family history of premature heart disease, myocardial infarction, or death of father/first degree male relative < 55, mother/female relative < 65
      c. Cigarette smoking
      d. Hypertension or on antihypertensive medication (defined as > 140/90 mm Hg in patients < 60 years of age and all patients with diabetes mellitus or chronic kidney disease and > 150/90 mm Hg in patients ≥ 60 years of age without diabetes mellitus or chronic kidney disease)
      e. Low HDL cholesterol < 40 mg/dL (> 60 mg/dL negative risk)
      f. LDL > 100 mg/dL
      g. Diabetes mellitus
   3. Obesity (20% above desirable weight)—mortality rates increase with weights 10% above desirable weights; obesity is associated with multiple attendant health risks (U.S. Preventative Services Task Force, 2014)
      a. Three times more prevalent in patients with hypertension and type 2 diabetes mellitus
      b. Increased risk of high cholesterol and coronary artery disease
      c. Increased risk of cancer (colon, rectal, prostate, gallbladder, biliary tract, breast, cervical, endometrial, and ovarian)
      d. Abdominal adiposity associated with increased risk of stroke and death from all causes
   4. Suicide risk factors
      a. Family history of psychiatric disorders (especially depression or suicide)
      b. Previous suicide attempts
      c. Family violence (verbal, physical, or sexual abuse)
      d. Family instability (frequent separation from, or loss of, loved one)
      e. Alcohol or substance abuse
      f. Availability and accessibility of firearms in the home

- Age-Related Health Monitoring (if asymptomatic)—specific health screenings are part of secondary prevention; see **Table 2-2**
   1. Screening guidelines
      a. Generalized screening indicated for diseases of high prevalence in the population and diseases with profound morbidity/mortality if not diagnosed
      b. Screening tests must be reliable with acceptable technical process; must include appropriate follow-up
      c. Tests should be sensitive (those with disease screen positive); may need confirmatory testing with high-specificity testing (those who are positive have the disease for which they are tested)
   2. Adolescence (12–19 years of age)—American Medical Association (AMA) recommends three visit intervals, 11–14 years, 15–17 years, and 18–21 years, unless more frequent examinations are indicated; information available on AMA website, "Guidelines for Adolescent Preventative Services (GAPS)"
      a. Complete physical examination including
         (1) Height/weight (use anthropometric chart)
            (a) Screen for eating disorders if indicated
            (b) Assess perception of food, weight
         (2) Complete skin examination
         (3) Assessment for gingivitis, caries, and malalignment
         (4) Assessment for signs of abuse or neglect
         (5) Hearing assessment (if exposed to excessive noise) and vision assessment
      b. Blood pressure (BP) every 2 years, normal 120/80 mm Hg or below
      c. Tuberculin skin test (PPD) every 2 years with any exposure or if at risk

TABLE 2-2 Adult Screening Guidelines (U.S. Preventive Services Task Force, American Cancer Society, NCEP ATP-III, NHLBI JNC VIII)

| Service | Who Needs | Frequency[a] | Risk Factors |
|---|---|---|---|
| Blood pressure | All adults | Every 2 years | Male, blk, fam hx |
| Cholesterol | All adults | Every 5 years | Male, tob, htn, fam hx |
| Dental | All adults | Annual | |
| ECG | Adults 40+ | Annual (only with cardiac risk factors) | |
| Pap smear | Women 3 years after onset of intercourse but no earlier than age 21 | Recommended every 3 years after two normal exams for women without risk factors[b] | New sexual partners; unprotected sex |
| Self-breast exam | No recommendation for or against (ACS) | | Fam hx of breast cancer |
| Clinical breast exam | Women 40+ | Annual (age 20–39 every 3 years) | Fam hx of breast cancer |
| Mammogram (ACS) | Women 40+ | Annual (ACS) (USPSTF every 1–2 years) | Fam hx of breast cancer |
| Colorectal screen (fecal testing annually, flexible sigmoidoscopy or double contrast barium enema every 5 years, or colonoscopy every 10 years) | Adults 50+ | Any positive FOBT, flexible sigmoidoscopy, or double contrast barium enema should be followed with colonoscopy | Fam hx of colorectal cancer |
| Prostate specific antigen (PSA) with or without digital rectal exam[c] | Men 50+; at age 45 if African American or have a father or brother who died of prostate cancer before age 65 | Annual (ACS) | Blk, fam hx |
| Glaucoma screen[c] | Adults 40+ | Annual (with risk factors)[d] | |
| Hearing | Only w/excessive noise exposure | | |
| Chest x-ray | Not recommended | | |
| Thyroid palpation[c] | Adults 20–39<br>Adults 40+ | Every 3 years<br>Annual | |
| Urinalysis | Controversy | | |
| Hgb/Hct | Controversy | | |
| Health education/promotion (nutrition, exercise, stress management, substance abuse, safety, safe sex, and cancer prevention) | All adults | Every encounter | |

Blk = African American; dm = diabetes mellitus; ECG = echocardiogram; fam hx = family history; FOBT = fecal occult blood test; htn = hypertension; STD = sexually transmitted disease; tob = tobacco use;
[a]Increased frequency in the presence of risk factors.
[b]Risk factors for cervical cancer—history of STD, multiple partners, tob, first intercourse before age 18.
[c]Insufficient evidence to recommend for or against screening; the patient and healthcare provider should have a conversation about risk versus benefit.
[d]Risk factors for glaucoma—myopia, dm, fam hx, blk > 40.
The term *controversy* indicates that the U.S. Preventive Services Task Force recommends against routine screening.
Source: Adapted from *Guide to Clinical Preventive Services 2007*, by U.S. Preventive Services Task Force, American Cancer Society, National Cholesterol Education Program ATP-III, and National Heart Lung and Blood Institute JNC VIII (2013). Consult full reports for details.

    d. Female
       (1) Teach self-breast examination (SBE)
       (2) Determine Tanner stage
          (a) Stage I— prepubertal, average age for girls 10 years
          (b) Stage II—breast bud, sparse pubic hair
          (c) Stage III—breast mound development, pubic hair becomes coarser, growth spurt

(d) Stage IV—menarche
(e) Stage V—mature stage
(3) If sexually active and > 21 years old—Papanicolaou (pap) smear
e. Male
(1) Teach self-testicular examination (STE)
(2) Determine Tanner stage
(a) Stage I—prepubertal
(b) Stage II—scrotum skin thins, reddens, testicular volume increases
(c) Stage III—growth spurt, penis lengthens
(d) Stage IV—male organ enlargement in length and width
(e) Stage V—mature stage
f. If high risk, counseling and test for human immunodeficiency virus (HIV) and venereal disease research laboratory (VDRL) test; assess knowledge of contraceptives and protective barriers
g. Immunization
(1) Tetanus-diphtheria booster (Td)
(2) Others if needed; see immunization guidelines, this chapter
h. Remain alert for depressive symptoms, any suicide risk factors
i. Dental checkup with cleaning annually
3. Young adult (20–39 years of age) (see Table 2-2)
a. Complete physical examination (age 20, then every 5–6 years)
b. BP every 2 years; normal systolic 110–130 mm Hg, diastolic 60–80 mm Hg
c. Fractionated cholesterol screening every 5 years (may substitute nonfasting total cholesterol screen in low-risk individuals)
d. Female
(1) Pap and pelvic examination every 3 years, gonorrhea (GC) and chlamydia tests
(2) Clinical breast examination (by health professional) every 3 years
e. Male—clinical testicular examination every 3 years
f. PPD if exposed to tuberculosis
g. Immunizations—Td every 10 years; substitute 1 Tdap
h. Self-skin examination
i. Dental checkup with cleaning annually
4. Middle-aged adult (40–59 years of age) (see Table 2-2)
a. Complete physical examination (every 5–6 years)
b. BP every 2 years; normal systolic 110–130 mm Hg, diastolic 60–80 mm Hg; goal < 140/90 mm Hg; < 140/90 mm Hg if comorbid diabetes mellitus or chronic kidney disease (National Heart, Lung, and Blood Institute, 2013)
c. Cholesterol screening every 5 years; low-risk screening option not indicated over age 40
d. ECG, age 40+ with cardiac risk factors
e. Female
(1) Clinical breast exam yearly (performed by a health professional)
(2) Mammogram annually (ACS), every 1–2 years (USPSTF)
(3) Pap and pelvic examination every 3 years if no risk factors
f. Male—discuss prostate screening age 50 and annually (high-risk begin age 45) (ACS)
g. Colorectal screen (fecal occult or sigmoidoscopy)—age 50 annually
h. Glaucoma screen, annually
i. Dental examination with cleaning every 6–12 months
j. Cancer screening yearly
k. Immunizations—tetanus every 10 years
5. Elderly adult (60+ years of age) (see Table 2-2)
a. Complete physical examination every 2 years with laboratory assessments
b. BP every 2 years, goal < 150/90 mm Hg
c. Fractionated cholesterol every 5 years
d. ECG annually with cardiac risk factors
e. Female
(1) Mammogram—annual (ACS); every 1–2 years (USPSTF)
(2) Pap and pelvic examination every 3 years until age 70—no routine screening after age 70
f. Male—clinical testicular examination annually
g. Colorectal screen (fecal occult or sigmoidoscopy) age 50—annually
h. Glaucoma screen—annually
i. Dental examination with cleaning every 6–12 months
j. Immunizations—tetanus every 10 years, pneumococcal vaccine once, annual influenza vaccine, varicella zoster vaccine

- Age-Related Anticipatory Guidance (Wilkinson et al., 2013)
1. Adolescence (12–19 years of age)
a. Leading causes of death—motor vehicle accidents (MVA), suicide, other accidents, homicide, cardiovascular disease, congenital disease
b. Normal growth and development
(1) Physical changes with puberty
(2) Need for increased self-responsibilities for own health—nutrition, exercise, adequate sleep and safety habits
c. Nutrition
(1) Variety of foods, including breakfast
(2) Nutritious snacks, limit sweets and fast food

     d. Skin care/skin protection
     e. Dental care (brushing and flossing)
        (1) Fluoride supplementation
        (2) Dental visits with cleaning every 6–12 months
     f. Injury prevention
        (1) Athletics, safety helmets, pads, mouth guards
        (2) Safety belts
        (3) Firearm safety
        (4) Defensive driving, driver education
        (5) Violent behavior/gangs
     g. Physical activity
        (1) Need for regular physical activity
        (2) Encourage team activities, peer interaction
        (3) Encourage participation in after school and/or church activities
     h. Substance abuse
        (1) Tobacco use avoidance or cessation emphasizing unattractive cosmetic effects (stained teeth and fingernails, foul-smelling breath and clothes) and athletic consequences (decreased endurance, shortness of breath)
        (2) Smokeless tobacco is not safer, can be addicting/life-threatening
        (3) Alcohol and other drugs
     i. Sexuality
        (1) Dating
        (2) Responsible sexual behaviors, abstinence, contraception
        (3) Risks, sexually transmitted diseases, unwanted pregnancy
2. Young adult (20–39 years of age)
     a. Leading causes of death—motor vehicle accidents, homicide, suicide, injuries, heart disease
     b. Nutrition and exercise
        (1) Weight management with changing basal metabolic rate
        (2) Selection of exercise program
     c. Dental care
     d. Sexuality
        (1) Family planning, contraception
        (2) Sexually transmitted diseases
     e. Cancer warning signs, skin protection
     f. Substance use/abuse
        (1) Tobacco cessation, primary prevention
        (2) Alcohol and other drugs
     g. Injury prevention
        (1) Athletics
        (2) Safety belts, safety helmets
        (3) Firearm safety
        (4) Defensive driving
        (5) Violent behavior
     h. Lifestyle choices
        (1) Family and parenting skills
        (2) Stress management
     i. Safety and environmental health
3. Middle-aged adult (40–59 years of age)
     a. Leading causes of death—heart and vascular disease; lung, breast, prostate, and colorectal cancer
     b. Nutrition and exercise
        (1) Weight management with changing basal metabolic rate
        (2) Selection of exercise program
     c. Dental care
     d. Sexuality
        (1) Menopause
        (2) Sexual changes due to aging
        (3) Sexually transmitted diseases
     e. Cancer warning signs, skin protection
     f. Substance use/abuse
        (1) Tobacco cessation, primary prevention
        (2) Alcohol and other drugs
     g. Injury prevention
        (1) Athletics
        (2) Safety belts, safety helmets
        (3) Firearm safety
        (4) Defensive driving
        (5) Violent behavior
     h. Midlife changes
        (1) Empty nest syndrome, grandparenting
        (2) Planning for retirement
        (3) Stress management
     i. Safety and environmental health
4. Elderly adult (age 60+ years of age)
     a. Leading causes of death—heart and vascular disease, cancers as described for 40–59 age group, and influenza and pneumonia
     b. Nutrition and exercise
        (1) Weight management with changing basal metabolic rate
        (2) Selection of exercise program
     c. Dental care
     d. Sexuality
        (1) Sexual changes due to aging
        (2) Sexually transmitted diseases
     e. Cancer warning signs, skin protection
     f. Substance use/abuse
        (1) Tobacco cessation, primary prevention
        (2) Alcohol and other drugs
     g. Injury prevention
        (1) Athletics
        (2) Safety belts, safety helmets
        (3) Firearm safety
        (4) Defensive driving
        (5) Violent behavior
     h. Life changes
        (1) Retirement
        (2) Loss of spouse, friends

(3) Physical changes (vision, hearing, reaction time, alterations of bowel and bladder habits)
   i. Safety and environmental health
      (1) Home safety
      (2) Personal safety

- Immunization Guidelines (Centers for Disease Control and Prevention, 2014)
  1. Td booster is recommended every 10 years; adolescents 14–16 years of age should receive booster if no dose in past 5 years; every adult should have one dose of Tdap in place of Td vaccine
  2. Measles-mumps-rubella vaccine (MMR)—recommended for adolescents who have not received two doses at or after 12 months of age; second dose is now given routinely as part of preschool immunizations or at age 12–14 years, or prior to postsecondary education or military service; adults without documentation of disease or immunization need only one dose; adults born prior to 1956 are considered immune due to prevalence of diseases before that time
  3. Varicella vaccine—recommended for individuals who have never had chickenpox; adolescents and adults need two doses 4–8 weeks apart
  4. Influenza vaccine—recommended annually for all adults
     a. Groups that can transmit influenza to high-risk persons should be prioritized for immunization (e.g., healthcare workers and household members)
     b. Optimal time for immunization (mid-October through mid-November)
     c. Contraindications—there are no identified contraindications; patients with a history of hypersensitivity to influenza vaccine should be considered on a case-by-case basis
  5. Pneumococcal vaccine—recommended for any person who is at increased risk of complications due to chronic illness (e.g., heart or lung disease and diabetes, alcoholism, Hodgkin's disease, cirrhosis, sickle cell disease) and individuals who work or live with high-risk individuals); anyone over age 65 and persons without a spleen; revaccination after 5 or more years is recommended for those at highest risk of antibody decline, e.g., those with renal disease or who have undergone organ transplant and persons vaccinated before age 65
  6. Human papillomavirus (HPV) vaccine—a 3-dose series recommended for males and females between the ages of 9 and 26 years regardless of sexual history or history of HPV diagnosis
  7. Meningococcal vaccine—MCV4 vaccine should be administered at age 11–12 years with a booster dose at age 16
  8. Hepatitis B vaccine (HBV)—three-dose regimen now recommended for all individuals at time 0, 1–2 months, and 4–6 months. Adults who are at increased risk of infection include healthcare workers, individuals at high risk of exposure to blood and blood products, and individuals at increased risk of exposure due to sexual practices. The timing and need for periodic boosters is determined by serologic testing. Immunization series is now recommended for all adolescents who were not previously immunized.
  9. Zostavax vaccine is a live, attenuated virus indicated for the prevention of herpes zoster (shingles) in adults > age 60. It is given as a single dose 0.65 cc subcutaneous injection. Should not be given to those who are immunocompromised or who have a history of allergic response to gelatin or neomycin.
  10. Hepatitis A vaccine (HAV)—two doses at time 0 and 6–12 months are recommended for individuals working in or traveling to countries with high levels of HAV infection; men who have sex with men, parenteral drug users, persons exposed to nonhuman primates, persons with chronic liver disease
  11. Polio—inactivated poliovirus vaccine-enhanced potency (IVP-e) is indicated for unimmunized adults who are traveling outside the United States and healthcare workers; partially immunized or unimmunized adults with close contact with children receiving OPV; the second dose is given 1 month after the first with a third dose 6 months later
  12. Lyme disease—people age 15+ working in endemic geographic areas may be at risk and should receive Lyme disease vaccine
  13. Catch-up schedule, contraindications and precautions
      a. For individuals with uncertain immunization histories (lacking documentation)
         (1) First visit—Td, IPV, MMR, HBV, HAV, varicella, influenza, pneumococcal are optional depending upon risk factors
         (2) Second visit (4–6 weeks after first visit)—Td, IPV, HBV, with second dose of HAV, varicella, if given initially
         (3) Third visit (6 months after second visit)—Td, IPV, HBV, with third dose of HAV for adolescents
      b. Contraindications

(1) Anaphylactic reaction to known component
    (a) MMR and influenza (eggs)
    (b) Hepatitis (baker's yeast)
    (c) IPV (streptomycin, polymyxin B or neomycin)
    (d) Varicella (gelatin or neomycin)
(2) Moderate to severe illness (fever > 100.4°F)
(3) Immunocompromised individuals (no live virus)
    c. Precaution with MMR—delay pregnancy for 3 months following immunization
14. Immunization schedule synopsis for adolescents and adults with documentation of immunizations during childhood
    a. Adolescents and adults
        (1) Hepatitis B series
        (2) Td booster, repeat every 10 years
        (3) Varicella, if needed, two doses 4–8 weeks apart
        (4) MMR if born after 1956
    b. Adults over 65, chronic disease (heart, lung, or diabetes; those who work or live with high-risk individuals)
        (1) Influenza vaccine each fall
        (2) Pneumococcal vaccine

## QUESTIONS

■ **Select the best answer.**

1. Using the Health Belief Model, determine which of the following individuals would be most motivated for behavior change:
    a. 42-year-old married female with excess weight for over 20 years
    b. 16-year-old female with poorly controlled sugar levels and poor dietary habits consistent with her friends
    c. 50-year-old male with recent myocardial infarction, whose prognosis is good with positive changes in diet and weight loss
    d. 40-year-old male who reports spouse wants him to lose weight

2. Which of the following activities would prepare an individual planning retirement to successfully resolve the final developmental tasks proposed by Erickson?
    a. Plan to simultaneously complete any community obligations
    b. Become involved with community activities
    c. Plan several extended trips early in retirement while able
    d. Avoid any commitments initially; wait for opportunities to present themselves

3. Screening for breast cancer is which level of prevention?
    a. Primary
    b. Secondary
    c. Tertiary
    d. Preliminary

4. Patient (age 70) comes into your clinic the first week of November for health screening. Her last immunization, Td (tetanus), was 10 years ago. Which immunization(s) will you recommend?
    a. Td, influenza, and pneumococcal vaccine
    b. Influenza and pneumococcal vaccine and schedule Td within 3 months
    c. Td and influenza
    d. Td only

5. A temporary certificate for school attendance is given following initial immunizations for a 14-year-old boy. When should the adolescent return for more immunizations?
    a. 6 months
    b. 4–6 weeks
    c. 1 year
    d. 4 months

6. A woman, age 19, will be entering college in January. She is not pregnant. Without evidence of recent immunization, she should receive which of the following today?
    a. Second MMR, Td, and polio boosters
    b. *Haemophilus influenzae* type b (HIB) and a tetanus booster
    c. Second MMR and Td
    d. Immunization for rubella, tetanus, and influenza

7. Joe, age 15, has just moved to your community and is staying in a temporary foster home. He has no record of any immunizations. Which of the following does Joe need today?
    a. MMR, Td, and varicella
    b. IPV, MMR, HBV, and Td
    c. Td only
    d. MMR and Td

8. According to research, which type of social support has the strongest relationship with health status?

   a. Emotional
   b. Instrumental
   c. Informational
   d. Appraisal

9. According to research, how much sleep is associated with a longer, healthier life?

   a. 5–6 hours
   b. 6–7 hours
   c. 7–8 hours
   d. 8–9 hours

10. Josh, age 32, is ready to start exercising and wants to jog. Guidelines should include which of the following?

    a. Jog 1 mile initially, then add distance daily until goal is reached
    b. Jog at least once a week for 30 minutes to condition his heart and lungs
    c. Begin with brisk walking and gradually replace with jogging for at least 20 minutes 2 times weekly
    d. Warm-up exercises before or after jogging

11. Several cups of coffee immediately prior to the clinic visit would likely elevate which of the following?

    a. Heart rate
    b. Respiratory rate
    c. Cholesterol
    d. Blood sugar

12. Jim asks why cooling down is necessary for an exercise plan. You tell him cooling down will:

    a. Allow the body temperature and heart rate to decrease slowly
    b. Loosen and strengthen muscles
    c. Maintain and increase flexibility
    d. Sustain heart rate for a longer period of time

13. According to the Transtheoretical Model, intervention at which level is most likely to result in behavior change?

    a. Maintenance
    b. Contemplation
    c. Precontemplation
    d. Preparation

14. Which stress management technique would be most appropriate for a newly diagnosed diabetic?

    a. Change avoidance
    b. Habituation
    c. Time blocking
    d. Imagery

15. According to the U.S. Preventive Services Task Force Recommendations, a woman age 21 needs which of the following annually?

    a. Blood pressure and cholesterol screen
    b. Clinical breast exam
    c. Pap and pelvic exam
    d. Dental screen

16. Your female patient, age 49, has had a normal baseline mammogram. She asks when she should get her next mammogram. You advise:

    a. Annually or every 1–2 years
    b. Every other year from age 50 to 59, then yearly
    c. Every 3 years until age 60
    d. Every 5 years for the rest of her life

## Answers

1. **c**   9. **c**
2. **b**   10. **c**
3. **b**   11. **a**
4. **a**   12. **a**
5. **b**   13. **d**
6. **c**   14. **c**
7. **b**   15. **d**
8. **a**   16. **a**

## BIBLIOGRAPHY

American Cancer Society. (2014). Guidelines for the early detection of cancer. Retrieved from http://www.cancer.org/healthy/findcancerearly/cancerscreening guidelines/american-cancer-society-guidelines-for-the-early-detection-of-cancer

American College of Sports Medicine. (2003). *American College of Sports Medicine fitness book* (3rd ed.). Champaign, IL: Author.

American College of Sports Medicine. (2011). Quantity and quality of exercise for developing and maintaining cardiorespiratory, musculoskeletal, and neuromotor fitness in apparently healthy adults: Guidance for prescribing exercise. *Medicine and Science in Sports and Exercise, 43*(7), 1334–1359. doi:10.1249/

MSS.0b013e318213fefb. Retrieved from http://journals.lww.com/acsm-msse/Fulltext/2011/07000/Quantity_and_Quality_of_Exercise_for_Developing.26.aspx

Armado, J., & Thomas, D. (2002). Early recognition of Marfan's syndrome. *Journal of the American Association of Nurse Practitioners, 14*(5), 201–204.

Bandura, A. (1986). *Social foundations of thought and action.* Englewood Cliffs, NJ: Prentice Hall.

Becker, M. (1972). The health belief model and personal health behavior. *Health Education Monographs, 2,* 326–327.

Bomar, P. (2004). *Promotion of health in families: Applying research and theory.* Philadelphia, PA: Saunders.

Centers for Disease Control and Prevention. (2014). Adult immunization schedules. Retrieved from http://www.cdc.gov/vaccines/schedules/hcp/adult.html

Clark, M. (2003). *Nursing in the community* (4th ed.). Norwalk, CT: Appleton & Lange.

Erikson, E. (1963). *Childhood and society* (2nd ed.). New York, NY: Norton.

Friedman, M., Bowden, V., & Jones, S. (2003). *Family nursing: Research, theory, and practice* (5th ed.). Upper Saddle River, NJ: Prentice Hall.

Green, L., & Kreuter, M. (1991). *Health promotion planning: An educational and environmental approach.* Mountain View, CA: Mayfield.

Hudgens, J., & Langkamp-Henken, B. (2004). The Mini Nutritional Assessment as an assessment tool in elders in long-term care. *Nutrition in Clinical Practice, 19*(5), 463–470.

Lewin, K. (1951). *Field theory in social science; selected theoretical papers* (D. Cartwright, ed.). New York, NY: Harper & Row.

Maslow, A. (1954). *Motivation and personality.* New York, NY: Harper & Row.

National Heart, Lung, and Blood Institute. (2013). 8th report of the Joint National Committee on Prevention, Detection, Evaluation, and Treatment of High Blood Pressure (JNC 8). *Journal of the American Medical Association.* [published online December 18, 2013]. JAMA. doi:10.1001/jama.2013.284427

National Heart, Lung, and Blood Institute Education Initiative. (2000). *The practical guide: Identification, evaluation, and treatment of overweight and obesity in adults.* Retrieved from http://www.nhlbi.nih.gov/guidelines/obesity/prctgd_c.pdf

Neuman, B., & Fawcett, J. (2002). *The Neuman systems model.* Upper Saddle River, NJ: Prentice Hall.

Pender, N. (2002). *Health promotion in nursing practice* (4th ed.). Upper Saddle River, NJ: Prentice Hall.

Prochaska, J., & Velicer, W. (1997). The Transtheoretical Model of health behavior change. *American Journal of Health Promotion, 12*(I), 38–48.

Selye, H. (1974). *Stress without distress.* Philadelphia, PA: Lippincott.

Swartz, M. (2009). *Textbook of physical diagnosis* (4th ed.). Philadelphia, PA: Saunders.

U.S. Department of Agriculture. (2011). MyPlate. Retrieved June 30, 2014 from http://www.choosemyplate.gov/information-healthcare-professionals.html

U.S. Department of Health and Human Services. (2011). *Healthy people 2020.* Washington, DC: U.S. Government Printing Office.

U.S. Preventive Services Task Force. (2014). *The guide to clinical preventive services: Recommendations of the United States Preventive Services Task Force.* Retrieved from http://www.uspreventiveservicestaskforce.org/adultrec.htm

von Bertalanffy, L. (1968). *General systems theory.* New York, NY: George Braziller.

Wilkinson, J., Bass, C., Diem, S., Gravley, A., Harvey, L., Maciosek, M., ... Institute for Clinical Systems Improvement. (2013). *Preventive services children and adolescents.* Retrieved from https://www.icsi.org/_asset/x1mnv1/PrevServKids.pdf

# Special Considerations in the Gerontological Patient

*Debbie Gilbert Kramer*

## DEMOGRAPHICS OF OLDER ADULTS

The elderly population in the United States is increasing rapidly. This population's rates are significantly higher than those of other segments of the population. A greater number of aged persons are living longer and healthier lives for a variety of reasons, including improved health care and healthier lifestyles. The average U.S. life span has increased appreciably since the beginning of the 20th century. The average life expectancy at birth increased by almost 2 years during the past decade. The term *elderly* is generally accepted as referring to persons 65 years of age and older. The World Health Organization further categorizes the elderly population as follows:

- Definitions of Late Adulthood
  1. Age 65–74 years—the young-old
  2. Age 75–84 years—the middle-old
  3. Age 85–100 the oldest-old
  4. Age ≥ 100 years—the elite old

- Population Statistics (U.S. Census Bureau, 2012)
  1. The years 2010 to 2030 will see a sharp increase in the > 65 years population because of the aging of baby boomers and decrease in mortality at older ages
  2. More people were > 65 years old than in any other census
  3. The Census Bureau projects the elderly population will more than double to 80 million, 1 in 4 persons, between now and 2050; in 2010 there were 40.4 million, up 5.4 million from the 2000 census
  4. The > 95 years population increased by 26%
  5. The > 65 years population increased by 15.1% as compared to a 9.7% increase in the overall population
  6. The 80–94 years age group was the third largest growing group
  7. The baby boomers will number 19 million in 2050 when they become the oldest-old, making them 24% of elderly Americans and 5% of all Americans
  8. The leading causes of death at age 65 and older are heart disease, cancer, stroke, chronic obstructive pulmonary disease, and pneumonia/influenza

- Gender Statistics
  1. Elderly women outnumber elderly men with a ratio of 100 to 82 between ages 65 and 74 years; ratio widens to 100 to 50 by age 85 years; however, this gap is narrowing
  2. The majority of elderly men live with a spouse or other relative; the majority of elderly women live alone
  3. Men have higher death rates at each age; additionally, the highest percentage of successful suicides in all populations is the elderly Caucasian male

- Ethnic Diversity
  1. Caucasians comprise the highest percentage of the U.S. population > 65 years of age at 83%, but this trend is narrowing
  2. Representation by other ethnic groups is on the rise; by 2030 it is projected that

a. Percentage of African Americans will increase from 8% to 11%
b. Percentage of Latinos will increase from 4.5% to 17%
c. Percentage of Asians and Pacific Islanders will increase from 2.3% to 7.4%

- Marital Status and Living Arrangements
  1. In 2010, more than half of older noninstitutionalized persons were living with a spouse
  2. The likelihood of living alone or in a residential care facility increases with age
      a. 73% of noninstitutionalized elderly men were married and living with their spouses; 41% of their female counterparts were married and living with their spouses
      b. 10% of the older population were divorced or separated
      c. 31% of noninstitutionalized elderly lived alone; half of women older than 75 years lived alone
      d. Older women were four times more likely than men to be widowed—46% versus 14%; 8 out of 10 elderly persons living alone are women
  3. Only 9% of noninstitutionalized persons aged 65–69 years needed assistance with their activities of daily living (ADLs), whereas 50% of the 85-and-older age group required such assistance
  4. Although a small number of the older-than-65-year population lived in nursing homes in 2000, the percentage increases dramatically with age from 1.1% at ages 65–74 to 18.2% for persons older than 85 years
  5. In 2010, almost 485,000 grandparents older than 65 years were the persons with primary responsibilities for their grandchildren who lived with them
  6. Most persons older than 65 years lived in metropolitan areas
  7. In 2010, more than half (56.5%) of persons 65 years or older lived in 11 states: California, Florida, New York, Pennsylvania, Texas, Ohio, Illinois, Michigan, North Carolina, Georgia, and New Jersey

- Income and Poverty
  1. Likelihood of living below the government-defined poverty level increases with age
  2. Older persons living alone are much more likely to be poor than are those living with families
  3. Older women (10.7%) have a higher poverty rate than older men (6.7%), and, in 2010, 10.4% of married couples were living below the poverty line
  4. Elderly African Americans (23.8%) and Hispanics (21.4%) outnumber Caucasians (8.3%) with low income levels
  5. Within each race/ethnic group, poverty is more prevalent in women than in men; income varies with differences in age, gender, race, ethnicity, marital status, living arrangements, education, former occupation, and work history
  6. In 2010, the median income of elderly men was $25,704 and $15,072 for women

- Educational Status
  1. Better education is correlated with a healthier, longer life
  2. In 2010, 79% of noninstitutionalized elderly had completed high school, a statistic that varied considerably by race and ethnicity
  3. The oldest-old were more likely to have only an eighth-grade education or less (24% versus 6%); the level of education decreases with increase in age
  4. 17% of the elderly have college degrees versus 20% of those aged 55–59 years and 27% of persons 45–49 years

- Health and Health Care
  1. 40% of noninstitutionalized elderly rated their health as excellent or very good as compared to 64.7% for adults aged 18–64 years; Caucasians had the highest percentage perception of good health (42.8%), followed by Asians (35.3%), Latinos (28.2%), African Americans (26%), and Alaskan and Native Americans (24.3%)
  2. In 2010, 63% of the elderly received an influenza vaccine and 59% received pneumococcal vaccine
  3. In 2010, persons > 65 years old averaged 7.1 outpatient visits as compared to 3.7 outpatient visits for adults < 65 years of age
  4. In 2010, 97% of elderly reported that they had a usual place to go for health care; only 3% reported failure to obtain medical care during the previous 12 months because of financial barriers
  5. In 2010, 93.1% of noninstitutionalized elderly were covered by Medicare
  6. 58% had some type of private health insurance
  7. 8% had military-based health insurance
  8. Among institutionalized Medicare beneficiaries, 46% also were covered by Medicaid

## THEORIES OF BIOLOGICAL AGING

Aging is a process that occurs to organisms with the passage of time that eventually results in death.

Whereas physiological theories of aging can be classified in various ways, all theories of aging are of three primary types. Science generally assumes that aging is a multifactorial phenomenon and that an intricate relationship among several aging processes is represented by the three types of theories. The theories of aging are not mutually exclusive and include

1. Genetic cellular theories—aging is a consequence of a built-in cellular biological clock
2. Nongenetic cellular theories—cellular damage occurs over time as a consequence of both intrinsic and extrinsic damage as opposed to a preprogrammed time frame
3. Physiological systems theories—aging occurs as a result of the failure of physiological systems (Bengston, Gans, Putney, & Silverstein, 2008).

- Genetic Cellular Theories
  1. Genes—process of aging is dictated by preprogrammed genetic components influenced by biological markers such as puberty and menopause; one or more genes control the cellular aging process, and specific genes may influence longevity; these are activated, and the organism dies
  2. Error-catastrophe—an early theory suggesting errors occur through somatic mutations, chromosomal rearrangements, or genetic material transcriptions, and as the errors accumulate the cell cannot survive
  3. DNA—mutations occur in the mitochondria of DNA and continually mount upward throughout an individual's lifetime, causing aging
  4. Hayflick limit or cell aging—cells will multiply and divide only a finite number of times; genetically preprogrammed
  5. Programmed—a senescence or aging factor accumulates in cells and dominates cellular function

- Nongenetic Cellular Theories
  1. Chemical—chemical reactions occur naturally and result in irreversible molecular defects; may occur from air, food, smoking, and the like; if insults and injuries outweigh the repairing process, the system fails
  2. Cross-linkage—atoms or molecules have chemical sites that may link to DNA in the cell; damaged DNA is repaired by body's defense mechanism; if cross-linkage impedes transport of nutrients and information, the damage cannot be repaired
  3. Free-radical—free radicals are oxygen metabolites produced by one-electron reduction of oxygen that can produce damage and lead to cell death

- Physiological Systems Theories
  1. Autoimmune—immune system loses its ability to distinguish normal material from foreign antigens and begins to destroy its host
  2. Gradual imbalance—brain, endocrine, or immune system begins to fail, possibly at different rates, causing an imbalance and decreased effectiveness
  3. Neuroendocrine regulatory system—enables body to adapt to real or perceived challenges such as changes in workload, temperature, or psychological threats
  4. Wear and tear—mechanical and biological features of aging; irreversible damage occurs over time

## THEORIES OF PSYCHOSOCIAL AGING

The elderly adult has approached the last stage of a life span that is characterized by psychosocial or developmental tasks, a feature of every phase of the life cycle. Successful socialization and adaptation in the last stages of life are characterized by successful resolution of what are often defined as developmental conflicts or tasks of aging.

- Developmental Theories
  1. Erik Erickson's resolution of psychological conflict—ego integrity versus despair
     a. The older adult must come to terms with who he has become as compared to what he hoped to be
     b. There is a realization that there is a finite end to the life cycle, and that many hopes, dreams, and plans will not be realized
     c. Some elderly do not accept this and are at higher risk for maladaptive responses, e.g., depression
  2. Robert Peck expanded on Erickson's conflict of aging—as with Erickson's theory, older adults who cannot resolve these conflicts or accept a new state of affairs are at higher risk for maladaptive responses
     a. Ego differentiation versus work role preoccupation—many adults whose entire identity was embodied in a professional or work role will lose that identity with retirement
     b. Body transcendence versus body preoccupation—older adults must learn to accept a body that does not look, act, or feel the way that it did in middle age—this can range from cosmetic to functional
     c. Ego transcendence versus ego preoccupation—older adults are healthiest who learn to accept themselves and enjoy the life they have left rather than become fixated on the limited years remaining

3. Daniel Levinson's Seasons of Life—individual must ultimately come to terms with the inevitability of death; focus is on the relationship of physical changes to personality
4. Developmental tasks theory
   a. Adjust to decreasing physical strength and health
   b. Adjust to retirement and reduced income
   c. Adjust to death of partner
   d. Establish affiliation with peers
   e. Adapt to social rules
   f. Establish satisfactory physical living arrangements

## INTERVIEW AND HEALTH HISTORY

Geriatric intervention goals include care and cure, improvement and maintenance of function, and quality of life. The goal of the interview is to obtain a complete and accurate health history, which is a subjective account of the individual's status. Much of the information obtained will be utilized to formulate diagnoses and a plan of care. The interview and health history are much like any patient interview and history, but there are issues to which the nurse practitioner should be particularly attentive.

- Develop a Relationship
  1. Develop a climate of trust
  2. Establish a caring relationship
  3. Identify the chief complaint
  4. Maintain a goal-directed interview because older adults may have long and complex histories
     a. Direct flow of conversation—avoid a "positive" review of systems, answering "yes" to all questions—it is helpful to point out that all people from time to time experience a symptom, but you are asking whether the patient experiences any of these symptoms to a remarkable degree
     b. Ask specific questions, but allow individual to elaborate
     c. Design questions to address one issue at a time
  5. Be aware that gender and age can influence the patient–provider relationship
  6. Family may be present to assist in the evaluation. The patient may rely on the family for answers to interview questions; however, be cautious that as a function of normal aging, information processing and response may be a bit delayed—allow the patient adequate time to answer a question
  7. Sensitive issues such as incontinence, abuse, failing cognition, sexual dysfunction, and alcohol abuse need to be addressed. It is critical that the patient not feel trust or confidence is betrayed
  8. Be alert to nonverbal cues. Patients may be concerned that admitting to a symptom, e.g., memory loss, falls, incontinence, may place them at risk for institutionalization. It is not uncommon for a patient to deny a problem the first time a question is asked.

- Communication
  1. Speak slowly; do not shout; lower octaves are generally heard more clearly because bilateral, symmetrical, high-frequency hearing loss is a common age-related change
  2. Help interpret patient's feelings; ask for clarification
  3. Convey warmth and concern through listening, appropriate touch
  4. Observe for signs of anxiety, exhaustion, nervousness
  5. Understand social mores, cultural differences, language barriers, personal biases

- Environment
  1. Provide a quiet, private setting
  2. Set time limit because the elderly may tire
  3. Sit face to face to ensure eye contact; exhibit a relaxed, but concerned, atmosphere
  4. Provide good lighting and ventilation; avoid light source shining from behind you because it creates shadows and glares

- Values Assessment
  1. Elderly patients may have different goals and values from those traditionally assumed during a health-related encounter
  2. *Assessing values and goals for care will determine the direction of the remainder of the encounter*
     a. Will the patient consider primary prevention strategies?
        (1) Sometimes elderly patients feel that quality of life is more important, e.g., an 80-year-old patient will not discuss smoking cessation
        (2) Short-term comfort strategies may be more valuable to the patient than actions that promote long-term survival
     b. Will the patient pursue secondary prevention activities?
        (1) Elderly patients may not be willing to discuss or consider vascular and cancer screenings
        (2) May not return for care if the provider pursues this agenda

  c.  Will the patient consider tertiary prevention, e.g., medication and other disease control activities?
    (1)  Often elderly patients have a very specific agenda
    (2)  Prioritize short-term comfort over improved long-term outcomes, e.g., antihypertensives make them feel unwell, so they prefer to risk target organ damage rather than to take medication
 3.  The primary goal of care for elderly patients may be conservative, short-term peace or comfort; recognizing goals should direct the care encounter

- Health History—format (assess reliability of historian)
  1. Biographical data—important to obtain name and phone number of closest relative
  2. Family history
     a. Parents' health history; cause of death (if applicable)
     b. History of diabetes, heart and kidney disease, cancer, alcoholism, drug abuse, mental illness, and other major medical problems in family
     c. Special attention should be given to neurodegenerative or mood disorders
  3. Occupation—any environmental or occupational exposure to pulmonary toxins; adjustment to retirement; source of income
  4. Medications—prescriptions, over-the-counter, nontraditional modalities, home remedies, herbal medications, use of medications prescribed to spouse and friends
  5. Smoking history, illegal drug use history
  6. Alcohol use or abuse
  7. Allergies, drug sensitivities, foods
  8. Mental health problems
  9. Nutrition evaluation
     a. General
        (1) Attitude toward eating—alone, with family or caregiver
        (2) Appetite
        (3) Change in ability to taste
        (4) Consumption, special dietary restrictions
        (5) Meal preparation
        (6) Shopping
     b. Significant weight loss (at least 5% of usual body weight)—sudden (days to weeks) versus gradual weight loss
     c. Common causes of weight loss
        (1) Cancer (lung, gastrointestinal, lymphoma, genitourinary)—up to 36% of cases
        (2) Diabetes and hyperthyroidism
        (3) Depression, anxiety, and dementia
        (4) AIDS—do not rule out high-risk behaviors in elderly such as homosexuality, IV drug abuse, history of blood transfusion, infected spouse, multiple sexual partners, paid sexual partners
  10. Sleep
      a. Note patterns—hour of bedtime/sleep, daytime fatigue/naps, insomnia
      b. Sleep aids—pharmacological and nonpharmacological
      c. Normal changes of sleep patterns with aging
         (1) Longer stage 1, light sleep
         (2) Shorter stages 3 and 4, decreased 20%—deep sleep shorter, therefore less restful nights
         (3) Increased sleep apnea of 10 seconds or more without awakening
         (4) Increased time awake during night
  11. Exercise patterns, recreational profile
  12. Review of systems
      a. Systematic review of elderly individual
      b. Subjective data collected
      c. Diseases may present atypically
  13. Preventive health practices—check frequency of screening tests such as Papanicolaou smear, testicular and prostate exams, stool guaiac test, sigmoidoscopy, cholesterol level, mammograms

- Past Medical History
  1. Hospitalization and operations
  2. Vaccinations—influenza, pneumonia, hepatitis, tetanus
  3. Accidents, injuries, falls
  4. Childhood and adult illnesses
  5. Communicable disease history
     a. Tuberculosis
     b. Influenza
     c. HIV status
     d. Sexually transmitted diseases
     e. Streptococcal infections
     f. Hepatitis

- Health Practices, Religious Implications
  1. Blood transfusion acceptance/denial
  2. Dietary restrictions
  3. Fasting on certain holidays
  4. Sabbath restrictions for procedures, activities

- Safety Assessment
  1. Environment
     a. Home—stairs, scatter rugs, electrical wires, telephone cords, locks on doors and windows

     b. Neighborhood—sidewalks, location of stores, banks, post office, pharmacy
     c. Community services
     d. Crime
2. Driving—loss of independence if taken away (difficult decision); must weigh the risks versus benefits of action
     a. Assessment of driver safety may be indicated
     b. Specific driving safety test not available
     c. American Medical Association makes some recommendations for driver safety assessment—see the *Physician's Guide to Assessing and Counseling Older Drivers*
        (1) Clock Drawing Test
        (2) Clinical Dementia Rating (CDR)—American Medical Association advocates on-road testing for those who score > 0.5
3. Elder abuse—recent and increasingly common form of domestic violence
     a. Estimated to be approximately 1 million persons
     b. Abuser frequently is caregiver or family member
     c. Physical or psychological abuse, neglect, financial abuse, or sexual abuse

- Patient Self-Determination Act (1990)—encourage patient to discuss this with family and healthcare provider and act on wishes. It is important to determine the patient's perception of the legality of any advance directive and the circumstances under which it may be implemented; only advance directives very specifically executed consistent with the laws of the state in which they are to be implemented will survive any legal contest.
  1. Advance directives—indicate intent of patient based on his or her wishes with right to refuse any or all interventions of medical care
  2. Living will—a contract specifying the patient's wishes concerning the end of his or her life; varies according to state in which the patient resides; a copy should be given to the healthcare provider and family member
  3. Durable power of attorney for health care—authorizes an agent to make medical decisions on behalf of the patient when the patient is unable
  4. Physician-assisted suicide may become an issue

## LIVING SITUATIONS AND INCOME STATUS

1. Socialization
2. Support systems in place such as family and friends
3. Available resources in the community
4. Effect of change in financial resources upon retirement or disability
5. Effect of change when spouse or important family member is institutionalized or dies
6. Assess role and status of caregiver; care of the caregiver

## FUNCTIONAL ASSESSMENT

- Definition—method used to measure an individual's ability to perform ADLs and instrumental activities of daily living (IADLs) through physical, emotional, cognitive, and social parameters
  1. Physical function identifies sensorimotor ability, gait, and mobility
  2. Emotional function focuses on coping mechanisms
  3. Cognitive function identifies intellectual and reasoning capabilities
  4. Social function evaluates ability to maintain social roles

- Certain deficits affect functional status
  1. Visual and auditory deficits may precipitate or worsen confusion; eye and ear examination should be performed when deteriorating function is the chief complaint
  2. Unfamiliar surroundings may cause confusion, sleep disturbances
  3. Musculoskeletal injury resulting in mobility impairment, dependence, loss of control, and sleep disturbances

- Determine ability to perform ADLs and self-care activities independently using the Index of Independence in Activities of Daily Living Scale (Katz, 1983)
  1. Elderly tend to overrate abilities; underrate disabilities
  2. Family members tend to underrate abilities
  3. Index ranks ability to perform basic functions such as bathing, dressing, feeding, and continence

- Determine ability to perform IADLs (Katz, 1983)
  1. More complex personal tasks such as cooking and shopping
  2. More complex independent functions such as taking care of finances, banking, and managing medications

- Cognitive status assessments are used to detect causes of cognitive impairment
  1. Short Portable Mental Status Questionnaire (SPMSQ) is used to identify the presence and degree of intellectual impairment by testing orientation, memory concerning self-care, remote memory, and math (Pfeiffer, 1975)

2. The Mini-Mental State Exam (MMSE) is used to identify cognitive aspects of mental functions such as orientation, attention, recall, and language (Folstein, Folstein, & McHugh, 1975)

- Other functional issues may be assessed such as medical conditions, communication, senses, resources, and behavior problems

## PHYSICAL ASSESSMENT

An essential component of the evaluation from which valuable information can be obtained; an organized, systematic approach such as head-to-toe or major organ system should be utilized. As with history taking, the mechanics of physical examination of the older adults are the same as for any adult. However, the nurse practitioner should be alert to particular nuances that will influence interpretation of findings.

- General Inspection
    1. Provide initial assessment of health status
    2. Identify specific characteristics—posture, gait, appearance
    3. Determine whether exhibiting altered concentration as a result of pain, memory loss, agitation, and other signs of focusing deficits
    4. Identify strengths, disabilities, and limitations
    5. Evaluate skin changes consistent with frequent accidental or purposeful injury that may provide information about declining functional abilities or abuse

- Normal Aging Changes in the Elderly: General Appearance
    1. Fat increases by 30% and water decreases by 53% by age 70; fat distribution shifts from extremities to trunk
    2. Weight increases until about age 50 and then begins to fall; longevity favors individuals who are "ideal" weight or slightly above
    3. Anatomic size and height—elderly lose 1–2 inches as a result of thinning of cartilage between vertebrae and poor posture; kyphosis; males and females lose approximately 1/16 inch each year beginning around age 30 years

- Integumentary System
    1. Anatomical and physiological changes
        a. Decreased elasticity—increased wrinkles, folds, sagging, dry skin resulting in poor turgor
        b. Decreased perspiration—increased heat tolerance, poor temperature regulation; tendency toward hypo-/hyperthermia
        c. Body and facial hair thins and grays; increased facial hair on women
        d. Nail growth slows, thickens; hypertrophy common
        e. Eyebrows coarse, bristle-like
        f. Cell regeneration slower
        g. Thinning of epithelial cells and subcutaneous fat layers
    2. Clinical implications
        a. Increased risk of infection
        b. Decreased wound healing
        c. Pruritus
        d. Poorly supported blood vessels rupture easily causing purpura
        e. Common benign skin lesions
            (1) Seborrheic keratosis—macular-papular, dark, warty areas seen on face, neck, and trunk
            (2) Cherry angioma—small, round, red, domed papules seen on trunk and proximal extremities
            (3) Cutaneous skin tags—pedunculated papillomas seen on neck, chest, and intertriginous sites
            (4) Common blue nevus—benign, firm, dark-blue/gray/black, well-defined papule, usually seen on hands and feet
        f. Sun exposure changes
            (1) Solar lentigo—flat, brown, pigmented macule on exposed areas only
            (2) Solar keratosis—single or multiple discreet, dry, rough, scaly lesions on face, neck, and hands
    3. Abnormal changes and disease
        a. Infections—viral, bacterial, fungal
        b. Skin ulcerations
        c. Ingrown toenails
        d. Bunions, corns, calluses
        e. Onychomycosis—fungal infection of nails
        f. Abnormal skin lesions
            (1) Actinic keratosis—precancerous macular, irregular, scaly lesions seen on sun-exposed areas, e.g., hands, arms, neck, and face; small (1:1,000), but present risk of progression to squamous cell carcinoma
            (2) Squamous cell carcinoma—malignant soft, red-brown lesion of skin and mucous membrane arises as result of exogenous carcinogens such as sunlight or x-rays; seen on exposed areas, especially face, ears, scalp, arms, lips, and genitalia; low but present risk of metastasis
            (3) Basal cell carcinoma—most common type of skin cancer; hard pearly-gray or pink, round, oval lesion with depressed center; usually on forehead, eyelids, nose, and lips—no risk of metastasis but may produce significant local, invasive damage

(4) Malignant melanoma—round, oval, brown, or tan irregular macular lesions seen mostly on trunk, arms, legs; familial tendency, not as common in older population, high risk of metastasis with lung as most common site

- Cardiovascular System
  1. Anatomical and physiological changes
     a. Slight decrease in heart size
     b. Decreased cardiac output by up to 30%; heart fills and expels blood less efficiently
     c. Increased peripheral vascular resistance due to arteriosclerotic calcification of the vascular endothelium
     d. Increased ectopic activity due to decreased threshold for cellular excitability
     e. Decreased resting heart rate; increased with exercise/stress, takes longer to return to baseline; decreased exercise tolerance
     f. Increased rigidity and thickness of valves—development of aortic stenosis may occur
     g. Decreased sensitivity of baroreceptors—patients are less responsive to changes in position and consequently at greater risk for orthostatic hypotension and near-syncope or syncope
  2. Clinical implications
     a. Hypertension leads to a significant increase in the risk of heart attack, stroke, and heart failure
     b. Orthostatic hypotension; near syncope with sudden position change
     c. Increased narrow or wide pulse pressure
     d. Unilateral or bilateral pain or swelling in lower extremities
     e. Varicosities—tortuous peripheral vessels
     f. Functional systolic murmurs increase with age; systolic heart murmurs are reported in one-third of 80-year-olds; assess to determine etiology
     g. $S_4$ commonly heard
     h. Heart rate < 60 or > 90 beats per minute may be diagnostically significant
     i. Dysrhythmia such as atrial fibrillation more common

- Respiratory System
  1. Anatomical and physiological changes
     a. Decreased vital capacity, decreased tissue elasticity, loss of elastic recoil of alveolar tissue
     b. Increased residual volume, decrease in functional alveoli
     c. Increased diameter of the chest
     d. Decreased ability to clear lungs, less efficient cough
     e. Decreased diffusion of gases
     f. Decreased strength of expiratory muscles, more rigid intercostal muscles
     g. Decreased clearance of congestion
     h. Kyphosis may be present
  2. Clinical implications
     a. Increased anteroposterior diameter
     b. Barrel chest, retraction
     c. Decreased ventilation at lung bases
     d. Pallor, cyanosis
     e. Nail clubbing
     f. Vesicular breath sounds, bilateral basilar crackles
     g. Decreased reserve
     h. Decreased response to exercise, stress, and disease

- Breasts
  1. Anatomical and physiological changes
     a. Atrophy of fatty tissue and glands, pendulous breasts
     b. May appear nodular
     c. Increased sagging
     d. Nipples are lower
     e. Elderly men may have increased breast size
  2. Clinical implications
     a. Wide variation of size, symmetry, contour, texture, pigmentation
     b. Development of fibrocystic breasts
     c. Gynecomastia for men

- Gastrointestinal System
  1. Anatomical and physiological changes
     a. Loss of taste-functional taste buds
     b. Loss of or "softening" of teeth
     c. Decreased saliva
     d. Decreased mastication
     e. Decreased peristalsis
     f. Weakening of lower esophageal sphincter
     g. Lower esophageal sphincter often fails to relax
     h. Decreased gastric acid secretion
     i. Decreased hepatic metabolism
     j. Decreased pancreatic secretion
     k. Decreased insulin release
     l. Decreased smooth muscle motility
     m. Decreased function of rectal stretch receptors
  2. Clinical implications
     a. Constipation, fecal impaction
     b. Indigestion
     c. Increased sensitivity to medication in GI tract
     d. Increased response to alcohol, nicotine, chocolate, peppermint, and caffeine
     e. Periodontal disease
     f. Malnutrition

- Genitourinary and Reproductive Systems
    1. Anatomical and physiological changes
        a. Renal changes
            (1) Decreased kidney function, number of nephrons, and glomerular filtration rate (GFR)
            (2) Decreased bladder capacity and muscle tone
            (3) Decreased sphincter control
            (4) Increased frequency, urgency, nocturia
        b. Hormonal changes
            (1) Decreased estrogen in females
            (2) Decreased testosterone in males
            (3) Atrophy of ovaries, uterus, and vagina
            (4) Development of firmer testes, may be smaller
            (5) Sclerosis of penile arteries and veins
            (6) Decreased seminal fluid, sperm number, motility
            (7) Pubic hair thins and grays
            (8) Prostate gland enlargement
            (9) Decreased vaginal secretions
    2. Clinical implications
        a. Asymptomatic urinary tract infections
        b. Urinary incontinence
        c. Atrophic vaginitis, foul-smelling vaginal discharge
        d. Dyspareunia
        e. Pelvic prolapse
        f. Benign prostatic hypertrophy
        g. Drug toxicity
        h. Urinary retention
        i. Impotency
        j. Testicular enlargement, nodules

- Endocrine System
    1. Anatomical and physiological changes
        a. Decreased size, number, and activity of sweat glands
        b. Decline in body's cooling mechanism
        c. Decreased ability to perspire
        d. Decreased ability to metabolize glucose
        e. Reduced insulin secretion
        f. Delayed insulin response
        g. Increased insulin resistance
    2. Clinical implications
        a. Dehydration
        b. Hyperthermia
        c. Hyperglycemia

- Musculoskeletal System
    1. Anatomical and physiological changes
        a. Bone demineralization
        b. Decreased strength and endurance, range of motion
        c. Joint and cartilage erosion
        d. Loss of flexibility in the joints
        e. Bony growths at joints
        f. Decreased muscle mass
        g. Bony prominences develop
    2. Clinical implications
        a. Gait disturbances
        b. Falls
        c. Loss of height
        d. Hallux valgus—bunions
        e. Hammer toes
        f. Valgus, varus deformities
        g. Lordosis, scoliosis, kyphosis
        h. Stiffness and decreased range of motion of joints

- Sensory System
    1. Vision
        a. Anatomical and physiological changes
            (1) Lens yellows and clouds
            (2) Pupils smaller, but remain equal
            (3) Decreased tear production
            (4) Lens stiffens
            (5) Decreased peripheral vision
            (6) Difficulty in color discrimination
            (7) Eyelids thinning, increased stretching, poor fit; entropion and ectropion
            (8) Conjunctiva pale and less white
            (9) Arcus senilis
        b. Clinical implications
            (1) Decreased visual acuity
            (2) Decreased adaptation to darkness
            (3) Corneal irritation
            (4) Decreased peripheral vision
            (5) Dry appearance
            (6) Progressive eyelid relaxation
    2. Hearing
        a. Anatomical and physiological changes
            (1) Decreased discrimination of pitch and acuity
            (2) Decreased sensitivity to higher frequency sounds
            (3) Excessive cerumen, drying of cerumen, hair growth in canal
            (4) Tympanic membranes may lose mobility
        b. Clinical implications
            (1) Vertigo, tinnitus
            (2) Diminished hearing
            (3) Auricle loses elasticity, lobe elongates
            (4) Conductive hearing loss
    3. Head/throat/neck/nose
        a. Anatomical and physiological changes
            (1) Decreased sense of smell; difficulty distinguishing specific odors
            (2) Decreased size of thyroid gland
            (3) Atrophy of pharynx, larynx
            (4) Nose sags, appears longer

(5) Lymph nodes may be noted—less than 1 cm in size; soft, discrete, and mobile considered normal variations
b. Clinical implications
(1) Marked asymmetry of face
(2) Increased size of lymph nodes
(3) Soft voice
(4) Difficulty swallowing
(5) Postnasal drip
4. Taste
a. Anatomical and physiological changes
(1) Decreased number of taste buds, papillary atrophy
(2) Difficulty distinguishing specific tastes
(3) Teeth yellow, increased space between teeth
(4) Decreased ability to chew
b. Clinical implications
(1) Loss of interest in eating
(2) Poor fitting dentures, loose or broken teeth
(3) Dental caries, gingival disease or decay, halitosis
(4) Dehydration
5. Touch
a. Anatomical and physiological changes
(1) Decreased receptors
(2) Lower ability to distinguish temperature and pain
(3) Increased pain tolerance
b. Clinical implications
(1) Decreased sensation
(2) Numbness, tingling
(3) Potential for burns, injury

- Neurological system
1. Anatomical and physiological changes
a. General decrease in cerebral blood flow
b. Global brain atrophy
c. Slowed response to heat and cold
d. General slowing of reaction time
e. Sluggish deep tendon reflexes
f. Loss of vibratory sensation
2. Clinical implications
a. Benign senile tremors
b. Decreased coordination and balance
c. Wide-based gait
d. Nystagmus
e. Decreased response to pain
f. Loss of balance

## PHARMACOTHERAPY AND THE ELDERLY

Age-related physiological changes result in the elderly being at high risk for side effects and toxic effects; compounded when chronic diseases are present.

- Important Issues
1. The average older adult is on six prescription medications and eight total medications
2. Approximately one-third of drug-related hospitalizations and one-half of all drug-related deaths occur in persons 60 years and older
3. 30% of all U.S. dollars spent on prescription medication annually and 40–50% of all U.S. dollars spent on over-the-counter medications annually are for elderly patients
4. More than $3 billion a year is spent by elderly on prescription and nonprescription drugs
5. Majority of elderly have one or more chronic conditions such as arthritis, hypertension, heart disease, and diabetes that are treated with multiple medications
6. Drug therapy for one condition may adversely affect another medical condition
7. Increased number of adverse drug reactions (ADRs); ADRs have occurred in 30% of elderly outpatients and account for up to 10% of hospital admissions
a. Reflective of number and type of medications taken
b. Frequent use of over-the-counter, self-prescribed medication, home remedies
c. Multiple healthcare providers with lack of coordination of care
d. Multiple pharmacies used with lack of ability to identify potential drug interactions
e. Do not assume that behavior change is age-related
8. Common ADRs in the elderly include edema, nausea, vomiting, anorexia, dizziness, diarrhea, constipation, confusion, and urinary retention or incontinence; should not be misinterpreted as signs and symptoms of illness or results of the aging process

- Physiological Changes—may lead to increased plasma concentrations of drugs
1. Decreased tolerance of standard dosages; toxic reactions occur at lower doses
2. Decreased metabolism—usually occurs in the liver, which is decreased in size with decreased blood flow
3. Decreased absorption—decreased liver enzyme activity and gastric emptying time; gastric pH and transit time increased
4. Variable distribution—lean muscle mass decreases and fat tissue increases; fat-soluble drugs have longer duration; water-soluble drugs have smaller volume of distribution and higher plasma concentrations; increased adipose tissue can cause increased storage of lipid-soluble drugs

5. Decreased ability to excrete drugs as a result of decreased GFR; results in decreased excretion time for medication; GFR declines 50% between third and ninth decades of life

- Potential Side Effects of Commonly Prescribed Drugs
    1. Confusion—digoxin, cimetidine, dopamine agents, antihistamines, hypnotics, sedatives, anticholinergics, anticonvulsants, fluoroquinolones
    2. Anorexia—digoxin
    3. Fatigue/weakness—diuretics, antidepressants, antihypertensives
    4. Ataxia—sedatives, hypnotics, anticonvulsants, antipsychotics
    5. Forgetfulness—benzodiazepines
    6. Constipation—anticholinergics, calcium channel blockers
    7. Diarrhea—oral antacids
    8. GI upset—iron, nonsteroidal anti-inflammatory drugs (NSAIDs), salicylates, corticosteroids, estrogens
    9. Tinnitus—analgesics, NSAIDs, some antibiotics
    10. Urinary retention—anticholinergics, alpha-agonists, antihistamines
    11. Orthostatic hypotension—antihypertensives, sedatives, diuretics, antidepressants
    12. Depression—benzodiazepines, beta-adrenergic antagonists
    13. Delirium—corticosteroids, sedatives, antihistamines
    14. Dizziness—sedatives, antihypertensives, anticonvulsants, diuretics

- Problems with Use of Medication
    1. Overuse—elderly feel when they seek care from a healthcare provider they should receive a prescription
    2. Misuse—self-prescribing habits, changing dosages, use of old prescriptions, use of friend's medication, poor history given to provider, outdated prescriptions
    3. Knowledge deficit—difficulty understanding as a result of educational level *or* misunderstanding due to hearing deficits *or* inadequate information provided by healthcare professional
    4. Memory deficit—forget purpose, dosage, frequency of taking medication; may accidentally repeat dosage
    5. Cost—may not purchase medication because of limited financial resources
    6. Visual deficit—inability to properly read label, may take wrong medication
    7. Mobility problems—difficulty opening bottles, small tablets hard to handle, splitting pills in half is sometimes necessary, difficulty manipulating inhalers
    8. Multiple providers, multiple pharmacies—conflicting/duplicate medications prescribed by various healthcare practitioners; generic and brand name prescriptions being taken concurrently

- Recommendations for Drug Use in the Elderly—identify factors that predispose the elderly to ADRs, e.g., multisystem disease, greater severity of disease, female gender, small body size, hepatic or renal disease, previous drug reactions; proceed cautiously with the following:
    1. Clear indication for use
    2. Reliably effective drug
    3. Shortest duration appropriate
    4. Lowest dosage—"start low, go slow"
    5. Cost-effectiveness
    6. Likeliness to enhance quality of life
    7. Avoid adverse outcomes
    8. Evaluate patient compliance
    9. Identify resource person to assist in administering if necessary
    10. Use calendars, pill boxes, and large print to assist
    11. Use of devices to aid administration such as spacers for inhalers

## Special Considerations in the Hospitalized Patient

- Illness Assessment in the Gerontological Population
    - Although the mechanics of assessment are the same as for any other patient, certain principles must be remembered to ensure accurate interpretation of history and physical examination findings in the older adult. Because of normal age-related changes, disease presentations may be different in the older adult as compared to a young or middle-aged population.
    - Principles to consider in geriatric illness assessment
        - Normal age-related changes must be differentiated from indicators of illness
            - An increased anterior-posterior chest diameter suggests chronic obstructive pulmonary disease (COPD) in a young or middle-aged adult; in the elderly it may be a normal finding

*(continues)*

### Special Considerations in the Hospitalized Patient (*continued*)

- A corneal ring suggests dyslipidemia in a young or middle-aged population; in the elderly it may be a normal finding
- Decreased skin turgor suggests volume contraction in a young or middle-aged adult; in the elderly this is normal as a consequence of increased fat-to-water ratio in body composition
- Recognize the effects of normal age-related physiological decline
  - Decreased cardiac output—up to 30% decrease from baseline is normal as people age
  - Short-term memory decrease is normal with aging and does not in itself indicate a dementing disorder
  - Loss of subcutaneous fat is normal with aging; in young or middle-aged adults it suggests a nutritional or metabolic problem
- Disease presentations are often atypical
  - Urinary tract infection may present as confusion and urinary incontinence
  - Myocardial infarction may present as confusion
  - Pneumonia may present as falling
- Atypical presentation of illness—because of the weakness in the four organ systems listed in the following table, the strain of disease in any body system tends to manifest in one of the four weak ones. Because of this, a limited number of symptoms tend to predominate regardless of what the underlying problem is. In the elderly patient, the organ system associated with the particular abnormality or problem is less likely to be the source of symptoms than in a younger adult

| Organ Systems Most Affected by Age-Related Decline |
|---|
| Neurological |
| Cardiovascular |
| Musculoskeletal |
| Lower urinary |

- Predominant symptoms of illness in the older adult
  - Acute confusion
  - Depression
  - Falls
  - Incontinence
  - Syncope
- Another atypical manifestation is that diseases usually present at an earlier stage as a result of normal, age-related decline in compensatory mechanism; as a result, they are generally easier to treat
  - Heart failure might be precipitated by mild hypothyroidism
  - Mild hyperparathyroidism may produce significant cognitive dysfunction
  - Mild prostate hypertrophy may result in urinary retention
  - Mild glucose intolerance may result in nonketotic coma

## QUESTIONS

### Select the best answer.

1. The greatest increase in ethnic representation in the elderly population by 2030 will be in which population category?
   a. African American
   b. Caucasian
   c. Latino
   d. Asian and Pacific Islander

2. By the year 2050, the elderly population will:
   a. Begin to decrease
   b. Level off at 50 million persons
   c. Include those persons 55 years and older
   d. More than double to 80 million

3. Elderly women outnumber elderly men:
   a. Three to two
   b. Four to three
   c. Five to two
   d. Two to one

4. Which of the following is a true statement with regard to elderly men?
   a. They comprise the poorest subgroup of the elderly population
   b. They are much more likely to live with a spouse than elderly women are
   c. They have the greatest incidence of unsuccessful suicides
   d. They are more likely to be institutionalized than elderly women are

5. Better education has been proven to improve one's life. Which of the following statements is true about noninstitutionalized adults?
   a. Seventy-nine percent of the elderly have completed high school
   b. The elderly are as likely to have completed only eighth grade as persons younger than 75 years of age are
   c. Middle-old have the highest percentage of college degrees
   d. Lack of education increases with age

6. What percentage of the older-than-85-year population lives in long-term care?
   a. Less than 5%
   b. More than 50%
   c. Almost 20%
   d. Between 30% and 35%

7. When performing a health history on an elderly patient, which of the following should the nurse practitioner avoid?
   a. Standing near the window so that the patient can see the interviewer more clearly
   b. Considering the implications of cultural differences and social mores
   c. Asking open-ended questions, but keeping conversation focused
   d. Observing for signs of fatigue

8. Which of the following is not a normal age-related physical change?
   a. Short-term memory loss
   b. Urinary incontinence
   c. Loss of 30% ejection fraction
   d. Joint degeneration

9. Which statement is most accurate about the sleep patterns of older persons?
   a. Sleep apnea of 10 seconds or more may occur, awakening the elderly
   b. The elderly fall asleep quickly but awaken frequently during the night
   c. The elderly have difficulty falling asleep, but then sleep soundly
   d. There are shorter stages 3 and 4 and longer stage 1 sleep cycles

10. Elder abuse is presently a problem in the United States. Which of the following statements regarding elder abuse is *not* true?
    a. The most common abusers are family members or caregivers
    b. Physical abuse is four times more common than psychological abuse
    c. It is a common form of domestic violence
    d. Up to 10% of the elderly may be subjected to one type of abuse

11. Which of the following is not included in the Patient Self-Determination Act of 1990?
    a. Durable power of attorney for health care
    b. Living will
    c. Organ donation
    d. Indication of patient's intent for medical care

12. In performing activities of daily living:
    a. The elderly overrate their own abilities
    b. The family members overrate the elder's ability
    c. The elderly cannot manage their finances well
    d. The elderly frequently pay for services such as cooking and cleaning

13. When observing general physical findings, the nurse practitioner is aware that:
    a. The elderly lose 1–2 inches in height due to the thickening of the cartilage
    b. The fat distribution shifts from the trunk to the extremities
    c. Fat decreases as body water decreases
    d. An increased AP chest diameter is a normal finding

14. The elderly are at increased risk for some skin cancers because they have been exposed to the sun for many decades. Which of the following is considered a precancerous skin condition?
    a. Solar lentigo
    b. Actinic keratoses
    c. Cherry angiomas
    d. Seborrheic keratoses

15. A decrease in threshold for cellular membrane excitability increases the elderly patient's risk for:
    a. Atrial fibrillation
    b. Orthostatic hypotension
    c. Constipation
    d. Thinning hair

16. Normal age-related changes of the cardiovascular system increase the elderly patient's risk for which of the following?
    a. Diastolic hypertension
    b. Tricuspid stenosis
    c. Ventricular fibrillation
    d. Orthostatic hypotension

17. Which of the following is not a normal age-related change of the head and neck?
    a. Hypertrophy of taste buds
    b. Bilateral high-frequency hearing loss
    c. Decreased saliva production
    d. Optic disk opacity

18. Which of the following age-related changes of the respiratory system is not typically found in the elderly?
    a. Decreased vital capacity and tissue elasticity
    b. Increased residual volume
    c. Decreased anterior-posterior diameter of the chest
    d. Less efficient cough and clearance of congestion

19. Normal age-related changes frequently result in atypical presentation of illness in the elderly client. Which of the following signs and symptoms of pneumonia is frequently not found in the elderly?
    a. High fever
    b. Tachypnea
    c. Confusion
    d. Chest pain

20. The elderly have breast-related variations. Which statement is true?
    a. Elderly men have a decrease in breast size
    b. There is atrophy of the fatty tissue and a nodular appearance
    c. Significantly unequal breast size is a normal variation
    d. Dimpling and milky discharge are not uncommon

21. Which of the following is not a normal age-related change of the GI tract?
    a. Decreased gastric acid secretions
    b. Decreased response to alcohol, caffeine, and nicotine
    c. Constipation and indigestion
    d. Weakening of the esophageal sphincter

22. Normal age-related changes of the skin may be confused with what clinical abnormality?
    a. Basal cell carcinoma
    b. Vitiligo
    c. Scabies
    d. Dehydration

23. Because of the normal changes of aging, abnormalities often present differently in an older adult. What is the most common cause of delirium in an elderly patient?
    a. Drug intoxication
    b. Hypoxia
    c. Infection
    d. Hospitalization

24. Abnormal disease processes of the musculoskeletal system include:
    a. Bone demineralization
    b. Bony growths at joints
    c. Decreased strength and endurance
    d. Decreased muscle mass

25. Aging results in a variety of normal, nonpathological changes in the body. Which of the following is a normal, age-related change in the structure or function of the ear?
    a. Decreased discrimination of pitch and acuity
    b. Increased sensitivity to low-pitched sounds
    c. Decreased hair growth in the canals
    d. Increased mobility of the tympanic membrane

26. Polypharmacy contributes to a variety of symptoms in the older adult. Which of the following can exacerbate depression?
    a. $H_2$ receptor antagonists
    b. Beta-adrenergic antagonists
    c. Benzodiazepines
    d. SNRIs

■ Answers

1. c
2. d
3. a
4. b
5. d
6. c
7. a
8. b
9. d
10. b
11. c
12. a
13. d
14. b
15. a
16. d
17. a
18. c
19. a
20. b
21. b
22. d
23. c
24. a
25. a
26. b

# BIBLIOGRAPHY

American Geriatric Society BEERS Update Criteria Expert Panel. (2012). American Geriatric Society Updated BEERS criteria for potentially inappropriate medication use in older adults. Retrieved from http://www.americangeriatrics.org/files/documents/beers/2012BeersCriteria_JAGS.pdf

American Medical Association & National Transportation Safety Board. (2010). *Physician guide to assessing and counseling older drivers.* Chicago, IL: Author.

Bengtson, V. L., Gans, D., Putney, N., & Silverstein, M. (2008). *Handbook of theories of aging* (2nd ed.). New York, NY: Springer.

Diegelman, N. M., Gilberston, A. D., Moore, J. L., Banou, E., & Meager, M. R. (2004). Validity of the Clock Drawing Test in predicting reports of driving problems in the elderly. *BioMed Central Geriatric, 4*(1), 10. Retrieved from http://www.biomedcentral.com/1471-2318/4/10

Duthie, E., & Katz, P. R. (2007). *Duthie: Practice of geriatrics* (4th ed.). Philadelphia, PA: Saunders.

Folstein, M. F., Folstein, S. E., & McHugh, P. R. (1975). Mini-Mental State: A practical method for grading the cognitive state of patients for the clinician. *Journal of Psychiatric Research, 12*, 189–198.

Fulton, M., & Allen, E. (2005). Polypharmacy in the elderly: A literature review. *Journal of the American Academy of Nurse Practitioners, 17*(4), 123–132.

Gallo, J. J., Bogner, H. R., Fulmer, T., & Paverza, G. J. (2006). *Handbook of geriatric assessment* (4th ed.). Sudbury, MA: Jones and Bartlett.

Gore, V. F., & Mouzon, M. (2006). Polypharmacy in older adults: Front line strategies. *Advance for Nurse Practitioners, 14*(9), 49–52.

Katz, S. (1983). Assessing self-maintenance: Activities of daily living, mobility, and instrumental activities of daily living. *Journal of the American Geriatrics Association, 31*, 721–727.

Pfeiffer, E. A. (1975). Short portable mental status questionnaire for the assessment of organic brain deficit in elderly persons. *Journal of the American Geriatric Society, 23*, 433–441.

Snyder, C. H. (2005). Dementia and driving: Autonomy versus safety. *Journal of the American Academy of Nurse Practitioners, 17*(10), 393–402.

U.S. Census Bureau. (2012). *Statistical briefs.* Washington, DC: Economics and Statistical Administration, U.S. Department of Commerce.

U.S. Department of Health and Human Services, Office on Aging. (2011). *A profile of older Americans: 2011.* Washington, DC: Author.

Williams, B. A., & Chang, A. (2014). *Current geriatric diagnosis and treatment: Geriatrics* (2nd ed.). New York, NY: McGraw-Hill Medical.

# Dermatological Disorders

*Sylvia Torres Fletcher*
*Susan E. Chaney*

## ACNE VULGARIS

- Definition—self-limited or chronic disorder characterized by development of open comedones (black heads) and closed comedones (white heads) due to an increase in sebum release by the sebaceous glands after puberty; if further inflammation is present, pustules, cysts, and nodules on erythematous bases may be present

- Etiology/Incidence
    1. Four primary pathogenic factors
        a. *Propionibacterium acnes*
        b. Increased sebum production
        c. Abnormal follicular keratinization
        d. Chemotactic factors
    2. Factors that predispose to comedone formation
        a. Cosmetics and hair products
        b. Coal tar and insoluble oils
        c. Corticosteroids (topical and systemic), oral contraceptives, lithium, phenytoin
    3. Contributing host factors
        a. Heredity
        b. Environment
        c. Stress
    4. May occur as a result of polycystic ovarian disease
    5. May be worse in fall and winter seasons
    6. Seen primarily in adolescents and young adults; may persist to fifth decade
    7. More common in males than females
    8. Circumstances characterized by increased androgen production increase risk

- Signs and Symptoms
    1. Lesions are nonpruritic, may be erythematous and tender
    2. Females may notice an increase in symptoms prior to menses

- Differential Diagnosis
    1. Acne rosacea
    2. Eosinophilic folliculitis (seen in HIV patients)
    3. Drug-induced folliculitis
    4. Pyogenic folliculitis

- Physical Findings
    1. Morphology
        a. Closed comedones, "white heads," are pustular lesions found in hair follicles due to blockage of sebum and keratinous materials
        b. Open comedones, "black heads," are dilated follicular orifices with easily expressed darkened oily debris
        c. Cysts, fluctuant closed lesions, containing any combination of blood, pus, and serous fluid
        d. Papules ($< 0.5$ cm) and nodules ($> 0.5$ cm), which are raised, solid lesions
    2. Distribution
        a. Forehead
        b. Cheek, nose, and chin
        c. Chest, upper arms, back, and buttocks

- Diagnostic Tests/Findings—none typically indicated; acne vulgaris is a clinical diagnosis based on history and physical examination

- Management/Treatment
  1. For mild or episodic cases
     a. Mild skin cleansing twice daily
     b. Benzoyl peroxide 2.5–10%—apply to affected area daily
     c. Topical benzoyl peroxide/antibiotic combinations (Benzaclin, Benzamycin)
     d. For moderate cases
        (1) Oral antibiotic therapy for at least 2 months (options include tetracycline 250–500 mg, initially 1 g/day, may increase to 2–3 g/day; minocycline 50–100 mg b.i.d.; whereas tetracycline class antibiotics are preferred, trimethoprim/sulfamethoxazole is also approved for management of acne vulgaris
        (2) Females—combination oral contraceptives with high estrogen component
  2. Prevent development of comedone with comedolytic agent
     a. Retinoic acid cream or gel
     b. Caution patient about photosensitivity
     c. Erythromycin/benzoyl peroxide gel in morning and topical retinoid at night 3 times a week most effective regimen
  3. Severe nodulocystic acne may require aggressive treatment to decrease sebum production—13-cis-retinoic acid (Accutane) 0.5–2 mg/kg/day for 16–20 weeks (typically prescribed by dermatologists or professionals who have completed manufacturer education)
     a. Teratogenic—use with extreme caution in females of child-bearing age; two forms of birth control required by manufacturer
     b. Multiple systemic side effects
     c. Monitor liver function tests (LFT), complete blood count (CBC), triglyceride levels
     d. Associated increase in suicide; monitor mood and suicide risk
  4. Patient education
     a. Noticeable improvement may not be apparent for 6 weeks
     b. Reassure patient, advise on stress reduction
     c. Skin care including mild skin cleansing twice daily; advise patient to not squeeze or pick lesions
     d. Be alert to changes in mood; seek help immediately if suicidal thoughts occur

## ALOPECIA

- Definition—the complete or partial loss of hair from areas where it normally is present; may be total, diffuse, patchy, or localized
- Etiology/Incidence
  1. Hair loss involving hair matrix or follicle destruction due to chemical agents, physical agents, or both, and by infectious or immunologically mediated inflammation; may also result from a slowing of hair growth due to metabolic diseases
  2. Cicatricial alopecia—scarring
     a. Destruction of hair follicles from inflammatory processes with healing resulting in scarring
     b. Permanent and irreversible
  3. Noncicatricial alopecia—nonscarring alopecia
     a. 95% of alopecia seen in primary care
     b. Most common is male or female baldness, which is genetic or developmental
     c. Considered an autoimmune disease
     d. Other causes include vitiligo, thyroid disease, familial autoimmune polyendocrinopathy syndrome
  4. Androgenetic alopecia
     a. Males after puberty, females after age 60
     b. Cause is combined effects of androgen on genetically predisposed hair follicles

- Signs and Symptoms
  1. Usually the patient is symptom free but verbalizes distress over hair loss
  2. Hair loss resulting from physical agents or infectious disease such as tinea capitis may cause pain or pruritus

- Differential Diagnosis
  1. Secondary syphilis
  2. Traction alopecia
  3. Early chronic systemic lupus erythematosus (SLE)
  4. Dermatomyositis
  5. Trichotillomania

- Physical Findings
  1. Genetic pattern baldness of
     a. Males—frontotemporal hairline recession with various amounts of hair loss at scalp vertex
     b. Females—diffuse or vertex hair loss
  2. Traumatic alopecia findings are patchy hair loss and breakage of hairs
  3. Infectious alopecia—patches of partial hair loss
  4. Alopecia areata (immunologic)—smooth, salmon-colored patches

- Diagnostic Tests/Findings
  1. Usually a clinical diagnosis
  2. Hair pull test of 10–20 grouped hairs; if more than 40% of shafts are removed, disease is more advanced
  3. KOH (potassium hydroxide) preparation—negative for fungus

4. ANA (antinuclear antibody) to rule out SLE
5. RPR (rapid plasma regain) to rule out secondary syphilis

- Management/Treatment
  1. Treatment for scarring alopecia areata—hair transplant
  2. Treatment for nonscarring alopecia areata
     a. Intralesional injection with triamcinolone acetate 3.5 mg/mL
     b. Systemic glucocorticoids
     c. Systemic cyclosporine
  3. Treatment of androgenetic alopecia
     a. Topical minoxidil 5% solution for 4–12 months
     b. Oral finasteride 1 mg daily for 6–12 months (cannot be used in pregnant women or women planning pregnancy; use is off-label in women)
     c. Antiandrogens for women (spironolactone, cimetidine)
  4. Patient education
     a. About 40% of patients have moderate hair growth within 1 year
     b. Discontinuation of treatment will result in regression to pretreatment levels of baldness within 2–3 months

## BACTERIAL INFECTIONS/PYODERMAS

- Definitions
  1. Impetigo—contagious and autoinoculable bacterial infection of skin; the two types are small vesicle and bullous
  2. Folliculitis—infection surrounding hair follicle caused by occlusion of ostium
  3. Furunculosis—deep-seated, autoinoculable infection involving entire hair follicle and adjacent subcutaneous tissue
  4. Carbuncle—several furuncles developing in adjoining hair follicles and coalescing to form deep mass with multiple drainage points
  5. Hidradenitis suppurativa—chronic suppurative disease of the apocrine gland-bearing areas of the skin
  6. Cellulitis—spreading infection of epidermis, subcutaneous tissue, and superficial lymphatic system

- Etiology/Incidence
  1. Impetigo
     a. Most frequent causative organisms—*Staphylococcus aureus* (*S. aureus*), group A beta hemolytic *Streptococcus pyogenes* (GAS)
     b. Seen primarily in children, bullous in children and young adults
     c. Predisposing factors
        (1) Humid, warm climate
        (2) Preexisting skin disease, especially atopic
        (3) Prior antibiotic therapy
        (4) Poor hygiene, crowded living conditions
        (5) Chronic staph carrier (nose, axilla, perineum, bowel)
  2. Folliculitis, furunculosis, carbuncle
     a. Most frequent causative organism—*S. aureus*
     b. Predisposing factors
        (1) Shaving hairy areas such as beard, axillae, legs
        (2) Occlusion of hair-bearing areas (plastic, clothing, positioning)
        (3) Topical glucocorticoid steroids, systemic antibiotics
        (4) Diabetes
  3. Hidradenitis suppurativa
     a. Pathogenesis unknown, mechanism plugging apocrine duct with subsequent ulceration, fibrosis, and sinus tract formation
     b. Males—anogenital involvement; females—axillary involvement although can occur in any anatomical location rich with apocrine glands
     c. Predisposing factors
        (1) Obesity
        (2) Family history of nodulocystic acne, hidradenitis suppurativa
  4. Cellulitis
     a. Most frequent causative organisms *S. aureus* and GAS
     b. Less common—*H. influenzae*, group B streptococci (GBS), pneumococci
     c. Diabetic/immunocompromised—*E. coli, Proteus mirabilis, Acinetobacter, Enterobacter, Pseudomonas aeruginosa*
     d. Predisposing factors
        (1) Multiple dermatoses—tinea, inflammatory, bullous, ulceration, pyodermas
        (2) Trauma
        (3) Surgical wounds
        (4) Infections
     e. Risk factors
        (1) Immunocompromised, cancer, and diabetes
        (2) Alcohol and drug abuse
        (3) Cancer, cancer chemotherapy

- Signs and Symptoms
  1. Localized pain, redness, swelling, or heat
  2. More severe infections (e.g., cellulitis)—systemic symptoms such as malaise, fever, chills

- Differential Diagnosis
  1. Contact dermatitis
  2. Allergic dermatitis
  3. Fungal dermatitis
  4. Herpes dermatitis

- Physical Findings
  1. Severe infections
     a. Regional lymphadenopathy
     b. Fever
     c. Skin tracking
  2. Morphology
     a. Impetigo—small vesicle caused by streptococcus
        (1) Small, red macules that progress to water-filled vesicles
        (2) Ruptured vesicles leave characteristic honey-colored crusted area
     b. Bullous impetigo caused by *S. aureus*
        (1) Large flaccid blister
        (2) Cloudy to purulent contents
     c. Folliculitis, furuncle, carbuncle
        (1) Abscess—tender, fluctuant nodule
        (2) Furuncle—firm, tender nodule with central necrotic plug
        (3) Carbuncle—multiple abscess/furuncles with sieve-like openings draining purulent material
     d. Hidradenitis suppurativa
        (1) Initial—inflamed nodule/abscess with serous/purulent drainage and sinus tracks; open, black comedones when active nodules are absent
        (2) Late phase—fibrous "bridge" scarring and contractures
     e. Cellulitis
        (1) Bright red plateau, erythema with indistinct margins
        (2) Lymphangitis (red streaking from the area of cellulitis toward proximal lymph nodes) may be present
  3. Distribution
     a. Impetigo—anywhere
     b. Folliculitis, furuncle, carbuncle
        (1) Hair-bearing area—beard, axilla, occipital scalp, back of neck
        (2) Any non-weight-bearing area, buttock, upper trunk, puncture wound site
     c. Hidradenitis suppurativa—regions rich with apocrine glands
        (1) Axilla
        (2) Inguinal area
        (3) Anogenital area
        (4) Buttocks, scalp
     d. Cellulitis
        (1) Any area where normal lymphatic drainage has been disrupted
        (2) Recent venous and lymphatic surgical sites
        (3) Previous cellulitis sites
        (4) Cheek or cheek bone and lower extremities

- Diagnostic Tests/Findings
  1. Gram's stain—may be positive for cocci
  2. Culture and sensitivity of exudate especially on immunocompromised patient
  3. KOH—negative
  4. Wood's lamp—no fluorescence
  5. Tzanck test—negative

- Management/Treatment
  1. GAS—small vesicular impetigo
     a. Small, localized affected area may be treated with topical Bactroban (mupirocin)
     b. Larger surface involvement requires systemic antistreptococcal treatment
        (1) Penicillin (PCN) VK 250 mg q.i.d. for 10 days
        (2) Benzethine penicillin 1.2 million units
        (3) Cephalexin 250–500 mg q.i.d. for 10 days
  2. *S. aureus*
     a. Small, localized affected area may be treated with topical Bactroban (mupirocin)
     b. Trimethoprim/sulfamethoxazole DS b.i.d. × 10 days
     c. Clindamycin 300–450 mg t.i.d. for 10 days
     d. Minocycline 100 mg b.i.d. for 10 days
     e. Linezolid 600 mg b.i.d. for 10 days
  3. Folliculitis, furuncle, carbuncle, and hidradenitis suppurativa
     a. Mild folliculitis
        (1) See impetigo
        (2) Terbinafine 250 mg daily for 14 days—fungal folliculitis
     b. Moderate infection
        (1) Warm moist compresses to promote spontaneous drainage
        (2) Incision and drainage (I & D) usually required
        (3) Culture recurrent abscesses
        (4) See impetigo
     c. Hidradenitis suppurativa—additional measures to reduce inflammation
        (1) Intralesional triamcinolone 3–5 mg/mL diluted with lidocaine
        (2) Prednisone 70 mg tapered over 14 days
  4. Cellulitis
     a. Facial involvement—consider inpatient management
     b. I & D may be required
     c. See impetigo

d. Rest, immobilization, elevation, moist heat, analgesia
e. Reevaluate in 48 hours

# DERMATITIS

- Definition—group of inflammatory pruritic skin diseases that have different etiologies but share common symptoms and clinical manifestations
  1. Atopic dermatitis—acute, subacute, but usually chronic, pruritic inflammation of the epidermis and dermis; term often used synonymously with eczema, IgE dermatitis
  2. Contact dermatitis—acute or chronic inflammatory reactions to substances that come in contact with the skin
  3. Stasis dermatitis—inflammatory response to extravasated blood in dermis and subcutaneous tissue resulting from stasis
  4. Seborrheic dermatitis—chronic dermatosis characterized by redness and scaling reaction where sebaceous glands are most active

- Etiology/Incidence
  1. Atopic dermatitis
     a. Thought to have genetic basis; often seen as part of an "atopy" triad; dermatitis, asthma, and allergic rhinitis
     b. Two-thirds of patients have personal or family history of respiratory atopy
     c. Seen in all populations and geographic locations
     d. More common in males than in females
     e. Highest incidence in childhood, usually resolves by third decade
     f. More prevalent in urban areas and developed countries
     g. Exacerbated by allergies, skin dehydration, emotional stress, hormonal changes, and infection
  2. Contact dermatitis
     a. Irritant contact dermatitis
        (1) More common than allergic contact dermatitis
        (2) Most irritants used daily in work and home environments
        (3) Accounts for high percentage of work-related skin disorders
           (a) Low-caustic irritants—soapy water, cleansers, rubbing alcohol, kerosene
           (b) High-caustic irritants—bleach, strong acids, alkalines
        (4) Higher incidence in those with compromised skin integrity
     b. Allergic contact dermatitis
        (1) Delayed (type IV) cell-mediated hypersensitivity to a substance
           (a) Substance (antigen) binds with epidermal protein
           (b) Antigen-protein complex presented to T-helper cells causing release of mediators
           (c) T-helper cell expansion occurs in regional lymph nodes producing T-effector lymphocytes
           (d) T-effector lymphocytes circulate in bloodstream and produce the epidermal response
           (e) Entire process occurs in 5–21 days
           (f) Reexposure—dermatologic response in 12–48 hours
        (2) Most common sensitizer in United States is oleoresin of Rhus family of plants—poison oak, poison ivy, and poison sumac
        (3) Other common sensitizers are nickel in jewelry, fragrances, and preservatives in topical preparations
  3. Stasis dermatitis
     a. Occurs as a result of chronic venous insufficiency
     b. Complicated by low-grade tissue ischemia associated with stasis at capillary level
     c. History of varicosities, thrombophlebitis, or postphlebitic syndrome
     d. Often complicated by allergic contact dermatitis and chronic infection
  4. Seborrheic dermatitis
     a. Etiology unknown, thought to have a genetic basis
     b. Overgrowth of naturally occurring yeast, *Pityrosporum ovale*
     c. Often begins in early adulthood, aggravated by stress
     d. Can be an early cutaneous sign of HIV infection
     e. Often severe in patients with chronic neurological diseases
     f. Seen in patients with severe acne
     g. More common in males

- Signs and Symptoms—pruritic scaly rash

- Differential Diagnosis
  1. Scabies
  2. Tinea
  3. Atopic/eczema dermatitis
  4. Contact dermatitis
  5. Nummular dermatitis
  6. Psoriasis (seborrheic dermatitis)
  7. Cellulitis (stasis dermatitis)

- Physical Findings
  1. Common clinical findings for all types of dermatitis
     a. Initial stage—erythema, papules, microvesicles, and excoriation
     b. Chronic stage—lichenification
  2. Atopic dermatitis
     a. Papules, erythema, excoriations, and lichenification
     b. Pustules represent secondary infections with staphylococci
     c. Distribution—flexural areas of neck, antecubital fossae, and popliteal fossae
     d. Other locations—face, wrist, and forearm
  3. Irritant contact dermatitis
     a. Mild irritants—erythema, chapped skin, dryness, and fissuring
     b. Severe cases—edema, serous oozing, tender, crusting, scaling
     c. Painful bullae may develop with potent irritant
     d. Distribution—hands most common, also face and eyes
  4. Allergic contact dermatitis
     a. Erythema, edema, papules, vesicles, serous oozing, crusting, scaling
     b. Distribution—corresponds to exposed area
     c. Lesions outline site of irritant, often linear pattern with plant exposure
  5. Stasis dermatitis
     a. Early stage—mottled pigmentation and slight erythema
     b. Evidence of varicosities, ankle edema
     c. Mild tenderness with deep palpation; pulses normal
     d. Chronic stage—subcutaneous tissue becomes thick, fibrous
     e. Distribution—lower legs
  6. Seborrheic dermatitis
     a. Ill-defined, greasy yellow scales overlying erythematous patches
     b. Distribution—scalp, within external ear, postauricular area, eyebrows, nasolabial folds, central chest, and at times axilla, groin, submammary folds
- Diagnostic Tests/Findings
  1. Serum IgE—levels elevated in patients with atopy
  2. KOH—negative for spores/hyphae
  3. Skin scrapings—negative for burrows
- Management/Treatment
  1. Three goals of therapy
     a. Treatment of inflamed skin
     b. Control of pruritus
     c. Control of exacerbating factors
  2. Treatment of inflamed skin
     a. Mild disease—low-potency steroid cream
        (1) Hydrocortisone 1–2.5% cream 2–4 times daily
        (2) Desonide 0.05% b.i.d. (face or areas resistant to hydrocortisone)
     b. Severe disease—medium potency steroid cream (2–4 weeks)
        (1) Triamcinolone acetonide 0.1% cream 2–4 times daily
        (2) Fluocinolone acetonide 0.025% cream b.i.d.
     c. Topical corticosteroid with occlusion may be helpful
        (1) Treat area with steroid cream and cover with plastic wrap
        (2) Leave on overnight and remove plastic wrap in morning
     d. Lesions resistant to medium potency steroids use ultra-high potency—betamethasone dipropionate 0.05% b.i.d., with or without occlusion
     e. Pimecrolimus 1%—apply twice daily for steroid-resistant cases or for cases requiring steroid cessation
     f. Acute flares may require short-term oral glucocorticoids
        (1) Prednisone 40–60 mg tapered over 14–21 days
        (2) Solu-Medrol Dosepak
     g. Ultraviolet light therapy and oral glucocorticoids for most severe cases
     h. Wet to dry compresses with water or aluminum acetate (Burow's solution) to dry vesicular lesions
     i. Bullous lesions—may be drained; do not remove top thin skin
  3. Control of pruritus
     a. Antihistamines—work best for histamine-induced pruritus but may be effective for other types
        (1) Cetirizine 10 mg q.d./b.i.d. prn
        (2) Desloratadine 5 mg q.d./b.i.d. prn
        (3) Hydroxyzine 25 mg t.i.d./q.i.d. prn
        (4) Diphenhydramine 25–50 mg every 4–6 hours prn
     b. Doxepin 10–25 mg, may titrate to 50 mg at hs
        (1) Effective for pruritus associated with anxiety or depression
     c. Tepid baths to cool and hydrate skin
     d. Mild soaps, avoid dry scaly areas
     e. Emollients
     f. Control of exacerbating factors
        (1) Treat secondary bacterial infections, usually staphylococcus
        (2) Maintain good hydration and integrity of skin

(3) Gently towel dry skin, no brisk rubbing
(4) Continued use of emollients to prevent skin drying
(5) Wear gloves to avoid contact irritants
(6) Identify and avoid offending irritants
(7) Stasis dermatitis—special measures
   (a) Elevate legs; support stockings
   (b) Exercise daily to help reduce venous pressure and edema
(8) Seborrheic dermatitis—special measures
   (a) Daily use of shampoos containing tar, sulfur, salicylic acid, or selenium
   (b) Ketoconazole 2% cream and shampoo (twice weekly) is an alternative to topical steroids
   (c) Low-potency topical steroid, hydrocortisone 1%
(9) Educate patient on stress reduction to avoid exacerbation
(10) Follow-up in 1–2 weeks

# FUNGAL AND YEAST INFECTIONS

- Definitions
  1. Tinea (dermatophytosis)—fungal infection of skin, nails, and hair; characteristic lesions varies by site
  2. Tinea (pityriasis) versicolor—chronic, asymptomatic, scaly dermatitis
  3. Candidiasis—yeast-like fungal infection of skin and mucous membrane

- Etiology/Incidence
  1. Tinea
     a. Causative organisms—*Trichophyton, Microsporum,* and *Epidermophyton*
     b. Transmitted by people through fomites, animals (pets), and, to a lesser extent, soil
  2. Tinea versicolor
     a. Causative organism—nondermatophyte fungus *Pityrosporum orbiculare*; normal inhabitant of skin
     b. Most common in young adults when sebum production is high
  3. Candidiasis
     a. Causative organism usually *Candida albicans*; normal saprophytic inhabitant of GI tract; overgrowth often due to antibiotic use
     b. Occurs in intertriginous, moist, cutaneous areas
  4. Contributing factors
     a. Warm, moist environments for fungal infections
     b. Obesity
     c. Altered immunity
        (1) HIV
        (2) Diabetes
        (3) Pregnancy
        (4) Inhaled or oral steroids
     d. Oral contraceptives
     e. Antibiotic therapy

- Signs and Symptoms (depends upon area of involvement)
  1. Mild pruritus
  2. Inflamed, tender rash
  3. Thickened nails
  4. Hair loss

- Differential Diagnosis
  1. Seborrheic dermatitis
  2. Psoriasis
  3. Alopecia
  4. Atopic dermatitis
  5. Contact dermatitis
  6. Pityriasis rosea
  7. Bacterial infection

- Physical Findings
  1. Morphology
     a. Tinea (dermatophytosis)—characteristic lesion varies by site
        (1) Tinea capitis—well-defined or irregular, diffuse areas of scaling and hair loss on scalp
        (2) Tinea corporis—annular appearance (ringworm), deep inflammatory nodules, or granulomas
        (3) Tinea cruris—sharply demarcated, erythematous, scaly patches
        (4) Tinea pedis—erythema/edema, scaling, and occasional vesiculation; fissured toe webs
        (5) Tinea unguium—opacified, thickened nails with subungual debris
        (6) Immunocompromised patient—may see abscess or granulomas
     b. Tinea (pityriasis) versicolor—oval scaly hyper- or hypopigmented macules
     c. Candidiasis
        (1) Skin (intertrigo)—erythematous macerated areas with satellite pustules
        (2) Mucous membranes—white friable patches on mucous membranes
        (3) Most common fungal infection of the penis and scrotum
  2. Distribution
     a. Tinea
        (1) Capitis—scalp
        (2) Corporis—non-hair-bearing skin

(3) Cruris—(males) groin and upper thigh sparing scrotum
(4) Pedis—feet, usually between 4th and 5th toes
(5) Unguium—nails, usually 1st and 2nd toenails
b. Tinea versicolor
(1) "Shawl-like" back, chest, and shoulders
(2) Less common—groin, thigh, genitalia
c. Candidiasis
(1) Body folds—axillae, submammary, groin, intergluteal, webspaces of fingers and toes
(2) Oral and vaginal mucous membranes

- Diagnostic Tests/Findings
    1. Direct microscopy of skin, hair, or nail samples
    2. Wood's lamp (tinea versicolor)—golden fluorescence
    3. KOH—positive for hyphae, pseudohyphae, and/or spores
    4. Fungal culture—may be useful for inflammatory tinea corporis and tinea capitis

- Management/Treatment
    1. Tinea
        a. Scalp
            (1) Prevention—ketoconazole or selenium sulfide shampoo, may eradicate carrier state
            (2) Terbinafine 250 mg daily 4–8 weeks
            (3) Itraconazole 200 mg daily 6–8 weeks
            (4) Griseofulvin microsized 250 mg daily 4–8 weeks
            (5) Fluconazole 200 mg daily 2 weeks
            (6) Ketoconazole 200–400 mg daily
            (7) Advise hair regrowth will be slow
        b. Body/feet
            (1) Prevention—apply powder containing miconazole to fungus-prone areas after bathing
            (2) Multiple topical imidazoles and triazoles applied b.i.d. until 1–2 weeks after clinical clearing
            (3) Terbinafine 1% cream b.i.d. 1–2 weeks after clinical clearing
            (4) If topical antifungals fail, use oral agents (see tinea capitis)
            (5) Avoid occlusive footwear for tinea pedis
        c. Nails
            (1) Ciclopirox (Penlac) 8% lacquer—limited efficacy
            (2) Itraconazole 200 mg daily or terbinafine 250 mg daily for 3 months (check liver function tests at 6 weeks)
                (a) Fingernails—6 weeks
                (b) Toenails—12 weeks
            (3) Poor results with topical agents; usually reserved for maintenance after successful systemic treatment
        d. Follow up in 2 weeks to reevaluate treatment
    2. Tinea versicolor (pityriasis versicolor)
        a. Selenium sulfide lotion 2.5%—apply and leave on for 10–15 minutes, and then rinse, for 1 week
        b. Ketoconazole shampoo (same as selenium sulfide)
        c. Terbinafine 1% solution b.i.d. for 7 days
        d. Imidazole or triazole creams b.i.d. for 1 week
        e. Retreat if no improvement in 1 month
        f. Recurrence common as organism is normal inhabitant of skin
    3. Candidiasis
        a. Nystatin cream or powder b.i.d. 2–4 weeks
        b. Ketoconazole cream daily for 2–4 weeks
        c. Fluconazole 150 mg orally once
        d. Dry intertriginous area—wet Burow's compresses 3–4 times daily
        e. Rule out HIV or diabetes in patients with multiple recurrences

# PAPULOSQUAMOUS DISORDERS

- Definition—group of disorders with unique scales due to abnormal keratinization process; these lesions are sharply delineated, which distinguishes them from scaling lesions of eczematous diseases
    1. Psoriasis vulgaris—genetically determined, chronic, epidermal proliferate disease of unpredictable course
    2. Pityriasis rosea—self-limited, mild, inflammatory skin disease lasting 3–8 weeks

- Etiology/Incidence
    1. Psoriasis
        a. Genetic predisposition, although not fully understood
        b. Autoimmune component
        c. Affects 2% of population in United States, Caucasians > African Americans
        d. Type 1, early onset, occurring in 2nd decade
        e. Type 2, late onset, occurring in 6th to 8th decades
        f. Approximately 5% of patients will develop psoriatic arthritis affecting primarily distal interphalangeal (DIP) joints
        g. Abrupt onset seen with early HIV infection
        h. Trigger factors
            (1) Physical trauma
            (2) Infection

(3) Stress
(4) Drugs—corticosteroids, lithium, antimalarial, interferon, beta-blockers
2. Pityriasis rosea
   a. Etiology unknown; herpes 7 is suspected
   b. Seen primarily in the spring and fall seasons
   c. Patients frequently report recent upper respiratory infection
   d. Equal incidence in males and females

- Signs and Symptoms
  1. Psoriasis
     a. Frequently asymptomatic, indolent lesion may be present for months
     b. Severe pruritus in body fold eruptions
     c. Constitutional symptoms, joint pain, acute fever, and chills
  2. Pityriasis rosea
     a. Mild pruritus, 50%
     b. Initial lesion precedes general eruption by 1–2 weeks
     c. Self-limiting—heals without scarring in 4–8 weeks

- Differential Diagnosis
  1. Psoriasis
     a. Seborrheic dermatitis
     b. Candidiasis
     c. Psoriasiform dry eruptions (beta blockers, methyldopa)
     d. Tinea corporis
  2. Pityriasis rosea
     a. Secondary syphilis
     b. Tinea infections
     c. Drug eruptions, e.g., captopril, barbiturates

- Physical Findings
  1. Psoriasis
     a. Cutaneous lesions reveal four prominent features
        (1) Sharply demarcated lesions with clear-cut borders
        (2) Erythematous plaque base
        (3) Overlapping silvery scales
        (4) Auspitz sign—removal of scales results in small blood droplets
     b. Fingers/nails
        (1) Stippling or pitting of nail plate
        (2) Yellow or brown-red staining of oncholytic patches with accumulation of yellow debris under nails
        (3) Swelling, redness, and scaling of paronychial margins
  2. Pityriasis rosea—classic disease pattern
     a. A single lesion termed *herald patch* precedes generalized eruption by 7–10 days
     b. Herald patch is found usually on neck or lower trunk; oval, slightly erythematous, rose or fawn-colored
     c. Oval patches seen in general eruption have an unusual fine, white scale located near the border of the plaques, forming a collarette
     d. Lesions follow skin cleavage lines in a "Christmas tree" pattern

- Diagnostic Tests/Findings
  1. Psoriasis
     a. Diagnosis generally based on clinical presentation
     b. Biopsy may be necessary
     c. HIV serology
     d. Serum uric acid
  2. Pityriasis rosea
     a. Diagnosis generally based on clinical presentation
     b. KOH—negative for spores/hyphae
     c. Throat culture or rapid strep test—**negative** for scarlatina
     d. RPR—negative for syphilis

- Management/Treatment
  1. Psoriasis—localized to palm/soles/scalp < 5% involvement
     a. Strong potency topical corticosteroid—adjunctive therapy for 2–3 weeks
        (1) Topical fluorinated high-potency glucocorticoids
        (2) Occlusion with plastic wrap
        (3) More effective if scales removed prior to application
     b. Tar-based preparations are useful adjuncts
     c. Anthralin cream 0.1–1% at bedtime
     d. Calcipotriene ointment or cream twice daily
     e. Goeckerman regimen—phototherapy ultraviolet B radiation (UVB), sun exposure 4–6 hours daily for 4 weeks
     f. Ingram regimen—phototherapy ultraviolet B radiation (UVB) used in combination with anthralin 0.1– 0.5% applied daily
  2. Psoriasis—generalized (> 30% body surface affected)
     a. Referral to dermatologist
     b. May include some combination of UVB, PUVA (psoralen with UVA), etretinate, methotrexate, cyclosporine, acitretin, immunomodulators
     c. Patient education for localized and generalized psoriasis—family issues, emotional support, stress reduction, National Psoriasis Foundation

3. Pityriasis rosea
   a. Treatment often not necessary
   b. UVB light treatments for 1 week
   c. Topical corticosteroids and antihistamines for control of pruritus

## SCABIES

- Definition—common highly pruritic transmissible ectoparasite infection

- Etiology/Incidence
  1. Caused by itch mite, *Sarcoptes scabiei*
  2. Adult female mite burrows into skin shortly after contact; lives for 4–6 weeks
  3. Incubation period 4 weeks from initial contact; generalized hypersensitivity eruption 1–2 weeks later
  4. Transmitted primarily by person-to-person or sexual contact
  5. Transmission via clothing, bedding less common—mite typically cannot survive more than 24–48 hours without host
  6. May affect entire families
  7. Frequently seen in institutionalized persons, such as homeless shelters, nursing homes, correctional facilities

- Signs and Symptoms
  1. Pruritus always present; most intense when individual is in bed or after a hot shower
  2. Pruritus frequently less intense in the HIV patient

- Differential Diagnosis
  1. Atopic dermatitis
  2. Contact or irritant dermatitis
  3. Adverse cutaneous drug reaction
  4. Pediculosis

- Physical Findings
  1. Burrows, small pruritic vesicles, or wavy dark lines a few millimeters to 1 cm in length with papule at open end
  2. May be difficult to visualize because patient scratching destroys burrows
  3. Lesions are believed to be due to a hypersensitivity reaction to the excreta deposited by mite
  4. Generalized excoriations surrounding vesicles and pustules on fingers, palms, wrists, elbows, axillae, feet, nipples in females, scrotum or penis in males, buttocks
  5. Usually spares the head and neck, except in the elderly or patients with AIDS—in the patient with HIV, hyperkeratotic plaques may be located on any area of the body

- Diagnostic Tests/Findings—microscopic examination of skin scraping in oil immersion detects presence of mite, eggs, or fecal pellets

- Management/Treatment
  1. Treatment of choice is 5% permethrin cream applied to all areas of the body from the neck down; left on for 8–14 hours and then removed with soap and water; may be repeated in 1 week
  2. Alternative is 1% lindane
     a. Lotion or cream applied from neck down to all areas of the body and removed with soap and water after 8 hours
     b. Not recommended for pregnant or lactating women, patients with extensive dermatitis, or infants
  3. Alternative is 10% crotamiton cream applied to the body from the neck down for 2 consecutive nights and then removed with soap and water 48 hours after the last application
  4. All household members and sexual partners should be evaluated and treated if necessary to prevent reinfection
  5. For persistent pruritus, triamcinolone 0.1% cream to affected areas b.i.d.
  6. Secondary pyoderma is generally due to staphylococcus; treat with topical mupirocin or oral erythromycin
  7. Patient education
     a. Launder all bedding and clothing in hot water and on hot dryer cycle
     b. Place clothing that cannot be laundered in plastic storage bags for at least 4 days—mites will not survive off the host longer than 4 days
     c. Advise patient that pruritus may continue for several weeks

## SKIN CANCER

- Definitions
  1. Basal cell carcinoma (BCC)—slow-growing locally destructive carcinoma of basal cell layer of epidermis; metastasis rarely seen but can occur
  2. Squamous cell carcinoma (SCC)—malignant, nodular, tumor arising from squamous cells in epithelium; hyperkeratotic growth
  3. Malignant melanoma (MM)—cancer that arises in melanocytes; accounts for 5% of all skin cancers; two most common types are superficial spreading melanoma (SSM) and nodular melanoma (NM)
  4. Kaposi's sarcoma (KS)—multisystem vascular neoplasm characterized by mucocutaneous and violet lesions and edema; involves nearly all body organs

- Etiology/Incidence
  1. Basal cell carcinoma
     a. Cause is multifactorial; cumulative sunlight exposure (UVB) is most significant factor
     b. Primarily affects fair-skinned persons with tendency to sunburn easily
     c. Most common form of human cancer
     d. More than 400,000 new cases in United States per year; mostly persons in 4th decade
     e. Additional risk factors
        (1) Extensive sun exposure as a youth
        (2) History of treatment with x-ray for facial acne
  2. Squamous cell carcinoma
     a. Causal/contributing factors
        (1) UVB light
        (2) Human papillomaviruses (HPV) have also been implicated
        (3) Immunocompromised
        (4) Chemical carcinogens—topical nitrogen mustard; oral PUVA (psoralens with UVA [used to treat psoriasis]); industrial carcinogens
        (5) Increased risk of oral and lip SCC in cigarette and cigar smokers
     b. Mainly seen on sun-damaged areas of fair-skinned persons, but can appear anywhere on the body
     c. Also found in brown- and black-skinned person on plantar surface of foot
     d. Frequency of metastasis is by location; SCC of the cutaneous tissue has an overall metastatic rate of 3–4%; invasive SCC arising from chronic osteomyelitis sinus tracts, burn scars, and sites of radiation dermatitis have metastatic rates of 31%, 20%, and 18%, respectively
  3. Malignant melanoma
     a. All causes not known
     b. Brief, intense exposure to long-wave ultraviolet radiation contributes to development
     c. Predisposing/risk factors
        (1) Presence of precursor lesions, e.g., Clark's dysplastic melanocytic nevus, congenital melanocytic nevus
        (2) Family history of melanoma
        (3) Fair complexion; red or blonde hair; freckles; tendency to sunburn easily
        (4) Excessive sun exposure
     d. Peak age distribution 30–50 years
     e. SSM more common in women, NM equal in women and men
     f. Incidence has increased 300% in 40 years
  4. Kaposi's sarcoma
     a. Human herpesvirus-8 present in all forms
     b. Epidemic clusters in United States predominantly found in HIV-infected individuals—incidence has decreased from 40% to 18% of HIV population
     c. Occurs when $CD4^+$ count < 500
     d. Non-HIV-related forms are less common but do occur
        (1) African-endemic—accounts for 8–12% of malignancies in Zaire
        (2) Classic (European)—occurs predominantly in elderly white males, rarely fatal
        (3) Iatrogenic immunosuppressive drug associated—occurs infrequently in patients on immunosuppressive or cytotoxic chemotherapy; resolves when drug withdrawn

- Signs and Symptoms
  1. BCC/SCC—painless sore that will not heal, especially on sun-damaged skin, lower lip, or on radiodermatitis
  2. Malignant melanoma—six signs (ABCDEE)
     a. **A**symmetry in shape
     b. **B**order is irregular
     c. **C**olor is mottled
     d. **D**iameter is usually large (> 6 mm)
     e. **E**levation is almost always present
     f. **E**nlargement or a history of an increase in size is perhaps the most important sign
  3. Kaposi's sarcoma—small reddish-purple to brown macule

- Differential Diagnosis
  1. BCC/SCC
     a. Seborrheic keratosis
     b. Malignant melanoma
     c. Actinic keratosis
     d. Psoriasis
     e. Nummular eczema
  2. Malignant melanoma
     a. Melanoma in situ
     b. Solar lentigo
     c. Dysplastic melanocytic nevus with marked atypia
     d. Recurring melanocyte nevus
     e. Hemangioma
     f. Pyogenic granuloma
     g. Pigmented BCC
  3. Kaposi's sarcoma
     a. Sclerosing hemangioma
     b. Ecchymosis
     c. Stasis dermatitis

- Physical Findings
  1. Basal cell carcinoma
     a. Most commonly found on face and head
     b. Types—nodular, ulcerated, sclerosing pigmented and superficial lesions

c. Pearly appearance with telangiectatic vessels is most diagnostic (nodular)
d. Lesions may have a central crust or erosion (sclerosing)
2. Squamous cell carcinoma
   a. In situ (Bowen's disease)
      (1) Sharply demarcated, scaling, or hyperkeratotic macule, papule, or patch
      (2) Red, sharply demarcated, glistening macule or plaque-like on genital and perineum
   b. Invasive squamous cell carcinoma
      (1) Highly differentiated SCC
         (a) Keratinization within or on surface of tumor
         (b) Firm or hard upon palpation
      (2) Poorly differentiated SCC
         (a) Shows no sign of keratinization
         (b) Fleshy, granulomatous; soft on palpation
3. Malignant melanoma
   a. SSM
      (1) Pigment variation of dark brown, black, pink, or gray; starts as flattened papule, progressing to plaques, and then nodules
      (2) Asymmetrical to 12 mm (early), to 25 mm (late)
      (3) Isolated single lesions found primarily on sun-exposed areas—back (men), legs (women)
      (4) Regional lymphadenopathy (later stages)
   b. NM
      (1) Dark blue, black uniformly elevated "blueberry-like" nodule ranging in size from 1 to 3 cm; oval or round with smooth sharply defined borders
      (2) Distribution and regional lymphadenopathy same as SSM
4. Kaposi's sarcoma
   a. Red, purple, or dark color palpable plaques or nodules on cutaneous or mucosal surfaces
   b. Oral lesions are often initial manifestation
   c. Lymph node involvement in 50% of patients with HIV-associated KS
   d. May also involve the lung, gastrointestinal tract, lymphatic system, or urogenital system

- Diagnostic Tests/Findings—total excisional biopsy with narrow margins for SSM and NM

- Management/Treatment
  1. Basal cell carcinoma
     a. Simple excision—5–10% recurrence
     b. Referral to oncology for therapy
        (1) Three cycles of curettage and electrodessication
        (2) Radiotherapy with 4,000–5,000 rads in 6–10 doses (cure 95%)
        (3) Mohs surgery—removal of tumor; 98% cure rate
  2. Squamous cell carcinoma
     a. Referral to oncologist for therapy
     b. Surgical excision, Mohs surgery, radiotherapy (invasion of SCC)
     c. Cryotherapy, 5-fluorouracil chemotherapy
  3. Malignant melanoma
     a. Refer to oncologist for therapy—initial excision to establish diagnosis
        (1) Total excisional biopsy with narrow margins where possible
        (2) If total excision not possible, punch biopsy followed by extensive surgery
     b. Close follow-up for evidence of recurrence of metastasis
  4. Kaposi's sarcoma
     a. Referral for cryotherapy, radiation, or laser surgery—treatment depends on underlying condition and location of sarcoma
     b. Supportive care, counseling for HIV-progressive disease

## VIRAL DERMATOSES

- Definitions
  1. Herpes simplex I (HS-I) ("fever blister")—recurrent cutaneous viral infection characterized by single or multiple clusters of small vesicles on an erythematous base; lesions appear on the lips, in the mouth, or in the pharynx
  2. Herpes (varicella) zoster ("shingles")—an acute central nervous system (CNS) cutaneous viral infection characterized by vesicular eruptions and neurological pain; involves primarily the dorsal root ganglia
  3. Human papillomavirus—cutaneous infections (HPV-CI), common contagious epithelial tumors; usually benign

- Etiology/Incidence
  1. Herpes simplex
     a. Caused by herpes simplex virus (HSV-I)
     b. Outbreaks typically follow a minor infection, trauma, stress, or sun exposure
     c. 90% of adults have serologic evidence of virus
     d. Incubation period 2–20 days
  2. Herpes (varicella) zoster
     a. Reactivation of varicella zoster virus (VZV) in chickenpox
     b. Proposed that VZV is dormant in dorsal root ganglia
     c. May occur at any age, but most common after age 50

d. May precede marked immunosuppression in patients with HIV or Hodgkin's disease
e. Post-transplant patients on immunosuppression medication are also at risk
3. HPV (cutaneous infections)
a. Caused by any of more than 150 human papillomaviruses
b. Squamous cell carcinoma associated with HPV infections in anogenital region
c. Common in young adults, but uncommon in the aged

- Signs and Symptoms
1. HS-I
a. Small umbilicated vesicles appear after a short prodrome of tingling, burning, or itching
b. Vesicles dry to a yellow crust within a few days
2. Herpes zoster
a. Pain along nerve root precedes eruption by 2–3 weeks
b. Characteristic crops of vesicles then appear in 3–5 days
3. HPV (cutaneous infections)—generally asymptomatic
4. Postherpetic neuralgia months to years

- Differential Diagnosis
1. HS-I
a. Aphthous stomatitis
b. Hand, foot, and mouth disease
c. Herpangina
2. Herpes zoster (local lesion and pre-eruptive pain)
a. Contact dermatitis
b. Herpes simplex
c. Migraine
d. Myocardial infarction
e. Acute abdomen
3. HPV (cutaneous infection)
a. Squamous cell carcinoma
b. Hypertrophic actinic keratosis
c. Molluscum contagiosum
d. Seborrheic keratosis

- Physical Findings
1. Regional lymphadenopathy may be seen with herpetic diseases
2. HS-I
a. Small, grouped vesicles on an erythematous base that progress to crusted erosion
b. Duration 5–7 days
c. Distribution—lips, mouth, pharynx
3. Herpes zoster
a. Prodrome (2–3 weeks); papules (24 hours); vesicles-bullae (48 hours); pustules (96 hours); crust (7–10 days)
b. Painful unilateral vesicular eruptions with crust formation within a dermatome lasting 3–5 days
c. Duration 2–3 weeks
d. Distribution—face and trunk
e. Regional lymph glands may be tender or edematous
f. Complication of postherpetic neuralgia involving trigeminal region
4. HPV
a. Common wart (verruca vulgaris)
(1) Solitary flesh-colored papule with scaly irregular surface 2–10 mm in diameter
(2) Appear most often on fingers, around nail plate, elbows, knees (site of trauma)
b. Flat wart (verruca plantaris)
(1) Groups of smooth flat-topped, flesh-colored lesions
(2) Distribution—face and extremities (site of trauma)
c. Plantar warts
(1) Endophytic (growing inward) with thick keratin surface
(2) Common on sole of foot, toes
(3) May be exquisitely painful

- Diagnostic Tests/Findings
1. HS-I and zoster
a. Direct immunofluorescent antibody (ELISA)—positive
b. Tzanck smear—multinucleated cells (least sensitive)
c. Viral culture—positive (not highly sensitive)
d. Consider testing for HIV or Hodgkin's if recurrence of herpes
2. HPV
a. Acetic acid 5%—lesions turn white
b. Biopsy—rule out squamous cell carcinoma

- Management/Treatment
1. HS-I
a. Immunocompetent patient
(1) Initial episode—7–10 days
(a) Acyclovir 400 mg 3 times/day for 7–10 days
(b) Valacyclovir 1,000 mg b.i.d. for 7 days
(c) Famciclovir 250 mg t.i.d. for 5–10 days
(2) Recurrent episodes—5 days
(a) Acyclovir 400 mg 3 times/day for 5 days
(b) Valacyclovir 1,000 mg b.i.d. for 5 days
(c) Famciclovir 125 mg b.i.d. for 5 days
(3) Topical acyclovir not recommended, minimally effective
b. Immunosuppressed patient
(1) Initial episode
(a) Acyclovir 200 mg 5 times/day for 7–10 days

                (b) Acyclovir 5 mg/kg/IV every 8 hours for severe cases
            (2) To prevent reactivation (i.e., immediate post-transplant)—acyclovir 400 mg 3–5 times/day
        c. Caution family—virus may remain on fomites for several hours
    2. Herpes zoster
        a. Immunocompetent
            (1) Immunization for those > 60 years old with Zostavax (zoster vaccine live)—not intended to treat existing disease
            (2) Acyclovir 800 mg 4 times/day for 7–10 days started within 48–72 hours
            (3) Famciclovir 500 mg t.i.d. for 7 days started within 48–72 hours
            (4) Valacyclovir 1,000 mg t.i.d. for 7 days started within 48–72 hours
            (5) Good hydration essential
            (6) Nerve block for analgesia may be necessary
            (7) Acute pain—prednisone 60 mg/day for 3 weeks
            (8) Monitor renal function in patient with renal disease
        b. Immunosuppressed patient
            (1) Consult with physician
            (2) Antiviral therapy as with immunocompetent except of longer duration until lesions have completely crusted
        c. Postzoster neuralgia
            (1) Capsaicin ointment 0.025–0.075% every 4 hours
            (2) Chronic regional nerve blockade
            (3) Antiepileptic or antidepressant medications (e.g., pregabalin, amitriptyline)
    3. HPV (cutaneous infection)
        a. Most are unresponsive to all therapeutic modalities
        b. Most will resolve spontaneously in 1–2 years
        c. Multiple keratolytic agents—salicylic acid or salicylic acid and lactic acid combination
        d. Imiquimod cream—apply, leave on for 6–10 hours, and then wash, 3 times a week
        e. Plantar warts—hyperthermia with hot water ½ to ¾ hour 3 times a week

### Special Considerations in the Hospitalized Patient

- Generalized principles of management of bacterial infection of the skin remain the same
    - Bacterial infection of the skin is presumed to be streptococcal or methicillin-resistant staphylococcal aureus (MRSA)
    - Conditions characterized by abscesses should undergo incision and drainage
    - Antibiotic choices are similar but are generally given parenterally and in higher doses
        - Penicillin G is the drug of choice for streptococcal infection at 5–10 million units daily in 4–6 divided doses
        - MRSA may be treated with Vancomycin 15–20 mg/kg q.8.hrs
            - Vancomycin resistant MRSA may be treated with linezolid not to exceed 600 mg 8.h.; other options include Clindamycin 600 mg IV t.i.d.
    - Consider gram negative infection (to include pseudomonas) in the immunocompromised patient
- Necrotizing fasciitis
    - Very rare in otherwise healthy patients; occurs when a burn, scrape, or other injury allows bacterial penetration beyond the skin barrier
    - Initial symptoms occur within hours of injury
    - Patient may complain of "sore muscle" type of pain
    - Areas of purple edema may spread rapidly with ulcer/blister development
    - Characteristic is the complaint of pain disproportionate to the appearance
    - Systemic symptoms, e.g., fever, chills, vomiting quickly occur
    - Three important types of necrotizing fasciitis include
        - Polymicrobial (type A)
        - Group A streptococcal (type B)
        - Gas gangrene (type C)
    - Laboratory assessment should include
        - CBC
        - Serum chemistries
        - Blood and tissue cultures
        - MRI preferred to assess extent of tissue damage
    - Management
        - This is a surgical emergency for the seriously ill patient

- Antibiotic coverage dependent upon cultures if available but may include
  - Penicillin G
  - Aminoglycosides
  - Clindamycin
  - Beta lactams (Penicillin and/or cephalosporins)
  - Vancomycin
- General sepsis management
- Palpable purpura
  - Defined as purpura (red discoloration) that does NOT blanch with pressure
  - Indicates damage to blood vessel wall that allows extravasation of erythrocytes
  - May be the primary disease process or a secondary symptom of something else
  - Palpable purpura is the hallmark lesion of leukocytoclastic (small vessel) vasculitis
    - Vasculitis may be small vessel, mixed, or large vessel
    - Palpable purpura always requires a thorough workup and the presumption of serious systemic disease
  - Laboratory assessment should include
    - CBC, ESR, ANA, ANCA, complement and UA
    - Based upon patient history consider HIV, HBV, HCV, stool, and throat cultures
    - Skin biopsy is often necessary for diagnosis
  - Palpable purpura is never a benign finding and may indicate any variety of vasculitis or systemic septic infection

## QUESTIONS

### Select the best answer.

1. Mrs. Trevino is a 35-year-old patient with patchy hair loss as a result of chronic systemic lupus erythematosus. You have determined that she has scarring or cicatricial alopecia. What is the most effective treatment you can offer?

   a. Topical minoxidil
   b. Intralesional corticosteroids
   c. Topical estrogen
   d. Referral for hair transplants

2. Mr. Johnson is a 45-year-old patient with diabetes who is homeless. He presents with tender fluctuant nodules on the skin around his beard. He has been previously treated with benzoyl peroxide 5% with minimal response. You order warm moist compresses and:

   a. Dicloxacillin 500 mg q.i.d. for 10 days
   b. Trimethoprim/sulfamethoxazole every day for 5 days
   c. Acyclovir topical
   d. Clotrimazole 1% b.i.d. for 10 days

3. Mr. Johnson returns to your office with his friend. His friend presents with multiple abscesses and "boils" on the back of his neck that have coalesced and developed sieve-like openings draining pus. Your diagnosis is:

   a. Scabies
   b. Folliculitis
   c. Carbuncle
   d. Contact dermatitis

4. To reduce inflammation in a hidradenitis suppurativa lesion, immediately prior to incision and drainage you would:

   a. Apply cold packs to axilla
   b. Order Solu-Medrol Dosepak
   c. Apply tretinoin topically
   d. Inject intralesional triamcinolone 3–5 mg/mL diluted with lidocaine

5. What is the most common sensitizer in the United States responsible for allergic contact dermatitis?

   a. Oleoresin
   b. Tinea
   c. Rubbing alcohol
   d. Bleach

6. Mrs. Waterman is a 64-year-old with a history of varicosities and a single episode of thrombophlebitis. On inspection of both lower extremities you note mottled pigmentation, erythema, varicosities, and ankle edema. What is your initial impression?

   a. Cellulitis
   b. Stasis dermatitis
   c. Atopic dermatitis
   d. Contact dermatitis

7. What is the most effective antifungal agent used in the treatment of tinea capitis?

   a. Terbinafine orally
   b. Clotrimazole 1% cream
   c. Triamcinolone 0.025% cream
   d. Nystatin cream

8. Janet is a 22-year-old white female who presents for evaluation of lesions on the palm of her right hand. The lesions consist of silvery scales on an erythematous base and are isolated by a sharply demarcated border. You remove the scales and minute drops of blood appear giving a positive Auspitz sign. Your diagnosis is:

   a. Pityriasis rosea
   b. Squamous cell carcinoma
   c. Psoriasis
   d. Eczema

9. Common mode(s) of transmission of scabies include:

   a. Moist fomites
   b. Person to person
   c. Household pets
   d. Soil

10. A 24-year-old presents to clinic with a 5-cm purple, palpable plaque on the upper right posterior chest. He admits to unprotected homosexual activity for the past 10 years. On further exam you note axillary and inguinal lymphadenopathy. You suspect this patient may have:

    a. Squamous cell carcinoma
    b. Malignant melanoma
    c. Basal cell carcinoma
    d. Kaposi's sarcoma

11. Initial laboratory evaluation(s) for this patient in question 10 should include:

    a. HIV antibody screening
    b. Complete blood count
    c. GC/chlamydia cultures
    d. Liver function tests

12. The common wart, verruca vulgaris, is characterized as:

    a. Solitary flesh-colored papule with scaly irregular surface
    b. Group of flat-topped flesh-colored papules
    c. Thick, endophylitic papules or plaques
    d. Papular, nodular, ulcerated sclerosing pigmented lesion

13. Joan is a 15-year-old with multiple closed comedones and a few pustules on her face and upper back. She has been on tretinoin for her face but is distressed at the progression of acne to her back. What would you prescribe?

    a. 13-cis-retinoic acid (Accutane)
    b. Erythromycin 500 mg b.i.d. for 10 days
    c. Benzoyl peroxide cleansing soap
    d. Amoxil 250 mg t.i.d. for 10 days

14. Janice is an 18-year-old who presents to your clinic with a scaly, pruritic rash on the dorsal aspect of her toes. This rash has occurred each winter for the past 8 years. Her family history is unremarkable except for her father who has asthma. What is the most likely diagnosis?

    a. Psoriasis
    b. Candidiasis
    c. Contact dermatitis
    d. Atopic dermatitis

15. Overgrowth of *Pityrosporum orbiculare* in the young adult results in:

    a. Tinea corporis
    b. Tinea versicolor
    c. Tinea capitis
    d. Tinea pedis

16. A 30-year-old male presents with multiple, scattered, discrete vesicular lesions on the right leg for 5 days. There are honey-colored "stuck-on" crusts and erosions in some of these lesions. The culture yields *Staphylococcus aureus*. What is the most likely diagnosis?

    a. Herpes simplex
    b. Herpes zoster
    c. Stasis dermatitis
    d. Impetigo

17. A 19-year-old female presents with small grouped vesicles on an erythematous base on her lower lip. The lesion is painful. She has had this before, and it has always gone away in a week or so. You suspect herpes simplex 1. You would confirm your diagnosis with which of the following laboratory tests?

    a. Direct immunofluorescent antibody (ELISA)
    b. KOH test
    c. Culture and sensitivity
    d. Wood's lamp

18. Mr. Smith, age 46, presents to the adult–gerontological nurse practitioner (ANP) with fever, malaise, and a painful, linear vesicular rash on just one side of his trunk. What is the most likely diagnosis?

    a. Tinea corporis
    b. Carbuncle
    c. Herpes simplex
    d. Herpes zoster

19. Mr. Thompson has chronic eczema. He presents with pruritic, dry, leathery patches with accentuated skin markings on his forearm. What is the most appropriate treatment?

a. Amoxicillin orally
b. Clotrimazole 1% cream
c. Desonide 0.05%
d. UVB with coal tar

20. Melissa, age 22, presents with a slightly pruritic red rash on her trunk and breast following the line of skin cleavage giving a "Christmas tree" configuration. She states that the rash started as a single red patch on her abdomen. Medical history is unremarkable, except for a recent upper respiratory infection. What is your initial diagnosis?

    a. Tinea versicolor
    b. Folliculitis
    c. Pityriasis rosea
    d. Seborrheic dermatitis

21. Mr. Kirk is a 45-year-old African American who presents with a sore on his lip that will not heal. Medical history includes psoriasis treated with oral PUVA. Upon inspection you note an erythematous plaque, slightly raised with sharp borders, and no sign of infiltration or telangiectatic vessels. You make a referral to the dermatologist for further evaluation of what you suspect is:

    a. Basal cell carcinoma
    b. Squamous cell carcinoma
    c. Kaposi's sarcoma
    d. Psoriasis refractory to treatment

22. Mrs. Summers presents with a complaint of red rash and large blister after wearing a new prosthetic leg for 3 days. This prosthesis has a new polyurethane material she did not have with her old prosthesis. Her leg was amputated below the right knee secondary to an accident as a child. Upon inspection you note a tender, erythematous, scaly, maculopapular rash. It is warm and edematous with a large bullous lesion on the posterior popliteal fossae. What is your initial diagnosis?

    a. Eczema
    b. Severe irritant contact dermatitis
    c. Herpes zoster
    d. Carbuncle

23. Your management of Mrs. Summers includes oral glucocorticoids steroids, UVB (sunlight exposure), and:

    a. Reducing bullae with sterile needle and syringe
    b. Leaving bullae alone and let rupture spontaneously
    c. Advising continued use of new prosthesis
    d. Removing top of bullae and applying high-potency steroid cream

24. Which of the following medications has no severe teratogenic properties and is safe for use in the sexually active young female with acne?

    a. Erythromycin
    b. Tretinoin
    c. Accutane
    d. Tetracycline

25. Mrs. Lopez is a 45-year-old who presents with a tender, mildly pruritic rash under both breasts and on her abdomen. She is a diabetic with poor control due to poor medication compliance and is at 160% ideal body weight (IBW). Upon inspection you note moist erythematous macerated areas with satellite pustules under both breasts. What is your initial impression?

    a. Candidiasis intertrigo
    b. Tinea corporis
    c. Herpes zoster
    d. Pityriasis rosea

26. Along with better control of Mrs. Lopez's diabetes and continued effort at weight modification, you would prescribe which of the following:

    a. Nystatin cream or powder
    b. Selenium sulfide lotion 2.5%
    c. Terbinafine 1% cream
    d. Hydrocortisone 1% cream

27. What is the most appropriate treatment for tinea versicolor?

    a. To apply selenium sulfide lotion 2.5% to the body and leave on for 10–15 minutes, and then rinse, for 1 week
    b. To apply topical steroids t.i.d. to the rash for 7 days
    c. To apply coal tar preparations such as estar gel
    d. To use psoralen with UV light

■ **Answers**

| 1. **d** | 10. **d** | 19. **c** |
| 2. **a** | 11. **a** | 20. **c** |
| 3. **c** | 12. **a** | 21. **b** |
| 4. **d** | 13. **b** | 22. **b** |
| 5. **a** | 14. **d** | 23. **a** |
| 6. **b** | 15. **b** | 24. **a** |
| 7. **a** | 16. **d** | 25. **a** |
| 8. **c** | 17. **a** | 26. **a** |
| 9. **b** | 18. **d** | 27. **a** |

## BIBLIOGRAPHY

Braunwald, E. (Ed.). (2011). *Harrison's principles of internal medicine* (18th ed.). New York, NY: McGraw-Hill.

Brodell, R. T., & Elewski, B. (2000). Antifungal drug interactions: Avoidance requires more than memorization. *Postgraduate Medicine, 107*(1), 41–43.

Campo, T. M., & Lafferty, K. (2010). *Essential procedures for practitioners in emergent, urgent, and primary care settings: A clinical companion.* New York, NY: Springer.

DiPiro, J. T., Talbert, R. L., Yee, G. C., Matzke, G. R., Wells, B. G., & Posey, L. M. (Eds.). (2008). *Pharmacotherapy: A pathophysiologic approach* (7th ed.). New York, NY: Lange Medical Books/McGraw-Hill.

Edlich, R. F. (2013). Necrotizing fasciitis treatment and management. Emedicine. Retrieved from http://emedicine.medscape.com/article/2051157-treatment

Hay, W. W., Levin, M. J., Deterding, R., & Sondheimer, J. M. (2008). *Current pediatric diagnosis and treatment* (19th ed.). New York, NY: McGraw-Hill.

McPhee, S. J., Papadakis, M. A., & Rabow, M. W. (Eds.). (2012). *Current medical diagnosis and treatment* (51st ed.). New York, NY: McGraw-Hill.

Ozgediz, D., Smith, E. B., Zheng, J., Otero, J., Tabatabi, Z. L., & Corvera, C. U. (2008). Basal cell carcinoma does metastasize. *Dermatology Online Journal, 14*(8), 5. Retrieved from http://dermatology.cdlib.org/148/case_reports/bcc/corvera.html

Uphold, C. R., & Graham, M. V. (2013). *Clinical guidelines in family practice* (5th ed.). Gainesville, FL: Barmarrae Books.

Wolff, K., & Johnson, R. A. (2009). *Fitzpatrick's color atlas and synopsis of clinical dermatology* (6th ed.). New York, NY: McGraw-Hill.

# Eye, Ear, Nose, and Throat Disorders

*Margaret Hadro Venzke*

## CONJUNCTIVITIS

- Definition—inflammation of palpebral and/or bulbar conjunctiva; classic description is "pink eye"

- Etiology/Incidence
  1. Bacterial
     a. *Staphylococcus aureus*
     b. *Streptococcus pneumoniae*
     c. *Haemophilus influenzae*
     d. *Neisseria gonorrhoeae*
     e. *Chlamydia trachomatis*
     f. Proteus species
  2. Viral
     a. Adenoviruses (most common)
        (1) Adenopharyngeal conjunctivitis (APC)—"swimming pool"
        (2) Epidemic keratoconjunctivitis (EKC)—highly contagious, corneal involvement
     b. Herpes simplex
     c. Herpes zoster
  3. Allergic
     a. Seasonal allergies—pollen, grass, trees
     b. Hypersensitivity
     c. Chemical irritants
  4. Other
     a. Trauma
     b. Contact lens wearer—more susceptible than general population
     c. Foreign body
     d. Drug induced—preservative in eye drops, antimicrobials
     e. Systemic illness
        (1) Measles
        (2) Varicella
        (3) Rocky Mountain spotted fever
        (4) Reiter's syndrome
     f. Contaminated contact lens solution
     g. Mascara/eyeliner, makeup
  5. Mode of transmission—direct contact with contagion or allergen
  6. Most common eye disease in primary care; usually benign, self-limiting disorder

- Signs and Symptoms
  1. Mild to moderate redness and irritation
  2. No change in visual acuity
  3. Absence of photophobia and eye pain
  4. Mild discomfort, often associated with itching, burning sensation, or excessive tearing
  5. Discharge may be watery, stringy, purulent; scant to copious
  6. Bacterial conjunctivitis
     a. Mucopurulent discharge (profuse exudate suggests *Neisseria gonorrhoeae*)
     b. Thick purulent crust of material on eyelids after night's sleep
     c. Unilateral (initially)
     d. Self-limiting—10–14 days without treatment, resolves in 2–4 days with treatment
  7. Viral conjunctivitis
     a. Redness, general discomfort, profuse watery discharge
     b. Preauricular adenopathy common
     c. Association with upper respiratory illness, fever, pharyngitis

## CHAPTER 5 Eye, Ear, Nose, and Throat Disorders

  d. Unilateral (initially)
  e. Symptoms last 2–3 weeks (contagious, viral shedding in tears for approximately 2 weeks)
 8. Allergic
  a. Moderate to severe bilateral itching
  b. Clear to stringy mucoid discharge
  c. Chronic hypersensitivity—vernal conjunctivitis associated with corneal ulceration
 9. Chlamydial conjunctivitis
  a. More often unilateral than bilateral
  b. Moderate exudate
  c. Enlarged, tender preauricular nodes
  d. Symptoms persist 3–9 months without treatment

- Differential Diagnosis
 1. Urgent ophthalmic conditions—prompt referral to avoid compromised eyesight. See **Table 5-1**.
  a. Acute uveitis/iritis
  b. Acute glaucoma
  c. Corneal trauma/infection
  d. Orbital cellulitis

- Physical Findings
 1. Injected conjunctiva
 2. Discharge (see Signs and Symptoms)
 3. Cornea—clear
 4. Pupillary response—equal and reactive to light
 5. Visual acuity (Snellen)—no acute change
 6. Preauricular adenopathy—often viral etiology

- Diagnostic Tests/Findings
 1. Typically none indicated; uncomplicated cases diagnosed based on clinical examination
 2. Fluorescein uptake staining—dye uptake suggests corneal involvement
 3. Culture—only if chronic problem or gonococcal conjunctivitis suspected
 4. Gram stain of discharge/scrapings—rarely done unless gonococcal conjunctivitis suspected
 5. Giemsa stain of scrapings—for *Chlamydia trachomatis* infection

- Management/Treatment
 1. Pharmacological
  a. Bacterial conjunctivitis—any variety of ophthalmic antibiotics including but not limited to:
   (1) Sodium sulfacetamide 10% ophthalmic solution
   (2) Bacitracin/polymyxin ophthalmic ointment
   (3) Erythromycin ophthalmic ointment
   (4) Tobramycin 0.3% or gentamycin 0.3% ophthalmic solution
  b. Gonococcal conjunctivitis—refer to ophthalmologist immediately
   (1) Topical antibiotics—erythromycin
   (2) Parenteral antibiotics
    (a) Ceftriaxone
    (b) Aqueous penicillin
   (3) Culture discharge
   (4) Report to health department
  c. Chlamydia conjunctivitis
   (1) Azithromycin 1 g orally × 1 dose
   (2) Doxycycline 100 mg orally b.i.d. for 21–30 days
   (3) May require concomitant treatment with ophthalmic antibiotics for chlamydia
  d. Viral conjunctivitis
   (1) Self-limiting
   (2) Topical antibiotics—to prevent secondary bacterial infection
   (3) Corticosteroids contraindicated
  e. Allergic conjunctivitis
   (1) Topical vasoconstrictors/antihistamines
    (a) Naphazoline HCL/pheniramine maleate
    (b) Ketotifen
   (2) Oral antihistamines

**TABLE 5-1** Characteristics of the Common Ophthalmic Conditions

|  | Conjunctivitis | Iritis | Acute Glaucoma |
|---|---|---|---|
| **Pain** | mild | moderate | severe |
| **Vision** | normal | slightly blurred | blurred |
| **Discharge** | clear, stringy, or mucopurulent | clear | clear |
| **Cornea** | clear | clear | cloudy |
| **Pupil** | normal | small irregular | mid-dilated and nonreactive |
| **Light response** | normal | poor | none |
| **Conjunctival injection** | diffuse toward fornices | circumcorneal | corneal/conjunctival hyperemia |

(3) Allergen avoidance
(4) Topical antihistamine mast cell stabilizer
    (a) Azelastine 0.05% drops
    (b) Olopatadine 0.1% drops
(5) Nonsteroidal anti-inflammatory drugs (NSAIDs)—ophthalmic (for ocular pruritus)—ketorolac tromethamine 0.5%
2. General measures
    a. Cool/warm compresses
    b. Frequent gentle eye wash to remove discharge
    c. Artificial tears
    d. Strict hand washing
    e. Use separate towels; avoid handshaking
    f. Contact lens care—clean contacts or change disposable lens, use new solutions, avoid "homemade" tap water solutions
    g. Avoid eye cosmetics during infection; change eye products frequently
    h. Refer if no improvement in 48 hours or if vision is impaired

# BLEPHARITIS

- Definition—inflammation of eyelid margins and eyelashes

- Etiology/Incidence
  1. Commonly affects elderly persons
  2. Associated with seborrheic dermatitis and acne rosacea
  3. Often a chronic condition
  4. Seborrheic blepharitis
     a. Erythematous lid margins
     b. Dry flakes, oily secretions
     c. Cosmetics and chemicals aggravate the condition
  5. Staphylococcal (ulcerative) blepharitis
     a. Acute/chronic inflammation of glands of lid margins
     b. *Staphylococcus aureus* and *Staphylococcus epidermidis*
     c. Mild ulceration of lid margin
     d. Loss of lashes
  6. Mixed blepharitis—most common (seborrheic with secondary staphylococcal infection)
  7. Infestation of eyelashes with lice

- Signs and Symptoms
  1. Gritty, burning sensation
  2. Crusted material on eyelids upon awakening
  3. Redness
  4. Swelling of lid margins
  5. Irritation and itching common
  6. Dry or greasy scales on lashes
  7. Mild conjunctival irritation and erythema
  8. Discomfort typically less than expected given appearance

- Differential Diagnosis
  1. Conjunctivitis
  2. Chronic chalazia
  3. Sebaceous cell carcinoma (rare)
  4. Keratitis

- Physical Findings
  1. Erythematous eyelid margins bilaterally
  2. Scaly lesions on lashes
  3. Sclera—white
  4. Conjunctivae—usually clear
  5. Masses on lids/lid margins (palpate with gloves)
  6. Preauricular adenopathy
  7. No change in visual acuity

- Diagnostic Tests/Findings—none indicated

- Management/Treatment
  1. Warm water compresses
  2. Eyelid margin gentle scrubs 2–4 times a day
     a. Use washcloth or cotton tip applicator, moisten with dilute solution of water and baby shampoo or commercial lid cleaner
     b. Rinse well
  3. Antibiotic ointment q.i.d. to lid margins for 7 days (erythromycin, sulfacetamide sodium)
  4. Systemic antibiotics for severe infection
  5. Coexisting seborrhea of face/scalp—treat with selenium sulfide shampoo
  6. Maintain hygiene (lid washes) to prevent recurrence of seborrheic and mixed blepharitis

# FOREIGN BODY IN EYE

- Definition—object or debris in eye causing irritation

- Etiology/Incidence
  1. Most common ocular injury in primary care
  2. Foreign body (FOB) often lodges in conjunctiva or cornea

- Signs and Symptoms
  1. Unilateral, acute onset
  2. Sensation of "something in the eye"
  3. Photophobia
  4. Redness
  5. Mild pain
  6. Mild decrease in visual acuity

- Differential Diagnosis
  1. Intraocular foreign body (penetrates eye globe)
  2. Corneal laceration

3. Corneal abrasion
4. "Contact lens wearer" keratitis

- Physical Findings
    1. Diagnosis based on physical findings
    2. Visual acuity may be normal
    3. Cornea—examine under magnification and bright light, FOB may show up as a dark speck
    4. Ring-shaped orange stain—embedded iron or steel body
    5. Observe for laceration, hyphema, irregular pupil, or absent red reflex—immediate ophthalmic referral
    6. Conjunctiva—instruct patient to look down, grasp lashes, evert eyelid, inspect upper eye and lid

- Diagnostic Tests/Findings—fluorescein stain highlights presence of foreign body and corneal abrasion

- Management/Treatment
    1. Remove simple (nonpenetrating) foreign body with moistened cotton applicator with water or sterile normal saline; reevaluate visual acuity
    2. Irrigation of eye—use only for chemical splash to eyes
    3. Antibiotic ophthalmic ointment
    4. Eye pad
    5. Follow up in 24 hours to evaluate
    6. Patient education
        a. Caution—no rubbing of eye
        b. Advise protective eye wear
    7. Refer
        a. Intraocular foreign body
        b. Change in visual acuity
        c. Acute ocular pain
        d. Large corneal abrasion

## CORNEAL ABRASION

- Definition—disruption in the epithelial surface of the cornea by mechanical or chemical factors

- Etiology/Incidence
    1. Common eye injury
    2. Direct trauma to eye; most commonly a scratch from contact lens, fingernail, or piece of paper
    3. Chemical splash
    4. Chronic dry eye
    5. Iatrogenic in patients with neuromuscular blockade, comatose states

- Signs and Symptoms
    1. Unilateral severe eye pain, progresses over period of hours
    2. Redness
    3. Tearing
    4. Photophobia
    5. Scratchy sensation that worsens with blinking
    6. Decreased visual acuity
    7. Difficulty keeping eye open

- Differential Diagnosis
    1. Keratitis (viral, bacterial, or acanthamoeba)
    2. Foreign body
    3. Corneal laceration

- Physical Findings
    1. Document visual acuity—often decreased
    2. Visualization of corneal lesion following fluorescein stain illuminated with cobalt blue light

- Diagnostic Tests/Findings
    1. Fluorescein dye; abraded or ulcerated areas will become stained and fluoresce yellow-green color
    2. Magnetic resonance imaging (MRI) of orbit if high-velocity injury or suspect embedded foreign body

- Management/Treatment
    1. Antibiotic ointment or sulfonamide drops to affected eye
    2. Ophthalmic nonsteroidal anti-inflammatory agent, e.g., ketorolac
    3. Oral analgesics or short-acting cycloplegic agent for pain relief
    4. Pain should be markedly improved in 48 hours; typically much better in 24 hours; if not, refer to ophthalmology
    5. Topical antibiotics q.i.d. for 24–48 hours
    6. Avoid topical anesthetic drops after initial examination; retard healing and mask symptom progression
    7. Topical steroids contraindicated; retard healing and increase risk of infection
    8. If chemical or thermal injury to eye, refer immediately to ophthalmology

## GLAUCOMA

- Definition—increased intraocular eye pressure resulting in atrophy of optic nerve, loss of visual fields and acuity; may be acute or chronic

- Etiology/Incidence
    1. Inadequate drainage of aqueous fluid in the anterior chamber of the eye
    2. Most common type is chronic open angle (wide angle)

3. Acute closed angle (angle closure, narrow angle) occurs in patients with an anatomically narrow angle
4. Chronic open angle
   a. Accounts for 90% of all cases
   b. Predominately seen in those older than age 40
   c. African Americans are affected more frequently
   d. Positive first-degree family history
   e. Diabetes mellitus and steroid use are risk factors
5. Primary angle closure (closed angle or narrow angle)
   a. Positive family history
   b. African Americans and Asians more affected than Caucasians
   c. Predominately age 55–75 years
   d. Females more than males
   e. Less common than open angle but more severe in presentation
   f. May be precipitated by stress, anxiety, darkness, increased fluid intake, or medications—anticholinergic medications are common triggers
6. Congenital glaucoma (developmental) in young children
7. Approximately 0.5% of total population

- Signs and Symptoms
  1. Chronic open angle glaucoma—obstruction to aqueous outflow
     a. Asymptomatic at onset
     b. Mid-peripheral vision affected in early stages
     c. Frequent change of glasses
     d. Central vision loss is a late sign
     e. Gradual, painless visual loss and ultimate blindness
  2. Primary angle closure—mechanical obstruction of flow of aqueous humor; iris may obstruct the trabecular meshwork at canal of Schlemm, resulting in elevated intraocular pressure
     a. Acute ocular pain
     b. Nausea, vomiting
     c. Photophobia
     d. Blurred vision
     e. Halos around lights at night
     f. Unilateral frontal headache
     g. Tearing
     h. Erythema

- Differential Diagnosis
  1. Uveitis
  2. Conjunctivitis
  3. Ocular trauma
  4. Neurological disease

- Physical Findings
  1. Visual acuity—decreased
  2. Cornea is clear
  3. Change in peripheral vision as measured by direct confrontation
  4. Chronic open angle glaucoma
     a. Cupping of optic disc
     b. Elevated intraocular pressure (IOP)
  5. Primary angle closure
     a. Lid edema
     b. Injected conjunctiva
     c. Fixed mid-dilated pupil
     d. Shallow anterior chamber, often cloudy
     e. Markedly elevated IOP
     f. Firm eye globe

- Diagnostic Tests/Findings
  1. Tonometry (normal range 10–20 mm Hg)
  2. Pressure reading 20 mm Hg or greater requires further evaluation
  3. U.S. Preventive Services Task Force reports insufficient evidence to recommend glaucoma screening; no consensus on frequency of screening
  4. May screen certain at-risk populations (African Americans, diabetes mellitus, or severe myopia)

- Management/Treatment
  1. Refer all patients with
     a. Elevated IOP
     b. Decreased visual acuity
     c. Visual field loss
     d. Nonreactive pupil
  2. Goal of therapy to stabilize IOP to prevent optic nerve damage and visual loss
  3. Pharmacological—chronic open angle glaucoma
     a. Parasympathomimetics—topical miotics (pilocarpine) facilitate aqueous outflow
     b. Beta blockers (timolol, betaxolol)—decrease aqueous production
     c. Carbonic anhydrase inhibitors (acetazolamide)—reduce aqueous production
     d. Hyperosmotics—reduce formation of fluid (mannitol)
     e. Alpha agonists—decrease aqueous production, increase outflow
  4. Pharmacological—primary angle closure
     a. Emergency treatment with IV acetazolamide, mannitol, and oral glycerol
     b. Maintenance therapy with additional miotic agents and corticosteroids
  5. Laser and surgical intervention are indicated for all patients with acute glaucoma after initial stabilization; may be indicated for chronic glaucoma after maximizing medication therapy

6. General measures
   a. Encourage frequent follow-up with ophthalmology
   b. Monitor side effects of medications
   c. Avoid over-the-counter cold preparations that may exacerbate glaucoma

# CATARACTS

- Definition—clouding/opacity of crystalline lens, causing disruption of visual acuity

- Etiology/Incidence
  1. Single largest cause of blindness
  2. 90% of cataracts due to aging process (senile cataract)
  3. Congenital cataract (rubella)
  4. Systemic disease (diabetes and thyroid)
  5. Drug induced, especially steroid use
  6. Ocular trauma
  7. Chronic uveitis
  8. Ultraviolet B light exposure

- Signs and Symptoms
  1. Painless
  2. Cloudy, fuzzy, blurred vision
  3. Change in refractive error
  4. Glare associated with bright lights (night driving)
  5. Alteration in color perception
  6. Unilateral or bilateral development

- Differential Diagnosis
  1. Senile macular degeneration (loss of central vision)
  2. Retinal detachment
  3. Diabetic retinopathy
  4. Ocular tumor

- Physical Findings
  1. Lens opacity
  2. Disruption of red reflex
  3. Visual acuity decreased
  4. Reduced color discrimination

- Diagnostic Tests/Findings—refer to ophthalmology

- Management/Treatment
  1. Refer to ophthalmologist
  2. Surgical intervention—lens implant is preferred treatment
  3. Follow up postoperatively to observe for hemorrhage or infection
  4. Nonsurgical treatment—frequent changes in glasses, bifocals, or contacts
  5. Optimize the environment of the inoperable patient with increased light sources, decreased glare; reorganize living space to prevent accidents/falls
  6. Prevention with protective eyewear to filter ultraviolet B exposure

# ACUTE OTITIS MEDIA (AOM)

- Definition—inflammation of middle ear

- Etiology/Incidence
  1. Eustachian tube dysfunction (ETD) or obstruction secondary to viral nasal pharyngitis—major pathogenic factors causing ineffective drainage of middle ear
  2. Bacterial pathogens
     a. *Streptococcus pneumoniae* (most common)
     b. *Haemophilus influenzae*
     c. *Moraxella catarrhalis*
     d. Occasional *Staphylococcus aureus*
  3. More frequent in young children (younger than age 7) than in adults
  4. Risk factors include
     a. Recent upper respiratory infection (URI)
     b. Congenital disorders—cleft palate, Down syndrome
     c. Active or passive smoking
     d. Native American/Eskimo heritage

- Signs and Symptoms
  1. Otalgia
  2. Fever
  3. Hearing loss (conductive)
  4. Otorrhea (if perforated eardrum)

- Differential Diagnosis
  1. Otitis externa
  2. Referred pain from jaw/teeth
  3. Dental abscess
  4. Mastoiditis
  5. Ear canal furuncle

- Physical Findings
  1. Bulging tympanic membrane (TM) uncommon; suggests imminent rupture
  2. Distorted light reflex/obscured landmarks
  3. Pneumatic otoscopy may show decreased TM mobility
  4. Erythema
  5. Bullae may form on TM—associated with *Mycoplasma pneumoniae* organism
  6. Postauricular or cervical adenopathy

- Diagnostic Tests/Findings
  1. Usually no tests ordered
  2. Pneumatic otoscopy reveals rigid or less flexible TM

3. Tympanometry—indicator of fluid posterior to TM
4. Complete blood count (CBC) with differential—if patient appears toxic; elevated white blood cell (WBC) count

- Management/Treatment
  1. Antibiotics
     a. Amoxicillin 500 mg orally t.i.d. for 10 days; alternative is amoxicillin 875 mg b.i.d. for 10 days—consider high-dose approach for patients at risk of drug-resistant *Streptococcus pneumoniae* (DRSP)
        (1) Advantage—inexpensive
        (2) Disadvantage—ineffective against beta-lactamase-producing pathogens
        (3) Contraindicated in those with penicillin allergy
     b. For recurrent otitis media with resistant pathogens or characterized by fever > 102°F and/or otalgia
        (1) Amoxicillin clavulanate
        (2) Cephalosporins—cefixime, cefaclor
        (3) Clindamycin if beta-lactam allergy
  2. If perforation is present, combined therapy of oral antibiotic and topical Cortisporin Otic Solution (neomycin and polymyxin B sulfates and hydrocortisone otic solution)—4 drops in each ear t.i.d. or q.i.d. for 10 days
  3. Pain management
     a. Acetaminophen
     b. Topical local anesthetic otic solution—pain reliever
        (1) A/B Otic 2 gtts t.i.d. for 4 days
        (2) Auralgan 2 gtts t.i.d. for 4 days
  4. Refer/consult with MD or otolaryngologist
     a. No response to treatment after 48–72 hours
     b. Persistent hearing loss after adequate treatment
     c. Complications
        (1) Mastoiditis
        (2) Facial nerve palsy
        (3) Chronic perforation
        (4) Recurrent infections
     d. Surgical procedures—myringotomy, tympanostomy tubes for recurrent infection

## SEROUS OTITIS MEDIA (SOM)

- Definition—effusion in middle ear—also known as chronic otitis media with effusion (OME)

- Etiology/Incidence
  1. Patency of Eustachian tube is impaired; prevents equalization of pressure
  2. Associated with
     a. Resolution of AOM
     b. Subacute infection
     c. Allergic manifestations
     d. Barotrauma
     e. Deviated septum
     f. Hypertrophic adenoids
     g. Benign or malignant neoplasms
  3. More common in children than in adults

- Signs and Symptoms
  1. Hearing loss
  2. Popping sensation with yawning/swallowing
  3. Fullness in ear
  4. Occasional dizziness
  5. Often asymptomatic

- Differential Diagnosis
  1. Acute otitis media
  2. Conductive hearing loss
  3. Meniere's disease

- Physical Findings
  1. Retracted tympanic membrane; distorted light reflex
  2. Air fluid level present, often with yellow/blue-tinged fluid posterior to TM or bubbles of air may be seen through tympanic membrane
  3. Decreased membrane mobility with insufflation
  4. Conductive hearing loss
     a. Weber test—lateralize to affected side
     b. Rinne test—bone conduction may be greater than air conduction, BC > AC

- Diagnostic Tests/Findings
  1. Audiometry—decreased hearing
  2. Tympanometry—shows middle ear effusion

- Management/Treatment
  1. If mild symptoms, may spontaneously resolve in 2–3 weeks
  2. Topical decongestants—phenylephrine 1–2 sprays to each nostril every 8–12 hours for 3 days only
  3. Oral decongestants may be helpful
  4. Antihistamines usually are ineffective
  5. Patient education on Valsalva maneuver or chewing gum—to relieve Eustachian tube blockage
  6. Follow up in 4–6 weeks
  7. Refer if persistent hearing loss

## OTITIS EXTERNA

- Definition—inflammation of external auditory canal; commonly known as "swimmer's ear"

- Etiology/Incidence

1. Infectious agents include
   a. *Pseudomonas aeruginosa* (most common)
   b. *Staphylococcus aureus* or streptococcus
   c. *Proteus mirabilis*
   d. Fungi
2. Inflammation develops from
   a. Frequent exposure to water (most common)
   b. Mechanical trauma from bobby pins, cotton applicators, ear plugs, hearing aids
   c. Eczema, skin disorders
3. Common in summer months, especially in hot, humid climates
4. More common in swimmers than in nonswimmers

- Signs and Symptoms
  1. Otalgia—gradual or acute onset
  2. Pruritus
  3. Purulent discharge
  4. Occasional hearing loss, "plugged ear"

- Differential Diagnosis
  1. Furuncle
  2. Otitis media
  3. Mastoiditis
  4. Foreign body
  5. Eczema
  6. Cellulitis

- Physical Findings
  1. Erythema and edema of ear canal
  2. Pain on manipulation of auricle or pressure on tragus
  3. Purulent or white "cheesy" exudate may be present
  4. Preauricular adenopathy
  5. Edema may impair visualization of tympanic membrane; TM usually not affected

- Diagnostic Tests/Findings—culture of discharge if no response to treatment or recurrent infection

- Management/Treatment
  1. Pharmacological
     a. Combined antibiotic, hydrocortisone, and propylene glycol will effectively treat infection and reduce inflammation—Cortisporin Otic Solution 4–5 gtts in ear(s) t.i.d. or q.i.d. for 7 days
     b. If unable to determine if TM is perforated or intact—ofloxacin 0.3% solution, instill 5–10 drops b.i.d. for 7–10 days
     c. Antifungal and antibacterial—acetic acid otic drops
     d. Saturated cotton wick with medication facilitates entry of medication in ear canal; moisten with antibiotic as directed
     e. Severe cases often require systemic antibiotics
     f. Analgesics
  2. General measures
     a. Protect ear from additional moisture
     b. Eliminate trauma to ear canal
     c. Prevent recurrences—instill 2% acetic acid 2–3 drops in ear canals b.i.d. after contact with water (commercial OTC products also available)
     d. Improvement in 48 hours after initiating treatment
     e. Instruction on proper technique to clean ears

## HEARING LOSS

- Definition—diminished ability to detect pure tones in decibels of 30 or greater

- Etiology/Incidence
  1. 10% of U.S. population has hearing problems
  2. Particularly common among elderly adults
  3. Hearing loss may result from interference in sound conduction (conduction loss) or impaired transmission through nervous system (sensorineural) or both (mixed hearing loss)
  4. Conductive loss—decreased ability of external and middle ear to conduct sound waves to inner ear due to
     a. Cerumen impaction
     b. Foreign body
     c. Otitis media
     d. Otosclerosis—hereditary, bony ankylosis of stapes
     e. Scarring or perforation of TM
     f. Congenital problems
     g. Cholesteatoma
  5. Sensorineural loss—results from changes to cochlea and/or involvement of the acoustic nerve; causes include
     a. Acoustic neuroma
     b. Meniere's disease
     c. Presbycusis—hearing loss associated with aging
     d. Excessive noise exposure
     e. Viral syndrome—rubella, mumps
     f. Drugs—acetylsalicylic acid (ASA), gentamicin, furosemide, erythromycin
     g. Syphilis
     h. Multiple sclerosis

- Signs and Symptoms
  1. Conductive hearing loss—decreased ability to detect low tones and vowels; often history of ear disease, patient speaks softly

2. Sensorineural—impaired high tone perception, poor speech discrimination, difficulty with background noise, and high-pitched female voice; patient speaks loudly
3. Presbycusis—hearing loss is bilateral; gradual in onset; loss of high frequencies first, then lower frequency sounds; tinnitus is common

- Differential Diagnosis—see Etiology/Incidence

- Physical Findings
  1. Otoscopic examination of ear—usually normal
  2. Gross hearing/whisper test—diminished (acoustic nerve)
  3. Rinne test—compares air to bone conduction
     a. Normal—AC > BC
     b. Conductive loss—decreased AC:BC ratio, BC may be > AC in affected ear(s)
     c. Sensorineural loss—AC > BC (remains normal)
  4. Weber test
     a. Normal—sound midline
     b. Conductive loss—lateralize to affected ear
     c. Sensorineural loss—lateralize to normal ear
  5. Red flags for immediate referral
     a. Cholesteatoma in conductive loss
     b. Acoustic neuroma in sensorineural loss

- Diagnostic Tests/Findings
  1. Speech discrimination testing
     a. Detects clarity of hearing—impaired in sensorineural loss
     b. Results recorded as percentage correct
     c. 90–100% is normal
  2. CT scan or MRI to detect tumors

- Management/Treatment—dependent on etiology
  1. Refer for formal audiogram
  2. Refer to otolaryngologist—particularly for sensorineural loss and conductive loss unresponsive to treatment
  3. Prevention
     a. Avoid loud music, machines (causes loss of high tones)
     b. Monitor ototoxic drugs carefully; if tinnitus or hearing loss, discontinue use
     c. U.S. Preventive Services Task Force recommends routine screening after 65 years of age
  4. Hearing aids—hearing amplification beneficial to patients with correctable hearing loss

# VERTIGO

- Definition—abnormal sensation of movement (may be peripheral or central); disturbances of peripheral/central vestibular system, which maintains spatial orientation/posture and is symptomatic of an underlying etiology

- Etiology/Incidence
  1. Peripheral vertigo (causes external to the brain stem and cerebellum) accounts for 85% of cases
     a. Benign paroxysmal positional vertigo (BPPV)—otoliths
     b. Recurrent vestibulopathy
     c. Labyrinthitis
     d. Positional vertigo
     e. Traumatic vertigo
     f. Perilymphatic vertigo
     g. Meniere's disease
     h. Infections—middle/inner ear, viral illness
     i. Medications—especially aspirin and alcohol
  2. Central vertigo
     a. Neoplasm
     b. Vascular disease
     c. CNS disease—multiple sclerosis, syphilis
     d. Cranial nerve VIII abnormality
  3. Incidence
     a. Approximately 50% of vertigo is benign positional
     b. Approximately 25% of vertigo is vestibular neuronitis
     c. Approximately 10% of vertigo is Meniere's disease
     d. Approximately 15% of vertigo is central vertigo

- Signs and Symptoms
  1. "Room spinning" or "head spinning"/weaving sensation—spinning is an essential characteristic that defines vertigo; other signs and symptoms may include:
     a. Nausea, vomiting, diaphoresis
     b. Imbalance
     c. Tinnitus
     d. Hearing loss
     e. Vague lightheadedness
  2. Signs and symptoms may occur in any position
  3. The more intense the vertigo, the more likely a peripheral cause

- Differential Diagnosis
  1. Ataxia
  2. Syncope or near syncope

- Physical Findings
  1. Nystagmus with testing of extraocular movements helps define central vs. peripheral causes
  2. Hearing loss
  3. Changes in blood pressure—associated with positional hypotension
  4. Carotid bruits—suggests impaired cerebral flow
  5. Cranial nerves—especially auditory changes, 5, 7, 8

6. Romberg test—often abnormal
7. Barany maneuver—stimulates vestibular system, reproduces vertigo
8. Additional findings consistent with specific cause
   a. Peripheral vertigo typically associated with
      (1) Hearing loss
      (2) Ear pain
      (3) Tinnitus
   b. Central vertigo typically associated with
      (1) Visual or sensory loss
      (2) Diplopia
      (3) Abnormalities in coordination

- Diagnostic Tests/Findings as indicated by remainder of history and exam
  1. Audiogram if hearing impaired
  2. CT scan/MRI—to rule out tumor/neurological dysfunction
  3. Venereal disease research laboratory (VDRL) test and FTA—reactive in syphilis
  4. Thyroid-stimulating hormone (TSH), CBC with differential, and glucose—to rule out infections and systemic disease
  5. Serum vitamin $B_{12}$ to rule out pernicious anemia

- Management/Treatment
  1. Immediate referral, if abnormal neurological signs
  2. Bed rest for acute episodes, e.g., viral labyrinthitis
  3. Epley maneuvers for suspected otoliths
  4. Antivertigo medications most helpful in central disease
     a. Meclizine—12.5–25 mg orally t.i.d.; causes dry mouth and sedation
     b. Dramamine 50 mg orally t.i.d.
     c. Scopolamine transdermal patch
  5. Antiemetic for nausea/vomiting—ondansetron orally disintegrating tablets (ODT) 4 mg t.i.d. prn.
  6. Do not perform tests for positional vertigo on geriatric patients
  7. Refer if vertigo persists

# EPISTAXIS

- Definition—bleeding from nostril, nasal cavity, or nasopharynx

- Etiology/Incidence
  1. Anterior epistaxis most common, occurring in the vascular plexus of septum (Kiesselbach plexus)
  2. Disruption of nasal mucosa due to
     a. Trauma
     b. Infection
     c. Allergies
     d. Dry environment
     e. Medications
     f. Cocaine use
     g. Neoplasm
     h. Occasionally systemic disease (hypertension, blood dyscrasia)
     i. Coagulopathy or anticoagulant therapy
  3. 10% of population will experience one significant nosebleed

- Signs and Symptoms
  1. Anterior epistaxis
     a. Unilateral bleeding from nostril
     b. Recurrent episodes last few minutes to ½ hour
     c. Venous source of blood
  2. Posterior epistaxis—occurs more in elderly adults, often difficult to correct
     a. Intermittent brisk bleeding
     b. Arterial source
     c. Blood flows into pharynx, may cause nausea and coffee ground emesis

- Differential Diagnosis—epistaxis is a sign/symptom, not a disease; assess for significant pathology
  1. Coagulation disorders
  2. Nasal malignancy
  3. Hereditary telangiectasia
  4. Malignant hypertension

- Physical Findings
  1. Visual site—usually bleeding from one nostril; bilateral bleeding suggests trauma
  2. Skin, mucous membranes, and conjunctivae with evidence of the following suggests a pathological condition:
     a. Rash
     b. Pallor
     c. Purpura
     d. Petechiae
     e. Telangiectasis

- Diagnostic Tests/Findings—dependent on suspected etiology
  1. Hemoglobin and hematocrit are decreased if severe blood loss
  2. Low platelet count and abnormal prothrombin time/partial thromboplastin time (PT/PTT) suggest a bleeding disorder

- Management/Treatment
  1. Position patient sitting up and leaning forward
  2. Apply continuous pinching pressure to anterior nasal septum for 10–15 minutes
  3. If inadequate blood clotting, place a small cotton pledget of 1:1,000 epinephrine or vasoconstrictor nasal drops (phenylephrine) into

vestibule of nose; apply pressure for 5–10 minutes; this will stop most anterior venous bleeds
4. Mechanical tamponade with nasal packing/nasal tampons
5. Application of ice may assist with clot formation
6. Refer to emergency room or otolaryngologist if bleeding persistent/continuous or if posterior bleed is suspected
7. General measures/prevention
   a. Warn against habitual nose picking, rubbing nose, forceful blowing
   b. Advise increased humidity, especially in winter months
   c. Use petrolatum-based ointment in nostril—promotes hydration
   d. Instruct patient on how to manage simple nosebleeds
8. Recurrent episodes of epistaxis require additional investigation

## NASOPHARYNGITIS

- Definition—minor, self-limiting viral infection of the upper respiratory tract

- Etiology/Incidence
  1. Rhinoviruses, coronaviruses, adenoviruses
  2. Incidence decreases with age
     a. Children average 6–8 colds per year
     b. Adults average 2–4 colds per year
  3. Transmission through hand-to-hand contact and airborne droplets

- Signs and Symptoms
  1. General malaise and fatigue
  2. Coryza
  3. Sore throat
  4. Low-grade fever
  5. Rhinorrhea and rhinitis
  6. Watery eyes
  7. Headache
  8. Nonproductive cough
  9. Symptoms typically of short duration—3–7 days on average
  10. Symptom progression predictable—migrate from one region to the next, e.g., nose to throat to cough

- Differential Diagnosis
  1. Influenza
  2. Atypical pneumonia
  3. Otitis media
  4. Sinusitis
  5. Rhinitis
  6. Allergies

- Physical Findings
  1. Mildly elevated temperature
  2. Conjunctivae clear, possible erythema
  3. Injected nasal and pharyngeal mucosa
  4. Lungs clear
  5. Clear rhinorrhea may progress to cloudy/purulent

- Diagnostic Tests/Findings—diagnosis based on clinical findings

- Management/Treatment—palliative
  1. Rest, maintain fluid hydration
  2. Acetaminophen or ibuprofen for fever and headache
  3. Topical decongestants for nasal congestion; use 3–4 days only to avoid "rebound congestion"
  4. Oral decongestants for congestion
  5. First-generation antihistamines/decongestant combination for cough
  6. OTC decongestants are used cautiously in diabetes, hypertension, and glaucoma patients
  7. Zinc, Echinacea, vitamin C—may reduce days of illness; begin within first day of symptoms for best results
  8. Frequent hand washing to prevent viral spread
  9. Symptoms lasting longer than 2 weeks or localizing unilaterally may indicate secondary bacterial infection

## INFLUENZA

- Definition—acute, contagious, febrile respiratory and systemic, viral infection

- Etiology/Incidence
  1. Influenza viral types A, B, C
  2. Type A influenza is most virulent, causing increased mortality
  3. Incubation 1–5 days
  4. Infections usually occur during epidemics in winter months
  5. Transmitted by airborne droplets

- Signs and Symptoms
  1. High fever, chills (sudden onset)
  2. Headache
  3. Myalgia (often severe)
  4. Malaise
  5. Sore throat
  6. Nonproductive cough
  7. Nausea and vomiting less common but may occur
  8. Coryza

- Differential Diagnosis
  1. Upper respiratory infection (URI)
  2. Bronchitis
  3. Pertussis
  4. Pneumonia
  5. Infectious mononucleosis

- Physical Findings
    1. Elevated temperature, rapid pulse
    2. Skin flushed
    3. Watery eyes
    4. Clear nasal discharge
    5. Occasional tender cervical lymph nodes
    6. Pharyngeal erythema
    7. Lungs—clear (occasional wheezes or rales)

- Diagnostic Tests/Findings
    1. Usually none
    2. Complete blood count (CBC) or white blood count (WBC)—mild leukopenia, lymphocytosis
    3. Chest radiography—normal
    4. Culture of nasopharyngeal secretions may confirm presence of influenza virus

- Management/Treatment—best treatment is annual influenza vaccination for primary prevention
    1. Supportive measures
        a. Increase fluid intake
        b. Humidified air
        c. Salt water gargles
        d. Analgesics and rest (for fever, headache, and myalgia)
    2. Antiviral medications
        a. Zanamivir 2 inhalations every 12 hours for 5 days
            (1) Effective against influenza types A and B
            (2) Administer within 48 hours of onset of symptoms
            (3) Contraindicated in patients with asthma, chronic obstructive pulmonary disease (COPD)
        b. Oseltamivir 75 mg orally b.i.d. for 5 days
            (1) Effective against uncomplicated cases of influenza types A and B
            (2) For patients 18 years of age and older
            (3) Administer within 48 hours of onset of symptoms
    3. Monitor for complications—especially in elderly adults
        a. Bacterial and viral pneumonia
        b. Otitis media
        c. Reye's syndrome
        d. Myocarditis (rare)
        e. Bronchitis
    4. Prevention
        a. Trivalent inactivated influenza vaccination (TIV) 0.5 cc IM deltoid
            (1) Administer every fall, prior to winter months
            (2) Centers for Disease Control and Protection recommends administration to everyone > 6 months old
            (3) Priority populations
                (a) Over age 65
                (b) Nursing home patients
                (c) Patients with chronic cardiac/respiratory disorders
                (d) Immunocompromised patients (i.e., asplenic persons, HIV infection)
                (e) Persons living in institutional settings
                (f) Pregnant females in second and third trimesters
                (g) Healthcare providers
            (4) Administer concomitantly with pneumococcal vaccine in high-risk patients
        b. Live attenuated influenza vaccine (LAIV)
            (1) Administer—½ dose in each nostril (intranasal route)
            (2) Approved for healthy persons, age 5–49 years
            (3) Contraindications—severe egg allergy, chronic medical and respiratory conditions (asthma, COPD), and immunosuppression
            (4) Expensive compared to injectable inactive influenza vaccine

# PHARYNGITIS

- Definition—inflammation of pharynx, tonsils, or both (sore throat)

- Etiology/Incidence
    1. Viral pharyngitis (most common)
        a. Respiratory viruses—adenovirus
        b. Rhinovirus
        c. Herpangina—due to Coxsackie virus
        d. Epstein-Barr virus (EBV), cytomegalovirus (CMV)—causes infectious mononucleosis
    2. Bacterial pharyngitis
        a. Groups A and B beta hemolytic streptococcus
        b. *Neisseria gonorrhoeae*
        c. *Corynebacterium diphtheriae*
        d. *Haemophilus influenzae*
        e. *Neisseria meningitidis*
    3. Other sources
        a. *Chlamydia trachomatis*
        b. *Mycoplasma pneumoniae*
        c. *Candida albicans*
        d. Trauma/irritating substance
        e. Mouth breathing/allergies
    4. Accounts for 10% of all office visits in primary care
    5. Occurs in all age groups

- Signs and Symptoms
    1. Throat pain
    2. Odynophagia
    3. Enlarged tonsils

4. Fever
5. Malaise

- Differential Diagnosis (see Etiology/Incidence section for pathogens)
  1. Peritonsillar abscess
  2. Pharyngeal abscess
  3. Epiglottitis
  4. Stomatitis
  5. Meningitis
  6. Thyroiditis

- Physical Findings
  1. Elevated temperature
  2. Viral presentation (respiratory)
     a. Tonsillar enlargement with or without exudate
     b. Injected "cobblestone" appearance postpharynx
     c. Rhinorrhea
  3. Bacterial—group A beta hemolytic *Streptococcus* (GAS)
     a. Erythema
     b. Often exudative tonsils
     c. Enlarged tender anterior cervical lymph nodes
     d. Occasionally petechiae
     e. Scarlatina rash

- Diagnostic Tests/Findings
  1. Viral (respiratory) pharyngitis—by clinical diagnosis *only*
  2. Throat culture—if suspect
     a. Group A beta hemolytic *Streptococcus*
     b. *Neisseria gonorrhoeae* (request separately)
  3. Rapid Strep Antigen Test—positive result, detects only GAS (5–10% false negatives)
  4. CBC with differential—WBC count elevated in bacterial infection
  5. Heterophil/monospot—negative

- Management/Treatment
  1. General measures
     a. Increase fluids
     b. Gargle with warm salt water
     c. Lozenges
     d. Acetaminophen or ibuprofen for pain relief
  2. Strep throat (GAS)
     a. Penicillin in the presence of a confirmed strep culture
        (1) Penicillin V 500 mg t.i.d. for 10 days
        (2) Benzathine penicillin 1.2 million units IM one time only
            (a) Advantage—full treatment completed
            (b) Disadvantage—5-fold to 10-fold increase in anaphylactic reaction
     b. Amoxicillin with suspicious clinical findings but negative culture or no culture available
     c. Alternative for penicillin allergy—erythromycin 250 mg orally q.i.d. for 10 days
     d. Post-treatment cultures—for recurrent strep infection or rheumatic fever
     e. Complications—if no or inadequate antibiotic treatment
        (1) Scarlet fever
        (2) Peritonsillar abscess (immediate referral)
        (3) Suppurative adenitis
        (4) Rheumatic fever
        (5) Acute glomerulonephritis
     f. Tonsillectomy—for recurrent severe infections
  3. Gonococcal pharyngitis
     a. Ceftriaxone 125 mg IM single dose *or* cefixime 400 mg orally single dose *or* ofloxacin 400 mg orally single dose
     b. Co-treat for chlamydia—doxycycline 100 mg orally b.i.d. for 7 days *or* erythromycin 500 mg orally q.i.d. for 7 days *or* azithromycin 1 g orally single dose

# INFECTIOUS MONONUCLEOSIS

- Definition—acute viral syndrome associated with fever, pharyngitis, and adenopathy; often known as "kissing" disease

- Etiology/Incidence
  1. Epstein-Barr virus—herpes-type virus causes 90% of cases
  2. Cytomegalovirus—rare
  3. Transmission via saliva
  4. Usually occurs in adolescents and young adults (ages 10–35 years) in middle- and upper-socioeconomic populations
  5. Prolonged period of communicability—approximately 2–6 months after infection

- Signs and Symptoms—variable, but typically include
  1. Fever
  2. Fatigue/malaise
  3. Nausea/anorexia
  4. Swollen lymph nodes
  5. Sore throat

- Differential Diagnosis
  1. Streptococcal pharyngitis
  2. CMV
  3. Toxoplasmosis
  4. Hepatitis A or B
  5. Lymphoma/leukemia
  6. HIV infection

- Physical Findings
    1. Marked erythema and edema of pharynx
    2. Tonsillar enlargement with exudate, occasionally palatal petechiae
    3. Enlarged lymph nodes—especially posterior cervical nodes
    4. Splenic enlargement—50% of cases
    5. Hepatomegaly
    6. Occasionally periorbital edema
    7. Maculopapular rash

- Diagnostic Tests/Findings
    1. Complete blood count with differential
        a. WBC—leukocytosis (range of 10,000–20,000/mm$^3$)
        b. Increased lymphocytes (greater than 50% of leukocyte count)
        c. Atypical lymphocytes—common characteristic
        d. Thrombocytopenia (range 100,000–140,000/mm$^3$) 2–4 weeks after onset of illness
    2. Positive monospot or elevations in heterophil titer—1:224 or greater is diagnostic
    3. Liver function tests—elevations in aspartate aminotransferase (AST), alanine aminotransferase (ALT), bilirubin, and lactic dehydrogenase (LDH)
    4. Throat culture—frequently secondary infection with streptococcus (GAS)
    5. CT scan imaging—may reveal splenomegaly and/or hepatomegaly
    6. EBV—antibody titers
        a. IgG—past infections
        b. IgM—recent infections

- Management/Treatment
    1. Supportive/palliative measures
    2. Rest during acute phase of illness
    3. Avoidance of contact sports for at least 1 month with splenomegaly; CT scan to determine resolution of splenomegaly
    4. Avoid alcohol (ETOH) with elevated liver enzymes/hepatomegaly
    5. Corticosteroids often prescribed for significant pharyngeal edema and obstructive tonsillar enlargement
    6. Analgesics for pain relief
    7. Antiviral medications not effective
    8. Ampicillin/amoxicillin should be avoided, as patients frequently develop a maculopapular rash
    9. Existence of chronic EBV infection (chronic fatigue syndrome) is very controversial

## ALLERGIC RHINITIS

- Definition—a noninfectious symptom complex that includes perennial or seasonal manifestations

- Etiology/Incidence
    1. Seasonal allergies—symptoms at same time each year, related to pollens
        a. Trees (April to July)
        b. Grasses (May to July)
        c. Ragweed (August to October)
    2. Perennial allergies—year-round symptoms related to molds, animal dander, feathers, dust mites, cockroaches
    3. Most common allergens—pollens, molds, dust mites, animal dander
    4. 8–12% of U.S. population affected; onset usually before age 30

- Signs and Symptoms
    1. Nasal congestion
    2. Sneezing
    3. Clear, watery nasal discharge
    4. Itchy nose, throat, eyes
    5. Cough from postnasal drip
    6. Mouth breather/snoring
    7. Loss/alteration of smell

- Differential Diagnosis
    1. Vasomotor rhinitis
    2. Foreign body
    3. Nasal polyps/tumor
    4. Sinusitis
    5. Medications—especially overuse of topical decongestants ("rebound"); oral contraceptives
    6. Deviated septum
    7. Hypothyroidism and pregnancy cause nasal congestion

- Physical Findings
    1. Pale, boggy nasal mucosa
    2. Enlarged turbinates
    3. Injected conjunctiva, tearing
    4. "Allergic shiner" under eyes
    5. No sinus tenderness

- Diagnostic Tests/Findings
    1. Typically a clinical diagnosis
    2. Nasal smear for eosinophils—elevated
    3. Serum IgE—elevated in 30–40% of patients
    4. Allergy testing—identify specific allergens

- Management/Treatment
    1. Preventive measures
        a. Allergen avoidance
        b. Air conditioning/air filters
        c. Environmental control—vacuum, dust, remove carpeting, feather pillows, stuffed animals
        d. Minimize contact with animals
        e. Avoid outside activities early in the morning or early in the evening

2. Pharmacological
   a. Antihistamines—mainstay of treatment for acute symptom relief
      (1) Both sedating and nonsedating available OTC and by prescription
         (a) Fexofenadine
         (b) Desloratadine
         (c) Cetirizine
         (d) Diphenhydramine
         (e) Also available in ophthalmic and otic forms
   b. Decongestants (oral or topical)—vasoconstriction; decrease mucosal edema
   c. Topical corticosteroids—mainstay of chronic control; up to 2 weeks before significant improvement occurs
      (1) Beclomethasone dipropionate—2 sprays each nostril b.i.d.
      (2) Flunisolide—2 sprays each nostril b.i.d.
   d. Leukotriene modifiers
   e. Omalizumab for serious refractory cases; required documented treatment failure to typical therapies, eosinophilia, and elevated IgE—prescribed by allergist
   f. Immunotherapy desensitization for management failures; patients receiving desensitization must know signs/symptoms of anaphylaxis

# SINUSITIS

- Definition—inflammation of one or more paranasal sinuses

- Etiology/Incidence
  1. Bacterial infections
     a. *Streptococcus pneumoniae*
     b. *Haemophilus influenzae*
     c. *Moraxella catarrhalis*
  2. Preceding sinus inflammation often a factor
     a. Viruses—majority of cases are either viral in origin or postviral URI inflammation
     b. Allergies
  3. Anatomical predisposition to bacterial collection—deviated septum
  4. Classified as acute or chronic based on duration of infection
  5. Maxillary sinuses most common site of infection, followed by ethmoid, sphenoid, and, last, frontal involvement

- Signs and Symptoms
  1. Nasal congestion and pressure
  2. Mucopurulent nasal discharge/postnasal drip
  3. Cough more prevalent in the a.m. because of increased posterior sinus drainage when supine
  4. Malaise and fever
  5. Headache
  6. Vertigo
  7. Pain—dull to throbbing
     a. Over cheeks, worse with bending (maxillary sinus)
     b. Above and behind eye—ethmoid sinus
     c. Above eyebrows—frontal sinus
  8. Periorbital edema

- Differential Diagnosis
  1. Rhinitis—viral or allergic
  2. Dental abscess
  3. Nasal polyp/tumor
  4. URI
  5. Migraine/cluster headache

- Physical Findings
  1. Mild to moderate elevated temperature
  2. May have purulent discharge in nasal cavity
  3. Percussion/palpation over frontal and maxillary sinuses—may exacerbate pain/tenderness
  4. Transillumination of sinuses—may show impaired light transmission
  5. Percussion of maxillary teeth—may reveal dental root infection

- Diagnostic Tests/Findings
  1. None for typical presentation
  2. Maxillofacial CT scan when diagnosis is in question or patient unresponsive to treatment—will demonstrate opacity, air fluid levels, thick mucosa
  3. Nasal culture—sinus fluid to determine actual organisms
  4. CBC with differential, if patient appears toxic—elevated WBC

- Management/Treatment
  1. Antibiotics
     a. Amoxicillin/clavulanate 500–875 mg b.i.d. for 10 days
     b. Several cephalosporin options for 14 days
     c. Alternative for PCN allergy
        (1) Macrolides—clarithromycin
        (2) Trimethoprim/sulfamethoxazole—1 double strength tablet b.i.d. for 14 days (PCN alternative)
     d. Respiratory fluoroquinolones for moderate/severe cases or those unresponsive to above therapies
  2. General measures
     a. Increase fluids
     b. Steam inhalation
     c. Avoid smoking
     d. Analgesics for pain relief
     e. Nasal decongestant—improves sinus drainage

3. Topical steroids—reduce mucosal inflammation
4. Refer to ENT if no improvement after 72 hours of appropriate treatment and maxillofacial CT scan supports diagnosis
5. Instruct patient to report symptoms of complications
   a. Stiff neck (meningitis)
   b. Periorbital edema (orbital cellulitis)
   c. Severe dental pain (abscess)

**Special Considerations in the Hospitalized Patient**

- Complications of Sinusitis
  - Orbital cellulitis
    - May follow untreated or inadequately treated sinusitis
    - More common in patients at risk for immunocompromise
    - Typically, the recent history includes treatment for or symptoms of sinusitis, but other causes include hematogenous spread of systemic infection or direct trauma
    - Presenting signs and symptoms of orbital cellulitis include:
      - Fever
      - Periorbital erythema and edema
      - Purulent discharge from the eye
      - Pain with eye movement
      - Orbital pain to palpation
      - Purulent nasal discharge
    - Diagnostic evaluation should include
      - Markers of systemic infection, e.g., CBC with differential, blood cultures
      - Culture of purulent drainage
      - High-resolution contrast CT to rule out brain abscess formation
    - Management
      - In-patient management includes general measures for infection—fluid replacement, antibiotic therapy to cover likely organisms
        - If extension of sinusitis is suspected in the immunocompetent patient, cover strep, *Haemophilus*, and *Moraxella*; immunocompromised patients should be covered for Gram negative infection to include *Pseudomonas*
      - Ear, nose, and throat (ENT) consultation
      - Surgical consultation if poor response to antibiotic therapy after 72 hours
      - Neurosurgical consultation if brain abscesses on imaging
  - Cavernous sinus thrombosis
    - *Staphylococcus aureus* accounts for 70% of cases
    - Very uncommon in patients properly treated for sinusitis with antibiotic therapy
    - May follow any infection of the sinus or midface; approximately 25% of cases involve a facial furuncle that has been manipulated
    - Presenting signs and symptoms (due to venous obstruction)
      - Headache often earliest symptom; sharp, progressive, and localized to the branches of the trigeminal nerve
      - Orbital pain and fullness
      - Periorbital edema
      - Visual disturbances
      - Lateral gaze palsy
      - Ptosis
      - Cranial nerve 3 dysfunction
      - Sluggish pupil response
      - Spread to the contralateral eye via intercavernous sinuses within 48 hours is pathognomonic
      - At end stage, rapid mental status changes, coma, death
    - Diagnostic evaluation
      - Laboratory studies not particularly helpful; D-dimer may be elevated
      - MRI with MR venogram is the preferred imaging study—will show the absence of venous flow to affected area
    - Management
      - Aggressive broad spectrum antibiotics to include coverage for (but not limited to) *Staphylococcus aureus*
      - Consider anticoagulation—no clear literature to support the practice universally but should be considered
      - Systemic corticosteroids as an adjunct to reduce inflammation
      - Consider infectious disease consult for appropriate antibiotic therapy
      - Consider surgical consult for sinus drainage

# QUESTIONS

**Select the best answer.**

1. The common cold is caused by:
   a. *Haemophilus influenzae*
   b. Rhinoviruses
   c. *Streptococcus*
   d. Herpes virus

2. Nasal congestion is a characteristic of upper respiratory infection (URI). It is best treated with:
   a. Antihistamines
   b. Nasal corticosteroids
   c. Topical decongestants
   d. Antibiotics

3. Prevention of influenza epidemics is best achieved by administration of annual "flu" vaccine. Contraindications to administering the vaccine include:
   a. Immunosuppressed patients
   b. History of anaphylaxis to vaccine
   c. Chronic respiratory disease
   d. Allergy to aspirin products

4. Zanamivir and osteltamivir are used in the treatment of influenza. Which of the following statements is true about these drugs?
   a. They are preferred to influenza vaccination in persons with penicillin allergy
   b. Both agents are effective against types A and B influenza
   c. Both agents are contraindicated in COPD
   d. They are contraindicated for those younger than the age of 5 and older than the age of 49

5. Group A beta hemolytic strep (GAS) is a common pathogen in bacterial pharyngitis. It is also an infectious agent in which of the following medical conditions?
   a. Acute pyelonephritis
   b. Rheumatic fever
   c. Viral meningitis
   d. Acute mononucleosis

6. What is the most common physical finding associated with strep pharyngitis?
   a. Unilateral tonsillar edema
   b. Exudative tonsils
   c. Ulcerations on buccal mucosa
   d. Injected uvula

7. Infectious mononucleosis is caused by:
   a. Coxsackie virus
   b. Herpes simplex
   c. Viral hepatitis A
   d. Epstein-Barr virus

8. Earl Thomas, an 18-year-old college student, presents with fever of 101°F, sore throat, dysphagia, and fatigue. Physical exam reveals periorbital edema, exudative tonsils, enlarged tender posterior cervical nodes, and no hepatosplenomegaly. Your preliminary diagnosis is infectious mononucleosis. What diagnostic tests would you order to confirm your diagnosis?
   a. Throat culture
   b. Heterophile antibody
   c. Electrolytes
   d. CMV titer

9. A 40-year-old male accountant presents with a 3-day history of left eye irritation. On physical examination, there is moderate conjunctival injection, watery discharge, palpable preauricular lymph nodes, and visual acuity, 20/20 both eyes. What is the most likely diagnosis?
   a. Acute glaucoma
   b. Bacterial conjunctivitis
   c. Blepharitis
   d. Viral conjunctivitis

10. In the history of a patient presenting with red eye, it is important to ask about:
    a. Photophobia
    b. Itchiness
    c. Cold symptoms
    d. Myopia

11. What are the two most important tests in assessment of a corneal abrasion?
    a. Pupillary reaction and extraocular movements
    b. Funduscopic exam and peripheral vision
    c. Visual acuity and fluorescein stain
    d. Cover/uncover test and accommodation

12. Miss Shell presents with sinus pain, pressure, and yellow nasal discharge. Your examination of this patient would include palpation and transillumination of the:
    a. Ethmoid and frontal sinuses
    b. Maxillary and sphenoid sinuses
    c. Frontal and maxillary sinuses
    d. Sphenoid and ethmoid sinuses

13. Which of the following conditions may predispose a patient to sinusitis?

    a. Tumor, gingivitis, deviated septum
    b. Nasal polyps, allergies, upper respiratory infection
    c. Temporomandibular joint syndrome, rhinitis, otitis
    d. Common cold, pharyngitis, meningitis

14. Ototoxic drugs are a potential cause of sensorineural hearing loss. Which of the following drugs may cause hearing loss?

    a. Gentamicin
    b. Penicillin
    c. Cephalexin
    d. Minocycline

15. A 60-year-old male suddenly develops headache, blurred vision, and severe eye pain upon entering a dark movie theater. What is the most likely diagnosis?

    a. Angle closure glaucoma
    b. Uveitis
    c. Giant cell arteritis
    d. Open angle glaucoma

16. Absent red reflex may indicate which of the following ophthalmological conditions:

    a. Foreign body
    b. Cataracts
    c. Glaucoma
    d. Uveitis

17. Presbycusis—hearing impairment associated with aging—is characterized by:

    a. Acoustic nerve damage
    b. Cerumen impaction
    c. High-frequency loss
    d. Conductive loss

18. Macular degeneration is manifested by:

    a. Loss of peripheral vision
    b. Irregular pupils
    c. Loss of central vision
    d. Excessive tearing

19. Which condition is most likely associated with conductive hearing loss?

    a. Syphilis
    b. Meniere's disease
    c. Acute otitis media
    d. Hypothyroidism

20. A physical characteristic that differentiates otitis externa from otitis media is:

    a. Hearing loss
    b. Pain with movement of pinna
    c. Excessive cerumen
    d. Enlarged submaxillary node

21. What is the most common pathogen of acute otitis media in adults?

    a. *Pseudomonas aeruginosa*
    b. *Streptococcus pneumoniae*
    c. *Mycoplasma pneumoniae*
    d. *Escherichia coli*

22. A 30-year-old housewife presents with long-standing nasal stuffiness, clear watery nasal discharge, and annoying sneezing. What is the most likely diagnosis?

    a. Chronic sinusitis
    b. Nasal polyps
    c. Common cold
    d. Allergic rhinitis

23. Microscopic examination of nasal secretions of a patient with allergic rhinitis may reveal:

    a. Lymphocytes
    b. Neutrophils
    c. Eosinophils
    d. Basophils

24. What is the primary treatment for allergic rhinitis?

    a. Allergy avoidance and antihistamines
    b. Systemic steroids and decongestants
    c. Topical nasal sprays and antibiotics
    d. Humidified air and cough suppressants

25. What is the most common cause of vertigo?

    a. Malignant neoplasm
    b. Otoliths
    c. Vascular disease of the cerebellum
    d. Benign positional vertigo

26. Topical steroids are contraindicated in patients with corneal abrasions because:

    a. They inhibit tearing
    b. They increase risk of bacterial infection
    c. They increase intraocular pressure
    d. They may lead to iritis

27. Which of the following is not a cause of epistaxis?

    a. Hypertension
    b. Diabetes mellitus
    c. Neoplasms
    d. Trauma

28. A special diagnostic test/procedure for vertigo is:

    a. Tonometry
    b. Barany maneuver
    c. Pneumatic otoscopy
    d. EEG

29. Mr. Jones, a 32-year-old salesman, presents with a complaint of frequent nosebleeds for the last 2 months. He states they occur spontaneously 3 times a week and usually stop within 10 minutes. He denies any other acute or chronic medical problems. Which of the following diagnostic tests is indicated at this time?

    a. CBC
    b. Hemoglobin electrophoresis
    c. Prothrombin time
    d. Clotting time

30. Upon further evaluation of Mr. Jones, you find he has nasal congestion, postnasal drip, and a scratchy throat. He uses an antihistamine at night for nasal symptoms and sleep. Your initial treatment plan for Mr. Jones should be:

    a. Add a decongestant to alleviate nasal congestion
    b. Increase humidity to moisten nasal mucosa
    c. Have patient elevate head of bed to promote sleep
    d. Discontinue antihistamine because of drying effect on nasal mucosa

31. Kyle Smith, a 21-year-old law student, presents with fatigue for 3–4 months, low-grade fever, and intermittent sore throat. You order a complete blood count. The result of the CBC is as follows: Hgb and Hct normal, elevated WBC, and atypical lymphocytes. What is the most likely diagnosis?

    a. Hepatitis A
    b. Infectious mononucleosis
    c. Herpangina
    d. Toxoplasmosis

32. Which of the following is not a common cause of vertigo?

    a. Otoliths
    b. Viral labyrinthitis
    c. Meniere's disease
    d. Transient ischemic attack

33. What is the antibiotic of choice in the treatment of gonococcal pharyngitis?

    a. Erythromycin
    b. Ampicillin
    c. Ceftriaxone
    d. Amantadine

34. Hearing loss caused by cerumen impaction is a:

    a. Conductive loss
    b. Sensorineural loss
    c. "Mixed" loss
    d. Congenital loss

35. Zeke Gilbert, a 72-year-old retired factory worker, has hearing loss in his right ear due to excessive noise exposure. When performing a Weber test, you would expect to find:

    a. Sound lateralizes equally to both ears
    b. Sound lateralizes to the left ear
    c. Sound lateralizes to the right ear
    d. Sound lateralizes to neither ear

36. What is the most sensitive test for diagnosing sinusitis?

    a. CBC
    b. Nasal culture
    c. CT scan
    d. Sinus radiography

37. What is the most common cause of otitis externa?

    a. Fungus
    b. *Staphylococcal epidermidis*
    c. Alpha streptococcus
    d. *Pseudomonas aeruginosa*

38. A physical finding that differentiates conjunctivitis from glaucoma is:

    a. Injected conjunctiva
    b. Excessive tearing
    c. Clear cornea
    d. Nystagmus

39. When prescribing topical corticosteroids for patients with allergic rhinitis, it is important to discuss that:

    a. Topical steroid use may predispose to infections
    b. It may take up to 2 weeks before they experience significant reduction in symptoms
    c. Steroids must be taken with antihistamines to be effective
    d. After 48 hours of use, patients will experience reduction in symptoms

40. It is important to highlight the short-term use of topical nasal decongestants because of this adverse effect:

   a. Rhinorrhea
   b. Confusion
   c. Somnolence
   d. Rebound congestion

### ■ Answers

| 1. b  | 21. b |
|-------|-------|
| 2. c  | 22. d |
| 3. b  | 23. c |
| 4. b  | 24. a |
| 5. b  | 25. d |
| 6. b  | 26. b |
| 7. d  | 27. b |
| 8. b  | 28. b |
| 9. d  | 29. a |
| 10. a | 30. d |
| 11. c | 31. b |
| 12. c | 32. d |
| 13. b | 33. c |
| 14. a | 34. a |
| 15. a | 35. b |
| 16. b | 36. c |
| 17. c | 37. d |
| 18. c | 38. c |
| 19. c | 39. b |
| 20. b | 40. d |

## BIBLIOGRAPHY

Andreoli, T. E., Carpenter, C. J., Griggs, R. C., & Ivor, B. (Eds.). (2007). *Cecil essentials of medicine* (7th ed.). Philadelphia, PA: Saunders.

Barker, L. R., Fiebach, N. H., Kern, D. E., Thomas, P. A., & Ziegelstein, R. C. (Eds.). (2006). *Principles of ambulatory medicine* (7th ed.). Baltimore, MD: Lippincott Williams & Wilkins.

Bickley, L. S., & Szilagyi, P. G. (Eds.). (2007). *Bates guide to physical examination and history taking* (9th ed.). Philadelphia, PA: Lippincott.

Centers for Disease Control and Prevention National Immunization Program. (2008). *The pink book: Epidemiology and prevention of vaccine-preventable diseases* (10th ed.). Washington, DC: Author.

Distelhorst, J. S., & Highes, G. M. (2003). Open-angle glaucoma. *American Family Physician, 67*(9), 1937–1944.

Johnson, T. D. (2008). *Control of communicable diseases manual* (19th ed.). Washington, DC: American Public Health Association.

Lustig, L. R., & Schindler, J. (2012). Ear, nose, and throat disorders. In S. J. McPhee, M. A. Papadakis, & M. W. Rabow (Eds.), *Current medical diagnosis and treatment* (51st ed., pp. 196–237). New York, NY: McGraw-Hill.

Riordan-Eva, P. (2009). Disorders of the eye and lids. In S. J. McPhee, M. A. Papadakis, & M. W. Rabow (Eds.), *Current medical diagnosis and treatment* (51st ed., pp. 164–193). New York, NY: McGraw-Hill.

Sinus and Allergy Health Partnership. (2004). Antimicrobial treatment guidelines for acute bacterial rhinosinusitis. *Otolaryngology, Head & Neck Surgery, 130*, 1–45.

Uphold, C. R., & Graham, M. V. (2003). *Clinical guidelines in family practice* (4th ed.). Gainesville, FL: Barmarrae Books.

Weber, P. C. (2010). Evaluation of hearing loss in adults. Retrieved from http://www.uptodate.com/contents/evaluation-of-hearing-loss-in-adults

# Respiratory Disorders

*Margaret Hadro Venzke*

## PULMONARY FUNCTION TESTS

Proper assessment of pulmonary disease requires the use of pulmonary function testing. Pulmonary function tests objectively measure the respiratory system's ability to perform gas exchange via assessment of ventilation, diffusion, and mechanical properties. Understanding these tests is important for correct interpretation of results and accurate patient diagnosis.

- Indications for use of pulmonary function tests (PFTs)
  1. Evaluation of dyspnea, cough, pulmonary dysfunction
  2. Early detection of lung dysfunction
  3. Disability assessment, including evaluation of risk factors in work settings
  4. Evaluation of response to therapy
  5. Reevaluation of progress of restrictive or obstructive disease
  6. Preoperative evaluation
  7. Contribute to diagnostic criteria for asthma and chronic obstructive pulmonary disease (COPD)

- Types of pulmonary function tests
  1. Spirometry—measures airflow rates and forced vital capacity (FVC)
     a. Forced vital capacity (FVC)—volume of air forcefully expelled from lungs after maximal inhalation
     b. Forced expiratory volume ($FEV_1$)—the volume of air expelled in the first second of FVC
     c. Forced expiratory flow 25–75 ($FEF_{25-75}$)—maximal midexpiratory airflow rate
     d. Peak expiratory flow rate (PEFR)—the maximum airflow rate on forceful expulsion after maximum inspiration
     e. Maximum voluntary ventilation (MVV)—maximum volume of gas that can be breathed in 1 minute
  2. Lung volumes
     a. Total lung capacity (TLC)—volume of air in the lungs after maximum inspiration
     b. Functional residual capacity (FRC)—air left in lungs after a normal unforced expiration
     c. Residual volume (RV)—air remaining in lungs after maximum forced expiration
     d. Slow vital capacity (SVC)—volume of gas slowly exhaled after maximal inspiration
     e. Expiratory reserve volume (ERV)—the gas volume difference between the FRC and RV

- General relationship of PFT to pulmonary disease
  1. Obstructive pulmonary disease is characterized by reduced airflow rates; causes include
     a. Asthma
     b. Chronic obstructive pulmonary disease (COPD)
     c. Cystic fibrosis
  2. Restrictive pulmonary disease is associated with reduced lung volumes; examples include
     a. Intrinsic
        (1) Asbestosis
        (2) Pneumonitis

(3) Sarcoidosis
(4) Idiopathic pulmonary fibrosis
(5) Acute respiratory distress syndrome
b. Extrinsic
(1) Neuromuscular disease (e.g., myasthenia gravis)
(2) Anatomical disorders (e.g., kyphosis)
(3) Volume restricting—obesity

## ACUTE BRONCHITIS

- Definition—acute inflammation of trachea, bronchi, and bronchioles

- Etiology/Incidence
  1. Common causes
     a. Viral cause in 90% of cases—usually short course of afebrile illness
        (1) Rhinovirus
        (2) Coronavirus
        (3) Adenovirus
     b. Bacterial infection possible in those with underlying airway disease or unimmunized
        (1) Atypical pathogens, *Mycoplasma pneumoniae, Chlamydia pneumoniae*
        (2) *Bordetella pertussis*
  2. Mucous membranes become hyperemic, edematous with increased bronchial secretions
  3. Frequency and severity increase with cigarette smoking

- Signs and Symptoms
  1. Cough—persistent, deep, and pervasive (hallmark symptom)
     a. Initially dry
     b. Later productive with mucopurulent sputum
  2. Fever (may be absent)
  3. Fatigue, malaise
  4. Chest burning or substernal pain
  5. Headache
  6. Occasional dyspnea
  7. Wheezing
  8. Generally self-limiting illness but may last several weeks or even months—longer in smokers

- Differential Diagnosis
  1. Pneumonia
  2. Asthma
  3. Influenza
  4. Pertussis
  5. Upper respiratory infection (URI)
  6. Allergies
  7. Cystic fibrosis
  8. Tuberculosis
  9. Postinfectious cough

- Physical Findings
  1. Temperature less than 101°F
  2. Chest and lungs—lung consolidation rules out diagnosis
     a. Clear to auscultation
     b. Resonant to percussion
     c. Wheezes
     d. Diffuse bronchi (often clear with coughing)
     e. Occasional crackles

- Diagnostic Tests/Findings
  1. Diagnosis based on clinical presentation
  2. If diagnosis uncertain or symptoms severe
     a. Chest radiograph—may be some pleural thickening but essentially normal in acute bronchitis
     b. Sputum cultures—not helpful in the diagnosis and not indicated
     c. Complete blood count (CBC)/white blood cell (WBC)—normal or slightly elevated
  3. Purified protein derivative (PPD)—clinical suspicion exists for tuberculosis exposure

- Management/Treatment
  1. Antibiotics not indicated unless clinical suspicion for bacterial infection
  2. Palliative measures
     a. Rest
     b. Increase fluid intake to thin secretions
     c. Humidity/steam
     d. Expectorants—not recommended, no demonstrable benefit
     e. First generation antihistamine/decongestant combination for cough
     f. Cough suppressants—dextromethorphan or codeine for patients who cannot tolerate cough without hypoxia or interference with activities of daily living
     g. Decrease environmental irritants
     h. Analgesics for pain/fever
  3. Smoking cessation
  4. Bronchodilator for wheezing/cough
  5. Recovery usually in 7–14 days; postinfectious cough may persist for weeks
  6. Follow-up visit if no improvement or worsening symptoms after 72 hours
  7. Secondary bacterial infections associated with higher fever; treat with antimicrobial therapy to cover atypical pathogens, more likely in patients who smoke cigarettes or have underlying chronic airway disease
     a. Azithromycin 500 mg orally once on first day followed by 250 mg daily for 4 days
     b. Doxycycline 100 mg b.i.d. for 10 days for coverage of *C. pneumoniae, M. pneumoniae* organisms

# PNEUMONIA

- Definition
    1. Acute inflammation of lung parenchyma, including alveoli and interstitial tissues; usually secondary to infection
    2. Categorized as either community acquired or hospital acquired (nosocomial) regardless of causative organism
        a. Hospital acquired occurs > 72 hours after admission
        b. Community acquired encompasses all others occurring as an outpatient or within first 72 hours of hospitalization

- Etiology/Incidence
    1. Community acquired—activation of colonized infection (*Streptococcus pneumoniae*) and inhalation of pathogens (atypical pathogens) most common
    2. Hospital acquired—aspiration of secretions, inhalation of pathogens and/or hematogenous dissemination
    3. Common pathogens in outpatient setting
        a. Bacteria
            (1) *S. pneumoniae* (pneumococcus)—most common
            (2) Atypical pathogens *M. pneumoniae* and *C. pneumoniae* second-most-common cause of bacterial pneumonia in the outpatient setting
            (3) *Haemophilus influenzae*—ranked second to streptococcal pneumonia in hospitalized patients; not as prevalent in outpatient setting
        b. Viruses (4–39% of adult pneumonias, more prevalent in children)
            (1) Influenza
            (2) Parainfluenza
            (3) Adenovirus
            (4) Varicella
    4. Common pathogens in inpatient setting in addition to *S. pneumoniae* and *H. influenzae*
        a. *Staphylococcus aureus*
        b. *Klebsiella pneumoniae*
        c. *Legionella pneumophila*—1–4% of community-acquired pneumonia
        d. *Moraxella catarrhalis*
        e. *Chlamydia pneumoniae*
        f. *M. pneumoniae* (most common in adolescents/young adults)
        g. *Pseudomonas aeruginosa*
        h. *Escherichia coli*
    5. Hospital-acquired pneumonia (nosocomial)—occurs more than 72 hours after hospital admission, more common in patients requiring intensive care and mechanical ventilation
    6. Increasingly common in elderly adults and patients with coexisting illness or disease
    7. Ranked first for cause of death from infectious disease
    8. Sixth leading cause of death in the United States
    9. Biological warfare pathogens such as anthrax, tularemia, plague
    10. Severe acute respiratory syndrome (SARS)—SARS coronavirus (first identified in 2002 in China)

- Signs and Symptoms
    1. Fatigue, malaise
    2. Pleuritic chest pain—worsens with inspiration
    3. Fever
    4. Chills
    5. Dyspnea
    6. Cough
    7. Purulent mucus production—more common in hospital acquired

- Differential Diagnosis
    1. Types of pneumonia (see Etiology/Incidence)
    2. Atelectasis
    3. Pneumothorax
    4. Lung abscess
    5. Congestive heart failure
    6. Neoplasms
    7. Chronic obstructive pulmonary disease (COPD)
    8. Tuberculosis

- Physical Findings
    1. Elevated temperature and pulse
    2. Observe respiratory status, may have
        a. Cyanosis
        b. Nasal flaring/grunting
        c. Tachypnea
    3. Diminished localized breath sounds
    4. Evidence of consolidation
        a. Dullness to percussion
        b. Increased fremitus
        c. Egophony "e to a" changes
        d. Whispered pectoriloquy
        e. Rales
    5. Fine crepitant rales—do not clear with cough

- Diagnostic Tests/Findings
    1. Chest radiograph essential to diagnosis and may show any variety of lower airway consolidation—different pathogens produce different patterns of consolidation, but consolidation in some form is present
    2. CBC with differential—WBC often elevated
        a. WBC differential with left shift (neutrophilia, bandemia)—bacterial origin

b. Differential useful in evaluating severity and prognosis
3. Gram stain and sputum culture—consider that atypical pathogens will not Gram stain; typically not useful unless induced via bronchoscopy
   a. Gram positive—*S. pneumoniae, S. aureus*
   b. Gram negative—*H. influenzae, K. pneumoniae*
4. Serum electrolytes, hepatic enzymes—important in severe cases (when considering hospitalization); hyponatremia
5. Blood cultures—severely ill, toxic patients
6. Thoracentesis if pleural effusion
7. PPD to rule out tuberculosis
8. Serum cold agglutinins—for mycoplasma
9. Pulse oximetry

- Management/Treatment
  1. General measures
     a. Increase fluid intake
     b. Analgesics for fever and headache
     c. Avoid cough suppressants and cigarettes
     d. Humidification
  2. Empiric antimicrobial treatment of community-acquired pneumonia (CAP)
     a. Patients without comorbidity
        (1) A macrolide antibiotic (erythromycin, azithromycin, or clarithromycin) *or*
        (2) Doxycycline
     b. Patients with comorbidity—hospitalized or outpatient
        (1) Beta lactam with macrolide or doxycycline *or*
        (2) Respiratory fluoroquinolone or beta lactam antibiotic + either an advanced-generation macrolide or doxycycline
        (3) Consider the need to cover drug-resistant streptococcus
        (4) Consider the need for hospitalization with CURB-65 criteria
     c. CURB-65 criteria—hospitalize for treatment if patient has at least three of the five criteria:
        (1) **C**onfusion
        (2) **U**remia (BUN > 19 mg/dL)
        (3) **R**espiratory rate > 30 bpm
        (4) **B**lood pressure < 90 mm Hg SBP or 60 mm Hg DB
        (5) **65** years old
     d. Hospitalized patients with community-acquired pneumonia are covered with the same antibiotic regimens as an outpatient with comorbidity
        (1) Patients in the intensive care unit or those who are intubated require coverage of *Pseudomonas aeruginosa*
        (2) Patients with high-risk methicillin-resistant *Staphylococcus aureus* (MRSA) or with a positive culture require coverage with an antistaphylococcal antibiotic
        (3) Hospitalized patients should have supportive oxygen therapy by the least invasive means possible to a $PaO_2$ > 60 mm Hg or $SaO_2$ > 90%
        (4) See supplement Special Considerations in the Hospitalized Patient for more detail on hospital-acquired pneumonias
  3. Prevention
     a. Pneumococcal 23 valent vaccine (Pneumovax) 0.5 cc IM—indicated for patients older than age 65 and those with immunosuppression or chronic disease
     b. Influenza vaccine annually—may administer with Pneumovax at the same time, at different sites
  4. Refer/consult with physician regarding
     a. Seriously ill, toxic patients
     b. Suspected biological warfare pathogens or SARS (infectious disease consult)

# ASTHMA

- Definition—complex disorder characterized by variable and recurring symptoms, airflow obstruction, bronchial hyperresponsiveness, and an underlying inflammation; airflow obstruction is widespread but variable and is reversible with an improvement of $FEV_1$ > 12% with a short-acting bronchodilator

- Etiology/Incidence
  1. Caused by a single or multiple triggers such as
     a. Allergies
        (1) Airborne pollens
        (2) Molds
        (3) House dust
        (4) Animal dander
        (5) Food additives/preservatives
        (6) Feather pillows
     b. Nonallergic factors
        (1) Smoke and other pollutants
        (2) Infections
        (3) Medications—acetylsalicylic acid (ASA), nonsteroidal anti-inflammatory drugs (NSAIDs), beta blockers
        (4) Exercise
        (5) Gastroesophageal reflux
        (6) Emotional factors
        (7) Hormones
        (8) Menses, pregnancy
        (9) Thyroid disease

2. Affects men and women equally, approximately 5% of the U.S. population
3. Chronic airway inflammation with exacerbations characterized by acute hyperresponsiveness

- Signs and Symptoms
  1. Cough—often the only symptom and increased by circumstance that challenges the airway; exercise, heat
  2. Diffuse, bilateral wheezing is common—may be absent in severe exacerbation when air movement is essentially absent
  3. Dyspnea
  4. Chest tightness
  5. Exercise intolerance
  6. URI symptoms
  7. Conditions associated with asthma
     a. Rhinitis
     b. Sinusitis
     c. Nasal polyps
     d. Eczema/atopic dermatitis

- Differential Diagnosis
  1. Heart disease—congestive heart failure
  2. Foreign body aspiration (FOB)
  3. Chronic obstructive pulmonary disease (COPD)
  4. Acute infection—bronchitis/pneumonia
  5. Pulmonary embolism
  6. Cough secondary to beta blockers or angiotensin-converting enzyme (ACE) inhibitors
  7. Gastroesophageal reflux disease
  8. Anaphylaxis due to allergen

- Physical Findings
  1. General appearance—note distress or decreased responsiveness but consider that physical appearance not a reliable indicator of level of obstruction
  2. Nasal flaring
  3. Use of accessory respiratory muscles, retraction
  4. Lungs
     a. Tachypnea
     b. Prolonged expiration
     c. Expiratory wheezing—unilateral wheezing suggests mechanical obstruction
     d. Generalized decreased or distant breath sounds
  5. Red flags—indicate potentially life-threatening severe exacerbation requiring immediate emergency treatment
     a. Pulsus paradoxus—an exaggerated fall in systolic blood pressure during inspiration
     b. Diaphoresis
     c. Inaudible breath sounds
     d. Inability to lie flat
     e. Cyanosis

- Diagnostic Tests/Findings
  1. Diagnosis is made based on a symptom assessment, frequency of bronchodilator use, pulmonary function testing, and number of exacerbations requiring hospitalization in the last year
  2. Pulmonary function tests/spirometry—forced expiratory volume 1 ($FEV_1$) at least < 80% of predicted norm for age, gender, height and reversible by at least 12% with bronchodilator use; degree of decrease correlates with staging of asthma
  3. CBC—eosinophil increase related to allergic response
  4. Chest radiograph—normal
  5. Arterial blood gases (ABG)
     a. Hypoxia in severe cases
     b. Hypocapnia
     c. Normal $pCO_2$ (35–45 mm Hg) indicates very ill patient
     d. Hypercapnia is a medical emergency; a $pCO_2$ > 42 mm Hg is an indication for intubation
  6. Sputum examination—positive for eosinophilia
  7. Nasal secretion—positive for eosinophilia
  8. Allergy testing

- Management/Treatment
  1. The treatment-naïve patient is classified based on the subjective and objective assessment as either intermittent or mild, moderate, or severe persistent asthma
  2. A six-step treatment algorithm is utilized to determine initial management strategies based on classification
     a. Step 1—short-acting beta-adrenergic agonists p.r.n.
     b. Step 2—low-dose daily inhaled corticosteroids (ICS) as preferred treatment; alternatives include mast-cell stabilizers and leukotriene receptor antagonists
     c. Step 3—medium-dose ICS preferred, may add long-acting beta-adrenergic agonists (LABA) to a low-dose ICS
     d. Step 4—medium-dose ICS with LABA; alternatives available
     e. Step 5—high-dose ICS with LABA
     f. Step 6—high-dose ICS with LABA and oral corticosteroid; consider omalizumab
  3. Patients are reassessed after treatment begins and classified as either well controlled, not well controlled, or very poorly controlled based on a quantitative symptom analysis, spirometry, and use of a validated asthma control questionnaire

4. Nonpharmacological interventions
   a. Avoidance of triggers
   b. Environmental management
      (1) Do not open windows before 10:00 a.m.
      (2) Remove carpets from sleeping rooms
      (3) Wash bed linens frequently in very hot water
      (4) Annual influenza vaccination
5. Goals of treatment
   a. Activity without symptoms; sleep through the night
   b. Prevention of chronic troublesome symptoms
   c. Sports and exercise participation
   d. Optimal pharmacotherapy with minimal/no adverse effects
   e. Maintain nearly normal pulmonary function
   f. Meet patient's/family's expectations of, and satisfaction with, asthma care

# CHRONIC OBSTRUCTIVE PULMONARY DISEASE (COPD)

- Definition—a common, preventable, and treatable disease characterized by persistent airflow limitation that is usually progressive and associated with an enhanced chronic inflammatory response in the airways and the lung due to noxious particles or gases. Chronic bronchitis may contribute to development of COPD, and its pathology may be characterized by emphysmatic changes
  1. Emphysema—permanent abnormal distention of the terminal air spaces due to loss of elastic recoil; characterized by destruction of alveolar walls and resultant air trapping
  2. Chronic bronchitis—excessive sputum production with chronic or recurring cough on most days for 3 months or more during 2 consecutive years

- Etiology/Incidence
  1. Exposure to irritants
  2. Heredity—alpha$_1$ protease inhibitor deficiency may cause emphysema; suspect in patients younger than age 35 who have COPD
  3. Risk factors
     a. Lung growth and development
     b. Asthma/bronchial hyperreactivity
     c. Low socioeconomic status
     d. Chronic bronchitis
     e. 10–15% of smokers develop COPD
  4. Affects 5% of the adult population in the United States
  5. Third leading cause of death in the United States
  6. Predominantly seen in those older than age 40
  7. 70-pack year smoking history is the best predictor of airflow obstruction
  8. Affects men more than women, but prevalence in women is rising

- Signs and Symptoms
  1. Key indicators to screen for COPD
     a. Chronic cough
     b. Chronic dyspnea
     c. Chronic sputum
  2. Early in disease patients may be asymptomatic
  3. As disease progresses, cough, dyspnea, and sputum may develop and worsen
  4. In later stages, systemic symptoms of chronic hypoxia will likely occur
  5. Objective symptom assessment by the COPD Assessment Test (CAT) or modified British Medical Research Council (mMRC) scale used to determine pharmacological treatment modality

- Differential Diagnosis
  1. Asthma
  2. Congestive heart failure (CHF)
  3. Tuberculosis (TB)
  4. Acute bronchitis
  5. Chronic sinusitis
  6. Lung cancer

- Physical Findings
  1. Hypertrophied accessory muscles
  2. Increased anteroposterior diameter of the chest wall with increased air trapping
  3. Hyperresonance to percussion
  4. Decreased tactile fremitus

- Diagnostic Tests/Findings
  1. FEV$_1$ to FVC ratio < 70% postbronchodilator therapy is required for diagnosis
  2. Once a diagnosis is established, patients are assigned treatment group A, B, C, or D based on a three-pronged assessment of
     a. Global obstructive lung disease (GOLD) stage
        (1) Stage I—FEV$_1$ > 80% predicted
        (2) Stage II—FEV$_1$ > 50% but < 80% predicted
        (3) Stage III—FEV$_1$ > 30% but < 50% predicted
        (4) Stage IV—FEV$_1$ < 30% predicted or chronic respiratory failure (PaO$_2$ < 60 mm Hg)
     b. Objective symptom assessment (CAT or mMRC score)
     c. Number of exacerbations in the last year
  3. Arterial blood gases
     a. Hypercapnia (PaCO$_2$ > 45 mm Hg)

b. Hypoxemia earlier in chronic bronchitis; present in later stages of both chronic bronchitis and emphysema
4. Increased hematocrit indicative of polycythemia
5. Chest radiograph
   a. Hyperinflation, occasional bullae/blebs
   b. Increased markings and cardiac enlargement
   c. Increased retrosternal airspace
   d. Flattened diaphragm
6. ECG may show right ventricular hypertrophy

- Management/Treatment
  1. Avoid irritants, discontinue smoking—consider pharmacological interventions if necessary
  2. Avoid airway irritants and temperature extremes
  3. Maintain hydration and indoor humidity
  4. Pharmacological therapy according to treatment group A, B, C, or D
     a. Group A—short-acting beta-adrenergic agonist or anticholinergic p.r.n.; if inadequate symptom control, change to daily long-acting option of one or the other
     b. Group B—daily long-acting beta-adrenergic agonist or anticholinergic; if inadequate symptom control, use both daily
     c. Group C—daily inhaled corticosteroid with either a long-acting beta-adrenergic agonist or a long-acting anticholinergic; if inadequate symptom control, discontinue the inhaled corticosteroid and add whichever long-acting bronchodilator is not already in use
     d. Group D—daily long-acting beta-adrenergic agonist and anticholinergic agonist; if inadequate symptom control, change regimen to include a phosphodiesterase (PDE) 4 inhibitor (roflumilast)
  5. All stages of COPD should have annual influenza immunization and a pneumococcal vaccination
  6. Exacerbations of COPD
     a. Are diagnosed subjectively based on a worsening of chronic symptoms
     b. Consider escalation to the next level of chronic pharmacotherapy
     c. Antibiotic therapy appropriate for most patients with COPD exacerbations
     d. If baseline COPD is < 50% predicted, include 5-day course of oral prednisone in the regimen

# TUBERCULOSIS (TB)

- Definition—chronic bacterial infectious disease most commonly infecting the lungs; may occur in lymph nodes, bones, kidneys, and meninges and can disseminate throughout body

- Etiology/Incidence
  1. Mycobacteria of "tuberculosis complex," primarily *Mycobacterium tuberculosis*, a Gram positive, acid-fast bacillus
  2. Usually spread by airborne droplet nuclei
  3. 10–15 million infected in the United States
  4. Incidence of TB is greatest in Asians, Pacific Islanders, American Indians, Alaska Natives, and Hispanics
  5. 90–95% of primary TB infections remain in a latent or dormant stage
  6. High-risk populations include
     a. HIV-infected individuals
     b. Close contacts of infected persons
     c. Low-income populations
     d. Alcoholics and IV drug abusers
     e. Elderly adults
     f. Immigrants from Asia and Central/South America
     g. Persons in correctional institutions and in long-term care facilities
     h. Individuals with chronic disease

- Signs and Symptoms (90% asymptomatic at the time of primary infection)
  1. Fatigue
  2. Anorexia, weight loss
  3. Fever
  4. Night sweats
  5. Productive cough with purulent sputum
  6. Hemoptysis
  7. Pleuritic chest pain

- Differential Diagnosis
  1. Pneumonia
  2. Malignancy
  3. Pleurisy
  4. Histoplasmosis
  5. Silicosis
  6. COPD

- Physical Findings
  1. Typically none early in disease
  2. Later may appear chronically ill, weak, and cachectic
  3. Lungs
     a. Auscultation—apical rales, often a positive whispered pectoriloquy
     b. Palpation—increased tactile fremitus over consolidated areas
     c. Percussion—dull

- Diagnostic Tests/Findings
  1. PPD
     a. Positive with active disease or prior exposure
     b. History of Bacillus Calmette-Guérin (BCG) vaccine does not affect interpretation of PPD

c. Patients with AIDS and other mechanisms of immunosuppression may have diminished reactivity
2. PPD interpretation (record induration, not erythema)
    a. A reaction of 5 mm is considered positive in patients with
        (1) Recent close contact with infected person
        (2) Evidence of inactive disease
        (3) HIV infection
    b. A reaction of 10 mm is considered positive in the following patients:
        (1) Those with diabetes mellitus, cancer, or end-stage renal disease
        (2) Immigrants from Asia, Africa, Latin America
        (3) Medically underserved, low-income populations
        (4) High-risk minorities
        (5) Residents of nursing homes and prisons
        (6) Healthcare workers
    c. A reaction of 15 mm is considered positive for all populations
    d. False-negative result
        (1) PPD administered after live virus vaccine (e.g., postponed for 4–6 weeks following measles vaccination)
        (2) Immunosuppressed
        (3) Elderly
    e. False-positive result—nontuberculosis mycobacterium
3. QuantiFERON-TB Gold
    a. May be used in all circumstances in which PPD screening currently indicated
    b. Requires venipuncture and processing within 12 hours
    c. Results not subject to reader bias
    d. Not affected by BCG vaccine
4. Sputum for acid-fast bacilli (AFB) provides presumptive diagnosis and is an indication to begin treatment; is not definitive diagnosis
5. Sputum culture
    a. Essential to confirm diagnosis of TB—three specimens advised
    b. Takes 3–6 weeks for results to be obtained
6. Gastric aspirate culture
    a. Alternative to bronchoscopy
    b. Use for culture only—not stained smear

- Management/Treatment
    1. Prevention
        a. Bacillus Calmette-Guérin (BCG) vaccine intended for prophylaxis of noninfected persons; not routinely used in the United States
        b. Positive PPD converter or QuantiFERON—prescribe isoniazid 300 mg orally and vitamin $B_6$ 50 mg orally every day for 9 months
    2. Pharmacotherapy—consult/refer to physician or health department for management
        a. Medication options include (for sensitive organisms)
            (1) Isoniazid daily 5 mg/kg up to 300 mg per day for 2 months, together with
            (2) Rifampin daily 10 mg/kg up to 600 mg per day for 2 months
            (3) Pyrazinamide 15–30 mg/kg up to 2 g per day for 2 months
        b. Order baseline liver function tests prior to initiating antituberculosis medications
        c. Perform baseline color vision (red-green) test prior to ethambutol therapy and an audiology examination prior to streptomycin treatment
    3. Follow up on contacts of persons with active disease
    4. Reportable disease—report to state and local health departments
    5. After therapy completion, follow up in 1 year; monitor for recurrence
    6. Stress importance of compliance; Directly Observed Therapy (DOT)—one method of ensuring adherence
    7. Review symptoms of drug side effects and toxicity
        a. Isoniazid
            (1) Peripheral neuropathy (prevent with daily pyridoxine)
            (2) Hepatitis
            (3) Hypersensitivity
        b. Rifampin
            (1) Orange discoloration of secretions and urine
            (2) Permanent orange stain to contact lenses
            (3) Nausea
            (4) Vomiting
        c. Pyrazinamide
            (1) Hepatotoxicity
            (2) Hyperuricemia
        d. Ethambutol
            (1) Fever
            (2) Rash
            (3) Optic neuritis
        e. Streptomycin—ototoxicity
    8. Stress importance of nutritious diet and education regarding selection of food

# LUNG CANCER

- Definition—primary malignant neoplasm of the lung; cell types involved include squamous cell, adenocarcinoma, large cell carcinoma, and small cell carcinoma

- Etiology/Incidence
    1. Cigarette smoking accounts for 95% of lung cancer in men and 85% of lung cancer in women
    2. Cigarette smoke in combination with other environmental pollutants (e.g., asbestos) associated with increased incidence
    3. Most common in 50- to 70-year-olds
    4. Occurs in males more frequently than in females
    5. Leading cause of cancer death in men and women in the United States

- Signs and Symptoms—depend on the area of tumor location and involvement of nodes or other organs; only 10–25% of patients are asymptomatic at time of diagnosis; symptoms occur with advanced disease
    1. "Smoker's cough"—most common early symptom
    2. Anorexia/weight loss
    3. Dyspnea—related to obstruction of major bronchus
    4. Hemoptysis—20% of all patients with hemoptysis have lung cancer
    5. Wheezing
    6. Fever
    7. Chest pain—related to extension beyond parenchyma
    8. Fatigue
    9. Hoarseness
    10. Bone pain
    11. Neurological deficits

- Differential Diagnosis
    1. Pneumonia
    2. Lung abscess
    3. Bronchitis
    4. Tuberculosis

- Physical Findings
    1. Examination may not reveal significant changes
    2. Tumor obstructing bronchus—may cause atelectasis or unilateral wheeze
    3. Visible or palpable supraclavicular lymph nodes
    4. Hepatomegaly

- Diagnostic Tests/Findings
    1. Chest radiograph
        a. Negative in 15% of patients with lung cancer
        b. Not diagnostic in itself, but indicates need for additional workup
        c. Manifestations—hilar or enlarging mass, infiltrate, atelectasis, cavitation, or pleural effusion
    2. Laboratory
        a. CBC
        b. Liver function tests
        c. Serum electrolytes and calcium
    3. Definitive diagnosis requires cytologic or histologic evidence
    4. Sputum for cytology—positive in 40–60% of patients
    5. Bronchoscopy with biopsy
    6. MRI/CT scan

- Management/Treatment
    1. Surgery—25% of patients with lung cancer are candidates for surgery
    2. Chemotherapy
    3. Radiation therapy—generally palliative
    4. Refer to physician when lung cancer suspected
    5. Encourage patient to stop smoking
    6. Decrease exposure to pollutants
    7. Realistic assessment for patient and family of prognosis, pros and cons of therapy—essential to patient's decision for treatment
    8. Discuss side effects of chemotherapy/radiation
    9. Encourage nutritious diet
    10. Effective pain control
    11. Hospice care

### Special Considerations in the Hospitalized Patient

- Management of asthma exacerbation—all patients with asthma should be given an asthma action plan at the time of diagnosis; this includes instruction to assess peak expiratory flow rate (PEFR) during an exacerbation and seek urgent or emergency care if < 70% of personal best
  - If patient presents with a PEFR of < 70% personal best
    - Order albuterol nebulizer treatments alternating with ipratroprium bromide nebulizer treatments
    - If after 1 hour of care the patient's PEFR remains < 70%, admit for inpatient management
    - If PEFR < 40% or $PaCO_2$ > 42 mm Hg, admit to intensive care and consider intubation
    - All patients who require hospital admission should have oxygen therapy to an $SaO_2$ of 90%
    - All patients who require hospital admission should have a systemic corticosteroid regimen initiated
    - Those who require ICU admission require hourly short-acting bronchodilator treatments
    - See attached algorithms per EPR-3:
      - **Table 6-1**: Formal Evaluation of Asthma Exacerbation Severity in the Urgent or Emergency Care Setting
      - **Figure 6-1**: Management of Asthma Exacerbations: Emergency Department and Hospital-Based Care
- *Hospital-acquired pneumonia* (HAP) is a collective term that includes healthcare-associated pneumonia (HCAP) and ventilator-associated pneumonia (VAP). HAP is often due to multi-drug-resistant (MDR) bacteria such as *Pseudomonas aeruginosa*, *Staphylococcus aureus*, and *Acinetobacter* species; goals of evidence-based guidelines include prevention by identifying risk factors, implementing preventive strategies, and selecting appropriate antibiotics in appropriate doses while avoiding excessive use
  - Risk factors for HAP, HCAP, and VAP include
    - Antibiotic therapy in the preceding 90 days
    - Current hospitalization of > 5 days
    - High frequency of antibiotic resistance in the community or hospital unit
    - Residence in a nursing home or extended care facility
    - Home infusion therapy
    - Chronic dialysis in the last 30 days
    - Home wound care
    - Immunosuppressive disease or therapy
    - Nasogastric tube
    - Prolonged invasive mechanical ventilation
  - Key points in diagnostic testing
    - Lower respiratory tract cultures
    - Chest radiography, PA and lateral when possible
    - Arterial blood gases
    - All patients with suspected VAP should have blood cultures
    - Diagnostic thoracentesis in all patients with large effusions and any effusion in which the patient appears toxic
  - Antibiotic selection
    - Late onset (> 5 days since admission) or high risk for MDR pathogens, broad spectrum therapy to target MDR is appropriate
    - HCAP with < 5 days or not high risk for MDR, limited spectrum is appropriate
    - Beta lactam antibiotics and respiratory fluoroquinolones are mainstays of therapy—specific agents, doses, and durations depend on spectrum of activity and patient risk
    - Inappropriate therapy is a major risk factor for extended morbidity and mortality—treatment in accordance with American Thoracic Society (ATS)/Infectious Diseases Society of America (IDSA) guidelines minimizes risk

### TABLE 6-1  Formal Evaluation of Asthma Exacerbation Severity in the Urgent or Emergency Care Setting

|  | Mild | Moderate | Severe | Subset: Respiratory Arrest Imminent |
|---|---|---|---|---|
| **Symptoms** | | | | |
| Breathlessness | While walking<br><br>Can lie down | While at rest (infant—softer, shorter cry, difficulty feeding)<br>Prefers sitting | While at rest (infant—stops feeding)<br>Sits upright | |
| Talks in | Sentences | Phrases | Words | |
| Alertness | May be agitated | Usually agitated | Usually agitated | Drowsy or confused |
| **Signs** | | | | |
| Respiratory rate | Increased | Increased | Often > 30/minute | |
| | | Guide to rates of breathing in awake children: | | |
| | | *Age* — *Normal rate* | | |
| | | < 2 months — < 60/minute | | |
| | | 2–12 months — < 50/minute | | |
| | | 1–5 years — < 40/minute | | |
| | | 6–8 years — < 30/minute | | |
| Use of accessory muscles; suprasternal retractions | Usually not necessary | Commonly | Usually | Paradoxical thoracoabdominal movement |
| Wheeze | Moderate, often only and expiratory | Loud: throughout exhalation | Usually loud; throughout inhalation and exhalation | Absence of wheeze |
| Pulse/minute | < 100 | 100–120 | > 120 | Bradycardia |
| | | Guide to normal pulse rates in children: | | |
| | | *Age* — *Normal rate* | | |
| | | 2–12 months — < 160/minute | | |
| | | 1–2 years — < 120/minute | | |
| | | 2–8 years — < 110/minute | | |
| Pulsus paradoxus | Absent < 10mm Hg | May be present 10–25 mm Hg | Often present > 25 mm Hg (adult)<br>20–40 mm Hg (child) | Absence suggests respiratory muscle fatigue |
| **Functional Assessment** | | | | |
| PEF | ≥ 70 percent | Approx. 40–69 percent or response lasts < 2 hours | < 40 percent | < 25 percent Note: PEF testing may not be needed in very severe attacks |
| $PaO_2$ (on air) | Normally (test not usually necessary) | ≥ 60 mm Hg (test not usually necessary) | < 60 mm Hg: possible cyanosis | |
| and/or $PCO_2$ | < 42 mm Hg (test not usually necessary) | < 42 mm Hg (test not usually necessary) | ≥ 42 mm Hg: possible respiratory failure | |
| $SaO_2$ percent (on air) at sea level | > 95 percent (test not usually necessary) Hypercapnia (hypoventilation) develops more readily in young children than in adults and adolescents. | 90–95 percent (test not usually necessary) | < 90 percent | |

Key: $PaO_2$, arterial oxygen pressure; $PCO_2$, partial pressure of carbon dioxide; PEF, peak expiratory flow; $SaO_2$, oxygen saturation

**Notes:** The presence of several parameters, but not necessarily all, indicates the general classification of the exacerbation. Many of these parameters have not been systematically studied, especially as they correlate with each other. Thus, they serve only as general guides (Cham et al., 2002; Chey et al., 1999; Gorelick et al., 2004b; Karras et al., 2000; Kelly et al., 2002b and 2004; Keogh et al., 2001; McCarren et al., 2000; Rodrigo and Rodrigo, 1998b; Rodrigo et al., 2004; Smith et al., 2002). The emotional impact of asthma symptoms on the patient and family is variable but must be recognized and addressed and can affect approaches to treatment and follow-up (Ritz et al., 2000; Strunk and Mrazek, 1986; von Leupoldt and Dahme, 2005).

*Source:* Reproduced from National Heart, Lung, and Blood Institute, Expert Panel Report 3 (EPR3): Guidelines for the Diagnosis and Management of Asthma. http://www.nhlbi.nih.gov/guidelines/asthma/asthgdln.htm

**FIGURE 6-1** Management of Asthma Exacerbations: Emergency Department and Hospital-Based Care

**Initial Assessment**
Brief history, physical examination (auscultation, use of accessory muscles, heart rate, respiratory rate), PEF or FEV$_1$, oxygen saturation, and other tests as indicated.

**FEV$_1$ or PEF ≥ 40% (Mild-to-Moderate)**
- Oxygen to achieve SaO$_2$ ≥ 90%
- Inhaled SABA by nebulizer or MDI with valved holding chamber, up to 3 doses in first hour
- Oral systemic corticosteroids if no immediate response or if patient recently took oral systemic corticosteroids

**FEV$_1$ or PEF < 40% (Severe)**
- Oxygen to achieve SaO$_2$ ≥ 90%
- High-dose inhaled SABA plus ipratropium by nebulizer or MDI plus valved holding chamber, every 20 minutes or continuously for 1 hour
- Oral systemic corticosteroids

**Impending or Actual Respiratory Arrest**
- Intubation and mechanical ventilation with 100% oxygen
- Nebulized SABA and ipratropium
- Intravenous corticosteroids
- Consider adjunct therapies

Admit to hospital intensive care (see box below)

**Repeat Assessment**
Symptoms, physical examination, PER, O$_2$ saturation, other tests as needed

**Moderate Exacerbation**
FEV$_1$ or PEF 40–69% predicted/personal best
Physical exam: moderate symptoms
- Inhaled SABA every 60 minutes
- Oral systemic corticosteroid
- Continue treatment 1–3 hours, provided there is improvement; make admit decision in < 4 hours

**Severe Exacerbation**
FEV$_1$ or PEF < 40% predicted/personal best
Physical exam: severe symptoms at rest, accessory muscle use, chest retraction
History: high-risk patient
No improvement after initial treatment
- Oxygen
- Nebulized SABA + ipratropium, hourly or continuous
- Oral systemic corticosteroids
- Consider adjunct therapies

**Good response**
- FEV$_1$ or PEF ≥ 70%
- Response sustained 60 minutes after last treatment
- No distress
- Physical exam: normal

**Incomplete response**
- FEV$_1$ or PEF 40–69%
- Mild-to-moderate symptoms

Individualized decision re: hospitalization (see text)

**Poor response**
- FEV$_1$ or PEF < 40%
- PCO$_2$ ≥ 42 mm Hg
- Physical exam: symptoms severe, drowsiness, confusion

**Discharge Home**
- Continue treatment with inhaled SABA.
- Continue course of oral systemic corticosteroid.
- Consider initiation of an ICS.
- Patient education
  – Review medications, including inhaler technique.
  – Review/initiate action plan.
  – Recommend close medical follow-up.

**Admit to Hospital Ward**
- Oxygen
- Inhaled SABA
- Systemic (oral or intravenous) corticosteroid
- Consider adjunct therapies
- Monitor vital signs, FEV$_1$ or PEF, SaO$_2$

**Admit to Hospital Intensive Care**
- Oxygen
- Inhaled SABA hourly or continuously
- Intravenous corticosteroid
- Consider adjunct therapies
- Possible intubation and mechanical ventilation

Improve

**Discharge Home**
- Continue treatment with inhaled SABAs.
- Continue course of oral systemic corticosteroid.
- Continue on ICS. For those not on long-term control therapy, consider initiation of an ICS.
- Patient education (e.g., review medications, including inhaler technique and, whenever possible, environmental control measures; review/initiate action plan; recommend close medical follow-up).
- Before discharge, schedule follow-up appointment with primary care provider and/or asthma specialist in 1–4 weeks.

Key: FEV$_1$, forced expiratory volume in 1 second; ICS, inhaled corticosteroid; MDI, metered dose inhaler; PCO$_2$, partial pressure carbon dioxide; PEF, peak expiratory flow; SABA, short-acting beta$_2$-agonist; SaO$_2$, oxygen saturation

*Source:* Reproduced from National Heart, Lung, and Blood Institute, Expert Panel Report 3 (EPR3): Guidelines for the Diagnosis and Management of Asthma. http://www.nhlbi.nih.gov/guidelines/asthma/asthgdln.htm

**FIGURE 6-2** VAP Prevention Strategies

Prior to intubation →
1) Address reversible causes of respiratory failure (e.g., fluid balance, bronchospasm, analgesia, sedation)
2) Noninvasive mechanical ventilation

Process of intubation →
1) Avoid gastric overdistention
2) Oroendotracheal route

After intubation (data supported) →
1) Gastric tubes inserted via oral route
2) Head of bed elevated 30–45 degrees
3) Good hand hygiene
4) HME use when appropriate
5) Change respiratory circuit only when necessary and good respiratory care hygiene
6) Closed suctioning system
7) Continuous subglottic suctioning
8) Rotational beds
9) Chlorhexidine oral rinse in cardiac surgery patients
10) Minimize sedation to reduce duration of mechanical ventilation
11) Weaning protocols

After intubation (controversial) →
1) Early vs. late enteral nutrition
2) Selective gut decontamination
3) Rotational antibiotic schema
4) Antibiotic-impregnated endotracheal tubes

*Source:* Reproduced from Clin Microbiol Rev., 2006, Vol. 19(4), p. 637–665, DOI and reproduced with permission from the American Society for Microbiology.

## QUESTIONS

### ■ Select the best answer.

1. Which of the following drugs is contraindicated in patients with severe asthma?

   a. Propranolol
   b. Theophylline
   c. Amoxicillin
   d. Albuterol

2. What is the most common organism causing community-acquired pneumonia?

   a. *Escherichia coli*
   b. *Staphylococcus aureus*
   c. *Streptococcus pneumoniae*
   d. *Klebsiella pneumoniae*

3. Which of the following is a risk factor for COPD?

   a. Tuberculosis
   b. Asthma
   c. Immobility
   d. High socioeconomic status

4. What is the most common side effect of isoniazid?

   a. Idiopathic splenomegaly
   b. Seizures
   c. Gynecomastia
   d. Peripheral neuropathy

5. The mMRC is used to quantify symptoms in which disease?
   a. COPD
   b. Asthma
   c. Tuberculosis
   d. Pneumonia

6. A 25-year-old nurse presents to employee health for her annual physical examination. Her previous PPD, 1 year ago, was negative. A PPD is repeated and results 3 days later show 14 mm of induration. The nurse is asymptomatic and her chest radiograph is normal. The most appropriate management at this time would be:
   a. Repeat chest radiograph yearly
   b. Prescribe isoniazid and vitamin $B_6$ for 9 months
   c. Prescribe ethambutol for 6–12 months
   d. Repeat PPD in 2 months

7. Which of the following statements is true in the treatment of persistent asthma?
   a. Inhaled corticosteroids are the cornerstone of therapy
   b. Beta blockers should be used vigorously
   c. Cromolyn is used during acute attacks
   d. Long-acting beta-adrenergic agonists are contraindicated

8. Which of the following is not part of CURB-65 criteria?
   a. Age
   b. Blood pressure
   c. Cough
   d. Uremia

9. What is the most important measurement of pulmonary function in asthma?
   a. The total lung capacity
   b. The forced vital capacity
   c. The residual volume
   d. The forced expiratory volume ($FEV_1$)

10. What is the most common cause of acute bronchitis?
    a. Pneumococcus
    b. Virus
    c. Varicella
    d. Chlamydia

11. Which of the following represents the best choice of antibiotic for outpatient treatment of pneumonia in a 50-year-old healthy male?
    a. Amoxicillin
    b. Trimethoprim/sulfamethoxazole
    c. Azithromycin
    d. Cephalexin

12. Physical findings in bacterial pneumonia would include:
    a. Hyperresonance to percussion
    b. Rales that clear with cough
    c. Decreased fremitus
    d. Positive egophony

13. Max Murphy is a 55-year-old postal worker who was recently diagnosed with COPD. He is classified as treatment group A. The best choice for initial therapy would be:
    a. A short-acting beta-adrenergic agonist
    b. A long-acting anticholinergic inhaler
    c. Annual influenza vaccination
    d. Pulmonary rehabilitation

14. Pneumococcal vaccine is considered a preventive measure for bacterial pneumonia. For which population(s) is it indicated?
    a. Patients with acute bronchitis
    b. Patients with COPD
    c. Adolescents and young adults
    d. Persons older than age 45

15. Indicators of a severe asthma attack requiring emergency treatment include:
    a. Prolonged expiration
    b. Bilateral rales
    c. Chest tightness
    d. Inaudible breath sounds

16. When ordering a CBC in a person with acute exacerbations of asthma, you would expect to see:
    a. Moderate elevation in WBCs and atypical lymphocytes
    b. Decrease in WBCs and lymphocytosis
    c. Increased hematocrit and increased platelets
    d. Mild elevation in WBCs and eosinophilia

17. Albuterol is an example of:
    a. Antihistamine
    b. Beta-2 adrenergic agonist
    c. Corticosteroid
    d. Antitussive

18. Which of the following is not a risk factor for lung cancer?

a. Radon exposure
b. Passive cigarette smoking
c. Allergen irritant
d. Asbestos exposure

19. What is the leading cause of cancer deaths in the United States?

    a. Gastric cancer
    b. Malignant melanoma
    c. Breast cancer
    d. Lung cancer

20. What is the drug of choice for acute management of asthma exacerbation?

    a. Theophylline
    b. Erythromycin
    c. Cromolyn sodium
    d. Albuterol

21. Pulsus paradoxus is:

    a. Increase in diastolic blood pressure on expiration
    b. Decrease in systolic blood pressure on inspiration
    c. Increase in systolic blood pressure on expiration
    d. Decrease in diastolic blood pressure on inspiration

22. Mary is a 24-year-old female with mild persistent asthma since she was 7. She has been maintained on low-dose inhaled corticosteroids for several years, but an assessment of asthma control reveals that her condition is not well controlled. Which of the following is the next step in her pharmacological management?

    a. A leukotriene receptor antagonist
    b. A medium-dose, inhaled corticosteroid
    c. A long-acting beta-adrenergic agonist
    d. Oral corticosteroids

23. Which of the following groups is *not* at high risk for tuberculosis?

    a. HIV-infected individuals
    b. Asian immigrants
    c. Homeless individuals
    d. College students

24. The serum cold agglutinins test is used to diagnose:

    a. *Haemophilus influenzae* pneumonia
    b. Legionella pneumonia
    c. Rickettsia infection
    d. Mycoplasma pneumonia

25. The problem with diagnosing early stage lung cancer is that:

    a. The CBC lab result is normal
    b. It mimics the symptoms of asthma
    c. Patients are often asymptomatic until late in the disease
    d. Pulmonary function tests are normal

26. Key indicators to screen for COPD include all of the following except:

    a. Cough
    b. Dyspnea
    c. Asthma
    d. Sputum

27. Assessment findings in a patient with COPD would include:

    a. Increased egophony and increased rhonchi
    b. Decreased tactile fremitus and hyperresonance to percussion
    c. Bilateral wheezes and pleuritic chest pain
    d. Fever during exacerbations

28. Diagnostic criteria for COPD must include:

    a. A history of smoking or other irritant exposure
    b. The presence of dyspnea, chronic cough, and sputum
    c. An $FEV_1/FVC$ ratio of 70%
    d. An FVC of < 80% predicted

29. Young Chow, an 18-year-old Chinese exchange student, presents to student health for an immunization update. He states he had BCG vaccine as a young child and therefore will never get tuberculosis. You administer a PPD and the result is positive. Your next best action would be to:

    a. Assume the positive result is due to BCG vaccine; no further evaluation needed
    b. Assume the positive result is related to TB exposure or infection; order a chest radiograph
    c. Begin isoniazid therapy immediately
    d. Repeat PPD test in 1 month to verify results

30. The most common side effect of the antituberculin drug rifampin is:

    a. Hepatotoxicity
    b. Optic neuritis
    c. Fever
    d. Orange discoloration of secretions

## ■ Answers

| | | | |
|---|---|---|---|
| 1. | a | 16. | d |
| 2. | c | 17. | b |
| 3. | b | 18. | c |
| 4. | d | 19. | d |
| 5. | a | 20. | d |
| 6. | b | 21. | b |
| 7. | a | 22. | b |
| 8. | c | 23. | d |
| 9. | d | 24. | d |
| 10. | b | 25. | c |
| 11. | c | 26. | c |
| 12. | d | 27. | b |
| 13. | a | 28. | c |
| 14. | b | 29. | b |
| 15. | d | 30. | d |

## BIBLIOGRAPHY

American Thoracic Society & Infectious Disease Society of America. (2005). Guidelines for the management of adults with hospital-acquired, ventilator-associated, and healthcare-associated pneumonia. *American Journal of Respiratory and Critical Care Medicine, 171*, 388–416.

American Thoracic Society, Centers for Disease Control and Prevention, & Infectious Disease Society of America. (2003). Treatment of tuberculosis. *Morbidity and Mortality Weekly Report, 52*(RR11), 1–77.

Braman, S. (2006). Postinfectious cough: ACCP evidence-based clinical practice guidelines. *Chest, 129* (1 Suppl.), 138S–146S.

Chestnutt, M. S., & Prendergast, T. J. (2012). Pulmonary disorders. In S. J. McPhee & M. A. Papadakis (Eds.), *Current medical diagnosis and treatment* (51st ed.). New York, NY: McGraw-Hill.

Global Initiative for Chronic Obstructive Lung Disease (GOLD). (2014). *Global strategy for the diagnosis, management and prevention of COPD*. Retrieved from http://www.goldcopd.org/guidelines-global-strategy-for-diagnosis-management.html

Hart, A. M. (2007). An evidence-based approach to the diagnosis and management of acute respiratory infections. *Journal for Nurse Practitioners, 3*(9), 607–611.

Mandell, L. A., Wunderink, R. G., Anzueto, A., Bartlett, J. G., Campbell, G. D., Dean, N. C., … Whitney, C. G. (2007). Infectious Diseases Society of America/American Thoracic Society consensus guidelines on the management of community-acquired pneumonia in adults. *Clinical Infectious Diseases, 44*, S27–S72.

National Asthma Education and Prevention Programs. (2007). *Expert Panel Report 3: Guidelines for the Diagnosis and Management of Asthma*. U.S. Department of Health and Human Services Publication No. NIH08-5846. Bethesda, MD: National Institutes of Health, National Heart, Lung, and Blood Institute.

Qassim, A., Wilt, T. J., Weinberger, S. E., Hanania, N. A., Criner, G., van der Molen, T., … Shekelle, P. (2011). Diagnosis and management of stable chronic obstructive pulmonary disease: A clinical practice guideline update from the American College of Physicians, American College of Chest Physicians, American Thoracic Society, and European Respiratory Society. *Annals of Internal Medicine, 155*, 179–191.

U.S. Preventive Services Task Force. (2014). *The Guide to Clinical Preventive Services: Recommendations of the United States Preventive Services Task Force*. Washington, DC: Agency for Healthcare Quality and Research. Retrieved from http://www.uspreventiveservicestaskforce.org/recommendations.htm http://www.ahrq.gov/clinic/pocketgd.pdf

# Cardiovascular Disorders

*Sally K. Miller*

## HYPERTENSION (HTN)

- Definition—the definition of hypertension has morphed over the years from a condition categorized in accordance with a numerical range. However, the most recent report of the Joint National Committee (JNC 8) does not so much emphasize assessment or definition of blood pressure as it does evaluate levels of blood pressure at which the benefits of pharmacological treatment outweigh the risks. The JNC 8, based on expert review of the evidence, recommends treating blood pressure to a goal of < 150/90 mm Hg in persons > 60 years and to a goal of < 140/90 mm Hg in adults < 60 years old as well as all adults of any age with diabetes or chronic kidney disease (James et al., 2013)

- Etiology/Incidence—more than 90% of cases due to unknown etiology—unknown etiology is defined as primary, essential, or idiopathic hypertension; remaining cases are attributable to secondary causes

    1.  | Theories of Etiology of HTN | Etiology of Secondary HTN |
        |---|---|
        | Volume-related | Chronic kidney disease |
        | Renin-mediated | Renal vascular disease |
        | Neurogenic | Hyperaldosteronism |
        |  | Cushing's syndrome |
        |  | Pheochromocytoma |
        |  | Coarctation of the aorta |
        |  | Pregnancy |
        |  | Sleep apnea |
        |  | Thyroid or parathyroid disease |

    2. Incidence
        a. 10–15% of Caucasian adults
        b. 20–30% of black adults
        c. Heredity
        d. Cigarette smoking
        e. Increased salt intake
        f. Obesity
        g. Affects more than 70 million Americans

- Signs and Symptoms
    1. Often no symptoms—known as "silent killer"
    2. Symptoms of underlying cause may present in secondary hypertension
        a. Flushing
        b. Palpitations
        c. Pallor
        d. Tremor
        e. Profuse perspiration
    3. Suboccipital pulsating headache occurring early in morning and improving throughout the day in severe hypertension
    4. Chronic hypertension may result in ventricular hypertrophy and associated symptoms of heart failure
    5. Oliguria, nocturia, or hematuria may be present
    6. Epistaxis in severe hypertension
    7. Severe hypertension may present with signs and symptoms of hypertensive encephalopathy
        a. Nausea and vomiting
        b. Somnolence and confusion
        c. Visual disturbances

- Differential Diagnosis—secondary causes of hypertension must be ruled out
    1. Renal disorders
        a. Medical renal disease
        b. Diabetic nephropathy
        c. Acute tubular necrosis
    2. Endocrine disorders
        a. Cushing's syndrome
        b. Hyperaldosteronism
        c. Pheochromocytoma
        d. Diabetes mellitus (DM)
        e. Acromegaly
        f. Hyperthyroidism
    3. Structural/anatomic disorders
        a. Coarctation of the aorta
        b. Carotid artery stenosis
        c. Renal artery stenosis
        d. Sleep apnea
    4. Pregnancy

- Physical Findings
    1. Most significant is elevated blood pressure noted in definition
    2. $S_4$ gallop due to decreased left ventricular compliance is common
    3. Displaced point of maximal impulse (PMI) when left ventricular hypertrophy present
    4. Diffuse anterior chest wall heave when right ventricular hypertrophy present
    5. Peripheral pulses may be abnormal in some secondary cases
        a. Coarctation of the aorta
        b. Stenosis of major arteries
    6. Systolic murmur of aortic stenosis may be heard
    7. Dependent edema in chronic, uncontrolled disease
    8. Renal artery bruit in cases of renal artery stenosis
    9. Neurological evidence of previous cerebral infarcts may be present
    10. Flame hemorrhages and/or fluffy exudate on ophthalmoscopic examination

- Diagnostic Tests/Findings
    1. Laboratory findings usually normal in uncomplicated essential hypertension
    2. Microalbuminuria is earliest indication of target organ damage
    3. Hematuria and/or proteinuria in secondary renal disease
    4. Rapid sequence intravenous pyelogram (IVP) to rule out renal vascular disease
    5. Chest radiograph
        a. Rule out coarctation of the aorta via chest radiograph
        b. Cardiac hypertrophy in chronic, uncontrolled disease
    6. Plasma lipids may be elevated
    7. Hormone levels to evaluate underlying endocrine cause
        a. Elevated serum aldosterone levels—primary hyperaldosteronism
        b. Elevated adrenocorticotropic hormone or serum cortisol—Cushing's syndrome
        c. Low thyroid stimulating hormone and elevated $T_3$—hyperthyroidism
        d. Elevated serum and urine catecholamines—pheochromocytoma
    8. Sleep studies as indicated by history

- Management/Treatment
    1. Assessment of baseline status
        a. All hypertensive and prehypertensive patients should have a thorough review of systems and a physical examination documented to assess for target organ damage
        b. Those requiring pharmacological therapy should have baseline diagnostic testing to assess for target organ damage
        c. Electrocardiogram/chest radiograph frequently performed; utility questionable absent clinical suspicion for target organ myocardial damage
        d. Basic metabolic panel with renal function tests
        e. Urinalysis and microalbuminuria
        f. Hemoglobin
        g. Fasting blood sugar
        h. Serum lipid profile
        i. Serum uric acid to rule out hyperuricemia if thiazide diuretics are a therapeutic option
    2. Assessment of medical history
        a. Screening for presence of chronic kidney disease, which dictates use of angiotensin-converting enzyme (ACE) inhibitors or angiotensin II receptor blockers (ARBs) as initial therapeutic agent
        b. Screening for presence of contraindications to specific pharmacological therapy
            (1) Thiazides—gout
            (2) Calcium channel blockade—congestive heart failure (CHF)
            (3) ACEI second-, third-trimester (TM) pregnancy, angioedema

- Goals of Therapy
    1. Reduction of cardiovascular and renal morbidity and mortality

2. Reduction of blood pressure to identified goal based on age or presence of chronic kidney disease (CKD)/diabetes mellitus (DM)

- Lifestyle Modifications
  1. Weight reduction—10-kg weight loss can reduce systolic blood pressure by 20 mm Hg
  2. Dietary Approaches to Stop Hypertension (DASH) diet—increase fruits, vegetables; decrease fats
  3. Dietary sodium restriction to < 2.4 g/day
  4. Physical activity—30 minutes of moderately vigorous activity (brisk walking) 5 days weekly or vigorous activity (jogging) 20 minutes 2 days weekly
  5. Moderate alcohol consumption; no more than 2 drinks/day men, 1 drink/day women

- Pharmacological Management
  1. Indicated for all patients not at goal blood pressure
  2. Initial pharmacological therapy chosen from among four agents: thiazide diuretics, calcium channel blockers (CCBs), angiotensin-converting enzyme (ACE) inhibitors, and angiotensin II receptor blockers (ARBs)
     a. All patients with chronic kidney disease (CKD) should be started on either ACE inhibitors or ARBs
     b. All black patients without CKD should be started on a thiazide diuretic or CCBs
     c. All non-black patients without CKD should be started on either thiazide diuretics, CCBs, ACE inhibitors, or ARBs
  3. Patients not responsive to initial therapy should have a second agent added
  4. If the patient does not reach goal with the second agent, add the third
     a. ACE inhibitors and ARBs are to be used, one or the other—there is no indication to use both together
  5. Counseling regarding medication side effects, compliance, follow-up, and lifestyle modifications
  6. Refer for specialty evaluation if the patient does not respond to lifestyle management, thiazide diuretics, CCBs, and ACE inhibitors, or ARBs

# CORONARY ARTERY DISEASE (CAD)

- Definition—clinical syndrome also known as angina pectoris that occurs from atherosclerotic changes to the coronary vasculature; the result is decreased blood flow through vessels either due to partial obstruction (sclerosis) or vasospasm (may happen in a nonsclerotic vessel); when tissue ischemia and pain occur as a result of decreased blood flow, angina occurs

- Etiology/Incidence
  1. Hypertension
  2. Tobacco use
  3. Serum lipid abnormalities
  4. Diabetes mellitus
  5. Insulin resistance and metabolic syndrome
  6. Family history with a first-degree relative (particularly when age of onset < 50 years)
  7. Endothelial dysfunction
  8. Use of hormonal contraception
  9. Gender prevalence depends on age
     a. Overall more prevalent in men by a 4:1 ratio
     b. Younger than age 40, ratio is 8:1
     c. Older than age 70, ratio is 1:1
  10. Obesity
  11. Personality type is less-certain risk factor

- Types of Angina
  1. Exertional—occurs with activity, generally subsides with rest
  2. Variant threshold—occurs at various times, including rest
  3. Prinzmetal's angina—occurs only at rest
     a. Chest pain occurs without the usual precipitating factors
     b. Often affects women younger than age 50
     c. Characteristically occurs in early morning, awakening patient from sleep
     d. Tends to involve right coronary artery
     e. More common in patients with precipitating factors
        (1) Nitric oxide deficiency
        (2) Nicotine
        (3) Cocaine use
        (4) Stimulation of alpha receptors

- Signs and Symptoms
  1. Characteristic chest discomfort
     a. Sensation of tightness, squeezing, burning, pressure
     b. In 80–90% of cases discomfort is felt behind or slightly to the left of the midsternum
     c. Radiates most often to left shoulder and upper arm, traveling down inner aspect of arm to elbow, forearm, wrist, and fourth or fifth finger
     d. May be felt in lower jaw, back of neck, or upper left side of back
     e. Typically lasts 15–20 minutes, may resolve more quickly but usually lasts at least several minutes; pain lasting > 30 minutes is unstable angina

2. Anxiety
3. Dyspnea

- Differential Diagnosis
  1. Gastroesophageal reflux (heartburn)
  2. Anxiety
  3. Depression
  4. Costrochondral pain
  5. Pneumothorax
  6. Congestive heart failure
  7. Pneumonia
  8. Pericarditis
  9. Asthma
  10. Aortic dissection
  11. Myocardial infarction

- Physical Findings
  1. Systolic and diastolic blood pressures usually elevated during attack
  2. May hear apical systolic murmur due to transient mitral regurgitation
  3. Transient $S_3$ and/or $S_4$ may be present
  4. May detect signs of disease that contribute to or accompany CAD
     a. Diabetes mellitus
     b. Hypertension
     c. Aortic stenosis
     d. Hypertrophic cardiomyopathy
     e. Mitral valve prolapse
  5. Pulse and respirations may be elevated
  6. May see tobacco-stained teeth or fingers
  7. May see signs of peripheral artery disease
     a. Diminished distal pulses
     b. Pale skin
     c. Poor hair growth
  8. Levine's sign (clenched fist over sternum) highly suggestive of angina
  9. May not have any remarkable physical findings

- Diagnostic Tests/Findings
  1. Serum lipid levels
     a. Low-density lipoprotein (LDL) cholesterol will ideally be lowered by at least 50% from pretreatment baseline; while a 50% reduction is preferable, a 30% reduction is acceptable in patients at higher risk of adverse outcomes with statin use
     b. High-density lipoprotein (HDL) cholesterol should be increased to > 40 mg/dL
  2. Electrocardiogram (ECG)
     a. Normal in 25% patients with angina
     b. Characteristic finding is downward sloping of ST segment or T wave peak or inversion during attack; reverses after attack
     c. May show signs of old myocardial infarction or hypertrophy
  3. Exercise electrocardiography (stress testing)
     a. Ischemic changes or angina during exercise test—clinically diagnostic
     b. Markedly positive test is any one of the following
        (1) ST segment depression after start of exercise
        (2) > 2 mm of new ST segment depression in multiple leads
        (3) New ST segment elevation
        (4) Decreased systolic blood pressure with exercise
        (5) Development of heart failure with exercise
        (6) Inability to exercise for > 2 minutes
        (7) Prolonged interval after exercise for return to normal ECG
  4. Nuclear medicine studies to evaluate presence, location, and extent of coronary disease
     a. Exercise thallium imaging
        (1) Especially useful in patients with preexisting ECG abnormalities and patients taking digoxin
        (2) Areas of diminished uptake indicate hypoperfusion
        (3) Should be conducted at experienced center
     b. Radionuclide ventriculography
        (1) Images left ventricle and measures ejection fraction
        (2) Resting abnormalities represent infarction
        (3) Abnormalities with exercise indicate stress-induced ischemia
     c. Coronary angiography
        (1) Definitive test for diagnosis of CAD
        (2) Indicated in high-risk patients
           (a) With refractory unstable angina
        (3) With spontaneous or exercise-induced ischemia after myocardial infarction

- Management/Treatment (see **Figure 7-1**)
  1. Treatment of acute attack
     a. Sublingual or buccal spray nitroglycerin
     b. Dose may be repeated 3 times at 5-minute intervals
     c. Pain unrelieved after 3 doses is unstable and should be evaluated in emergency room
  2. Prevention of further attacks
     a. Reduction of risk factors when possible
        (1) Weight reduction
        (2) Smoking cessation
        (3) Exercise program
        (4) Daily acetylsalicylic acid (ASA)

## FIGURE 7-1 Treatment Algorithm for Stable Angina

```
                    History of overt heart failure
                         /              \
                       No                Yes
                       /                  \
        Contraindication to beta-blocker?   Nitrates
             /        \                       |
           No          Yes                 Control?
           /            \                   /    \
      Beta-blocker?   Calcium channel  →  Control? → Yes   No
           |            blocker              |              |
       Control?                             No           Angiography
        /    \                               |              |
      Yes    No                              ↓        Angioplasty or CABG
              |
       Calcium channel blocker
              |
          Control?
           /    \
         Yes    No  →  Add nitrate
                          |
                       Control?
                        /    \
                       No    Yes
                       |
                   Angiography
                       |
              Angioplasty or CABG
```

b. Lowering LDL cholesterol ideally to < 50% baseline—hydroxymethylglutaryl coenzyme A (HMG CoA) reductase inhibitors are the drug of choice for LDL reduction unless contraindicated
c. All patients whose risk for CAD warrants pharmacological therapy should also take aspirin daily
d. Beta blockers prevent angina by reducing myocardial oxygen requirements
   (1) Metoprolol 50–200 mg daily in 2 divided doses
   (2) Atenolol 25–200 mg once daily
   (3) Major contraindications are bronchospastic disease, bradydysrhythmias, and heart failure
e. Calcium channel blockers prevent angina by reducing myocardial oxygen demand and inducing coronary vasodilation
   (1) Nifedipine 30–120 mg daily
   (2) Verapamil 180–480 mg in 1 or 2 doses daily
   (3) Diltiazem 360 mg in 2 daily doses
f. Long-acting nitrates prevent angina by inducing coronary vasodilation
   (1) Isosorbide dinitrate 10–40 mg 3 daily
   (2) Sustained release nitroglycerin 6.25–25 mg daily in 2–4 divided doses
g. Coronary revascularization is indicated in the following
   (1) Unacceptable symptoms despite medical therapy to its tolerable limits

(2) Left main coronary artery stenosis greater than 50% with or without symptoms
(3) Three-vessel disease with left ventricular dysfunction
(4) Unstable angina with ischemia on exercise stress test after symptom control
(5) Post–myocardial infarction with continued angina or ischemia on noninvasive testing
h. Counseling regarding medication side effects

## DYSLIPIDEMIA

- Definition
  1. A general term used to describe any one or combination of lipid abnormalities that serve as a marker for coronary artery disease risk; although elevated total cholesterol (TC) and low levels of high-density lipoproteins (HDL) are linked to increased incidence of coronary artery disease, and conversely high HDL appears to be cardioprotective, elevated low-density lipoproteins (LDL) remain the primary target of lipid-lowering strategies in all levels of prevention
  2. In accordance with the 2013 American College of Cardiology (ACC)/American Heart Association guidelines (Stone et al., 2013), four population groups are identified as candidates for lipid-lowering therapy based on risk for atherosclerotic cardiovascular disease (ASCVD)
     a. Patients with LDL-C > 190 mg/dL
     b. Patients age 40 to 75 years with DM and an LDL-C between 70 and 190 mg/dL
     c. Patients with a history of clinical ASCVD
     d. Patients age 40 to 75 years with a 10-year risk of ASCVD > 7.5%

- Etiology/Incidence
  1. Familial hypercholesterolemia
  2. Endocrine disease
     a. Thyroid disorders
     b. Hypercortisolism
     c. Diabetes
  3. Nephrotic syndrome
  4. Hepatic disease
  5. Sedentary lifestyle
  6. Obesity
  7. Malignancy

- Signs and Symptoms
  1. Asymptomatic in most cases
  2. Diagnosis occurs as a function of screening or the laboratory evaluation of patients with heart disease

- Differential Diagnosis (of underlying causes)
  1. Familial syndrome
  2. Endocrine disease
  3. Liver disease
  4. Malignancy
  5. Obesity

- Physical Findings
  1. No specific findings in most cases
  2. May show findings consistent with vascular disease
  3. May show findings of underlying endocrine disease
  4. In extreme dyslipidemias
     a. Corneal arcus
     b. Xanthomas
     c. Lipemia retinalis
     d. Earlobe crease

- Diagnostic Tests/Findings
  1. LDL-C for targeted reduction based on four risk groups identified previously
  2. HDL < 40 mg/dL is a cardiac risk factor
  3. HDL > 60 mg/dL is cardioprotective and negates another risk factor
  4. Serum triglycerides > 150 mg/dL—no direct link to heart disease, but may cause pancreatic disease
  5. As indicated to rule out underlying secondary causes

- Management/Treatment
  1. Cholesterol-lowering diet
     a. Total fat < 25–30% of intake
     b. Saturated fat < 7% of intake
     c. Dietary cholesterol < 200 mg/day
  2. Pharmacological therapy—for patients in four risk groups
     a. HMG CoA reductase inhibitors
        (1) Initial drug of choice for patients who are candidates for risk reduction
        (2) Stratified to high-intensity statin therapy (reduce LDL-C by > 50%) or moderate-intensity statin therapy (reduce LDL-C by 30–50%)
        (3) Rosuvastatin and atorvastatin in higher doses for high-intensity therapy
        (4) Rosuvastatin and atorvastatin in lower doses and other statins for moderate-intensity therapy
        (5) Contraindicated in severe liver disease

# CONGESTIVE HEART FAILURE (CHF)

- Definition—clinical syndrome that results when cardiac output is insufficient to meet metabolic demands of body; any condition that affects heart rate or contractile function can precipitate CHF

- Etiology/Incidence
  1. Acute myocardial infarction; dysrhythmia
  2. Chronic hypertension
  3. Valvular stenosis or regurgitation
  4. Cardiomyopathy
  5. Medication toxicity
  6. 5 million estimated cases in the United States—500,000 new cases diagnosed annually

- Types of CHF
  1. Acute
     a. Abrupt onset usually follows acute myocardial infarction or valve rupture
     b. Also known as "left-sided failure"
     c. Symptoms are produced by acute diffusion of water into the pulmonary air spaces
  2. Chronic
     a. Develops as a result of inadequate compensatory mechanisms that have been employed over time to improve cardiac output
     b. Also known as "right-sided failure"
     c. Symptoms are produced by increased hydrostatic pressure in the venous system and subsequent diffusion of water into the interstitium
  3. Systolic—contractile dysfunction results in decreased cardiac output
  4. Diastolic—inability to relax and fill with blood results in decreased cardiac output; accounts for half of all cases of CHF

- Signs and Symptoms
  1. Acute CHF—symptoms typically related to acute pulmonary edema
     a. Dyspnea at rest
     b. Frothy cough worse in the recumbent position
     c. Feeling of anxiety and/or impending doom
  2. Chronic CHF—symptoms typically related to redistribution of fluid excess in systemic circulation
     a. Dyspnea on exertion; easily fatigued
     b. Chronic nonproductive cough
     c. Abdominal fullness
     d. Weight gain
     e. Paroxysmal nocturnal dyspnea
     f. Oliguria, nocturia
     g. Peripheral cyanosis

- Differential Diagnosis
  1. Acute MI
  2. Pulmonary embolus
  3. Pneumonia
  4. Asthma
  5. Chronic venous insufficiency

- Physical Findings
  1. Acute
     a. Coarse rales over all lung fields
     b. Wheezing over all lung fields
     c. $S_3$ gallop very common
     d. Appears generally healthy except for the acute event
     e. Systolic murmur of mitral regurgitation
     f. Usually no edema or systemic signs of fluid overload
  2. Chronic
     a. Lungs may be clear or may exhibit rales at the bases
     b. Dependent edema
     c. Appears chronically ill
     d. Jugular venous distention
     e. Hepatosplenomegaly
     f. Point of maximal impulse displaced to the left
     g. Diffuse anterior chest wall heave
     h. $S_3$ and/or $S_4$
     i. Any variety of stenotic or regurgitant murmurs

- Diagnostic Tests/Findings
  1. Acute
     a. B-type natriuretic peptide (BNP) levels above 80 pg/mL—may be as high as > 1,000 pg/mL (reference ranges vary among laboratories—interpretation should always be based on individual laboratory reference ranges)
     b. Hypoxemia and hypocapnia on arterial blood gas
     c. Basic metabolic panel 7 (sodium, potassium, chloride, carbon dioxide, blood urea nitrogen, creatinine, and glucose) usually normal
     d. Urinalysis usually normal
     e. Chest radiograph shows pulmonary edema, Kerley's lines, effusions
     f. Echocardiogram will show contractile, relaxation, and valve function
  2. Chronic
     a. Basic metabolic panel (BMP) may show electrolyte abnormalities
     b. Mild hypoxemia on arterial blood gas—$pCO_2$ usually normal
     c. Chest radiograph shows redistribution of flow, enlarged heart
     d. Echocardiogram will show contractile, relaxation, and valve function

- Management/Treatment
  1. Of primary importance is identification and treatment of underlying cause
  2. Nonpharmacological interventions
     a. Sodium/fluid restriction
     b. Rest/activity balance
     c. Weight reduction in the obese
  3. Pharmacological interventions
     a. Diuretics for all symptomatic patients and those who are not adequately managed with an ACE inhibitor/beta-adrenergic antagonist combination
        (1) Furosemide 20–160 mg in 1 or 2 daily doses, treatment of choice
        (2) Hydrochlorothiazide more questionable utility; may augment loops in doses ≥ 25 mg daily
     b. ACE inhibitors are mainstays of chronic management
        (1) Captopril 6.25–50 mg 3–4 times daily
        (2) Enalapril 2.5–40 mg daily in 2 divided doses
        (3) Lisinopril 2.5–10 mg daily
     c. Beta-adrenergic antagonists are mainstays of chronic management
        (1) Carvedilol to 25 mg b.i.d.
        (2) Toprol XL to 190 mg q.d.
        (3) Improve function by blocking excessive adrenergic stimulation
     d. Inotropic
        (1) Beneficial in moderate to severe systolic failure
        (2) Digoxin 0.125–0.25 mg daily
     e. Neurohormonal antagonists
        (1) Spironolactone 25 mg daily
        (2) Mediate major effects of renin-angiotensin-aldosterone activation, e.g., remodeling
     f. Vasodilators—useful as adjunct therapy in heart failure refractory to initial therapies
  4. Application of interventions according to stage
     a. Stage A
        (1) Patients at risk because of disease, cardiotoxins, or family history, but no structural disease
        (2) Manage underlying disease
        (3) Control other risk factors
        (4) ACE inhibitors as indicated
     b. Stage B
        (1) Patients with structural disease, but no symptoms
        (2) All interventions under stage A
        (3) ACE inhibitors and beta-adrenergic antagonists as indicated
     c. Stage C
        (1) Patients with structural heart disease and symptoms of failure
        (2) All measures under stage B
        (3) Inotropic agents as indicated
        (4) Dietary sodium restriction 2–2.5 g/day
     d. Stage D
        (1) Refractory heart failure
        (2) All measures under stage C
        (3) Assist devices, heart transplant, hospice as indicated
  5. Patient counseling
     a. Lifestyle modification
     b. Medication toxicities and side effects
  6. Physician consultation
     a. When pharmacological therapy initiated
     b. When patient unresponsive to initial medications

# PERIPHERAL ARTERIAL DISEASE (PAD)

- Definition—narrowing and eventual obstruction of the arterial lumen usually caused by atherosclerosis; occlusion tends to be segmental; result is decreased blood supply to limbs

- Etiology/Incidence—same as those for coronary artery disease

- Signs and Symptoms
  1. Intermittent claudication usually presenting symptom
  2. Distance patient can walk is indicative of degree of circulatory impairment
  3. Cold and/or numbness of the extremity
  4. Pain or ache at night/rest suggestive of severe disease

- Differential Diagnosis
  1. Sciatica
  2. Myopathies
  3. Acute arterial emboli

- Physical Findings
  1. Reduced or absent pulses distal to obstruction
  2. Dependent rubor
  3. Skin pallor or cyanosis
  4. Poor hair/nail growth
  5. Dry ulceration/gangrene in severe disease

- Diagnostic Tests/Findings
  1. Radiography of affected extremity may show calcification
  2. Doppler ultrasound will demonstrate reduced pressures distal to occlusion
  3. Arteriography will show location and extent of block

- Management/Treatment
  1. Control risk factors as much as possible
  2. Tobacco cessation

3. Walk daily to develop collateral circulation—walking to point of pain followed by a 3-minute rest should be done 8 times daily
4. Aspirin 80–325 mg has theoretical value and should be given to all patients with severe disease
5. Cilostazol 100 mg orally b.i.d.—contraindicated in heart failure
6. Pentoxifylline 400 mg orally t.i.d.
7. Surgical revascularization

## THROMBOPHLEBITIS

- Definition—partial or complete occlusion of a vein by a thrombus with secondary inflammation of venous wall—may be superficial or deep

- Etiology/Incidence
    1. Virchow's triad
        a. Vessel injury
        b. Venous stasis
        c. Hypercoagulation states
    2. Prolonged bed rest
    3. Use of oral contraceptives (particularly in smokers)
    4. Postoperative period
    5. More prevalent in females
    6. Occurs in 800,000 new patients annually

- Signs and Symptoms
    1. Sudden onset of pain (superficial)
    2. Pain, tenderness, ache, or tightness especially with activity (deep)

- Differential Diagnosis
    1. Muscle strain or contusion
    2. Cellulitis
    3. Arterial disease
    4. Lymphatic obstruction

- Physical Findings
    1. Localized heat and erythema (superficial)
    2. Edema distal to occlusion (deep)
    3. Distention of superficial venous collateral vessels
    4. Low-grade temperature
    5. Cool skin
    6. Palpable cords

- Diagnostic Tests/Findings
    1. Doppler ultrasound and impedance plethysmography to evaluate venous flow
    2. Contrast venography is definitive study to identify location and extent

- Management/Treatment
    1. Prevention
        a. Elevation of lower extremities 15–20 degrees
        b. Leg exercises when immobility required
        c. Compression stockings
        d. Anticoagulation
            (1) Low-dose unfractionated heparin
            (2) Low-molecular-weight heparin
    2. Elevation of extremity and warm compress (superficial)
    3. Bed rest with extremity elevated (deep)
    4. Anticoagulation therapy for deep thrombosis
        a. Low-molecular-weight heparin
        b. Factor Xa inhibition (rivaroxaban)
        c. Direct thrombin inhibition (dabigatran)

## CHRONIC VENOUS INSUFFICIENCY

- Definition—impaired venous return with resultant chronic lower-extremity edema

- Etiology/Incidence
    1. Destruction of valves in deep venous channels of lower legs secondary to deep thrombophlebitis
    2. Neoplastic obstruction of pelvic veins
    3. Leg trauma
    4. Sustained elevation of venous pressure
    5. More common in women than in men

- Signs and Symptoms
    1. Aching of lower extremities relieved by elevation
    2. Edema at end of day or after prolonged standing
    3. Night cramps

- Differential Diagnosis
    1. Lymphedema
    2. Congestive heart failure
    3. Renal disease
    4. Liver disease

- Physical Findings
    1. Edema of lower extremities
    2. Trophic changes with brownish discoloration
    3. Cool to touch
    4. Thin, shiny, atrophic skin
    5. Wet ulcerations on the medial or anterior aspect of the leg

- Diagnostic Tests/Findings
    1. Blood urea nitrogen (BUN)/creatinine to rule out renal disease
    2. Liver function tests to rule out liver disease
    3. Chest radiograph to rule out congestive heart failure
    4. Doppler ultrasound to rule out thrombosis

- Management/Treatment
    1. Bed rest with legs elevated to diminish chronic edema
    2. Use of elastic stockings

3. Weight reduction in the obese
4. Hydrocortisone cream for stasis dermatitis

## PERICARDITIS

- Definition—inflammation of the membrane lining the pericardium

- Etiology/Incidence
  1. Viral
  2. Bacterial
  3. Postmyocardial infarction
  4. Post open heart procedure
  5. Uremia
  6. Autoimmune disease, e.g., systemic lupus erythematosus

- Signs and Symptoms
  1. Pleuritic, knife-like stabbing chest pain over the precordium
  2. Dyspnea

- Differential Diagnosis
  1. Pleuritis
  2. Costochondritis
  3. Angina or MI
  4. Pneumonia
  5. Pneumothorax

- Physical Findings
  1. Appears acutely uncomfortable; worse with inspiration
  2. Pericardial friction rub
  3. Improvement in pain with sitting forward

- Diagnostic Tests/Findings
  1. None, clinical diagnosis based on symptom presentation in the outpatient setting
  2. 12-lead ECG may demonstrate diffuse concave ST elevation in all or near all leads

- Management/Treatment
  1. Nonsteroidal anti-inflammatory drugs are the mainstay of treatment
  2. Manage underlying cause if indicated, e.g., uremia
  3. Short dose of steroids if refractory to NSAIDs

## ENDOCARDITIS

- Definition—an infection of the endocardial surface of the heart that may include the valves, mural endocardium, or septum

- Etiology/Incidence
  1. Bacterial infection most common; 70% of cases are *Streptococcus* species, 25% *Staphylococcus* species
  2. Gram negative and fungal infections may occur in immunocompromised patients
  3. Prosthetic valves increase risk
  4. Intravenous drug abuse (IVDA) increases risk
  5. Previous surgical intervention to pacemaker system increases risk

- Signs and Symptoms
  1. Fever
  2. Fatigue
  3. Delirium
  4. Generally feels "sick"

- Differential Diagnosis
  1. Systemic infection
  2. CHF
  3. Physiological murmur

- Physical Findings
  1. Osler's nodes
  2. Janeway lesions
  3. Subungal hemorrhages
  4. Petechiae
  5. Cardiac murmur
  6. Roth spots

- Diagnostic Tests/Findings
  1. Duke criteria
     a. Two major criteria
     b. One major and three minor criteria
     c. Five minor criteria
  2. Major criteria
     a. Positive echocardiogram with specific findings
     b. Positive blood cultures with specific parameters (e.g., 3 separate sets)
     c. Myocardial abscess
     d. Partial dehiscence of prosthetic valve
     e. New onset valvular regurgitation
  3. Minor criteria
     a. Predisposing cardiac condition or IVDA
     b. Fever > 100.4°F
     c. Associated vascular phenomenon
     d. Positive blood culture or echocardiography not meeting major criteria

- Management/Treatment
  1. Antibiotic therapy to cover appropriate organisms
     a. Native valve disease—penicillin (PCN) G and gentamycin
     b. IVDA—cover methicillin-resistant *Staphylococcus aureus* (MRSA)
     c. Immunocompromised—cover Gram negative infection, consider *Proteus* species

## Special Considerations in the Hospitalized Patient

- Acute coronary syndrome (ACS)
  - Definition—a general term used to describe a spectrum of acute and unstable myocardial events to include unstable angina, non-ST elevation MI (NSTEMI), and ST elevation MI (STEMI). It is most often caused by rupture of an atherosclerotic plaque and results in partial or complete occlusion of a coronary artery
  - Etiology/Incidence
    - Same as those for coronary artery disease (see earlier)
    - May occur in the setting of an increased oxygen demand in the patient with a pre-existing high-grade lesion
    - When ACS occurs without increased oxygen demand, suspicion should be high for thrombosis or plaque hemorrhage
    - 720,000 Americans have a myocardial infarction each year; more than two-thirds of them are first MIs
    - Coronary heart disease kills 380,000 people each year
  - Signs and Symptoms
    - One-third of patients give history of alteration in typical pattern of angina
    - Palpitations
    - Diaphoresis, dyspnea, cough, and wheeze
    - Anxiety
    - Nausea and vomiting
    - Weakness or light-headedness
    - Often prefer not to lie quietly—continuously seek comfortable position
    - Women may present with atypical symptoms, i.e., burning sensation in chest, indigestion, weakness
  - Differential Diagnosis
    - Angina
    - Gastroesophageal reflux
    - Pulmonary embolus
    - Costochondral pain
    - Pericarditis
    - Dissecting aortic aneurysm
    - Anxiety
  - Physical Findings
    - Heart rate may range from bradycardia to tachycardia
    - Dysrhythmias common
    - Low-grade fever may appear after 12 hours and persist for several days
    - $S_4$ and murmur of mitral regurgitation common
    - $S_3$ less common—when present, indicates severe left ventricular dysfunction
    - Blood pressure may be elevated or abnormally low
    - May see findings consistent with heart failure; jugular vein distention, rales
    - Cyanosis and cold temperature indicate low cardiac output
  - Diagnostic Tests/Findings
    - ECG is essential—most patients have ECG changes in a regional distribution
      - Convex ST segment elevation with peaked upright or inverted T waves indicative of transmural (ST elevation) MI (STEMI)
      - ST segment depression may indicate subendocardial MI (NSTEMI); develops inverted T waves in chronic phase
      - Development of clinically significant Q waves (at least 1-mm deep and 1-mm wide) generally considered diagnostic of MI; develops in chronic phase of STEMI
      - Regional distribution
        - Inferior wall—leads II, III, aVF
        - Lateral wall—leads I, aVL
        - Anterior wall—leads $V_1$ through $V_6$
    - Leukocytosis 10,000–20,000/mL on second day
    - Cardiac isoenzymes progressively increase as necrosis evolves
      - Creatine kinase muscle-brain (CK-MB) increases within 4–6 hours of pain onset, peaks in 10–20 hours, returns to baseline in 36–48 hours
      - Troponin T and troponin I demonstrate high specificity and sensitivity and remain elevated for 5–7 days post MI
      - Lactic dehydrogenase elevations detectable 12 hours after pain onset, peak in 24–48 hours, and remain elevated for 10–14 days—$LDH_1$:$LDH_2$ ratio > 1 consistent with MI

*(continues)*

## Special Considerations in the Hospitalized Patient (*continued*)

- Echocardiography for assessment of cardiac wall motion and valvular/structural defects post MI
- Technetium-99m pyrophosphate scintigraphy used in diagnosis of MI for patients hospitalized late in the course
- Radionuclide ventriculography allows assessment of regional wall motion and ejection fraction
- Coronary angiography is definitive test to visualize the coronary vasculature
  - Management/Treatment—immediate hospitalization
    - Immediate goals are to provide oxygen, relieve pain, and treat dysrhythmia
      - Oxygen by nasal cannula, face mask, or endotracheal tube
      - Morphine sulfate 2–4 mg at 5- to 10-minute intervals p.r.n.
      - Nitroglycerin sublingual or intravenously
      - Heparin
      - Chewable aspirin
      - Treat dysrhythmia as indicated
    - Pharmacological anti-ischemic therapy
      - Nitrates
      - Beta-adrenergic antagonists—for all patients unless contraindicated
    - Pharmacological antithrombotic therapy
      - ASA
      - Platelet aggregate inhibitors
      - Glycoprotein IIb/IIIa inhibitors
    - Pharmacological anticoagulant therapy
      - Unfractionated heparin
      - Low-molecular-weight heparin
      - Factor Xa inhibitors
    - STEMI patients who are candidates for reperfusion
      - To catheterization lab for assessment—percutaneous coronary intervention is preferred intervention
      - Administer fibrinolytics if expected first medical contact > 120 minutes
    - NSTEMI elevation or high-risk unstable angina pectoris stratified according to risk
      - High-risk patients treated aggressively with anti-ischemics, anti-thrombotics, anticoagulants
      - Low-risk patients treated more conservatively with optimum medical management of CAD
    - Patient education regarding cardiac rehabilitation and risk factor reduction
- Indications and contraindications to fibrinolytic therapy
  1. Patient has been symptomatic (chest pain) for longer than 15 minutes but less than 12 hours
  2. ECG is diagnostic for ST elevation indicating an MI or a new left bundle branch block
  3. If any of the following are present, consider transfer to a PCI-capable facility
     a. Heart rate over 100 beats per minute in the presence of a systolic blood pressure less than 100 mm Hg
     b. Presence of signs that might indicate pulmonary edema, e.g., rales
     c. Cool and clammy skin that might indicate shock
     d. Contraindication to administration of fibrinolytics as listed in item 4 below
  4. If any of the following are present, fibrinolytics are contraindicated
     a. Systolic blood pressure over 180 mm Hg
     b. Diastolic blood pressure over 110 mm Hg
     c. Difference in systolic pressure more than 15 mm Hg between the right and left arms
     d. History of structural central nervous system (CNS) disease
     e. Any significant head or face trauma in the previous 90 days
     f. Major trauma, surgery, or gastrointestinal or genitourinary bleed in the last 6 weeks
     g. History of bleeding or clotting disorders
     h. On anticoagulants
     i. CPR has been implemented for more than 10 minutes
     j. Pregnancy in a female
     k. Any serious chronic disease such as liver or kidney disease or advanced cancer

# QUESTIONS

## ■ Select the best answer

1. When is it appropriate to diagnose and treat hypertension based on one blood pressure reading?
   a. When there is a strong family history
   b. When the diastolic pressure is > 100 mm Hg
   c. When there is target organ damage
   d. When there is suboccipital headache

2. Which of the following is not a cause of secondary hypertension?
   a. Exercise
   b. Thyroid disease
   c. Sleep apnea
   d. Coarctation of the aorta

3. What is the percentage of Caucasian adults afflicted with hypertension?
   a. < 10%
   b. 10–15%
   c. 20–30%
   d. > 50%

4. The patient with chronic hypertension presents with lower-extremity edema, abdominal pain, and fatigue. Physical exam findings reveal a diffuse chest wall heave and displaced point of maximal impulse. This makes you suspicious that the patient has:
   a. Biventricular hypertrophy
   b. Renal vascular stenosis
   c. Hypertensive encephalopathy
   d. Malignant hypertension

5. Which of the following endocrine disorders is not a cause of secondary hypertension?
   a. Cushing's syndrome
   b. Diabetes mellitus
   c. Hyperthyroidism
   d. Addison's disease

6. Pharmacological therapy should be started in any patient who is diagnosed with hypertension and has end organ damage. According to JNC 8 guidelines, pharmacological therapy may begin with all of the following *except*:
   a. Beta blockers
   b. Calcium channel blockers
   c. Diuretics
   d. Angiotensin-converting enzyme inhibitors

7. Which of the following medications is the drug of choice for the patient with hypertension and comorbid chronic kidney disease?
   a. Lisinopril 5 mg p.o. q.d.
   b. Furosemide 20 mg p.o. q.d.
   c. Metoprolol 50 mg p.o. b.i.d.
   d. Diltiazem 90 mg p.o. b.i.d.

8. Which of the following is not a risk factor for coronary artery disease?
   a. Stage 2 hypertension
   b. Serum cholesterol of 300 mg/dL
   c. A parent with history of myocardial infarction
   d. African American ancestry

9. Prinzmetal's angina typically occurs:
   a. During periods of emotional stress
   b. Early in the morning
   c. In men younger than age 50
   d. In extremes of temperature

10. Your patient complains of chest pain just to the left of the midsternal area that occurred while mowing the lawn. As you pursue the history of present illness in an effort to rule out angina, which of the following characteristics of the pain experience makes angina less likely?
    a. The pain was also felt in the back of the neck
    b. The pain felt like a burning sensation
    c. The pain lasted 15 minutes
    d. The pain was a stabbing, knife-like sensation

11. Aortic stenosis can be a contributing cause of coronary artery disease. Which of the following heart sounds is suggestive of aortic stenosis?
    a. A systolic murmur loudest at the second intercostal space, right sternal border
    b. A diastolic murmur loudest at the second intercostal space, left sternal border
    c. An extra heart sound heard early in diastole
    d. An extra heart sound heard early in systole

12. Exercise electrocardiography (ECG) is clinically diagnostic for coronary artery disease. Which of the following is not a positive finding on exercise ECG?
    a. > 2 mm of new ST segment depression in multiple leads
    b. Decreased systolic blood pressure with exercise
    c. ST segment depression after start of exercise
    d. Inability to exercise for > 5 minutes

13. You have diagnosed atherosclerotic coronary vascular disease in Mrs. J. Her LDL cholesterol is 130 mg/dL. According to the ACC/AHA guidelines, the most appropriate intervention is to:
    a. Initiate high-intensity statin therapy and reevaluate in 2 months
    b. Begin diet modification and reevaluate in 3 months
    c. Begin enteric-coated aspirin 325 mg q.d. and reevaluate in 1 month
    d. Begin cholestyramine 12 g b.i.d. and reevaluate in 3 months

14. Which of the following pharmacological agents prevents angina by reducing myocardial oxygen demand and inducing coronary vasodilation?
    a. Diltiazem
    b. Isosorbide dinitrate
    c. Atenolol
    d. Aspirin

15. Mr. L. is a 64-year-old patient with difficult-to-control angina. His initial therapy was atenolol 25 mg q.d., and his dose was increased until it was 100 mg daily. When angina persisted, diltiazem 180 mg b.i.d. was added to the regimen, but even the combination of medications is not controlling symptoms. At this point the next appropriate step would be to:
    a. Recommend cardiac angiography
    b. Begin nifedipine 30 mg q.d.
    c. Begin isosorbide dinitrate 10 mg t.i.d.
    d. Recommend radionuclide ventriculography

16. Patients having a myocardial infarction (MI) may report that the chest pain they are experiencing is different from their usual anginal pain. Which of the following is also suspicious for MI rather than angina?
    a. Pain lasting > 15 minutes
    b. Nausea and vomiting
    c. Elevated systolic blood pressure
    d. Presence of $S_3$ or $S_4$ heart sounds

17. Which of the following diagnostic findings is most suggestive of a history of myocardial infarction?
    a. 15,000/mL leukocytes
    b. Development of Q waves
    c. ST segment elevation
    d. Hypoxia on arterial blood gas (ABG)

18. Acute congestive heart failure produces symptoms as a function of the diffusion of water into the pulmonary air spaces. Acute failure is most commonly caused by:
    a. Chronic hypertension
    b. Valvular stenosis
    c. Medication toxicity
    d. Myocardial infarction

19. When increased hydrostatic pressure in the venous system causes water to diffuse into the interstitium, resultant physical findings would most likely include:
    a. Weight gain
    b. $S_3$ gallop
    c. Coarse rales in all lung fields
    d. Dyspnea at rest

20. Kerley's lines on chest radiography are suggestive of:
    a. Inadequate compensatory mechanisms when cardiac output fails
    b. Hydrostatic pressure increase in the peripheral vascular system
    c. Diffusion of water into interlobular septa
    d. Prinzmetal's angina

21. Congestive heart failure is a syndrome that results when the cardiac output is insufficient to meet the metabolic demands of the body. This can be either an acute or chronic state. Causes of chronic failure include:
    a. Hypertension
    b. Mitral valve rupture
    c. Myocardial infarction
    d. Cardiac ischemia

22. Typical laboratory findings in acute CHF include:
    a. Red blood cells in urinalysis
    b. Blood urea nitrogen (BUN) 70 mg/dL; serum creatinine 2 mg/dL
    c. $PaO_2$ 64 mm Hg by arterial blood gas
    d. Redistribution of flow by chest radiography

23. Cardiac glycosides may be useful therapy in congestive heart failure when:
    a. Failure is unresponsive to angiotensin-converting enzyme inhibitors
    b. Failure is severe and refractory to first-line therapies
    c. Failure is due to cardiomyopathy
    d. Failure is severe and refractory to vasodilators

24. Dependent rubor is a physical finding associated with:
    a. Chronic venous insufficiency
    b. Arteriosclerotic occlusive disease
    c. Deep vein thrombosis
    d. Superficial thrombophlebitis

25. Which of the following physical findings is not associated with thrombophlebitis?
    a. Low-grade temperature
    b. Cool skin
    c. Heat and erythema
    d. Reduced or absent peripheral pulses

26. Edema of the lower extremities is a physical finding associated with a variety of medical conditions. A diagnosis of chronic venous insufficiency is made when other causes are ruled out. When chronic venous insufficiency is diagnosed, the appropriate treatment includes:
    a. Heparin infusion for 7–10 days
    b. Use of elastic stockings
    c. Aspirin 325 mg daily
    d. Surgical revascularization

27. Mr. H. is a 32-year-old male who presents for a job-related physical. Cholesterol screening reveals serum LDL of 190 mg/dL. The appropriate action would be:
    a. Implement diet and lifestyle changes and reevaluate in 3 months
    b. Begin drug therapy with an HMG coenzyme A reductase inhibitor
    c. Repeat the lipid panel in 1 week before beginning interventions
    d. Begin drug therapy with niacin

## ■ Answers

| | | |
|---|---|---|
| 1. c | 10. d | 19. a |
| 2. a | 11. a | 20. c |
| 3. b | 12. d | 21. a |
| 4. a | 13. a | 22. c |
| 5. d | 14. a | 23. b |
| 6. a | 15. c | 24. b |
| 7. a | 16. b | 25. d |
| 8. d | 17. b | 26. b |
| 9. b | 18. d | 27. a |

## BIBLIOGRAPHY

Adams, K. F., Lindenfeld, J., Arnold, J. M. O., Baker, D. W., Barnard, D. H., Baughman, K. L., . . . Wagoner, L. E. (2006). Executive summary: HFSA 2006 comprehensive heart failure practice guideline. *Journal of Cardiac Failure, 12*(1), 10–38.

Bashore, T. M., Granger, C. B., Hranitzky, P., & Patel, M.R. (2014). Heart disease. In S. J. McPhee & M. A. Papadakis (Eds.), *Current medical diagnosis and treatment* (53rd ed.). New York, NY: McGraw-Hill.

Chobanian, A. V. (2007). Isolated systolic hypertension in the elderly. *New England Journal of Medicine, 357*, 780–796.

Crawford, M. H. (2009). *Current diagnosis and treatment in cardiology* (3rd ed.) New York, NY: McGraw-Hill.

Gey, D. C., Lesho, E. P., & Manngold, J. (2004). Management of peripheral arterial disease. *American Family Physician, 69*, 525–533.

Hunt, S. A., Abraham, W. T., Chin, M. H., Feldman, A. M., Francis, G. S., Ganiats, T. G., . . . Heart Rhythm Society. (2005). ACC/AHA 2005 guideline update for the diagnosis and management of chronic heart failure in the adult: A report of the American College of Cardiology/American Heart Association Task Force on Practice Guidelines (writing committee to update the 2001 guidelines for the evaluation and management of heart failure): Developed in collaboration with the American College of Chest Physicians and the International Society for Heart and Lung Transplantation: Endorsed by the Heart Rhythm Society. *Circulation, 112*(12), e154–235.

James, P. A., Oparil, S., Carter, B. L., Cushman, W. C., Dennison-Himmelfarb, C., Handler, J., . . . Ortiz, E. (2013). 2014 evidence-based guideline for the management of high blood pressure in adults: Report from the panel members appointed to the Eighth Joint National Committee (JNC 8). *Journal of the American Medical Association, 311*(5), 507–520. doi:10.1001/jama.2013.284427. Retrieved from http://jama.jama-network.com/article.aspx?articleid=1791497

Levy, P. J. (2002). Epidemiology and pathophysiology of peripheral arterial disease. *Clinical Cornerstone, 4*, 1–15.

Mann, S. J. (2004). Interview—an overlooked cause of refractory hypertension. *Clinical Advisor, 7*(2), 28–36.

National Cholesterol Education Program. (2004). Third report of the Expert Panel on Detection, Evaluation, and Treatment of High Blood Cholesterol in Adults (Adult Treatment Panel III) 2004 update. Retrieved from http://www.nhlbi.nih.gov/guidelines/cholesterol/index.htm

Stone, N. J., Robinson, J., Lichtenstein, A. H., Bairey Merz, C. N., Blum, C. B., Eckel, R. H., . . . Wilson, P. W. F. (2013). 2013 ACC/AHA guideline on the treatment of blood cholesterol to reduce atherosclerotic cardiovascular risk in adults: A report of the American College of Cardiology/American Heart Association Task Force on Practice Guidelines. *Journal of the American College of Cardiology*. Retrieved from http://circ.ahajournals.org/content/early/2013/11/11/01.cir.0000437738.63853.7a

Sutters, M. (2014). Systemic hypertension. In S. J. McPhee & M. A. Papadakis (Eds.), *Current medical diagnosis and treatment* (53rd ed.). New York, NY: McGraw-Hill.

# Hematological and Oncological Disorders

*Sister Maria Salerno*

## COMMON ANEMIAS

- Anemia is a clinical condition characterized by a low circulating hemoglobin. The World Health Organization defines it in terms of peripheral blood hemoglobin < 13 g (hematocrit < 45%) for men and < 12 g (hematocrit < 37%) for women. Anemia may occur as a function of abnormal red blood cell development and division, abnormal hemoglobin synthesis, or accelerated red blood cell destruction. Anemias are classified based on red cell morphology (microcytic, normocytic, or macrocytic) and are further described based on the amount of pigment red blood cells contain (hypochromic, normochromic) and/or underlying etiology.

## MICROCYTIC ANEMIAS (MCV < 80 M³)

- Because the majority of the mature RBC volume is hemoglobin, abnormalities of hemoglobin cause a low mean cell volume (MCV); consequently, microcytic anemias are anemias characterized by hemoglobin abnormalities. The two microcytic anemias commonly encountered are iron deficiency anemia and thalassemia.

## IRON-DEFICIENCY ANEMIA

- Definition—a microcytic, hypochromic anemia with an MCV < 80 m³ caused by insufficient iron for hemoglobin synthesis

- Etiology/Incidence
  1. Slow, persistent blood loss is the most common cause of iron-deficiency anemia in adults; specific causes include menorrhagia, gastritis, aspirin ingestion, polyps, gastrointestinal (GI) neoplasms, peptic ulcer disease, and esophageal varices
  2. Inadequate iron intake (< 1–2 mg/day), e.g., persons on vegetarian diets, alcoholics, pregnant women, or adolescents whose demand is increased
  3. Impaired absorption of iron, e.g., after gastrectomy, in celiac disease
  4. Slow, persistent blood loss, e.g., menorrhagia, gastritis, aspirin ingestion, polyps, GI neoplasms, peptic ulcer disease, esophageal varices, hemorrhoids; in adult males and postmenopausal females, acute or chronic hemorrhage is most common cause
  5. The most common anemia throughout the world; particularly prevalent in women of childbearing age; estimated 20% of adult women, 50% of pregnant women, and 3% of adult males in the United States have iron deficiency

- Signs and Symptoms
  1. Depend on
     a. Rate at which anemia develops
     b. Age of the individual
     c. Individual's compensatory mechanisms
     d. Activity level
     e. Underlying disease state
     f. Severity of the anemia

2. General signs and symptoms
    a. Easily fatigued
    b. Dyspnea on exertion
    c. Dizziness
    d. Listlessness
    e. Pallor (conjunctiva, nail beds, mucous membranes)
    f. Weakness
    g. Headaches
    h. Tachycardia
    i. Wide pulse pressure
    j. Heart murmurs
    k. Myocardial hypertrophy
3. Findings specific to iron-deficiency anemia
    a. Pica
    b. Brittle, dry hair
    c. Flat or concave nail beds

- Differential Diagnosis
  1. Thalassemia
  2. Sideroblastic anemia
  3. Anemia of chronic disease
  4. Lead poisoning

- Physical Findings
  1. May be normal without overt findings in mild anemia
  2. General appearance—pale, lethargic
  3. Vital signs—pulse and respirations may be increased in moderate to severe anemia; in severe cases postural hypotension may be evident
  4. Integumentary—pallor and dryness of skin and mucous membranes; brittle, flattened, ridged, concave, or spoon-shaped nails (koilonychia); brittle, fine hair
  5. Cardiovascular—tachycardia, mild cardiac enlargement; functional systolic murmurs in severe anemias
  6. Abdominal—may be some hepatic enlargement
  7. Neurological—usually within normal limits

- Diagnostic Tests/Findings
  1. See **Tables 8-1** and **8-2** for laboratory tests used in diagnosis of common anemias
  2. Routine complete blood count (CBC) (with peripheral smear)
      a. Hemoglobin—< 13 g/dL in males; < 12 g/dL in females
      b. Hematocrit (Hct)—< 45% in males; < 37% in females
      c. Low MCV (microcytic) and mean corpuscular hemoglobin concentration (MCHC) (hypochromic)
      d. Increased red cell distribution width (RDW) (> 15%)
  3. Iron status determinants—serum ferritin is considered the most sensitive and most specific for iron deficiency; bone marrow studies are done if the diagnosis is unclear and/or there is a lack of response to a 3-week therapeutic trial
      a. High total iron binding capacity (TIBC)—usually normal or low in anemia of chronic disease (ACD)
      b. Low serum ferritin < 12 mg/L—infection, chronic disease, and liver disease may raise ferritin levels and mask coexisting iron deficiency; in these cases a serum ferritin level < 30 mg/L is consistent with iron deficiency
      c. Serum iron—low < 50 mg/dL; may be normal in early stages (oral contraceptives may cause false elevation)
      d. Low serum transferrin saturation—< 20%
      e. Bone marrow studies
          (1) Show depletion of iron (on staining), normocytic hyperplasia
          (2) Usually not part of initial workup

- Management/Treatment
  1. Diagnostic
      a. Once diagnosis is established, underlying cause must be identified and, if possible, corrected; bleeding must be suspected in the absence of clearly identifiable nutritional intake deficiency or increased body need
      b. Search for infection, trauma, neoplasm, GI disorders
      c. Stool guaiac, bilirubin, and additional studies may be needed to establish etiology
      d. Obtain physician consult on any patient with
          (1) Hct < 25%
          (2) Positive stool guaiac or history of bleeding
          (3) Family history of anemia
          (4) Suspected underlying inflammatory, infectious, or malignant disease
          (5) Failure to respond to iron supplementation
  2. Therapeutic
      a. Oral iron replacement
          (1) Oral is safer and much less expensive than intramuscular (IM) or intravenous (IV)
          (2) Begin 6-month trial of ferrous sulfate tablets, 325 mg up to 3 times a day after meals
          (3) Determine effectiveness of iron replacement therapy during the first 2 weeks of therapy (increased reticulocyte count)

Iron-Deficiency Anemia 119

**TABLE 8-1 Common Laboratory Tests Used in Diagnosing Anemia**

| | |
|---|---|
| Hematocrit (Hct) | Relative amount of plasma to total red blood cell mass; measure of RBC concentration. Normal 40–54% males; 38–47% females (Hct typically 3 x Hgb, e.g., Hgb 12 g/dL = Hct 36%) |
| Hemoglobin (Hgb) | Basic screening test for anemia; main component of erythrocytes; vehicle for transport of $O_2$ and $CO_2$; normal 13–18 g/100 mL males; 12–15 g/100 mL females |
| Red blood cell count (RBC) | Measure of number of Hgb-carrying red blood cells (RBCs, erythrocytes); needed to calculate other RBC indices |
| Mean corpuscular volume (MCV) | Mathematical measure of average RBC size; expressed in micro cubic millimeters; value classifies cells as microcytic, normocytic, macrocytic; normal 80–100 $m^3$ |
| Mean corpuscular Hgb (MCH) | Mathematical measure of hemoglobin concentration of average RBC; expressed in picograms; calculated by dividing Hgb in grams by number of RBCs; allows for classification of RBCs as hypochromic, normochromic; normal 27–31 pg/cell |
| Mean corpuscular Hgb concentration (MCHC) | Mathematical measure of concentration of Hgb in grams per 100 mL of RBCs; normal 32–36 g/dL or 32–36%; little help in identifying hypochromia or microcytosis |
| Red cell distribution width (RDW) | Mathematical coefficient of width variation in red cell size—RDW increase indicates greater variation in cell size; normal RDW 11–15% |
| Serum iron (SI) | Concentration of iron bound to transferrin; inverse correlation with TIBC; normal 50–150 mg/dL in adults; insensitive to early iron deficiency |
| Total iron binding capacity (TIBC) | Measures amount of iron that transferrin can still bind; inverse correlation with serum iron; normal 250–450 mg/dL in adults |
| Bilirubin (indirect) | Fractionation of total bilirubin; reflects breakdown of hemoglobin; elevated levels indicate hemolysis |
| % Transferrin saturation w (% SAT) | 100 x SI/TIBC; low sensitivity for iron deficiency; normal 20–50% |
| Serum ferritin | Correlates roughly with total iron stores; no diurnal variation; not affected by exogenous ingestion or injection, or specimen contamination; most sensitive and specific for iron deficiency; normal males 12–300 mg/L; females 12–150 mg/L (McPherson & Pinkus, 2007) |
| Coombs indirect | Detects free antibodies in patient's serum and certain RBC antigens |
| Peripheral blood smear | Smear of whole blood stained with Wright's stain; variations in cell morphology and staining characteristics important to diagnosis of hematological conditions |
| Bone marrow | Marrow aspirated for microscopic examination; indicated when anemia not obviously due to iron deficiency; iliac crest preferred to sternum site |

*Note*: Laboratory reference ranges differ among laboratories. Check normal values in each laboratory where tests are conducted.

(4) Refer those on oral iron replacement therapy to a physician if 2 g/100 mL increase in Hgb is not seen in 3–4 weeks; in uncomplicated iron deficiency, a 1 g per week increase is expected

(5) Levels return to normal within 2 months, 3–6 months more needed to replace stores
(6) Response failure usually due to nonadherence

**TABLE 8-2** Select Morphological and Etiological Categories of Anemia and Related Laboratory Findings

|  | Macrocytic (MCV > 100) |  | Microcytic (MCV < 80) |  | Normocytic (MCV 80–100) |
| --- | --- | --- | --- | --- | --- |
|  | B$_{12}$ Deficiency | Folate Deficiency | Iron Deficiency | Thalassemia | Anemia of Chronic Disease |
| MCH | normal | normal | low | low | normal |
| Fe | high | high | normal/low | normal/slightly high | low–high |
| TIBC | normal | normal | high | normal | normal/low |
| Ferritin | high | high | low | normal | normal/high |
| Vitamin B$_{12}$ | low | normal | normal | normal | normal |
| Folate | normal | low | normal | normal/low | normal/low |

b. Parenteral iron is indicated if patient cannot tolerate or absorb oral iron or if iron loss exceeds oral replacement; IM or IV iron dextran is used (very rarely needed or used)
   (1) More expensive
   (2) Associated with significant side effects
      (a) Anaphylaxis
      (b) Phlebitis
      (c) Regional lymphadenopathy
      (d) Serum-sickness-type reaction
      (e) Staining of IM injection sites
   (3) Dose based on the patient's weight
3. Education
   a. Cause of iron deficiency and treatment plan
   b. Purpose, dosage, side effects, toxic effects of iron replacement
      (1) Side effects of nausea, GI irritation, constipation, diarrhea, and black stools
      (2) Food and fluid taken concurrently may interfere with absorption but may be warranted to alleviate gastric distress
      (3) Taking with orange juice or other source of vitamin C (ascorbic acid) will enhance absorption
      (4) Milk and antacids will interfere with absorption
      (5) Monitor and discuss with patients concurrent use of over-the-counter medications—some products such as urine and stool deodorizers often used by elderly with incontinence problems can lead to iron overdose and heart failure
      (6) Therapy should continue for 6 or more months to replenish tissue stores
   c. Nutrition—foods high in iron include organ and lean meats, egg yolk, shellfish, apricots, peaches, prunes, grapes, raisins, green leafy vegetables, iron-fortified breads and cereals

## THALASSEMIA

- Definition—thalassemia is a group of genetic inherited syndromes of abnormal hemoglobin synthesis

- Etiology/Incidence
  1. Inherited, autosomal recessive disorder that results in impaired synthesis of either one or more of the alpha or beta chain of adult hemoglobin; four genes control alpha chain production, two control beta chain production
  2. Second most common cause of microcytic anemia
     a. Alpha thalassemia more common in African Americans, Chinese, Vietnamese, Cambodians, and Laotians
     b. Beta thalassemia more common in those of Mediterranean descent (Italians, Greeks, some Arabs, and Sephardic Jews)
  3. In United States more common than iron deficiency in African Americans, Asian Americans, and Italian Americans

- Signs and Symptoms—the severity of the anemia can range from mild to severe depending on the number of hemoglobin-controlling genes involved; forms seen in adults include
  1. Alpha trait (carrier state) (one of four alpha chain-forming genes affected)—usually asymptomatic
  2. Alpha thalassemia minor (two of four alpha chain-forming genes affected) and betathalassemia minor (heterozygous form)—both are usually asymptomatic and have mild presentations with mild to moderate microcytic, hypochromic anemia, enlarged liver and spleen, bronze coloring of the skin, and bone marrow hyperplasia
  3. Beta thalassemia major (homozygous form affecting both beta chain-forming genes) also called Cooley's anemia—severe anemia

with significant cardiovascular burden; high output congestive failure is common; fractures related to bone marrow expansion; retarded growth and maturation; in addition to general signs and symptoms presented in section on iron-deficiency anemia earlier in this chapter
   4. Hemoglobin H disease (three of four alpha hemoglobin chain-forming genes affected)—occurs predominantly in Chinese; moderate to severe microcytic anemia with splenomegaly

- Differential Diagnosis
  1. Iron-deficiency anemia
  2. Sideroblastic anemia
  3. Anemia of chronic disease

- Physical Findings—will generally be within normal limits unless the more severe forms of thalassemia are encountered
  1. General appearance—pallor or bronze appearance; mild listlessness
  2. Abdominal—enlarged liver, enlarged spleen
  3. Cardiovascular—tachycardia, widened pulse pressure, systolic murmur if anemia is moderate or severe
  4. Respiratory—may have increased respiratory rate
  5. Musculoskeletal—some bone deformity of the face (chipmunk deformity) related to expansion of bones caused by hyperplastic marrow
  6. Neurological—within normal limits

- Diagnostic Tests/Findings
  1. Hgb—decreased
  2. MCV—markedly low; comparatively lower than in iron deficiency
  3. Serum iron—normal or increased
  4. TIBC—normal
  5. Ferritin—normal or increased
  6. RDW—normal
  7. Hemoglobin electrophoresis—demonstrates decreased alpha or beta hemoglobin chains
  8. Peripheral smear will show microcytosis, variable hypochromia, target cells (thin, fragile RBC), basophilic stippling
  9. Skull and skeletal radiographs—widened marrow spaces in skull and long bones; osteoporosis

- Management/Treatment
  1. No specific treatment for mild to moderate forms
  2. Iron supplementation generally contraindicated in all thalassemias because iron overload can result—patients with alpha trait and coexisting iron deficiency should be referred to physician for iron supplementation
  3. Chronic folate supplementation is used in certain circumstances; should be initiated by hematology
  4. Severe forms should be referred to a hematologist for treatment, which often includes transfusions and chelation therapy to avoid fatal iron overload (hemochromatosis)
  5. Refer for genetic counseling
  6. Stress overall good nutrition without additional iron supplementation
  7. Discuss signs and symptoms of iron overload
     a. Weakness/lassitude
     b. Loss of body hair
     c. Weight loss
     d. Palmar erythema
     e. Gynecomastia
     f. Loss of libido
     g. Abdominal pain
     h. Thinning, darkening skin
     i. Pain and or stiffness in joints
     j. Blurred vision or other symptoms related to onset of diabetes
     k. Shortness of breath
     l. Swelling in ankles

## MACROCYTIC ANEMIAS (MCV > 100 M³)

- Unlike microcytic anemias, macrocytic anemias are not characterized by hemoglobin abnormalities—hemoglobin synthesis is unimpaired; the etiology centers around inadequate red blood cell synthesis, and consequently macrocytic anemias are typically characterized by a low red blood cell count—each existing red blood cell is packed to excess with hemoglobin, resulting in macrocytosis.

## PERNICIOUS ANEMIA

- Definition—a megaloblastic, macrocytic, normochromic anemia caused by a deficiency of intrinsic factor produced by the stomach that results in malabsorption of vitamin $B_{12}$ necessary for DNA synthesis and maturation of RBCs

- Etiology/Incidence
  1. Typically occurs secondary to other factors, which lead to decreased production of intrinsic factor or decreased absorption of vitamin $B_{12}$
     a. Loss of parietal cells postgastrectomy
     b. Overgrowth of intestinal organisms
     c. Ileal resection or abnormalities
     d. Fish tapeworm
     e. Congenital enzyme deficiencies
  2. Less commonly due to an autoimmune reaction involving the gastric parietal cell that results in nonproduction of intrinsic factor and atrophy of gastric mucosa

3. Vegans with no vitamin B$_{12}$ supplementation
4. Common in Caucasians of northern European descent
5. Both sexes equally affected
6. Usually presents around age 60
7. Increased incidence in those with other autoimmune disease, e.g., hypothyroidism

- Signs and Symptoms
    1. Weakness
    2. Sore tongue or glossitis
    3. Peripheral paresthesia—numbness, burning, tingling
    4. Palpitations
    5. Dizziness
    6. Swelling of legs
    7. Anorexia
    8. Diarrhea
    9. Mucositis
    10. Dementia and spinal cord degeneration in advanced stages

- Differential Diagnosis
    1. Folate deficiency
    2. Anemia of liver disease
    3. Myelodysplastic syndromes

- Physical Findings
    1. General appearance—premature aging; premature graying of hair
    2. HEENT—smooth beefy red tongue (glossitis); sclera and skin may be slightly icteric
    3. Cardiovascular—systolic flow murmur (hemic murmur), tachycardia, and cardiomegaly if anemia is severe
    4. Abdomen—hepatomegaly and splenomegaly may be evident
    5. Neurological—deep tendon reflexes increased or decreased; diminished position sense; poor or absent vibratory sense in lower extremities; ataxia; poor finger–nose coordination; positive Romberg and Babinski; mental status changes ranging from mild forgetfulness and irritability to psychotic behavior (only form of anemia to produce neurological findings early in disease; neurological changes may precede anemia)

- Diagnostic Tests/Findings
    1. Hgb and Hct—decreased
    2. RBC—decreased
    3. Reticulocytes—normal or low with anisocytosis and poikilocytosis
    4. MCV—increased > 100 m$^3$ (usually markedly increased)
    5. MCHC—normal
    6. Serum vitamin B$_{12}$—may be decreased < 100 pg/mL; however, normal serum vitamin B$_{12}$ does not preclude diagnosis
    7. Increased lactic acid dehydrogenase (LDH)
    8. Serum folate and/or RBC level—normal or decreased
    9. Elevated methylmalonate (MMA) levels
    10. Parietal cell antibodies may be present
    11. Urinalysis—increased urobilinogen
    12. White blood cell (WBC) and platelet count decreased in severe cases

- Management/Treatment
    1. Correct underlying cause if possible
    2. Medication
        a. Vitamin B$_{12}$ (cyanocobalamin) 100 mg IM daily for 1 week; decrease frequency and administer a total of 2,000 mg during the first 6 weeks of therapy; maintenance treatment requires lifelong administration of 100 mg IM monthly
        b. In select cases, oral cobalamin in high doses (1,000 mg per day) can replace parenteral for maintenance, but must be taken daily and consistently
        c. If anemia is severe, may need K$^+$ supplementation to avoid hypokalemia
        d. Follow up elderly adults and those with cardiovascular symptoms 48 hours after initiating therapy; rapid increase in RBC production can lead to hypervolemia in these persons
        e. Consider concomitant iron supplementation during first month of therapy; rapid blood cell regeneration increases iron requirement and may lead to iron deficiency
    3. Education
        a. Teach client about etiology and nature of the disease
        b. Discuss need for lifelong vitamin B$_{12}$ replacement by injection
        c. Provide information on side effects of vitamin B$_{12}$ injections
            (1) Pain and burning at injection site
            (2) Peripheral vascular thrombosis
            (3) Transient diarrhea
        d. Central nervous system (CNS) symptoms/signs are reversible if present < 6 months prior to treatment
    4. Follow-up—check initial hematological response in 4–6 weeks; then every 6 months for Hct and stool for occult blood; endoscopy every 5 years; incidence of gastric cancer increased in persons with pernicious anemia

# FOLIC ACID–DEFICIENCY ANEMIA

- Definition—macrocytic, normochromic, megaloblastic anemia caused by a deficiency of folic acid needed for DNA synthesis, RBC maturation, and maintenance of gastric mucosa

# Folic Acid–Deficiency Anemia

- Etiology/Incidence
    1. Inadequate intake may be relative to malabsorption syndrome or increased demand as in pregnancy and infancy; body stores depleted more rapidly than vitamin $B_{12}$
    2. Drugs that may cause decreased folic acid levels include oral contraceptives, phenytoin, antimalarials, estrogen, chloramphenicol, phenobarbital, trimethoprim/sulfamethoxazole, and sulfasalazine
    3. Found in all races and in all age groups
    4. More common than pernicious anemia, especially in alcoholics and other chronically malnourished persons, e.g., anorexics, many elderly adults, and those who do not eat fresh fruits and vegetables (especially green leafy) or who overcook them

- Signs and Symptoms
    1. Similar to those of vitamin $B_{12}$ deficiency but more severe; neurological signs are absent
    2. General signs and symptoms
        a. Easily fatigued
        b. Dyspnea on exertion
        c. Dizziness
        d. Listlessness
        e. Pallor (conjunctiva, nail beds, mucous membranes)
        f. Faintness
        g. Weakness
        h. Headaches
        i. Tachycardia
        j. Wide pulse pressure
        k. Heart murmurs
        l. Myocardial hypertrophy
        m. Angina
        n. Anorexia
        o. Pica

- Differential Diagnosis
    1. Pernicious anemia
    2. Anemia of liver disease
    3. Myelodysplastic syndromes

- Physical Findings—similar to those found in most anemias
    1. General appearance—pale, lethargic, or no overt signs if anemia is mild
    2. Vital signs—pulse and respirations may be increased in moderate to severe anemia; in severe cases postural hypotension may be evident
    3. Integumentary—pallor and dryness of skin and mucous membranes; brittle nails; brittle, fine hair
    4. HEENT—glossitis, angular stomatitis or cheilitis; pale conjunctiva and gums
    5. Cardiovascular—tachycardia; mild cardiac enlargement; functional systolic murmurs in severe anemias
    6. Abdominal—may be some hepatic enlargement
    7. Neurological—usually within normal limits

- Diagnostic Tests/Findings
    1. Hct—decreased
    2. MCV—elevated
    3. MCHC—normal
    4. RBC folate level—< 150 ng/mL and/or RBC level decreased
    5. Serum folate—< 3 ng/mL; less reliable than RBC folate
    6. MMA—normal
    7. Serum vitamin $B_{12}$—normal
    8. Parietal cell antibodies absent

- Management/Treatment
    1. Correct underlying cause if able
        a. Improve dietary intake
        b. Change medications that may inhibit vitamin $B_{12}$ absorption if possible
    2. Folate 1 mg orally or parenterally per day
        a. Duration of treatment dependent on etiology and its elimination
        b. If related to malabsorption (e.g., sprue) up to 5 mg/day—very high doses of folate may be toxic and should be ordered only by hematology
        c. Large doses of folic acid will correct hematological abnormalities of vitamin $B_{12}$ deficiency, but not arrest neurological abnormalities
    3. Education—especially important for women of childbearing age because deficiency during first trimester is associated with neural tube defects in the fetus
        a. Nature and cause of anemia
        b. Need for and purpose of therapeutic replacement
        c. Teach dietary sources of folic acid, which include asparagus, bananas, fish, green leafy vegetables, peanut butter, oatmeal, red beans, beef liver, wheat bran
            (1) Encourage daily intake from these foods
            (2) Instructions in preparation because overcooking can destroy folic acid
            (3) Provide client with list of foods high in folic acid
        d. Need for frequent rest periods until anemia is corrected
    4. Follow-up
        a. Check initial hematological response with Hct and in 4–6 weeks
            (1) Hct begins to rise after the second week

(2) Total correction expected within 2 months
   b. Individuals with a good response can be followed every 6–12 months if they must continue therapy

## NORMOCYTIC ANEMIAS (MCV 80–100 M³)

- Normocytic anemias are characterized neither by hemoglobin or red blood cell abnormalities; therefore cell volume is normal.

## ANEMIA OF CHRONIC DISEASE (ACD)

- Definition—a chronic, normochromic, normocytic, hypoproliferative anemia associated with chronic inflammatory disease, e.g., systemic lupus, rheumatoid arthritis; infection, e.g., bacterial endocarditis, tuberculosis, AIDS, Crohn's disease, and some malignancies; *often progresses to a hypochromic anemia*

- Etiology/Incidence
  1. Etiology not fully understood but involves decreased erythrocyte life span, ineffective erythropoiesis, and disturbances of the iron cycle
  2. Most common cause of hypoproliferative, normocytic anemia
  3. Most common anemia in the elderly population

- Signs and Symptoms
  1. General symptoms common to all anemias such as fatigue, weakness, exertional dyspnea, lightheadedness, and anorexia
  2. Usually fewer and milder than most other anemias; Hgb rarely drops below 9 g/dL
  3. Other signs and symptoms are usually related to the specific underlying disease and may be more overt than those of anemia

- Differential Diagnosis
  1. Aplastic anemia
  2. Pure red blood cell aplasia
  3. Infiltration marrow diseases
  4. Exclude reversible causes

- Physical Findings
  1. General appearance—may appear thin, pale, toxic, or chronically ill
  2. Signs of underlying chronic disorder may dominate
  3. Vital signs—increased pulse and respirations
  4. Skin—pale, jaundiced, moist
  5. HEENT—sclera icteric, tongue coated
  6. Cardiovascular—cardiomegaly, tachycardia, systolic murmurs
  7. Abdomen—splenomegaly, hepatomegaly

- Diagnostic Tests/Findings
  1. Hct—low
  2. Hgb—low (if < 9 g/dL, consider other causes)
  3. MCV—normal or slightly reduced
  4. Serum iron—low
  5. TIBC—normal or low
  6. Serum ferritin—normal or increased
  7. Percentage of iron saturation (Fe/TIBC)—30% or more rules out iron deficiency

- Management/Treatment
  1. Treatment of associated disease
  2. Adequate nutritional intake; use of vitamin $B_{12}$, folic acid, and liver extract have not been effective in treatment of this type of anemia
  3. Adequate rest
  4. Erythropoietin alfa intravenous or subcutaneous is reserved for those who are transfusion dependent or those for whom the quality of life would be greatly improved by the hematological response

## SICKLE CELL ANEMIA

- Definition—a chronic hemolytic anemia characterized by sickle-shaped RBCs

- Etiology/Incidence
  1. Autosomal recessive genetic disorder; individual is homozygous for hemoglobin (Hb SS)
  2. Abnormal hemoglobin (Hb S) develops in place of hemoglobin A (Hb A)
  3. Some individuals may have sickle cell trait (heterozygous with about one-fourth of their hemoglobin in abnormal S form and remainder as normal A)
  4. Mutation that causes Hb S to develop involves one amino acid; one valine amino acid is substituted for a glutamic acid
  5. Prevalent in black persons of African or African American ancestry; also found at a lower frequency in persons of Mediterranean ancestry

- Signs and Symptoms
  1. Sickle cell trait
     a. Asymptomatic except in extreme conditions
     b. Symptoms from vaso-occlusion occur only in cases of severe hypoxia
  2. Sickle cell anemia
     a. Manifestations due to anemia, vaso-occlusive events, and secondary end organ damage
        (1) Osteomyelitis

(2) Retinopathy
(3) Renal disease—hematuria
(4) Cardiomegaly
(5) Nonpalpable spleen in adults
b. Increased susceptibility to infection
c. Vaso-occlusive crises
(1) Due to an increased rate of sickling
(2) Precipitating factors include conditions that cause hypoxia or deoxygenation of the RBCs, e.g., viral or bacterial infections, high altitudes, emotional or physical stress, surgery, blood loss, dehydration; occasionally, crisis occurs spontaneously
(3) Episodes characterized by sudden onset of excruciating pain in back, chest, or extremities
(4) Occasionally low-grade fever may occur 1–2 days following attack
(5) Pain may last from hours to days
(6) Severe abdominal pain with vomiting may be present

- Differential Diagnosis
    1. Acute pulmonary infarction without sickle beta thalassemia
    2. Anemia from other causes
        a. Sickle thalassemia
        b. Hemoglobin C disorders
            (1) Milder onset and course than sickle cell anemia
            (2) No Hb S on electrophoresis
    3. Acute hepatitis
    4. Choledocholithiasis
    5. Cholecystitis

- Physical Findings
    1. During vaso-occlusive crises, there may be no external findings such as heat, swelling, or tenderness over the affected bones; if bone infarction occurs close to a joint, an effusion can develop
    2. Chronic findings
        a. Skin ulcers/jaundice
        b. Mild scleral icterus; retinal hemorrhage or detachment, neovascularization
        c. Cardiomegaly, systolic murmur
        d. Hepatomegaly
        e. Degenerative arthritis

- Diagnostic Tests/Findings
    1. Peripheral smear
        a. Sickle cell trait—normal
        b. Sickle cell anemia—partially or completely sickled cells
    2. Sickle cell preparation/sickledex
        a. Sickle cell trait—sickle cells
        b. Sickle cell anemia—sickle cells
        c. Used for initial screening
        d. Cannot differentiate between anemia/trait
    3. Hemoglobin electrophoresis
        a. Sickle cell trait—Hb S and Hb A
        b. Sickle cell anemia—Hb S
        c. Used for confirmation and discrimination between anemia/trait
    4. MCV normal (low if beta thalassemia is also present)

- Management/Treatment
    1. Physician referral for suspected cases and consultation for management
    2. Therapeutic—primarily supportive
        a. Chronic folic acid supplementation
        b. Use of cytotoxic agents to reduce frequency of painful episodes
        c. Antibiotic prophylaxis
    3. In acute painful episodes
        a. Analgesia
        b. Large volume IV fluids
        c. Oxygen to treat hypoxia
        d. Antibiotics to treat associated bacterial infections
        e. Blood transfusions reserved for aplastic or hemolytic crises and during third trimester of pregnancy
    4. Referral for genetic counseling of identified heterozygotes (sickle cell trait) and prenatal diagnostic services for pregnancies at risk for sickle cell anemia

# LEUKEMIA

- Definition—acquired, neoplastic, myeloproliferative disorder of hematopoietic stem cells

- Etiology/Incidence
    1. In most cases no known cause can be found
    2. Possible causes include
        a. Exposure to ionizing radiation and certain chemicals, e.g., benzene, prior exposure to alkylating agents
        b. Genetic and congenital factors
    3. Incidence of all leukemias is approximately 13 per 100,000 per year
    4. More frequent in males than in females

- General features of the four common forms of leukemia are shown in **Table 8-3**

- Differential Diagnosis
    1. Viral-induced cytopenia, lymphadenopathy
    2. Immune- or drug-induced cytopenia
    3. Aplastic anemia

## TABLE 8-3 Comparison of Most Common Types of Leukemia

| Type | Age of Onset | Signs and Symptoms and Physical Findings | Diagnostic Tests/Findings | Prognosis |
|---|---|---|---|---|
| Acute lymphocytic (ALL) | Childhood; more gradual rise in frequency in later life; 20% of acute adult | Fever; pallor, bleeding; anorexia; fatigue; generalized lymphadenopathy and infection, joint pain, etc. | Cytopenia, pancytopenia WBC—H, L, or N RBC, Hgb, Hct—L Platelets—L Bone marrow—lymphoblasts | Good response to treatment; 80% of adults have complete remission |
| Acute myelogenous (AML) or nonlymphocytic (ANLL) | Increase with age; 50% younger than age 50 years | Fatigue; weakness; headache; mouth sores; bleeding; fever; sternal tenderness; occasional lymphadenopathy | RBC, Hgb, Hct—L Platelet ct—very low WBC—H to L Myeloblasts—many | Remission rates range from 50% to 85%; patients > 50 years are less likely to achieve complete remission |
| Chronic lymphocytic (CLL) | Mean age of onset 65 years | May be asymptomatic; may have fatigue, anorexia, weight loss, dyspnea on exertion; splenomegaly; lymphadenopathy; hepatomegaly | Hallmark is sustained absolute lymphocytosis 40,000–150,000/mL; bone marrow—increased lymphocytes | Median survival—approximately 10 yrs |
| Chronic myelogenous (CML) or chronic granulocytic (CGL) | Occurs most often at median age of 42 | May be asymptomatic; or insidious onset of nonspecific symptoms, e.g., fatigue, weakness, anorexia, weight loss, fever, night sweats, splenomegaly; blurred vision; respiratory distress; priapism, sternal tenderness | RBC, Hgb, Hct—L Platelet count—H early, L later WBC—H; leukocytosis with immature granulocytes WBC—about 150,000–200,000/mL in symptomatic patient; bone marrow—Ph[1] chromosome presence is significant | No advantage to early therapy if asymptomatic; 60% of young adults with allogeneic bone marrow transplants complete cure; median survival in nontransplanted patients is 3–4 years |

H = high; L = low; N = normal.

- Diagnostic Tests/Findings (see Table 8-3)
    1. CBC/differential—subnormal RBC, neutrophils, and occasionally subnormal platelets
    2. Sedimentation rate—elevated
    3. Reticulocyte count—< 0.5%
    4. Bone marrow studies—confirmatory for final diagnosis
    5. Chest radiograph—identification of mediastinal mass
    6. Ultrasound or CT—organomegaly

- Management/Treatment
    1. Physician referral for suspected cases
        a. Goal of treatment is remission
        b. Chemotherapy
        c. Bone marrow transplantation
    2. Assistance in meeting psychosocial needs
    3. Assistance for patient and families in adjusting to chronic effects of illness, e.g., dependence, withdrawal, changes in role responsibilities, alterations in body image
    4. Patient education
        a. Importance of compliance with chemotherapy regimens; side effects and management
        b. Disease process and rationale for treatment
        c. Adaptation to any physical limitations

## NON-HODGKIN'S LYMPHOMA

- Definition—heterogeneous group of lymphocytic malignancies with absence of giant Reed–Sternberg cells characteristic of Hodgkin's disease; characterized as indolent or aggressive

- Etiology/Incidence
    1. Etiology unclear; animal studies have suggested a viral etiology
    2. Other factors associated with increased incidence include
        a. Ionizing radiation
        b. Hereditary predisposition
        c. Congenital or acquired immunodeficiency
        d. Exposure to pesticides
    3. Approximately 55,000 new cases occur each year in the United States and appear to be increasing
    4. Most common neoplasm between ages of 20 and 40 years; with increased incidence of AIDS, number of cases has sharply increased

- Signs and Symptoms
    1. More than two-thirds of patients present with persistent painless peripheral lymphadenopathy
    2. Some patients may present with persistent cough and chest discomfort (mediastinal involvement)
    3. If abdominal contents involved, chronic pain, abdominal fullness, early satiety, or viscus obstruction may be presenting symptom
    4. Diffuse disease may present with skin lesions, testicular masses
    5. Fever, night sweats, weight loss

- Differential Diagnosis
    1. Infectious mononucleosis
    2. Cytomegalovirus infection
    3. Human immunodeficiency virus involvement
    4. Toxoplasmosis
    5. Other malignant tumors
    6. Cat scratch disease
    7. Tuberculosis
    8. Syphilis
    9. Sarcoidosis

- Physical Findings
    1. Painless peripheral lymphadenopathy may be initial finding
    2. May present with abdominal mass, massive splenomegaly
    3. Early systemic findings usually absent

- Diagnostic Tests/Findings
    1. Requires skilled interpretation of adequate tumor tissue to determine tumor architecture and cell type
    2. B cell and T cell typing—complements pathological interpretation
    3. Bone marrow biopsy—pathological confirmation of disease process
    4. Staging procedures conducted once diagnosis established—no perfect classification system exists; various types include the Rappaport classification, Luke-Collins classification, the International Working Formulation National Cancer Institute (NCI), Ann Arbor staging system is most popular
    5. Chest radiograph may show mediastinal mass

- Management/Treatment—based on grade and extent of disease
    1. Radiotherapy
    2. Chemotherapy
    3. Bone marrow transplantation
    4. Newer modalities include monoclonal antibodies (MAbs) alone and combined with radionuclides or toxins to produce cytotoxic effects; cytokines, e.g., interferons, tumor necrosis factor, and interleukin 2 are currently under study
    5. General considerations
        a. Prognosis not usually as good as with Hodgkin's disease
        b. Both family and patient require supportive therapy during diagnosis and treatment stages
        c. Education and necessity of drug compliance important factor
        d. Increased susceptibility to infection

# HODGKIN'S DISEASE

- Definition—malignant disorder with lymphoreticular proliferation

- Etiology/Incidence
    1. Cause is unknown
    2. People with a history of infectious mononucleosis due to Epstein-Barr virus are at greater risk; virus may activate a cellular pathway that leads to proliferation
    3. Approximately 8,000 new cases are diagnosed each year in the United States
    4. Most common malignancy in the 10–30 age group; average age is 28 years; peaks at 15–24 years and again after age 55
    5. More common in males
    6. Siblings have a three times higher risk than the general population
    7. Mortality in the United States has fallen more rapidly for adult Hodgkin's lymphoma than for any other malignancy; largely related to improved treatment

- Signs and Symptoms
    1. Most patients present with a painless, enlarging mass, most often in the neck or occasionally in axilla or inguinal region; often the only manifestation at time of diagnosis

2. Older patients may present with
   a. Fatigue
   b. Weight loss
   c. Persistent fever and/or night sweats
3. Pruritus—may be mild and localized, but may also be progressive; rarely occurs in the absence of fever
4. An unexplained symptom is immediate pain in diseased areas after consuming alcoholic beverages

- Differential Diagnosis
  1. Infectious mononucleosis
  2. Toxoplasmosis
  3. Cytomegalic inclusion disease
  4. Non-Hodgkin's lymphoma
  5. Leukemia
  6. Bronchogenic carcinoma
  7. Sarcoidosis
  8. Cat scratch disease

- Physical Findings
  1. Initial findings are usually enlargement of cervical, axillary, or inguinal lymph nodes (movable, nontender)
  2. Other findings may include hepatomegaly and splenomegaly; usually not present unless the disease is advanced

- Diagnostic Tests/Findings
  1. Presence of characteristic Reed–Sternberg giant cell on biopsy of lymph node tissue or other sites (needle aspiration not sufficient)
  2. WBC—polymorphonuclear leukocytosis may be present
  3. CBC—hypochromic, microcytic anemia in advanced disease
  4. Low serum iron, low iron binding capacity
  5. Chest radiological examinations—to determine mediastinal involvement

- Management/Treatment
  1. Physician referral for suspected cases
     a. Radiotherapy
     b. Chemotherapy
     c. Autologous bone marrow transplant for chemotherapy failures
  2. More than 75% of all newly diagnosed patients with adult Hodgkin's lymphoma can be cured with combination chemotherapy and/or radiation therapy
  3. Once patient is in remission, ongoing maintenance treatment is usually not needed; patients need to be instructed in the importance of returning for follow-up visits
  4. Patient education
     a. Gonadal side effects of treatment
     b. Consideration of sperm banking for males
     c. Risk of secondary malignancy

**Special Considerations in the Hospitalized Patient**

- Immune Thrombocytopenia Purpura
  - Definition—an autoimmune condition characterized by accelerated platelet destruction as a consequence of immune-mediated pathogenic antibody formation. In addition to the presence of autoantibodies that destroy platelets, many patients have a coincident inability to compensate
  - Etiology/Incidence
    - Idiopathic autoimmune disease
    - Infection, e.g., HIV and hepatitis C
    - Connective tissue disease
    - Lymphoproliferative disease
    - Numerous medications, e.g., heparin, may produce thrombocytopenia
  - Signs and Symptoms—typically do not occur until platelets count < 30,000/mcL
    - Spontaneous bruising
    - Epistaxis
    - Gingival bleeding
    - Hematuria
  - Differential Diagnosis
    - Bone marrow failure
    - Thrombocytic thrombocytopenia purpura
    - Heparin-induced thrombocytopenia
    - Drug-induced thrombocytopenia
    - von Willebrand disease
  - Physical Findings
    - Symptoms of underlying disease, e.g., HIV or hepatitis
    - Ecchymoses
  - Diagnostic Tests/Findings
    - Isolated thrombocytopenia is hallmark finding (platelets < 50,000/mcL)
    - Low Hgb/Hct if patient bleeding
    - Consider bone marrow analysis
    - Megakaryocyte abnormalities not likely
  - Management/Treatment
    - If other cause of thrombocytopenia identified, manage as able
    - If platelet count > 30,000/mcL, no treatment indicated; monitor for progression
    - When platelet count < 30,000/mcL:

- High-dose steroid pulse therapy
- Consider intravenous infusion of immunoglobulins (IVIG) or anti-D
- For recurrence, resume steroids and initial options or rituximab or thrombopoetin receptor agonist
- All bleeding patients should be transfused with platelets
- Splenectomy for those refractory to second-line agents
- Disseminated Intravascular Coagulation (DIC)
  - Definition—uncontrolled activation of the clotting cascade leading to depletion of coagulation factors and ultimately inability to clot in the setting of vascular insult
  - Etiology/Incidence
    - Sepsis
    - Malignancy
    - Labor and delivery
    - Trauma
    - Vascular stasis
    - Other forms of overwhelming systemic insult
  - Signs and Symptoms
    - Bleeding at multiple sites
      - Catheter insertion
      - Incisions
      - Vaginally
      - Sclera
    - DIC associated with malignancy (Trousseau syndrome) may present with multiple thrombi/emboli
  - Differential Diagnosis
    - Consumptive coagulopathies
    - Thrombotic thrombocytopenia purpura—hemolytic uremic syndrome
    - Heparin-induced thrombocytopenia (HITS)
    - Liver disease
    - Primary clotting disorders, e.g., hemophilia
  - Physical Findings
    - Bleeding from three unrelated sites
    - Ecchymoses at sites of puncture
    - Physical findings associated with underlying trigger
    - Hypotension, tachycardia, and other findings associated with volume contraction
    - Petechiae
    - Purpura
    - Thrombosis
  - Diagnostic Tests/Findings
    - No single test available to confirm DIC
    - Supportive tests—emphasis is that repeat measures are more useful than isolated values are
      - Platelet count < 50,000/mcL with a trend downward
      - aPTT or PT prolonged in > 50% of patients, but normal values cannot rule out DIC
      - Protein C may be decreased
      - Antithrombin may be decreased
      - Elevated D-dimer
      - Elevated fibrin degradation products (FDP)
      - Peripheral blood smear may demonstrate schistocytes
    - Scoring system for DIC by International Society on Thrombosis and Haemostasis
      - Score > 5 is a strong indicator of DIC
      - Score < 5 does not rule out DIC
        - Platelet count < 50,000/mcL = 2 points; 50,000 – 100,000/mcL = 1 point; > 100,000/mcL = 0 points
        - Elevated fibrin markers (FDP) strong increase = 3 points; moderate increase = 2 points; no increase = 0 points
        - Prolonged PT > 6 seconds = 2 points; 3 to 6 seconds = 1 points; < 3 seconds = 0 points
        - Fibrinogen level < 1 g/L = 1 point; > 1 g/L = 0 points
  - Management/Treatment
    - Underlying condition must be managed—in most cases treatment is supportive pending successful resolution of underlying disease process
    - Transfusion of blood products and coagulation factors depends on specific underlying deficiencies if severe bleeding has occurred or is likely to occur
    - Heparin use is controversial but may be beneficial in specific clinical circumstances; contraindicated if platelets cannot be maintained > 50,000/mcL or if imminent surgery is likely
    - Recombinant thrombomodulin in severe sepsis and malignancy

## QUESTIONS

■ Select the best answer.

### Questions 1 through 7 refer to the following scenario.

A 50-year-old male of Italian descent presents for a routine work-related health assessment. He has no complaints. His history and physical examination are unremarkable. A routine CBC reveals the following: Hgb 11.2 g/dL, MCV 72m$^3$, WBC 5.7 x 10$^3$, Hct 35%, and MCH 25.

1. Based on this information, how would his anemia be classified?

    a. Normocytic, normochromic
    b. Microcytic, hypochromic
    c. Macrocytic, hypochromic
    d. Microcytic, normochromic

2. Which aspect of this patient's history would provide the least useful information for diagnostic decision making?

    a. Diet (including alcohol use)
    b. Social history
    c. Family history
    d. Medical history

3. The patient in the preceding questions has a diet with regular daily intake of lean red meats, vegetables, and fruits and alcohol use once or twice a year. He admits to taking Maalox (calcium carbonate) almost daily for indigestion. He says that weak blood runs in his family, although he has never had this problem. He has no surgical history and has never been treated for any medical problems except high cholesterol, which was treated with diet and exercise. This information helps rule out which of the following as cause for his anemia?

    a. Folate deficiency
    b. Inadequate dietary intake
    c. GI bleeding
    d. Malabsorption of vitamins and minerals

4. This patient's lack of abnormal physical signs and symptoms:

    a. Probably indicates a lab error in the blood work
    b. Is not unusual given the degree of his anemia
    c. Is not unusual in a patient of this age
    d. May be masked by use of Maalox

5. Your next step would be to:

    a. Order vitamin B$_{12}$ and folate serum levels
    b. Order serum iron and TIBC
    c. Obtain a urine culture
    d. Order MMA test

6. What other test would be essential at this point?

    a. Stool guaiac
    b. GI series
    c. Bilirubin
    d. Liver function tests

7. Which is the most likely etiology of the type of anemia exhibited in this patient?

    a. Vitamin B$_{12}$ or folate deficiency
    b. Chronic disease
    c. Dehydration
    d. GI bleeding

8. If you obtain a negative stool guaiac in a male patient with a microcytic, hypochromic anemia who has a low serum iron and a high TIBC, you would:

    a. Begin ferrous sulfate 300 mg orally t.i.d.
    b. Order a Schilling test
    c. Repeat the stool guaiac
    d. Refer to a hematologist

### Questions 9, 10, and 11 refer to the following scenario.

Mrs. M. is a 30-year-old graduate student from Morocco with a family and personal history of "weak blood" who presents with a complaint of abdominal pain, increasing fatigue, and weight loss. She has never needed treatment for her blood problem but has been supplementing her usually well-balanced diet with high-potency vitamin and mineral supplements because of the increased stress of graduate studies in a foreign country. A routine CBC indicates a mild microcytic, hypochromic anemia.

9. It is likely that this patient's "weak blood" is:

    a. Thalassemia minor
    b. Thalassemia major
    c. Related to an unidentified chronic disease
    d. Related to an iron deficiency from gastrointestinal bleeding

10. Which of the following do you need to consider as a strong etiology for her current symptoms?

    a. Vitamin B$_{12}$ deficiency
    b. Folate deficiency
    c. Peptic ulcer
    d. Iron overload

11. If further blood studies indicate a decreased TIBC and increased serum iron, your next step should be which of the following?

    a. Tell Mrs. M. to discontinue her vitamin/mineral supplements; obtain hematological consult
    b. Refer her for genetic counseling
    c. Refer for hemoglobin electrophoresis
    d. Begin chelation therapy and refer for a GI consult

**Questions 12, 13, and 14 refer to the following scenario.**

Ms. Z. is a 26-year-old African American female who comes in complaining of fatigue, shortness of breath, and lightheadedness. Her history reveals no significant medical problems but several years of fad dieting without vitamin supplementation. Physical findings are unremarkable except for pallor of the mucous membranes, tachycardia, and a systolic flow murmur.

12. Your next step would be to:

    a. Start vitamin $B_{12}$ injections
    b. Order a CBC
    c. Order a TIBC and serum iron
    d. Start on multivitamins with iron

13. Ms. Z.'s CBC reveals a MCV of 110 and Hgb of 10.2 g/dL. Your next step should be to:

    a. Start vitamin $B_{12}$ injections
    b. Order serum iron and TIBC
    c. Order RBC-folate and vitamin $B_{12}$ levels
    d. Order an MMA level

14. Which of the following would help in your differential diagnosis?

    a. Patient's history of ice pica
    b. A + Romberg test and distal paresthesias on physical examination
    c. A confirmed diagnosis of sickle cell trait
    d. Family history of iron deficiency

15. The anemias most often associated with pregnancy are:

    a. Folic acid and iron deficiency
    b. Folic acid deficiency and thalassemia
    c. Iron deficiency and thalassemia
    d. Thalassemia and vitamin $B_{12}$ deficiency

16. Neural tube defects in the fetus have been primarily associated with which type of deficiency in the mother?

    a. Iron
    b. Folic acid
    c. Vitamin $B_{12}$
    d. Vitamin E

17. Most common causes of megaloblastic, macrocytic anemia are:

    a. Folate and or vitamin $B_{12}$ deficiency
    b. Chronic disease
    c. Iron deficiency and infection
    d. Hemolysis of blood cells

18. Patients with iron-deficiency anemia should be instructed that:

    a. Return of normal blood values will occur within a week of oral iron supplementation
    b. Iron supplements will need to be taken for the rest of their lives
    c. Taking iron preparations with milk will enhance absorption
    d. Iron preparation may be taken with meals

19. Elderly persons with pernicious anemia should:

    a. Be instructed to increase their dietary intake of foods high in vitamin $B_{12}$
    b. Be told they will not need to return for follow-up for at least a month after initiation of treatment
    c. Be told that oral vitamin $B_{12}$ is safer and less expensive than parenteral replacement
    d. Be told that diarrhea can be a transient side effect of vitamin $B_{12}$ injections

20. Which of the following would be included in a diet rich in iron?

    a. Peaches, eggs, beef
    b. Cereals, kale, cheese
    c. Red beans, enriched breads, squash
    d. Legumes, green beans, eggs

21. A woman taking folic acid supplements for folic acid deficiency will need to know that:

    a. It will take several months before she will feel better
    b. Folic acid should not be taken with meals and may cause diarrhea
    c. Iron supplements are contraindicated while one is on folic acid
    d. Oral contraceptives, pregnancy, and lactation increase dietary requirements for folic acid

22. In alcoholics with anemia:

    a. Pernicious anemia is more common than folic acid deficiency

b. Iron deficiency and folic acid deficiency may coexist
c. Alcohol interferes with iron absorption
d. Oral vitamin replacement is contraindicated

23. Which statement best characterizes macrocytic anemias?
    a. The underlying problem is usually an RBC deficiency
    b. They are most commonly hereditary
    c. They may produce neurological findings
    d. The pathophysiology includes abnormalities of hemoglobin synthesis

24. In normocytic anemia of chronic disease:
    a. Treatment is purely symptomatic
    b. Long-term supplementation of folic acid and vitamin $B_{12}$ is needed
    c. Treatment is focused on the associated disease
    d. Serum iron and TIBC are the most specific and sensitive diagnostic tests

25. Which of the following is true of anemia of chronic disease?
    a. An Hgb of < 9 g/dL confirms the diagnosis
    b. Symptoms associated with the anemia may be masked by the symptoms of the underlying disease
    c. Is manifested by more severe signs than most of the other common anemias
    d. Is never associated with reversible causes

26. Sickle cell anemia is caused by:
    a. Abnormalities in one or more hemoglobin chains
    b. Transposition of glutamic acid on hemoglobin A molecule
    c. Abnormal hemoglobin S in place of hemoglobin A
    d. In utero deficiency of folate

27. The test used to differentiate sickle cell anemia from sickle cell trait is:
    a. Sickle cell preparation
    b. Peripheral smear
    c. Sickledex
    d. Hemoglobin electrophoresis

28. Chronic myelogenous leukemia usually presents with the following:
    a. Increased platelets and leukocytosis
    b. Presence of Reed–Sternberg cells in bone marrow aspirate
    c. Ph[1] chromosome in bone marrow
    d. Typical fatigue, weakness, anorexia, and frequent nosebleeds

29. A 32-year-old male presents in the office with concerns about a painless lump in the area of his collar bone. He says that he feels well, but someone told him that it might be a sign of some kind of cancer. Your best response at this time would be to:
    a. Examine him and tell him to come back in 2 weeks to be reevaluated
    b. Inquire whether he has any cats that might cause cat scratch fever
    c. Work him up for a possibility of infectious mononucleosis
    d. Examine him with referral to physician for possible lymphoma disease workup

30. Diagnosis of Hodgkin's disease is based on:
    a. Hepatomegaly with fatigue, weight loss, pruritus, and night sweats
    b. Presence of Ph[1] chromosome in lymphoid tissue
    c. Extensive lymphadenopathy with elevated WBC count
    d. Presence of Reed–Sternberg cells in lymph node tissue

■ **Answers**

1. **b**        16. **b**
2. **b**        17. **a**
3. **b**        18. **d**
4. **b**        19. **d**
5. **b**        20. **a**
6. **a**        21. **d**
7. **d**        22. **b**
8. **c**        23. **a**
9. **a**        24. **c**
10. **d**       25. **b**
11. **a**       26. **c**
12. **b**       27. **d**
13. **c**       28. **c**
14. **b**       29. **d**
15. **a**       30. **d**

## BIBLIOGRAPHY

Advani, P. (2014). Thalassemia, beta. Retrieved from http://www.emedicine.com/med/TOPIC2260.htm

Amin, N. M. (2003). What's wrong with this picture: Diagnostic images, treatment issues … iron deficiency anemia. *Consultant, 40,* 2333, 2335, 2339.

Balducci, L. (2003). Epidemiology of anemia: Information on diagnostic evaluation. *Journal of the American Geriatric Society, 51*(3 Suppl.), 52–59.

Behrens, R. J., & Cymet, T. C. (2000). Sickle cell disorders: Evaluation, treatment, and natural history. *Hospital Physician, 36*(9), 17–18, 21–28.

Cheerva, A. C. (2013). Thalassemia, alpha. Retrieved from http://www.emedicine.com/med/TOPIC2259.htm

Fogarty, P. F., & Minichiello, T. (2014). Disorders of hemostasis, thrombosis, and antithrombotic therapy. In S. J. McPhee & M. A. Papadakis (Eds.), *Current medical diagnosis and treatment* (53rd ed.). New York, NY: McGraw-Hill.

Gilliland, D. G. (2001). Hematologic malignancies. *Current Opinion in Hematology, 8*(1), 189–191.

Goldberg, M. (2001). The diagnostic challenge ... non-Hodgkin's lymphoma. *Emergency Medicine, 33*(3), 77–78.

Goldman, D. (2000). Test your knowledge: Chronic lymphocytic anemia and its impact on the immune system. *Clinical Journal of Oncology Nursing, 4,* 233–234, 236.

Linker, C. A., & Damon, L. E. (2014). Blood disorders. In S. J. McPhee & M. A. Papadakis (Eds.), *Current medical diagnosis and treatment* (53rd ed.). New York, NY: McGraw-Hill.

Maakaron, J. E. (2013). Anemia. Retrieved from http://emedicine.medscape.com/article/198475-overview

McPherson, R. A., & Pincus, M. R. (2007). *Henry's clinical diagnosis and management by laboratory methods* (21st ed.). Philadelphia, PA: Saunders.

Russel, L. C. (2000). Hereditary hemochromatosis: Should clinicians screen for this common disease? *Journal of the American Academy of Nurse Practitioners, 12,* 273–279.

Streiff, M. B., Smith, B., & Spivak, J. L. (2002). The diagnosis and management of polycythemia vera in the era since the Polycythemia Vera Study Group: A survey of American Society of Hematology members' practice patterns. *Blood, 99,* 1144–1149.

# Gastrointestinal Disorders

*Sister Maria Salerno*

## PEPTIC ULCER DISEASE (PUD)

- Definition—ulceration of the gastrointestinal (GI) mucosa in areas bathed by acid pepsin; stomach, duodenum, and esophagus are common sites

- Etiology/Incidence
  1. Infection with *Helicobacter pylori* leading to imbalance between mucosal protective factors and corrosive effects of acid and pepsin is considered primary cause
  2. Steroidal and nonsteroidal anti-inflammatory drug (NSAID) therapy is the second most common cause
  3. Other causes include processes or factors leading to
     a. Hypersecretion of gastric mucosa
     b. Increased parietal cell mass
     c. Increased secretion of gastrin and hydrochloric acid
     d. Increased gastric emptying time
  4. Precipitating or aggravating factors include
     a. Steroidal and NSAID therapy, particularly aspirin
     b. Physiological stress—severe trauma, burns, shock
     c. Alcohol and nicotine use; caffeine, coffee
     d. Presence of alcoholic liver cirrhosis, chronic pancreatitis, chronic lung disease, hyperparathyroidism, rheumatoid arthritis
  5. Lifetime prevalence about 10% for adult population
     a. Duodenal
        (1) 80% are duodenal
        (2) Higher incidence in males
        (3) Without antibiotic treatment 80% recur in year following initial healing
        (4) Incidence decreasing in United States
        (5) Familial disposition—more frequent in persons with type O blood
        (6) Peak incidence between 25 and 55 years of age
     b. Gastric
        (1) Occur with about the same incidence in males and females
        (2) About 5% are malignant
        (3) Peak incidence—age 55–65 years of age; rare < 40 years of age

- Signs and Symptoms
  1. Intermittent epigastric discomfort—gnawing, burning, boring, nagging
  2. Pain begins 1–3 hours after eating, duodenal ulcers frequently awaken patients at night; gastric ulcers less so
  3. Pain relieved by food or antacids, particularly with duodenal ulcer
  4. Food sometimes aggravates pain of gastric ulcer
  5. Weight loss frequent in persons with gastric ulcer
  6. Dyspepsia (bloating, nausea, anorexia, excessive flatulence)

- Differential Diagnosis
  1. History of typical pain-food-relief pattern is an important criterion for clinical diagnosis
  2. Rule out other causes of epigastric pain
     a. Functional dyspepsia
     b. Gastroesophageal reflux disease (GERD)

c. Pancreatitis
d. Biliary tract disease
e. Neoplasms
f. Liver disease
g. Gastritis
h. Pneumonia
i. Cardiovascular disease

- Physical Findings
  1. Usually none
  2. Epigastric tenderness in advanced disease

- Diagnostic Tests/Findings
  1. Endoscopy
     a. Preferred diagnostic test in suspected PUD and should always be performed when alarm symptoms present and considered early on in patients > 50 years of age
        (1) Dysphagia
        (2) Unplanned weight loss
        (3) GI bleeding
        (4) Odynophagia
        (5) Early satiety
     b. Expensive but more sensitive and specific than barium radiographs; test of choice in most settings
     c. Rule out malignancy in gastric ulcers—should be performed if gastric ulcer suspected
        (1) Age of symptom onset > 55 years
        (2) Pain worsened with food
        (3) Typical symptoms do not respond to standard course of therapy
  2. Stool for occult blood—positive if bleeding is present
  3. Complete blood count (CBC)
     a. Hemoglobin (Hgb) and hematocrit (Hct) may be decreased
     b. With chronic slow bleeding—hypochromic, microcytic anemia is likely
     c. If bleeding is acute—normocytic, normochromic anemia
  4. Tests for *Helicobacter pylori*
     a. Urea breath test
        (1) 95–98% sensitivity and specificity; results comparable to endoscopic biopsy
        (2) Ingested drugs can cause false negatives; perform 4 weeks after last antibacterial treatment; 7 days after use of proton pump inhibitor
     b. Serological tests
        (1) IgA, IgG antibodies, enzyme-linked immunosorbent assay (ELISA)
        (2) Inexpensive; sensitivity and specificity about 95%
        (3) Not useful for follow-up testing because of slow decline after treatment
        (4) High serum lipid levels can interfere with results
     c. Histological evaluation
        (1) Requires endoscopic biopsy
        (2) Invasive and expensive
     d. Fecal antigen test
        (1) Sensitive to reinfection
        (2) Can be used to indicate response to treatment
     e. Culture of biopsy
        (1) Grows slowly and requires selective medium and environment
        (2) Primary use in research

- Management/Treatment
  1. Goals
     a. Relief of symptoms
     b. Healing
     c. Prevention of recurrence
     d. Eradication of bacteria
  2. Nonpharmacological
     a. Stop smoking
     b. Avoid nonsteroidal anti-inflammatory drugs
     c. Reduce stress
     d. Reduce use of alcohol and caffeine (conflicting data, but still recommended until healing is documented)
  3. Pharmacological
     a. Antimicrobials to eradicate *H. pylori*
        (1) Options include
            (a) Preferred treatment includes a 10- to 14-day course of combination antibiotic and antisecretory therapy including amoxicillin, clarithromycin, levofloxacin, tetracycline, metronidazole, and bismuth
            (b) Sequential therapy consisting of a proton pump inhibitor (PPI) and amoxicillin for 5 days followed by a PPI, clarithromycin, and tinidazole for an additional 5 days as an alternative to treatment failure with initial therapies
            (c) Levofloxacin-based salvage therapy for patients with treatment failure on regimens containing clarithromycin
        (2) Bismuth compounds act as topical antimicrobial, complementing antibiotics
        (3) Compliance with combination therapies a problem
        (4) Acquired resistance of microbe to metronidazole and, to a lesser extent clarithromycin, often occurs with either if given alone
        (5) Standard therapy currently least expensive
     b. Proton pump inhibitors to reduce gastric pH and provide environment to heal existing ulcer
        (1) Taken for 4–8 weeks

- (2) Should be administered 30 minutes before meals (usually breakfast)
- (3) Consider cytochrome P450 implications
- (4) Create less acidic environment suppressing, but not eradicating, *H. pylori*
- (5) Particularly useful in prevention/treatment of NSAID-induced ulceration
- (6) Available in parenteral and enteral forms
- c. H$_2$ receptor antagonists as an alternative to proton pump inhibitors
  - (1) Cimetidine—300 mg orally t.i.d. with meals and at bedtime for 4–6 weeks (more recent studies indicate similar healing with 400 mg b.i.d. or 800 mg at bedtime)
    - (a) Side effects
      - i. Frequently associated with acute confusional states in elderly adults or very ill patients
      - ii. Muscular pain; mild, transient diarrhea; impotence; gynecomastia; leukopenia; mildly elevated creatinine and transaminase levels are rare and tend to be seen only with long-term use
    - (b) Interferes with metabolism and increases blood levels of benzodiazepines, lidocaine, metronidazole, phenytoin, theophylline, and warfarin
    - (c) Should not be taken within an hour of taking antacids
  - (2) Ranitidine—150 mg orally b.i.d. or 300 mg orally at bedtime for active PUD; 150 mg orally at bedtime for maintenance
    - (a) Side effects—rise in transaminase levels alanine aminotransferase (ALT); dizziness; headache; tachycardia; malaise; constipation; diarrhea; rash; and, rarely, confusion
    - (b) No significant drug interactions
    - (c) May cause false-positive protein on urinary dip-stick analysis
  - (3) Famotidine—20 mg orally twice a day or 40 mg at bedtime
    - (a) As efficacious as other H$_2$RAs
    - (b) Least risk of drug interaction
  - (4) Nizatidine—150 mg orally twice a day or 300 mg at bedtime for up to 8 weeks
    - (a) No safer than cimetidine
    - (b) More expensive than cimetidine
- d. Antacids (used primarily as supplement to antisecretory agents)
  - (1) Primarily aluminum-, calcium-, or magnesium-containing agents; sodium bicarbonate very short acting and systemic absorption can cause alkalosis (not recommended)
  - (2) Length of effect dependent on gastric emptying time; 30 minutes on an empty stomach, longer when taken with meals
  - (3) Side effects
    - (a) Diarrhea with magnesium hydroxide–based agents
    - (b) Constipation with aluminum hydroxide-containing agents
    - (c) Hypophosphatemia in aluminum-containing agents due to aluminum phosphate binding and decreased GI absorption
    - (d) Osteopenia with long-term use of agents containing aluminum
    - (e) Rebound acid secretion and hypercalcemia with calcium-containing agents
  - (4) Drug interactions
    - (a) Interfere with taste; absorption of iron, digoxin, and some antibiotics, e.g., tetracyclines
    - (b) Interfere with effectiveness of oral contraceptives
- e. Treatment of NSAID-induced ulcers
  - (1) Antibiotic therapy not indicated
  - (2) Antisecretory therapy with a PPI or histamine 2 receptor antagonists (H$_2$RA) as described previously
  - (3) Discontinue NSAID during acute therapy
  - (4) If NSAID must be reintroduced, consider preventive/prophylactic therapy with an antisecretory agent
- f. Sucralfate (mucosal protectant)—1 g orally q.i.d. on an empty stomach
  - (1) No significant side effects
  - (2) Drug interaction
    - (a) Decreases absorption of digoxin, tetracycline, phenytoin, cimetidine, theophylline, and other drugs
    - (b) Antacids interfere with effectiveness and should not be given within 1 hour of sucralfate administration
- g. Treatment with antacids, H$_2$ receptor antagonists, or sucralfate results in 90–95% cure rate in 8–12 weeks

4. General considerations
  - a. Specialty consultation in atypical circumstances:
    - (1) Additional diagnostic studies for persons with suspected underlying disease or failure to respond to treatment in 2–4 weeks
    - (2) Patients with concurrent weight loss
    - (3) Patients with indications of peritonitis (rigidity, rebound tenderness, fever)

**138 CHAPTER 9** Gastrointestinal Disorders

(4) Clinical indicators of gastrointestinal bleeding or perforation
(5) Gastric outlet (pyloric) obstruction as suggested by vomiting of undigested food; dehydration; hypokalemia; and metabolic alkalosis
b. Patient education
(1) Disease and therapeutic management
(2) Purpose, dosage, side effects of medications
(3) Diet
(a) No evidence to support need for bland diet or small, frequent meals
(b) Encourage avoidance of known gastric acid stimulants, e.g., coffee, cola, and other caffeine-containing beverages
(c) Avoidance of any foods or beverages that aggravate symptoms
(d) Avoid eating within 3 hours of bedtime to avoid nocturnal stimulation of acid secretion
(4) Stress reduction
(5) Need to report to healthcare provider lack of response to medications, rectal bleeding, weight loss, increased weakness or dizziness, increasing pain
(6) Advise that smoking will delay gastric healing
c. Follow-up
(1) In 2–4 weeks to review
(a) Symptom response to medications
(b) GI bleeding
(c) Side or toxic effects of medications
(2) For those with gastric ulcers, document healing with upper GI barium radiograph or endoscopy—in 6 weeks for small ulcers; 12 weeks for large; imperative in gastric ulcers; unnecessary in uncomplicated duodenal ulcers

## GASTROESOPHAGEAL REFLUX DISEASE

- Definition—a condition that develops when the reflux of stomach contents causes troublesome pyrosis; pyrosis is considered troublesome if it affects a person's well-being after assurance of its benign nature

- Etiology/Incidence
  1. Most often related to inappropriate relaxation of the lower esophageal sphincter (LES), which allows reflux of gastric acid and pepsin into the distal esophagus
     a. Idiopathic
     b. Foods and other agents (see **Table 9-1**)
  2. Inflammation can also be caused by ingestion of caustic agents such as lye or infectious agents such as *Candida*, herpes simplex, or cytomegalovirus, which directly attack esophageal mucosa
  3. Infectious agents most often noted in immunosuppressed individuals, e.g., persons with AIDS or diabetes, and persons receiving chemotherapy
  4. Incidence not known; however, a monthly prevalence rate of heartburn, the major symptom of gastroesophageal reflux disease (GERD), has been estimated to be 40% in adult population

**TABLE 9-1** Foods and Other Substances That Decrease Lower Esophageal Sphincter Tone

| Anticholinergics | Alcohol |
|---|---|
| Benzodiazepines | Caffeine |
| Calcium channel blockers | Nicotine |
| Diazepam | Chocolate |
| Meperidine | Fatty foods |
| Narcotics | Peppermint |
| Progesterone | Yellow onions |

- Signs and Symptoms
  1. Retrosternal aching or burning heartburn (pyrosis) occurring 30–60 minutes after eating; associated with large meals, aggravated by lying down or bending over, and relieved with antacids
  2. Chest heaviness, pressure radiating to neck, jaw, or shoulders
  3. Regurgitation of fluid or food particles
  4. Nocturnal aspiration
  5. Extraesophageal symptoms may occur, but role is less certain
     a. Bronchospasm
     b. Pharyngeal discomfort
     c. Dysphonia
     d. Chronic cough

- Differential Diagnosis
  1. Myocardial infarction/angina
  2. Esophageal spasm
  3. Cholelithiasis
  4. Neoplasms
  5. Chemical or infectious esophagitis
  6. Conditions leading to gastric dysmotility, e.g., scleroderma, diabetes

- Physical Findings—generally insignificant

- Diagnostic Tests/Findings
  1. Not indicated in typical cases that respond to once- or twice-daily PPI therapy
  2. Endoscopy has become standard for documenting the type and extent of tissue damage
     a. Should be initiated at any time that alarm symptoms become present
        (1) Dysphagia
        (2) Unplanned weight loss
        (3) GI bleeding

b. Is indicated for the evaluation of patients with GERD who do not respond clinically to b.i.d. PPI therapy
3. Manometry for patients who have not responded to b.i.d. PPI therapy and have normal endoscopic findings
4. pH monitoring for patients who remain symptomatic on b.i.d. PPI therapy and have normal endoscopic and manometry findings; should be performed only after PPI therapy has been withheld for 7 days

- Management/Treatment
    1. Nonpharmacological measures should be targeted to specific patient circumstances; no evidence to suggest that across-the-board lifestyle interventions are effective
        a. Weight reduction if obese
        b. Elevation of head of bed if symptoms worse when supine
        c. Avoid large meals and carbonated beverages, particularly 3 hours prior to going to bed if nocturnal symptoms predominate
        d. Limit fats and carbohydrates
        e. Avoid straining with bowel movements
        f. Discontinue agents that decrease lower esophageal sphincter (LES) tone if the patient is using them—nicotine, alcohol, chocolate, caffeine, theophylline, calcium channel blockers, anticholinergics
        g. Antacids—may be effective for those with infrequent heartburn; however, with a diagnosis of GERD they are not indicated for routine therapy
    2. Pharmacological therapy
        a. PPI 30 minutes before breakfast
        b. If unresponsive to a.m. therapy, add second PPI 30 minutes before dinner
        c. No evidence that additional therapies, e.g., hour of sleep (h.s.) $H_2RA$, promotility agents, improve outcomes—not routinely indicated
        d. PPI clearly superior to $H_2RA$ for GERD management
        e. If unresponsive to b.i.d. PPI, refer to GI for endoscopy
    3. Currently there is no indication for management of extraesophageal symptoms without concomitant pyrosis
    4. Surgical intervention reserved for patients with stricture, bleeding, pulmonary aspiration, or severe refractory symptoms

## CHOLECYSTITIS

- Definition—acute or chronic inflammation of the gallbladder

- Etiology/Incidence
    1. About 90% related to presence of pigmented or cholesterol calculi, which can vary in diameter from 1 mm to 4 cm; when a stone becomes impacted in the cystic duct, inflammation develops behind the obstruction; if not relieved, pressure builds up in the gallbladder and leads to distention, ischemic changes, gangrene, and perforation with subsequent abscess formation and less frequently generalized peritonitis
    2. Occurs subsequent to bile stasis, bacterial infection, or ischemia
    3. Most common form of gallbladder disease; affects more than 20 million Americans
    4. Risk factors include being female, older than 40 years, obesity, and western European descent
    5. Pregnancy, sedentary lifestyle, low-fiber diet, use of oral contraceptives or antilipemics also associated with the development of cholecystitis

- Signs and Symptoms
    1. Episodic occurrences of postprandial fullness, heartburn, nausea, flatulence, regurgitation of bitter fluid, vomiting often precipitated by a large or fatty meal
    2. Anorexia (inability to finish an average-size meal)
    3. Recurrent episodes of biliary colic—sudden appearance of severe pain in the epigastrium or right hypochondrium, which subsides relatively slowly (12–18 hours)
        a. Tenderness of the same area may persist for days
        b. Accompanied by vomiting in 75% of the cases
    4. Constant aching pain or pressure in the right upper quadrant or epigastrium that radiates to the back or right shoulder

- Differential Diagnosis
    1. Perforated peptic ulcer
    2. Acute pancreatitis
    3. Appendicitis
    4. Salpingitis
    5. Diverticulitis
    6. Perforated hepatic carcinoma
    7. Liver abscess
    8. Hepatitis
    9. Pneumonia with right-sided pleurisy
    10. Myocardial infarction

- Physical Findings
    1. General appearance—unremarkable between attacks; ill during attack
    2. Vital signs—mild temperature elevation, tachycardia, and increased respiratory rate during acute attack
    3. Integument—mild jaundice occurs in about 20% of cases
    4. Abdomen—guarding, rebound tenderness in right hypochondrium; palpable, tender

sausage-shaped mass in right upper quadrant (RUQ) during acute attack in 20–30% of cases
  5. Positive Murphy's sign—inspiratory arrest secondary to extreme tenderness when subhepatic area is palpated during deep inspiration

- Diagnostic Tests/Findings
  1. CBC—mild leukocytosis with increased bandemia
  2. ECG—normal, important in ruling out myocardial infarction as cause of symptoms
  3. Chest radiograph—normal, important in ruling out pneumonia as cause of symptoms
  4. Flat plate radiograph of abdomen—gallstones
  5. Ultrasound (study of choice with 95% sensitivity, 98% specificity for stones)—gallstones, thickened gallbladder wall stones, but not as sensitive in acute cases
  6. Technetium $T_c 99_m$ PIPIDA (HIDA) scan—cystic duct occlusion and nonvisualized gallbladder; has high reliability if bilirubin < 5 mg/dL
  7. Alkaline phosphatase—elevated
  8. Serum amylase—elevated, > 1,000 suspect concomitant pancreatitis
  9. Serum aspartate aminotransferase (AST) and serum alanine aminotransferase (ALT) may be transiently elevated
  10. Bilirubin—mildly increased
  11. Old age, lymphoma, malnutrition, and immunosuppression may alter laboratory tests
  12. CT scan has no advantage over ultrasound in diagnosis of acute attack
  13. Oral cholecystography not used for acute attack

- Management/Treatment
  1. Elective cholecystectomy recommended for
     a. Symptomatic patients with radiological or ultrasound evidence of gallbladder disease
     b. Those at high risk for complications such as those with
        (1) A calcified gallbladder
        (2) Gallstones > 2 cm in diameter
        (3) Diabetes
        (4) Symptoms present for > 48 hours
  2. Conservative treatment for those who are asymptomatic
     a. Eliminate offending medications, e.g., clofibrate, oral contraceptives
     b. Avoid foods that precipitate symptoms; otherwise, no need to alter diet or restrict fats
     c. Treat dyspeptic symptoms with antacids (25–50% of patients will respond)
     d. Some patients may be put on a trial of chenodiol 750 mg orally per day
        (1) Best results are obtained in patients with small floating cholesterol stones
        (2) Contraindicated in patients with inflammatory bowel disease or peptic ulcer disease
        (3) Approximately 50% recurrence rate within 5 years after treatment
        (4) Side effects—hepatotoxicity, diarrhea, and increased low-density lipoprotein (LDL) cholesterol
        (5) Expensive
  3. Lithotripsy or destruction of stones with extracorporeal shock waves has limited application at present
  4. General considerations
     a. Patient education
        (1) Disease course, expected outcomes, and treatment
        (2) Changes in symptoms that necessitate contact of health professional, e.g., change in pain pattern or pain accompanied by fever, chills
        (3) Teach purpose, dosage, side effects of medications
        (4) Nutrition
           (a) If fatty foods seem to precipitate symptoms, a low-fat diet may be helpful
           (b) Some research has shown that increased fiber in the diet reduces incidence of gallstone formation
           (c) If obese, a reducing diet is indicated; avoid rapid weight loss and fad diets that may actually increase risk of gallstone formation and precipitate acute symptoms
        (5) Encourage regular physical exercise; sedentary lifestyle is associated with stone formation as well as obesity
     b. Complications include empyema, gangrene, and perforation

# APPENDICITIS

- Definition—inflammation of the vermiform appendix

- Etiology/Incidence
  1. Obstruction of the appendix with hardened feces (fecalith), stricture, inflammation, foreign body, or neoplasm
  2. Occurs in all age groups, but more common in males between 10 and 30 years of age
  3. Higher mortality rate because of complications in children, adolescents, and persons older than 55 years of age
  4. One of the leading causes for abdominal surgery

- Signs and Symptoms
  1. Acute onset of periumbilical or epigastric pain that ranges from mildly diffuse to severe
  2. Anorexia, nausea—vomiting not typical; if patient has several episodes of vomiting, consider alternate diagnosis
  3. Shifting of pain to right lower quadrant (McBurney's point) after several hours; aggravated by walking or coughing
  4. Occasional radiation of pain into the ipsilateral testicle or labia
  5. Spasm of abdominal muscles
  6. Constipation usual; diarrhea rare
  7. Elderly clients may present with mild symptoms of unexplained weakness, anorexia, tachycardia, and abdominal distention with little pain
  8. After 24 hours may progress to perforation with sudden cessation of pain and subsequent peritonitis manifested by
     a. Abdominal rigidity
     b. Generalized abdominal tenderness
     c. High fever
     d. Vomiting
     e. Dehydration
     f. Decreased bowel sounds
     g. Shock

- Differential Diagnosis
  1. Gastroenteritis
  2. Pneumonia
  3. Ruptured ovarian cyst
  4. Tubal pregnancy
  5. Acute cholecystitis
  6. Neoplastic perforation of the colon
  7. Renal calculi
  8. Pyelonephritis of the right kidney

- Physical Findings
  1. General appearance—may or may not appear ill
  2. Vital signs—fever 100–102° F
  3. Slight tachycardia related to pain and fever
  4. Abdominal—point and rebound tenderness in right lower quadrant (McBurney's point); decreased or absent bowel sounds
  5. Positive psoas, obturator (hip flexion maneuvers that stretch the inflamed peritoneum producing pain), and Markle (stand on tiptoe and drop quickly—produces pain in the right lower quadrant) signs
  6. Rectal/pelvic exams—tenderness in the right perirectal area
  7. Musculoskeletal—abdominal pain (right lower quadrant [RLQ]) with hip extension and with straight leg raise

- Diagnostic Tests/Findings
  1. CBC with differential—leukocytosis with increased band cells (shift to the left); in elderly adults shift may be present without leukocytosis
  2. CT scan of the abdomen
     a. Enlarged appendix
     b. Appendiceal wall thickening and enlargement
     c. Periappendiceal fat stranding

- Management/Treatment
  1. Refer immediately for surgical evaluation
  2. Begin antibiotic therapy to cover enteral flora
  3. IV hydration with isotonic fluids

## DIVERTICULITIS

- Definition—inflammation of one or more diverticula in the bowel wall with microperforation and abscess formation in the pericolic fat

- Etiology/Incidence
  1. Inflammatory process similar to etiologic agents in appendicitis
  2. Occurs in about 33% of persons with diverticula (estimated to be 5–20% of the adult population)
     a. Incidence increases after age 40
     b. More frequent in females
     c. Higher incidence in persons with low-fiber dietary habits
     d. Diverticula found most often in the sigmoid colon but may occur anywhere in the GI tract

- Signs and Symptoms
  1. Acute left lower quadrant pain—steady and severe, lasting for several days or crampy and intermittent
  2. Constipation more common than diarrhea
  3. Pain increased with defecation
  4. Flatulence
  5. Nausea
  6. Low-grade fever

- Differential Diagnosis
  1. Appendicitis
  2. Carcinoma of the colon
  3. Inflammatory bowel disease
  4. Ischemic colitis
  5. Gynecological disorders, including
     a. Ectopic pregnancy
     b. Ovarian abscess

- Physical Findings
  1. Vital signs—mild fever, tachycardia

2. Abdomen—guarding, rebound tenderness, rigidity especially over left lower quadrant (LLQ); if abscess has formed, a tender palpable mass may be noted
3. Rectal examination—tender painful mass may be present

- Diagnostic Tests/Findings
  1. CBC—mild to moderate leukocytosis
  2. Sedimentation (sed) rate—elevated
  3. Stool guaiac—positive in about 25% of cases
  4. Urine—normal unless colovesicular fistula present, then bacteriuria, leukorrhea, hematuria
  5. CT scan of the abdomen and pelvis is preferred diagnostic modality
  6. Colonoscopy after resolution of acute symptoms to confirm diagnosis and rule out other disorders
  7. Plain radiograph film of the abdomen in all hospitalized patients to identify free air, ileus, or obstruction in acute phase
  8. Barium enema may confirm presence of diverticulosis; greatest utility in ruling out other etiologies
  9. Stool for ova/parasites—negative

- Management/Treatment—for most patients with mild disease, outpatient treatment will be indicated and includes
  1. Clear liquids for 1–2 days followed by a bland diet once symptoms have subsided
  2. Broad-spectrum antibiotics with anaerobic activity for 7–10 days or until symptoms abate; for example:
     a. Amoxicillin/clavulanate potassium 875 mg/125 mg twice a day
     b. Metronidazole 500 mg 3 times a day plus ciprofloxin 500 mg twice a day or trimethoprim-sulfamethoxazole 160/800 mg twice a day
     c. Ciprofloxacin 500 mg 2 times a day or levofloxacin 500 mg once daily plus metronidazole 500 mg 3 times a day
  3. Bed rest to promote colon rest recommended until symptoms subside
  4. Low-fiber diet in acute phase
  5. Bowel rest—clear liquids, slowly advance as tolerated
  6. Chronically avoid nuts and seeds in diet
  7. General considerations
     a. Consider hospitalization for:
        (1) Those who fail to improve in 72 hours
        (2) Those with a temperature > 102° F
        (3) Need for additional testing
        (4) Those in advanced age
     b. Patients with severe disease require hospitalization, antibiotics, bowel rest, and IV hydration; approximately 20–30% of patients with diverticulitis will require surgical management
     c. Patient education
        (1) Etiology/incidence and usual clinical course of the disease and rationale for recommended treatment
        (2) Instruction on recommended dietary guidelines
           (a) After acute phase, high-fiber diet to include foods such as bran; whole grains; cereals; raw, cooked, or dried fruit; raw vegetables; cooked high-residue vegetables
           (b) High-fiber diet may cause bloating and flatulence during the first 2 weeks of use; this resolves with continued high-fiber intake
        (3) Avoid laxatives, enemas, antidiarrheal agents, and uncooked high-residue foods
        (4) Report fever, bleeding, increasing pain to healthcare provider immediately
        (5) Bulk forming agents such as psyllium hydrophilic mucilloid and use of stool softeners such as docusate sodium may help prevent frequent recurrence
     d. Follow-up—return visit or phone follow-up in 24–48 hours to verify relief with initiating therapy; and then again after completion of antibiotic therapy

# VIRAL HEPATITIS

- Definition—inflammation of the liver

- Etiology/Incidence
  1. Type A (infectious)
     a. Infection with hepatitis A virus (HAV), a small RNA enterovirus
        (1) Spread primarily by fecal-oral route; also parenterally
        (2) Found in infected water, food, shellfish
        (3) Intimate contact and poor sanitation and personal hygiene seem to be contributing factors
        (4) Incubation period 2–6 weeks
        (5) Infectivity—2–3 weeks in late incubation and early clinical phase
     b. Common in crowded situations such as low-income housing, school, military, and prison dormitories; can occur in any age group; common in immigrants from underdeveloped countries, school-age children, and young adults
        (1) Self limiting in > 99% of cases
        (2) No carrier state or chronic infection
        (3) Severity increases with age

(4) In United States seroprevalence of anti-HAV in adults indicates 40–50% have had the disease
2. Type B (serum)
    a. Infection with hepatitis B virus (HBV), a DNA virus with core and surface components
        (1) HBsAg (hepatitis B surface antigen) found in serum, saliva, semen, stool, and urine
        (2) Core contains HBcAg (hepatitis B core antigen) and, sometimes, HBeAg (secretory form of HBcAg present only in HBsAg positive sera); HBeAg associated with high virus titer and high infectivity
        (3) Incubation period 6 weeks to 6 months
        (4) Transmission by blood, blood products, and other body fluids, such as saliva and semen
        (5) Mother–infant transmission if mother infected during third trimester
        (6) Approximately 10% of infected individuals become chronic carriers
    b. Common in drug addicts, homosexual males, those with multiple sexual partners and densely populated urban neighborhoods; higher-risk individuals include persons exposed to needle punctures and blood products such as IV drug abusers; those on hemodialysis; those requiring blood transfusions or IV chemotherapy; and healthcare personnel such as nurses, laboratory workers, surgeons, and hemodialysis personnel
        (1) Considered to be a sexually transmitted disease
        (2) Accounts for about 40% of acute hepatitis cases/annually
3. HDV (hepatitis delta virus) incomplete RNA virus
    a. Requires antecedent or simultaneous HBV infection
    b. Common in IV drug users and recipients of multiple transfusions
    c. Concomitant infection usually results in more severe manifestations than HBV alone
    d. Immunity to HBV protects against HDV
    e. Associated with increased risk of hepatic cancer
4. Hepatitis C
    a. Infection with hepatitis C virus (HCV), an RNA virus
        (1) Incubation variable—6 weeks to 6 months
        (2) Chronic liver disease develops in 70%
        (3) Related to development of hepatocellular carcinoma in 10%
    b. High-risk population—IV drug users, hospital personnel, male homosexuals, those receiving multiple transfusions, intranasal cocaine users, and those with body piercings
5. Type E (enteral non-A)
    a. Infection with hepatitis E virus (HEV), a single-stranded RNA virus
        (1) Viral particles found in stool of infected persons
        (2) Does not progress to chronic liver disease
        (3) Incubation—2–9 weeks
        (4) Usually mild disease in adults > 15 years
        (5) Mortality as high as 10–20% in pregnant women
    b. Rare in the United States
6. Type G (HGV)
    a. Infection with a flavivirus
        (1) Transmitted percutaneously
        (2) Most infections asymptomatic
        (3) May result in chronic viremia, but chronic disease rare
    b. Risk groups include transfusion recipients, IV drug users
    c. Frequent coinfection with HCV

- Signs and Symptoms—clinical manifestations for type A, B, D, and E are similar and can vary from a minor flu-like illness to fatal liver failure; type C does not typically present in an acute state
    1. HAV may present with nonspecific or "flu" syndrome
    2. HBV clinical course more variable than HAV and associated with extrahepatic manifestations, e.g., urticaria, other rashes, arthritis—acute infection subsides and asymptomatic chronic state may ensue
    3. HCV may rarely produce acute flu-like illness that subsides spontaneously; however, most cases asymptomatic and discovered via routine screening of high-risk individuals
    4. Prodromal phase or preicteric phase in types A and B (lasts approximately 2 weeks)
        a. Fatigue, malaise
        b. Anorexia
        c. Nausea/vomiting
        d. Headache
        e. Hyperalgia
        f. Cough, coryza, pharyngitis
        g. Changes in taste with aversion to alcohol and smoking
        h. Right upper abdominal pain
        i. Weight loss of 2–4 kg

5. Active or icteric phase (lasts 2–6 weeks)
   a. Jaundice—sclera and skin (never manifested in some patients); not an indication of severity
   b. Dark urine
   c. Clay-colored stools; often precedes jaundice
   d. Enlarged tender liver
   e. Pruritus, urticarial rash more often associated with HBV
6. Posticteric or recovery phase
   a. Resolving jaundice, increasing sense of well-being, and decrease in symptomatology
   b. Chronic active hepatitis in those with HBV may begin at this point and is manifested by persistence of symptoms

- Differential Diagnosis
  1. Infectious mononucleosis
  2. Choledocholithiasis
  3. Hepatotoxic drugs, e.g., chloramphenicol, acetaminophen, methyldopa
  4. Carcinoma of the head of the pancreas
  5. Alcoholic cirrhosis
  6. History and serological tests assist in differentiating type

- Physical Findings
  1. General appearance—mildly ill to generally debilitated
  2. Vital signs—mild fever
  3. Integumentary—slight jaundice; rash
  4. Head, ears, eyes, nose, throat (HEENT)—yellow sclera, lymphadenopathy
  5. Abdomen—enlarged, tender liver; splenomegaly (in about 10% of cases); normal bowel sounds

- Diagnostic Tests/Findings
  1. CBC with differential—WBC low to normal, lymphocytosis, mild anemia
  2. Urinalysis—proteinuria; bilirubinuria
  3. Abnormal liver function tests
     a. Elevated AST and ALT typically 500–2,000 IU/L
     b. Rise 7–10 days before jaundice
     c. Begin to fall shortly after onset of jaundice; should return to normal after 6 months
     d. Degree of increase does not necessarily parallel disease severity
     e. LDH, serum bilirubin, alkaline phosphatase, prothrombin time normal or slightly increased
  4. Serology tests—refer to **Table 9-2**

- Management/Treatment
  1. Approach is primarily supportive in uncomplicated cases
     a. Activity/rest
        (1) Rest recommended during active phase
        (2) Resumption of full activities during the recovery period does not appear to prolong illness or cause relapse or development of chronic disease
        (3) Avoidance of activity that might cause trauma to liver or spleen

### TABLE 9-2 Serology Tests for Viral Hepatitis

| |
|---|
| **IgM** antibody to HAV—appears during acute or early convalescent phase and disappears in about 8 weeks; implies recent infection and acute infection as well as infectivity |
| **IgG** antibody to HAV—remote exposure and either a chronic state or immunity |
| **HBsAg** (hepatitis B surface antigen)—positive throughout the active phase of illness; first test to obtain if acute HBV infection is suspected; will remain positive in asymptomatic carriers and in chronic hepatitis |
| **Anti-HBs (HBsAg)** (antibody specific to HBsAg [hepatitis B surface antigen])—positive indication of noninfectious state and recovery, and immunity; appears after HBsAg disappears |
| **Anti-HBc** (antibody to HBcAg [hepatitis B core antigen])—present at onset of acute illness; remains present for years and is found in asymptomatic carriers; in many patients there is a period (window) between the disappearance of HBsAg and the appearance of anti-HBs antibody, usually during late stages of acute phase or early convalescence; during this period, anti-HBc will be the only serological marker of the infection; presence of anti-HBc indicates immunity due to natural infection (not present in immunized individual) |
| **Anti-HDV** (antibody to hepatitis D)—marker of co- or superinfection by hepatitis D in persons with hepatitis B; appears late and is short lived |
| **HBeAg** (protein derived from HBV core)—indicates active viral replication, circulating HBV, and highly infectious sera |
| **Anti-HBe** (antibody to HBeAg)—appears weeks to months after HBeAg and HBV are no longer detectable in blood; presence indicates substantially less infectious sera |
| **Anti-HCV** (antibody to HCV)—appears 6 months after initial infection, remains elevated indefinitely, considered infectious and capable of transmission |
| **HCV-RNA** (hepatitis C RNA)—can detect circulating virus in 1–2 weeks after infection; becoming the gold standard for HCV detection |

b. Adequate fluid and dietary intake
      (1) 3,000 to 4,000 mL fluid per day; high-carbohydrate fluids such as fruit juices and carbonated beverages are encouraged, but not always well tolerated
      (2) Foods high in protein, carbohydrates, and calories
      (3) Low-fat diet not shown to be beneficial
      (4) Most important to eat whatever is tolerated
   c. Antiemetics may be prescribed 30 minutes before meals to control nausea and vomiting; rectal administration may be better tolerated than oral
   d. Patients with elevated prothrombin time (PT) may be given vitamin K
   e. Symptomatic relief of pruritus with colloidal baths, soaps, and lotions
   f. Avoid alcohol and other drugs detoxified or metabolized by the liver
2. For HCV—combination therapy with pegylated interferon and ribavirin; treatment is complex and guidelines change frequently; consultation with a specialist for newly diagnosed cases is recommended
   a. Exact mechanism of action unknown
   b. Combination therapy can get rid of the virus in up to 5 out of 10 persons for genotype 1 and in up to 8 out of 10 persons for genotypes 2 and 3
   c. Most positive response with
      (1) Low serum titer HCV RNA
      (2) Younger age
      (3) Female
      (4) Absence of cirrhosis
   d. No data to date showing better survival rates or inhibition of progress to chronic active hepatitis
3. General considerations
   a. Refer for possible hospitalization and further testing
      (1) Complicated cases
      (2) Severely ill patients
      (3) Persons with signs of fulminating hepatitis or encephalitis
      (4) Dehydrated persons
      (5) Those with a PT > 15 seconds
      (6) Those suspected of having another underlying disease process
      (7) Avoid cephalosporins in those with acute disease or significantly elevated liver function tests (LFTs)
   b. Newly diagnosed cases reported to health department
   c. Patient education
      (1) Disease course and expected outcomes
      (2) Verify any drug use including over-the-counter medications and vitamin supplements with the healthcare provider until completely recovered
      (3) Maintain proper hygiene; proper hand washing, disposal of all body wastes
         (a) Should not donate blood
         (b) Close personal contacts, family members, and sexual contacts should be evaluated for active disease and may receive immune serum globulin for passive immunity (not useful once disease is clinically evident)
   d. Follow-up
      (1) Follow weekly for the first 2–3 weeks; monthly thereafter if symptoms subside and LFTs improving
      (2) Closer follow-up in those > 40 years of age
   e. Complications
      (1) HBV infection tends to be longer and more severe than HAV
      (2) Carrier states and chronic hepatitis are associated with HBV and HCV, but not with HAV
      (3) Chronic HBV treatment includes recombinant interferon a-2b and direct inhibitors of HBV replication, but treatment rarely produces permanent remission of the disease
      (4) Fulminant liver failure occurs in less than 1% of those with HAV and in about 5% of those with HBV
      (5) Chronic hepatitis can be associated with hepatic cancer
      (6) 70% of patients with hepatitis C will develop chronic hepatitis
   f. Prophylaxis—see **Table 9-3**

## ACUTE GASTROENTERITIS

- Definition—acute inflammation of the gastrointestinal mucosa

- Etiology/Incidence
  1. Commonly due to infectious agents—viruses, bacteria, and parasites (*Giardia*, amoebae)
     a. Exotoxins produced by some organisms (e.g., *Staphylococcus*) induce hypersecretion or increased peristalsis resulting in diarrhea or vomiting
     b. Bacteria such as *E. coli* and salmonella penetrate and invade the gastric mucosa and lead to diarrhea accompanied by fever and fecal leukocytes
     c. See **Table 9-4** for characteristics of some etiologic agents in gastroenteritis
  2. Among the top 10 leading causes of morbidity in the United States

**146** CHAPTER 9 Gastrointestinal Disorders

TABLE 9-3  Adult Prophylaxis for Viral Hepatitis

| Time of Exposure | Agent | Dose | Time |
|---|---|---|---|
| **Preexposure** | | | |
| Hepatitis A<br>Persons traveling to or working in endemic areas; men who have sex with men; drug users; those who work with nonhuman primates with HAV infection or in labs with HAV; persons with chronic liver disease; those with clotting factor disorders; and some food handlers | HA vaccine (preferred over serum) | 1 mL IM | 2 doses separated by 6–12 months depending on brand; protection begins 4 weeks after first dose; both doses needed for long-term protection |
| If travel or exposure expected in less than 4 weeks after 1st HAV vaccine dose | Immune serum globulin | 0.02 mL/kg once | |
| Hepatitis B<br>Recommended for healthcare personnel especially laboratory personnel; surgeons; dialysis personnel; also recommended for adolescents in areas with high incidence of HBV, drug abuse, sexually transmitted disease, teen pregnancies, and for homosexually active men | HB recombinant vaccine | 1 mL IM | Usually given in 3 doses; 2nd and 3rd given approximately 1 mo and 6 mo after the 1st dose; need all 3 doses for adequate protection |
| **Postexposure** | | | |
| Hepatitis A<br>Close contacts; family members; sexual partners | Immune serum globulin | 0.02 mL/kg | Once, not more than 2 weeks postexposure |
| Hepatitis B<br>Percutaneous needlestick or mucosal exposure if unvaccinated and source HBsAg + | HB immune globulin and HB vaccine 3 × | 0.06 mL/kg 1 mL IM | Within 24–48 hours of exposure; at same time as HBIg, then at 1 and 6 mo |
| Sexual exposure | Globulin and HB vaccine | 0.6 mL/kg 1 mL IM | Within 14 days of last sexual contact; at same time as HBIg, then at 1 mo and 6 mo |

Contact Centers for Disease Control and Prevention hotline for most current and more specific information: 1-404-332-4555 or www.cdc.gov.

   a. Occurs universally in all age groups
   b. Epidemic outbreaks of bacterial enteritis occur in groups of persons who have ingested contaminated food
   c. Viral gastroenteritis occurs more frequently in the winter months
   d. Primarily a self-limiting disease (1–2 weeks)
   e. The very young, elderly, and those with concomitant chronic debilitating disease are at higher risk for mortality

- Signs and Symptoms
   1. Abrupt onset of nausea, vomiting
   2. Explosive flatulence
   3. Crampy abdominal pain
   4. Frequent, watery diarrhea
   5. Myalgia
   6. Headache
   7. Fever
   8. Generalized weakness/malaise

- Differential Diagnosis
   1. Acute appendicitis
   2. Cholecystitis
   3. Inflammatory bowel disease, e.g., colitis
   4. Bowel obstruction
   5. Fecal impaction with overflow
   6. Pelvic inflammatory disease

- Physical Findings
   1. General appearance—ill
   2. Vital signs—fever moderate to high 101–102° F in bacterial; up to 103° F in viral
   3. Abdomen—diffuse tenderness; no spasm or rebound tenderness except with *Salmonella* infection; hyperactive bowel sounds; slight

**TABLE 9-4** Characteristics of Select Etiological Agents in Gastroenteritis

|  | Incubation or Onset | Fever | Fecal Leukocytes | Other |
|---|---|---|---|---|
| *E. coli* | 24–72 hrs | + | + | Common cause of travelers' diarrhea; doxycycline, bismuth subsalicylate used preventively; treatment with rifaximin |
| *Campylobacter* | 2–5 days | + | + | Erythromycin and tetracycline used in treatment |
| *Staphylococcus* | 1–6 hrs | – | – | Grows in meats; dairy foods |
| *Shigella/Salmonella* | 8–24 hrs | + | + | Highly infectious |
| Botulism | 12–36 hrs | – | – | Neuro. signs—diplopia, vertigo, dysphagia; respiratory support may be needed |
| *Giardia lamblia* | 7–21 days | – | – | Rifaximin used in treatment; cause of travelers' diarrhea |

distention; absent or hypoactive bowel sounds common with botulism
4. Neurological—dizziness, difficulty in swallowing, and other neurological deficits are indications of botulism and require emergency intervention; with other etiologies findings are expected to be normal

- Diagnostic Tests/Findings
  1. Normally not indicated unless symptoms > 72 hours in duration
  2. CBC—normal indices
  3. Stool guaiac—usually negative in viral infections; positive with invasive bacterial infections
  4. Stool examination—if etiologic agent is an invasive bacteria, leukocytes will be present
  5. Stool culture—diagnostic for bacteria
     a. Done in suspected cases of bacterial infection and food poisoning and if symptoms do not begin to abate in 72 hours
     b. Special cultures needed for suspected *Campylobacter*, cholera

- Management/Treatment
  1. Most can be treated for 72 hours without laboratory testing with
     a. Bed rest as needed progressing to regular activity
     b. NPO except for cracked ice while nausea and vomiting are present, then restriction to clear liquids for 24 hours; follow with addition of toast and crackers, proceeding to a bland then regular diet
     c. Antiemetics and antidiarrheals are usually not indicated and may prolong the problem; treatment of salmonella has been noted to prolong the carrier state
     d. Provide for parenteral administration of prescription medications if necessary
  2. General considerations
     a. Consider more aggressive diagnostic evaluation if symptoms do not abate in 72 hours; approach may include stool for ova and parasites, specialized stool cultures, and proctosigmoidoscopy
     b. Report bacterial infections and food poisoning to the health department
     c. Routine use of antibiotics is not recommended; consider use in those with
        (1) Symptoms lasting > 3 days
        (2) Impaired immune response
     d. Patient education
        (1) Disease course and expected outcome; symptoms usually resolve in 72 hours, but mild diarrhea may persist for a week or 2
        (2) Explain proper food preparation and storage
        (3) Appropriate dosage and side effects of medications
        (4) Proper methods of hygiene including hand washing and disposal of stool and vomit
        (5) Signs of dehydration; neurological involvement that requires contacting healthcare professional

e. Follow-up
    (1) Usually self-limiting; return visit warranted if symptoms (other than mild diarrhea) do not abate in 72 hours or if they worsen
    (2) Diarrhea may continue for 1–2 weeks with *Salmonella* infection

# IRRITABLE BOWEL SYNDROME (IBS) (FUNCTIONAL BOWEL SYNDROME)

- Definition—idiopathic clinical syndrome characterized by abdominal pain or discomfort occurring in association with altered bowel habits for at least 3 days per month for the last 3 months; because IBS is a functional motility disorder, it is characterized by an absence of systemic symptoms outside of the GI tract—fever, blood in stool, weight loss, or any other systemic symptom rules out IBS and requires a more aggressive diagnostic evaluation

- Etiology/Incidence
  1. Disturbance in bowel motor activity thought to include a normal response to severe stress and learned visceral response to stress leading to
     a. Nonpropulsive colonic contractions that lead to constipation
     b. Increased contraction in the small bowel and proximal colon with diminished activity in the distal colon leading to diarrhea
  2. May be influenced by emotional factors
  3. Common GI disorder
     a. Accounts for about 50% of most GI complaints seen by healthcare professionals and a major cause of morbidity in the United States
     b. Onset usually occurs before age 35
     c. Women affected more often than men
     d. More common in those with other functional disorders

- Signs and Symptoms
  1. Aching or cramping periumbilical or lower abdominal pain often precipitated by meals and relieved by defecation; does not awaken patient at night
  2. Pain may radiate to left chest or arm (gas in splenic flexure)
  3. Changes in bowel function
     a. Diarrhea
        (1) 4–6 movements/day
        (2) Small watery stools with clear mucus
        (3) Nocturnal diarrhea (rare)
     b. Constipation with irregular passage of small hard stools
     c. Alternating episodes of diarrhea and constipation
  4. Flatulence
  5. Exaggerated response to and preoccupation with bowel symptoms
  6. Bleeding, weight loss, and nocturnal diarrhea are not characteristic of IBS

- Differential Diagnosis
  1. Inflammatory bowel disease
  2. Viral or bacterial gastroenteritis
  3. GI neoplasms
  4. Parasitic infections
  5. Lactose deficiency
  6. Laxative abuse
  7. Side effects of drugs affecting bowel motility
  8. Rome III criteria for diagnosis requires 3 days per month for at least 3 months of continuous or recurrent abdominal pain or discomfort plus at least two of the following:
     a. Improvement with defecation
     b. Change in stool frequency (diarrhea or constipation)
     c. Change in stool form or appearance (loose, watery, mucus, or pellet-like)
     d. Symptom onset at least 6 months prior to diagnosis

- Physical Findings
  1. General appearance—"worried well," anxious, depressed
  2. Vital signs—normal
  3. Abdomen—mild abdominal tenderness, normal or mildly hyperactive bowel sounds, distention
  4. Rectal examination—normal
  5. Systemic symptoms, e.g., fever and weight loss, are absent

- Diagnostic Tests/Findings
  1. Stool examination—negative for blood, ova, parasite, pathogenic bacteria, and *Giardia*-specific antigen
  2. CBC, thyroid screen, chemical analysis—normal
  3. Barium enema—decreased motility; otherwise, normal
  4. Proctosigmoidoscopy—normal

- Management/Treatment
  1. Provide emotional support, reassurance, information on stress reduction
  2. Dietary changes may improve symptoms
     a. High-fiber diet
     b. Avoid lactose-containing and gas-producing foods
     c. Fiber supplement may be indicated in addition to high-fiber diet
  3. Pharmacological agents
     a. Bulk laxatives—psyllium hydrophilic mucilloid
     b. Narcotics, depressants, and long-term pharmaceutical use to be avoided

c. Anticholinergics
   (1) Dicyclomine hydrochloride 20–40 mg orally q.i.d. or propantheline 15 mg orally q.i.d.
   (2) Usually given only after nonpharmacological measures have failed
   (3) Side effects—dry mouth, tachycardia, orthostatic hypotension
   (4) Contraindicated if history of glaucoma, urinary retention, cardiac arrhythmia
   (5) Loperamide or other opiate-derived antidiarrheals are reserved for only very severe cases; potential for abuse in these patients is great
d. Tricyclic antidepressants
e. 5-HT$_3$ antagonists and 5-HT$_4$ agonist (suspended from general use but available under certain circumstances via certified providers in extreme cases)
f. Chloride channel activator (lubiprostone) for IBS-C
g. Rifaximin (nonabsorbable antibiotic) not yet approved for IBS but may be appropriate for refractory patients
h. Probiotic data are conflicting but present a safe, well-tolerated option in refractory patients
i. Zofran primarily used for management of severe nausea and vomiting

4. Patient education
   a. Disease course and expected outcomes
   b. Rationale for treatment
   c. High-fiber diet
5. Planned exercise (may help in stress reduction)
6. Need for annual rectal examination and sigmoidoscopy after age 40
7. Some patients may benefit from psychological counseling and/or relaxation techniques

## INFLAMMATORY BOWEL DISEASE

Definition—a term used to describe two systemic autoimmune inflammatory diseases with primary gut involvement, both of which are characterized by diffuse inflammation of the mucosal lining of the gut. Ulcerative colitis involves the rectum and part of the distal colon; Crohn's disease typically involves small intestine but may attack any part of the gastrointestinal tract. Both disorders are chronic and recurring and may involve any number of extraintestinal manifestations. Inflammatory bowel disease (IBD) should not be confused with irritable bowel syndrome (IBS), which is a functional motility disorder.

- Etiology/Incidence
  1. Etiology is characterized by three features:
     a. Genetic predisposition—first-degree relatives have up to 20% increased risk as compared to the general population
     b. Dysregulated immune response
     c. Abnormal response to normal gut flora
  2. Studies of environmental triggers are inconsistent
  3. Affects 1 to 2 million people in the United States
  4. Peak age of onset is 15–30 years

- Signs and Symptoms
  1. Primary symptoms are in the gastrointestinal tract
     a. Irregular bowel habits
     b. Passing of mucus with stool
     c. Blood in stool
     d. Cramping abdominal pain
     e. Tenesmus
  2. Systemic symptoms
     a. Weight loss
     b. Fever
     c. Fatigue and malaise
  3. Extraintestinal symptoms
     a. Arthralgias
     b. Ocular symptoms (episcleritis, uveitis)
     c. Delayed growth and/or sexual maturation in children
     d. Liver disease
     e. Back pain
     f. Thromboemolic events

- Differential Diagnosis
  1. Irritable bowel syndrome
  2. Celiac disease
  3. Lactose intolerance
  4. Functional diarrhea
  5. Colorectal cancer

- Physical Findings
  1. Fever, tachycardia
  2. Dry mucous membranes, poor skin turgor
  3. Pallor
  4. Underweight, poor nutrition
  5. Abdominal distention
  6. Abdominal tenderness (RLQ in Crohn's disease)
  7. Perianal abscess and/or fissures
  8. Prolapsed rectum
  9. Physical findings consistent with extraintestinal manifestations if present

- Diagnostic Tests/Findings
  1. CBC—consistent with anemia of chronic disease or iron deficiency anemia
  2. Nutritional markers may suggest poor gastrointestinal absorption
     a. Decreased vitamin B$_{12}$
     b. Decreased folate
     c. Decreased albumin or prealbumin

3. ESR and CRP may be elevated due to inflammation but not specific to IBD
4. Stool studies to rule out infectious disease
   a. Ova and parasites
   b. *Clostridium difficile*
   c. Yersinia
5. Radiographic studies may support diagnosis but none are diagnostic
   a. Barium enema when colonoscopy not available
   b. Specific studies as indicated to rule out complications, e.g., obstruction abscess, fistula
6. Colonoscopy is definitive diagnostic study
7. Fecal calprotectin may be a useful serological marker in children

- Management/Treatment
  1. Varies to some extent with specific disease
  2. Includes symptom control and mucosal healing
  3. Symptomatic therapy
     a. Antidiarrheal agents
     b. Bile acid sequestrants
     c. Antispasmodics
     d. Proton pump inhibitors
     e. H$_2$R antagonists
  4. Stepwise therapies for mucosal healing
     a. Step I—Aminosalicylates
        (1) Oral mesalamine
        (2) Sulfasalazine
        (3) Topical mesalamine inserts, enemas
     b. Step I—Corticosteroids (prednisone 10–60 mg daily; steroid enemas may be used
     c. Step III—Immune-modifying agents
        (1) Mercaptopurine
        (2) Azathioprine
        (3) Methrotrexate
     d. Step III—Biological therapies
        (1) Anti-TNF therapies, e.g., infliximab, adalimumab, certolizumab, golimumab
        (2) Anti-integrins, e.g., natalizumab, vedolizumab
  5. Antibiotics when abscess present, e.g., metronidazole, ciprofloxacin
  6. In some cases surgical diversion may be necessary for bowel rest
  7. Patient education
     a. Increased risk of colorectal malignancies
     b. Increased risk for extraintestinal manifestations
     c. Direction to support groups

## COLORECTAL CANCER

- Definition—malignancy of gastrointestinal tract, primarily colon or rectum
- Etiology/Incidence
  1. Causes remain unclear
  2. Risk factors include history of colonic polyps, breast or female genital tract cancer, chronic inflammatory bowel disorders, positive family history; high-fat, low-fiber, high-caloric diet
  3. Third leading cause of cancer morbidity and mortality in the United States

- Signs and Symptoms—vary by location
  1. Right-sided colon cancer
     a. Usually asymptomatic
     b. Vague or crampy, colicky abdominal pain
     c. Unexplained weight loss, fatigue, weakness
     d. Occult blood in stool
     e. Anemia
  2. Left-sided colon cancer
     a. Alternating constipation with diarrhea
     b. Change in stool caliber (narrow, ribbon-like)
     c. Lower abdominal pain
     d. Red blood in stool
     e. Sensation of incomplete evacuation
  3. Rectal cancer
     a. Tenesmus
     b. Rectal bleeding (bright red)
     c. Mucous discharge

- Differential Diagnosis
  1. Diverticular disease
  2. Lymphoma
  3. Irritable bowel syndrome
  4. Inflammatory bowel disease

- Physical Findings
  1. Palpable mass primarily in right colon
  2. Lymphadenopathy
  3. Rectal mass found on rectal examination
  4. Stools positive for occult blood

- Diagnostic Tests/Findings
  1. Colonoscopy—diagnostic study of choice; allows for biopsy of lesions
  2. Barium enema radiograph used much less commonly but may reveal lesions when evaluating other bowel symptoms
  3. Testing of stools for occult blood—effective for early detection, positive findings to be followed with colonoscopy
  4. Carcinoembryonic antigen (CEA) test—often performed, although not specific for colon cancer; normal level of CEA does not exclude possibility of malignancy
  5. CBC can demonstrate an iron-deficiency anemia; should be followed with endoscopic assessment in middle-aged and older adults
  6. Chest radiograph may reveal metastases

- Management/Treatment
  1. Referral for surgical excision or resection depending on the depth of invasion of tumors
  2. Patients with metastatic lesions, noted at the time of diagnosis, have a poor prognosis; palliative treatment is then indicated
  3. Patients with a resection often require a temporary colostomy
  4. General considerations
     a. American Cancer Society recommendations for colon cancer screenings for persons of average risk begin at age 50 and include
        (1) Testing for fecal occult blood annually
        (2) Flexible sigmoidoscopy every 5 years or
        (3) Double-contrast barium enema every 5 years or
        (4) CT colonography (virtual colonoscopy) every 5 years or
        (5) Colonoscopy every 10 years
     b. Monitor for signs of dehydration during colon preps
     c. Instruct patient on possibility of a colostomy after procedure and begin patient teaching on care of colostomy preoperatively
     d. Encourage patient and family to ventilate feelings regarding the diagnosis
     e. Make referrals to pastoral care or mental health liaison as indicated
     f. Refer to community agencies for assistance after discharge, i.e., American Cancer Society, United Ostomy Associations of America

## Special Considerations in the Hospitalized Patient

- Acute Gastrointestinal Bleeding
  - Definition—acute blood loss from a site originating in the GI tract; may present as either hematemesis, coffee-ground emesis, or melena if upper GI (UGI); mild anorectal bleeding to massive hematochezia in the lower GI (LGI) tract—both types self-limiting in most circumstances
  - Etiology/Incidence
    - Upper GI
      a. Peptic ulcer disease
         □ Portal hypertension
         □ Mallory–Weiss tears
         □ Vascular anomalies
         □ Neoplasms
         □ Erosive esophagitis or gastritis
    - Lower GI
      □ Diverticulosis
      □ Neoplasms
      □ Inflammatory bowel disease
      □ Anorectal disease
      □ Ischemic colitis
      □ Mesenteric ischemia
  - Signs and Symptoms
    - Hematemesis, coffee-ground emesis in UGI tract
    - Bright red blood or maroon stools in LGI tract
    - Painless large-volume bleeding typically diverticular
    - Bloody diarrhea with cramping or tenesmus suggests IBD, infection, or ischemia
    - Nausea
    - Fatigue
    - Palpitations
    - General symptoms of volume loss
  - Differential Diagnoses
    - Diagnosis is not typically in dispute
    - Diagnosis of underlying problem is primary issue (see Etiology/Incidence)
  - Physical Findings
    - Vomiting of frank blood or coffee ground emesis
    - Hematochezia in profound bleed
    - Melena
    - Hypotension
    - Tachycardia
    - Orthostasis
  - Diagnostic Tests/Findings
    - Decreased Hgb and Hct if > 1 L volume loss
    - Normal MCV
    - PT/aPTT to assess for underlying coagulopathy
    - Comprehensive metabolic panel to assess for hepatic or renal disease
    - Blood type and screen
    - Crossmatch for 2–4 units of packed red blood cells (PRBCs)
    - Endoscopy is required to identify cause
  - Management/Treatment
    - Assess hemodynamic status—systolic blood pressure (SBP) < 90 mm Hg or heart rate 100 bpm suggests unstable patient

*(continues)*

### Special Considerations in the Hospitalized Patient (*continued*)

- Two 18-gauge IV catheters inserted at minimum in unstable patients; central venous access preferred
- Aggressive volume replacement with isotonic fluid—normal saline solution (NSS) or lactated Ringer's (LR)
- Nasogastric tube placement
- Erythromycin 250 mg IV to promote gastric emptying when suspected blood clots in stomach
- Transfuse PRBC to maintain Hgb > 6 to 10 g/dL or in any patient with brisk and active bleeding regardless of Hgb
- Transfuse platelets when platelet count < 50,000/mcL—may need platelet transfusion regardless of count if on acetylsalicylic acid (ASA) or clopidogrel
- Desmopressin acetate tablets (DDAVP) 0.3 mcg/kg q.12.h. in uremic patients
- Fresh frozen plasma (FFP) in actively bleeding patients with international normalized ratio (INR) > 1.8
- 1 unit FFP for each 5 units of PRBC in massive bleed
- IV proton pump inhibitor (PPI)
- Curative treatment addresses underlying cause—surgical intervention is uncommon in both UGI and LGI bleeding
- Bowel Obstruction
    - Definition—anything that interferes with the passage of gut contents from the proximal to distal end of the GI tract; may be functional, mechanical, or pseudo-obstruction. Appropriate management always requires rapid identification and treatment of cause. All patients with bowel obstruction should be maintained NPO with intravenous fluid support until the obstruction is relieved.
    - Etiology/Incidence
        - Obstructing tumors
        - Adhesions
        - Paralytic ileus
            - Drug-induced
            - Volume-contraction related
            - Immobility
            - Malignancy
        - Pseudo-obstruction—gas obstructions due to excessive laxative use
    - Signs and Symptoms
        - Crampy, colicky, cyclic abdominal pain consistent with smooth muscle of the gut contracting forcibly to move its contents around an obstruction
        - Specific symptoms depend on location
        - Small bowel obstruction (SBO)
            - Nausea and vomiting of undigested contents
            - Onset of pain within hours of eating
            - Altered bowel habits—diarrhea early, constipation late
        - Large bowel obstruction (LBO)
            - Constipation
            - Onset of pain may take days or weeks to occur
            - Constipation early; vomiting of bile and feces late
    - Differential Diagnosis
        - Other GI pain causing conditions
        - Gastroenteritis
        - Functional motility disorders
        - Consider underlying cause
    - Physical Findings
        - May be absent in small bowel obstruction
        - Distended abdomen—more common in large bowel obstruction
        - Fever
        - Tachycardia
    - Diagnostic Tests/Findings
        - Plain film radiography is diagnostic study of choice in simple small bowel obstruction; two views at minimum—enteroclysis if radiographs negative and clinical suspicion high
            - Dilated horizontal loops of small bowel
            - Air fluid levels
            - Absent or minimal colonic gas
        - CT scan is study of choice if large bowel obstruction is suspected
            - Contrast CT helps differentiate partial from complete
            - Differentiates SBO from LBO
            - Differentiates ileus
    - Management/Treatment
        - Relief of obstruction
        - Decompress gut with nasogastric tube (NGT) placement
        - Support volume with isotonic fluids
        - Surgical consult when surgical cause or perforation suspected

## QUESTIONS

■ Select the best answer.

### Questions 1–4 refer to the following scenario.

Mr. P., a 55-year-old Irish male, complains of pain in his chest and stomach for the past 2 weeks. He has been taking Alka-Seltzer, which seems to give him temporary relief. The pain is intermittent but has awakened him at night. The pain has a burning quality and radiates up into his chest. He has hypertension, which is controlled with diuretics.

1. Which of the following would least likely be the cause of his pain?
   a. Coronary artery insufficiency
   b. Diverticulitis
   c. Duodenal ulcer
   d. Esophageal reflux

2. Your next step would be to:
   a. Start Mr. P. on antacids and a proton pump inhibitor
   b. Discontinue his diuretic and switch to another class of antihypertensive
   c. Order an endoscopy
   d. Obtain additional medical history data

3. The fact that Mr. P.'s pain is not increased with activity and is unrelieved by rest makes it less likely that his problem is:
   a. Coronary artery insufficiency
   b. Gastric ulcer
   c. Duodenal ulcer
   d. Esophageal reflux

4. Which fact favors a diagnosis of gastric ulcer in this case?
   a. The patient's gender
   b. The patient's age
   c. The patient's ethnic origin
   d. The use of diuretics

5. Which of the following would be most beneficial in distinguishing a duodenal ulcer from a gastric ulcer?
   a. A history of a confirmed healed duodenal ulcer in the past year
   b. Reported unexplained weight loss in the past 6 months
   c. Pain aggravated by food intake
   d. An endoscopy or upper GI barium radiograph

6. Causative factors for duodenal ulcer include:
   a. High-fat diet
   b. Stress
   c. Use of anti-inflammatory drugs
   d. ETOH ingestion

7. Bleeding from a duodenal ulcer:
   a. Usually causes increased pain
   b. In large amounts can cause diarrhea
   c. Is associated with constipation
   d. Indicates perforation

8. The physical examination of most patients with peptic ulcer disease:
   a. Is noncontributory
   b. Reveals epigastric discomfort to deep palpation
   c. Should be performed after an 8-hour fast
   d. Differentiates gastric from duodenal ulcer

9. A 55-year-old male with a peptic ulcer and mild anemia has a negative stool guaiac. You need to:
   a. Start iron supplementation
   b. Start a proton pump inhibitor and reschedule for return visit in 2–4 weeks
   c. Repeat the stool guaiac
   d. Refer for hematological workup

10. After 2 weeks of treatment for *H. pylori* ulcer disease, all symptoms of a small nonbleeding duodenal ulcer have abated in your 35-year-old patient. You:
    a. Need to confirm healing with an upper GI barium radiograph or endoscopy
    b. Instruct her that she may discontinue medications
    c. Instruct her to stop all medication and get a urea breath test
    d. Stop these medications and put her on $H_2$ antagonists

11. A major side effect of cimetidine that would be of special concern when prescribing for an elderly patient is:
    a. Confusion
    b. Decreased digoxin levels
    c. Hypophosphatemia
    d. Osteopenia

### Questions 12, 13, and 14 refer to the following scenario.

Mr. J. is an overweight 38-year-old who has had intermittent heartburn for several months. He has been taking Tums, which do provide temporary relief. During the past week, he has been awakening during the night with a burning sensation in his chest. He is on no medication and has had no other major health problems.

12. Which additional information would lead you to believe that gastroesophageal reflux is the cause of his pain?

    a. The pain seems better when he smokes to relieve his nerves
    b. Constipation has been a chronic problem and he uses over-the-counter laxatives at least weekly
    c. He often awakens at night with coughing and a bad taste in his mouth
    d. Coffee and fried foods never bother him

13. J. had no weight loss or dysphagia and his physical examination is unremarkable. Your next step would be to:

    a. Order an endoscopic exam
    b. Refer him to a gastroenterologist
    c. Start him on a proton pump inhibitor
    d. Tell him to eat a snack before bedtime

14. If you diagnose GERD, you will tell him:

    a. He probably has a hiatal hernia causing the reflux
    b. He will probably require surgery
    c. He should avoid all fruit juices
    d. Smoking, alcohol, and caffeine can aggravate his problem

15. The standard for documenting tissue damage in gastroesophageal reflux is:

    a. Stool guaiac
    b. Upper GI barium radiograph
    c. Cardiac and abdominal examination
    d. Endoscopy

**Questions 16–19 refer to the following scenario.**

Mary L. is 26 years old, slightly overweight, and 2 months postpartum. She is complaining of heartburn, flatulence, and anorexia. During her pregnancy she had experienced similar symptoms, but they have become more severe in the last week and she vomited twice. She has an intermittent pain in her right hypochondrium. She also thinks she pulled a shoulder muscle because she has an almost constant dull ache there.

16. Your first step is to:

    a. Order liver function tests
    b. Obtain a more detailed history
    c. Refer her back to her obstetrician
    d. Refer her to a gastroenterologist

17. Mary's physical examination is unremarkable except for RUQ tenderness and a positive Murphy's sign. Which of the following becomes your primary differential diagnosis?

    a. Appendicitis
    b. Salpingitis
    c. Cholecystitis
    d. Diverticulitis

18. Which would be the most helpful diagnostic test at this point?

    a. CBC and liver function studies
    b. Ultrasound
    c. Liver scan
    d. Chest radiograph and ECG

19. Mary's ultrasound is negative, but she remains symptomatic and you still think cholecystitis is likely. What is the next step in your assessment?

    a. Refer for surgical evaluation
    b. Obtain a CT scan of the abdomen with contrast
    c. Obtain a CT scan of the abdomen without contrast
    d. Order a HIDA scan

20. A 22-year-old male student comes to the student health service complaining of generalized abdominal pain and nausea. He had been out with a group of friends the night before and had been eating pizza and drinking beer. He awoke with generalized abdominal pain this morning and took some Alka-Seltzer without much effect. The pain has gotten steadily worse throughout the day, and he now feels nauseated. He wonders if he might have food poisoning. Examination reveals hypoactive bowel sounds and some tenderness in the RLQ. There is no guarding or rebound tenderness. His temperature is 100° F. The absence of guarding and rebound tenderness:

    a. Suggests a psychogenic cause of his pain
    b. Rules out appendicitis
    c. Makes peritonitis unlikely
    d. Indicates irritable bowel syndrome

21. When a patient has abdominal pain accompanied by several episodes of vomiting:

    a. It is not likely to be a surgical problem
    b. Stopping the vomiting becomes the primary priority
    c. Diarrhea is likely to occur within 6 hours

d. An antiemetic is contraindicated until the cause is definitively identified

22. Diverticulitis is most often characterized by:

    a. Left lower quadrant discomfort
    b. Bloody diarrhea
    c. Rebound tenderness in the LLQ
    d. Associated vomiting

23. When should a patient with GERD be referred for endoscopy?

    a. At the time of diagnosis
    b. When he is older than 55 years of age at symptom onset
    c. When he has symptoms despite b.i.d. PPI therapy
    d. When manometry is not consistent with GERD

24. In elderly patients which of the following would not be an expected indication of appendicitis?

    a. Mild fever
    b. Abdominal distention with little pain
    c. Flatulence and hyperactive bowel sounds
    d. Shift to the left without leukocytosis

**Questions 25, 26, and 27 refer to the following scenario.**

Ms. J. is a 29-year-old accountant who comes in complaining of frequent crampy abdominal pain after meals. She is often constipated and takes over-the-counter laxatives, which are followed by a couple of days of diarrhea. She does feel better after having a bowel movement but only temporarily. She has also been embarrassed by flatulence and has noticed some abdominal distention. She has had no weight loss and has not noticed any blood in her stool. This problem has gone on for at least 6 months.

25. Your next step would be to:

    a. Obtain a complete history
    b. Order a barium enema
    c. Order a Bernstein test
    d. Suggest a trial of antispasmodics

26. Which of the following makes diverticulitis an unlikely diagnosis in this patient?

    a. Her age
    b. Frequent constipation
    c. Flatulence
    d. Crampy, intermittent pain

27. Which of the following would not be expected to occur with irritable bowel syndrome?

    a. Anxiety
    b. Nocturnal diarrhea
    c. Pain radiating to the left chest and arm
    d. Bloating

28. Which of the following would be the reason for hospitalizing a patient with acute diverticulitis?

    a. LLQ tenderness
    b. Advanced age
    c. Leukocytosis
    d. Increased pain with defecation

29. Which of the following is not indicated for treatment of acute diverticulitis?

    a. Bed rest
    b. Liquid diet
    c. Antibiotics
    d. High-fiber diet

30. A positive stool guaiac in a person suspected of having diverticulitis is:

    a. Expected in 25–30% cases
    b. An ominous sign indicating need for hospitalization
    c. Often accompanied by more pronounced pain
    d. An indication of pending perforation

31. Bacteriuria in persons with acute diverticulosis may indicate:

    a. Abscess formation
    b. Bowel–bladder fistula
    c. Free perforation into the abdomen
    d. Reason for leukocytosis

32. Ms. S., a 19-year-old college freshman, has just completed exam week. She comes in complaining of fatigue, headache, anorexia, and a runny nose. Symptoms began about 2 weeks ago. She has been taking vitamins and over-the-counter cold preparations but feels worse. "Just the smell" of food makes her nauseated. Her boyfriend had mono about a month ago, and she wonders if she might have it. Physical examination reveals cervical lymphadenopathy, a slightly enlarged, tender liver, and enlarged spleen. Which laboratory tests in addition to a CBC, throat culture, and mono spot test would be most helpful in the differential diagnosis at this point?

    a. HAV IgG antibody test
    b. Anti-HBsAg
    c. Liver enzymes
    d. Stool culture

33. There is no indication in Ms. S.'s history to indicate IV drug abuse or exposure to blood products. Given the duration of her symptoms and a confirmed increase in her liver enzymes, which test would be most helpful in confirming your diagnosis?

    a. IgM antibody to HAV
    b. IgG antibody to HAV
    c. Anti-HDV
    d. Anti-HBs

34. A 30-year-old male with a history of acute hepatitis C over 1 year ago who was treated with interferon still tests HCV-RNA positive. He should be considered:

    a. Infectious
    b. Incapable of transmitting the virus
    c. Fully recovered
    d. To have high serum viral levels

35. Infection with HDV requires antecedent or simultaneous infection with:

    a. HAV
    b. HBV
    c. HCV
    d. HGV

36. When jaundice occurs with hepatitis infection, it:

    a. Indicates a more severe infection
    b. Increases the risk of acute liver failure
    c. Indicates development of chronic active hepatitis
    d. Usually resolves in 2–6 weeks

37. A normally healthy young adult diagnosed as having *Salmonella* food poisoning should be told:

    a. To take doxycycline 100 mg t.i.d.
    b. That antidiarrheal drugs may decrease his diarrhea temporarily but may also prolong the problem
    c. That he should try to force fluids despite his nausea and vomiting to prevent dehydration
    d. That the diarrhea should abate in about 24 hours

38. Which is the next laboratory test to obtain if diarrhea and vomiting persist for more than 48 hours?

    a. Stool guaiac
    b. Sigmoidoscopy
    c. Flat plate of the abdomen
    d. Stool culture and microscopic examination

39. Blurred vision and dizziness in a patient with suspected food poisoning require

    a. Gastroenterological consult
    b. Antibiotic therapy
    c. Immediate hospitalization
    d. Follow-up in 24 hours

40. An 18-year-old previously healthy female presents with a case of a sudden onset of nausea, vomiting, generalized crampy abdominal pain followed by explosive diarrhea. The stools are uniformly thin and watery, without blood or pus. Physical exam reveals hyperactive bowel sounds and bilateral lower quadrant tenderness but no guarding or rebound. Rectal exam is negative, and she is afebrile. The hypothesis that best explains these findings is:

    a. Acute appendicitis
    b. Acute salpingitis
    c. Acute gastroenteritis
    d. Ruptured ovarian cyst

# ■ Answers

1. **b**
2. **d**
3. **a**
4. **b**
5. **d**
6. **c**
7. **b**
8. **a**
9. **c**
10. **b**
11. **a**
12. **c**
13. **c**
14. **d**
15. **d**
16. **b**
17. **c**
18. **b**
19. **d**
20. **c**
21. **a**
22. **a**
23. **c**
24. **c**
25. **a**
26. **a**
27. **c**
28. **b**
29. **d**
30. **a**
31. **b**
32. **c**
33. **a**
34. **a**
35. **b**
36. **b**
37. **b**
38. **d**
39. **c**
40. **c**

# BIBLIOGRAPHY

AGA Institute Medical Position Panel. (2008). American Gastroenterological Association medical position statement on the management of gastroesophageal reflux disease. *Gastroenterology, 135,* 1383–1391.

Boche, S. P., & Kobos, R. (2004). Jaundice in the adult patient. *American Family Physician, 69*(2), 299–304.

Brunton, S. (2004). Irritable bowel syndrome: New perspectives on treatment. *Female Patient, 29*(4), 15–20.

Chey, W. D., Wong, B. C. Y., & Practice Parameters Committee of the American College of Gastroenterology (ACG). (2007). The American College of Gastroenterology guidelines on the management of *Helicobacter pylori* infection. *American Journal of Gastroenterology, 102,* 1808–1825.

Field, S. (2003). Approaches to diverticular disease. *Clinical Advisor,* 25–31.

Friedman, L. S. (2014). Liver, biliary tract, and pancreas. In S. J. McPhee & M. A. Papadakis (Eds.), *Current medical diagnosis and treatment* (53rd ed.). New York, NY: McGraw-Hill.

Lin, K. W., & Kirchner, J. T. (2004). Hepatitis B. *American Family Physician, 69*(1), 75–82.

McQuaid, K. R. (2014). Gastrointestinal disorders. In S. J. McPhee & M. A. Papadakis (Eds.), *Current medical diagnosis and treatment* (53rd ed.). New York, NY: McGraw-Hill.

National Digestive Diseases Information Clearinghouse. (2006). *Chronic hepatitis C: Current disease management.* NIH publication no. 07-4230. Bethesda, MD: Author. Retrieved from http://permanent.access.gpo.gov/lps80481/chronichepc.pdf

Salzman, H., & Lillie, D. (2005). Diverticular disease: Diagnosis and treatment. *American Family Physician, 72,* 1229–1234, 1241–1242.

Sherman, C. (2007). Dyspepsi a guidelines emphasize *H. pylori. Clinical Advisor, 69,* 73–74.

Trowbridge, R. L., Rutkowski, N. K., & Shojania, K. (2003). Does this patient have acute cholecystitis? *Journal of the American Medical Association, 289*(1), 80–86.

U.S. Preventive Services Task Force. (2014). *The guide to clinical preventive services: Recommendations of the United States Preventive Services Task Force.* Retrieved from http://www.ahrq.gov/professionals/clinicians-providers/guidelines-recommendations/guide/index.html

Vakil, N., van Zanten, S. V., Kahrilas, P., Dent, J., & Jones, R. (2006). The Montreal definition and classification of gastroesophageal reflux disease: A global evidence-based consensus. *American Journal of Gastroenterology, 101,* 1900–1920.

Wilkins, T., Pepitone, C., Biju, A., & Schade, R. R. (2012). Diagnosis and management of IBS in adults. *American Family Physician, 86*(5), 419–426.

Yoshida, E. M. (2003). Abnormal liver function tests: What to do for the patient. *Consultant, 43*(4), 505–513.

# Endocrine Disorders

*Sister Maria Salerno*

## DIABETES MELLITUS (DM)

- Definition—metabolic disorder of carbohydrate, fat, and protein storage characterized by abnormally high blood glucose levels due to inadequate or absent insulin production and/or impaired insulin action

- Etiology/Incidence
  1. Type 1—immune mediated
     a. Genetic susceptibility (*HLA-DR3* gene) with environmental exposure to virus or other infectious processes leading to abnormal autoimmune response and destruction of insulin-producing pancreatic beta cells is suspected
        (1) Family history of autoimmune disorders
        (2) Islet cell antibodies
        (3) Insulin autoantibodies
        (4) Absence of C-peptide
     b. Occurs more often in those < 20 years of age; those with European ancestry
     c. 10–15% of diabetics are of this type
     d. < 10% of patients with type 1 diabetes are idiopathic; no immune component appreciated
  2. Type 2—impaired peripheral insulin receptors (obese type) to predominantly insulin secretory defect (nonobese type); most patients have both features at time of diagnosis
     a. Obese type 2
        (1) Intracellular fat accumulation results in distended cell membranes with change in insulin receptor morphology
        (2) Insulin resistance as a result of altered insulin receptor morphology in target cells
        (3) Post cell receptor defect impairing glucose transport into the cells
        (4) Hyperinsulinemia results; precedes hyperglycemia by years
        (5) Eventual beta cell burnout results in decreased insulin production; hyperglycemia ensues
        (6) Most type 2 diabetes is of this type
     b. Nonobese type 2
        (1) Beta cells lose responsiveness to insulinogenic stimuli, e.g., glucose, glucagon
        (2) Decreased beta cell production of insulin leads to hyperglycemia
        (3) Insulin receptor abnormalities not a problem initially
     c. No specific human leukocyte antigen (HLA) or islet cell antibodies
     d. Risk factors include
        (1) Family history of diabetes
        (2) Being previously identified as glucose intolerant
        (3) African American, Asian American, Hispanic American, Native American, or Pacific Islander race
        (4) Age > 45
        (5) Physical inactivity/obesity
        (6) Having given birth to an infant weighing > 9 lbs
        (7) Metabolic syndrome

3. Diabetes associated with certain conditions or syndromes
    a. Includes endocrinopathy, infection, drug/chemically induced
    b. Genetic syndromes
4. Prediabetes
    a. Glucose levels fall between normal and overt diabetes
    b. May worsen over time, remain unchanged, or revert to normal
    c. Characterized by impaired fasting glucose, impaired glucose tolerance, or both
5. Gestational diabetes mellitus (GDM)
6. Latent autoimmune diabetes of adults (LADA)
    a. Presents as profound hyperglycemia without ketosis
    b. Often characterized by classic weight loss, polydypsia, polyuria, and polyphagia, but no acidosis
    c. Antibody markers such as GAD-65 often present
    d. C-peptide levels low suggesting decreased beta cell insulin release
7. Approximately 8 million diagnosed cases and estimated 8 million undiagnosed; after thyroid disease and obesity, most common metabolic disorder encountered in primary care settings; third leading cause of death in United States

- Signs and Symptoms
    1. Type 1
        a. Usually sudden and severe in onset
        b. Early
            (1) Polyuria
            (2) Polydipsia
            (3) Polyphagia
            (4) Weight loss with normal or increased appetite
            (5) Blurred vision
            (6) Fatigue/weakness
            (7) Nausea/vomiting
        c. With advanced disease and long-term complications
            (1) Loss of appetite
            (2) Bloating
            (3) Dehydration
            (4) Decreased level of consciousness
            (5) Neurogenic and microvascular changes
                (a) Paresthesias
                (b) Progressive visual impairment
                (c) Cold extremities
                (d) Decreased or absent pedal pulses
                (e) Constipation, nocturnal diarrhea
                (f) Nocturia, neurogenic bladder, uremia, impotence
    2. Type 2
        a. Onset more insidious
        b. Early disease typically not symptomatic; discovered incidentally or as a result of secondary screening
        c. With advanced disease and long-term complications
            (1) Similar to type 1, but macrovascular changes more prominent than microvascular
                (a) Atherosclerosis
                (b) Vascular insufficiency
                (c) Coronary heart disease
                (d) Recurrent vaginal or genital infection, fungus
                (e) Poor wound healing, skin rashes
                (f) Target organ damage to include microalbuminuria, cardiac hypertrophy, retinopathy
            (2) Hyperosmolar, nonketotic syndrome (HNS)

- Differential Diagnosis
    1. Pancreatitis
    2. Cushing's syndrome
    3. Pheochromocytoma
    4. Acromegaly
    5. Cirrhosis
    6. Secondary effects of drug therapy
        a. Oral contraceptives
        b. Corticosteroids
        c. Thiazides
        d. Phenytoin

- Physical Findings
    1. Type 1
        a. Early
            (1) Thin, decreased weight
            (2) Ill appearance
            (3) Orthostatic hypotension
            (4) Volume contraction
            (5) Paresthesias
            (6) Mental status changes as diabetic ketoacidosis (DKA) occurs
        b. With more advanced disease
            (1) Skin—ulcerations of feet and legs, "shin spots" over tibial bones; loss of hair over lower legs and toes
            (2) Eyes—retinopathy, including microaneurysms; yellow hard or fluffy "cotton wool" exudates; neovascularization, cataracts, glaucoma
            (3) Cardiovascular—diminished or absent pedal pulses; decreased capillary filling, pretibial edema, cool extremities
            (4) Neurological—sensory loss, absent knee and ankle jerks, deficits in extraocular movements
    2. Type 2
        a. Early

(1) Usually obese
(2) Hypertension
b. With advanced disease similar to type 1

- Diagnostic Tests/Findings
  1. Plasma blood sugar—criteria for confirmation
     a. The diagnosis of diabetes will be made if fasting blood sugar (FBS) > 126 mg/dL and is > 126 mg/dL on repeat testing *or*
     b. HgbA1c > 6.5% *or*
     c. Random plasma glucose (RPG) level is > 200 mg/dL *and*
        (1) Symptoms of polydipsia, polyuria, and weight loss are present *or*
        (2) On a subsequent day the FBS is > 126 mg/dL or oral glucose tolerance test (OGTT) glucose level at 2 hours is > 200 mg/dL
     d. It is advised that the OGTT not be used routinely
     e. If fasting glucose level is > 100 mg/dL but < 126 mg/dL, a diagnosis of "prediabetes" is made
     f. Pregnant women should be screened for gestational diabetes at 24–28 weeks gestation with a 50-g glucose load
        (1) A 1-hour glucose level < 140 mg/dL is negative
        (2) A 1-hour glucose level > 200 mg/dL is diagnostic
        (3) A 1-hour glucose level between 140 mg/dL and 200 mg/dL requires confirmation by a 100-g OGTT—the diagnosis is confirmed if two of four values meet or exceed recommended cutoff points
           (a) Fasting 105 mg/dL
           (b) 1-hour 190 mg/dL
           (c) 2-hour 165 mg/dL
           (d) 3-hour 145 mg/dL
        (4) Those with known risk factors such as race/ethnicity do not need the screening level 50-g exam but should receive the diagnostic 100-g exam at the 24–28 week point
  2. Urinalysis—presence of glucose, acetone (in type 1), and, in advanced stages, protein
  3. Blood urea nitrogen and urine creatinine—elevated in acute dehydration and with renal involvement
  4. Serum cholesterol and triglyceride levels—often elevated, especially in type 2
  5. Electrocardiogram and chest radiography—for coronary and pulmonary pathology
  6. Hemoglobin A1c—predominately used as a measure of glycemic control; indicates average plasma glucose level for previous 60–90 days; tested every 3–6 months, < 7% considered good control
  7. Glycated serum protein (GSP), serum fructosamine
     a. Index of glycemic status over past 1–2 weeks
     b. Clinical utility still under study; best used for those with hemoglobinopathies that render HgbA1c inaccurate

- Management/Treatment
  1. Goals of therapy are to attain best possible metabolic control while avoiding potential side effects—see **Table 10-1**
  2. Unless acutely ill, treatment can be instituted on an outpatient basis
  3. Give consideration to work schedule, lifestyle, economic, social, and cultural aspects in management approach, e.g., persons who are homeless, persons working a night shift
  4. Diet along with exercise is cornerstone of therapy
     a. Refer newly diagnosed to registered dietician
     b. Consistent dietary schedule; ideally three meals and three snacks; especially important for persons on insulin
     c. Avoid refined carbohydrates and simple sugars
     d. Total carbohydrate intake should be 50–60% of total caloric intake
     e. Limit fats to 20–30% of total calories; saturated at < 8–9%
     f. Increase fiber to 25 g/1,000 calories
     g. Moderate protein intake, 0.8 g/kg/day or 20% of total caloric intake
     h. Total caloric intake to maintain or achieve ideal body weight (IBW)
        (1) Calculation of IBW

**TABLE 10-1** Glycemic Control for Diabetics

| Glycemic Index | Target | Nondiabetic | Therapeutic Action Suggested |
|---|---|---|---|
| Fasting and preprandial glucose (mg/dL) | 80–120 | < 115 | < 80<br>> 140 |
| Bedtime glucose (mg/dL) | 100–140 | < 120 | > 160<br>< 100 |
| HbA1c (%) | < 7 | < 6 | > 8 |

(a) Females—allow 100 lbs for first 5 feet of height plus 5 lbs for each additional inch of height
(b) Males—allow 106 lbs for first 5 feet of height and add 6 lbs for each additional inch of height
(c) Small frame subtract 10%
(d) Large frame add 10%
(2) Caloric requirement
(a) Multiply IBW by 10 = baseline calories
(b) Add 3 × IBW if activity level is sedentary (most fall in this category); 5 × IBW if moderate; and 10 × IBW if strenuous
(c) IBW = 125 lbs
125 × 10 = 1,250 (baseline calories)
125 × 3 = 375 (activity calories)
1,250 + 375 = 1,625 (total calories needed per day)
(d) In type 2—obese, where weight reduction is primary treatment, subtract 500 calories from the total number needed per day
5. Exercise
a. Planned daily exercise is an essential component for all diabetics, at least 30 minutes 5 days weekly of moderately intense exercise or 20 minutes 2 days weekly of vigorously intense exercise
b. Older persons with diabetes may be limited in types of exercise because of other concurrent problems such as arthritis, retinopathy
c. Diminishes need for insulin by enhancing oxidation of sugar and facilitating absorption of insulin from injection sites
d. Those on insulin should be instructed to inject insulin furthest from site of intensive exercise, e.g., abdomen rather than arms or thighs
e. Additional carbohydrate should be ingested prior to exercise
f. Contributes to weight and lipid control, reduces risks of cardiovascular disease (CVD), improves insulin action
6. Examples of oral pharmacological agents
a. Beta cell stimulants (secretagogues)
(1) Sulfonylureas
(a) First generation potent with long duration of action, increased risk of hypoglycemia, especially in elderly adults
(b) Contraindicated in pregnancy, for those with sulfa allergy, gestational diabetes, or type 1 diabetes, or in ketoacidosis
(c) Few side effects, but special precautions in those with renal, liver, or cardiovascular disease
(d) Risk of hypoglycemia and weight gain
(2) Meglitinides cause brief but rapid pulse of insulin secretion
(a) Fast acting
(b) Taken just before each meal
(3) D-phenylalanine derivatives
(a) Nateglinide
(b) Fast acting
(c) Taken 1–30 minutes before each meal
b. Insulin receptor sensitizers
(1) Biguanide (metformin) 2 g daily in two divided doses
(a) Increases peripheral insulin sensitivity and inhibits hepatic gluconeogenesis
(b) Causes moderate weight loss
(c) Improved lipid profile regardless of glycemic effect
(d) Low risk of hypoglycemia
(e) Side effects of flatulence, diarrhea; metallic taste minimized by taking with meals and increasing doses more slowly
(f) Contraindicated in renal, liver, or advanced cardiovascular disease (cannot be used if serum creatinine level is > 1.5 m/dL in males and above 1.4 m/dL in females)
(g) Rare incidence of lactic acidosis; check pharmacology reference for precautions
(2) Thiazolidinediones (pioglitazone, rosiglitazone)
(a) Used for type 2 diabetes as monotherapy or in combination with insulin, metformin, or a sulfonylurea
(b) Pioglitazone 15–45 mg/day; rosiglitazone 4–8 mg/day
(c) Monitor liver function every 2 months for first 12 months and periodically thereafter
(d) Increased risk of hypoglycemia with combination therapy
(e) May induce postmenopausal ovulation/risk of unintended pregnancy
(f) May cause or potentiate congestive heart failure or myocardial infarction
(g) Potential for multiple drug interactions
(h) Adverse reactions include upper respiratory infections, sinusitis, headache, pharyngitis, anemia, and edema
c. Alpha-glucosidase inhibitor (acarbose and miglitol)

(1) Lowers postprandial blood glucose levels
(2) Low risk of hypoglycemia or weight gain
(3) Somewhat less efficacious than sulfonylureas or biguanides
(4) Flatulence, bloating, diarrhea frequent but abate with continued use

d. Incretin mimetics (exentide and liraglutide)
(1) Stimulates glucose-dependent insulin secretion and lowers glucagon concentrations during periods of hyperglycemia
(2) Inhibits postprandial glucagon release
(3) Slows gastric emptying
(4) 40% incidence of nausea; high dropout rate because of this effect
(5) Used as adjunct to sulfonylurea or metformin
(6) Maximal HgbA1c reduction 1–2%
(7) Used for type 2 only; intact beta cell function required

e. Amylin analogs (pramlintide)
(1) Modulates gastric emptying
(2) Used in both type 1 and type 2 diabetes when response to therapy is inadequate
(3) Contraindicated in gastroparesis
(4) Strict warning about hypoglycemia; diet requirements include 250-kcal meal with 30 g carbohydrate

f. Dipeptidyl peptidase-4 (DPP-4) inhibitors (sitagliptin, saxagliptin, linagliptin)
(1) Incretin stimulates synthesis and release of insulin from beta cells
(2) This drug increases endogenous incretin by blocking inactivating enzyme DPP-4
(3) Maximal HgbA1c reduction 0.4–0.6%
(4) Does not cause hypoglycemia

7. Insulin (categorized as basal or bolus based on duration of action) (see **Table 10-2**)
a. Indicated
(1) Confirmed or suspected type 1 or gestational diabetes
(2) Type 2 dietary and/or oral agent management fails to control glucose levels, or in times of stress
(3) For those for whom oral agents are contraindicated
(4) At time of diagnosis of type 2 if plasma glucose > 250 mg/dL

b. Some may need more than three injections per day and/or need to use an insulin pump to maintain control
c. Weight gain and need for frequent glucose monitoring can be problems
d. Insulin replacement and augmentation
(1) No medical contraindications to insulin use and glycemic control can be obtained with exogenous insulin replacement
(2) Replacement therapy is indicated with glucose toxicity (fasting plasma glucose [FPG]) > 250 mg per dL with ketosis, weight loss; pregnancy or planning pregnancy and in poor control; during acute illness, infection, or cardiovascular disease
   (a) Total daily insulin replacement in type 1 diabetes approximates 0.5 u/kg/day
      (i) Typical starting regimen would be 2/3 daily dose as long acting

### TABLE 10-2 Insulins

| Type | Onset | Peak (Hours) | Duration (Hours) |
|---|---|---|---|
| **Bolus/Mealtime** | | | |
| **Ultra short acting** aspart (NovoLog, Novo Nordisk) | 5–10 minutes | 1–3 | 4–6 |
| lispro (Humalog) | < 15 minutes | 0.5–1.5 | 4–6 |
| **Short acting** regular (Humulin R, Novalin R) | 30 minutes | 2–3 | 6–10 |
| **Basal Insulins** | | | |
| **Intermediate** NPH (Humulin N, Novolin N) | 2–4 hours | 4–10 | 14–18 |
| lente | 3–4 hours | 4–12 | 16–20 |
| **Long acting** ultralente | 6–10 hours | peakless | 20–24 |
| glargine | 1–6 hours | peakless | 24 |
| **Premixed** | | | |
| %NPH/regular 70/30 50/50 | 30–60 minutes | dual | 14–18 |
| 75% NPL/25% lispro (Humalog 75/25) | < 15 minutes | dual | 14–18 |
| 70% NPH/30% aspart (NovoLog 70/30) | 5–10 minutes | dual | 14–18 |

Note: Pork, beef-pork, and human synthetic insulin available in rapid, intermediate, and long acting. Onset and duration values are highly variable among individuals and may vary within patients depending on the site of injection and tissue blood flow, among other factors. Duration also depends on dose size and is increased in renal failure.
NPH = neutral protamine Hagedorn; NPL = neutral protamine lispro

basal and the remaining ⅓ as premeal short acting
- (ii) A 70-kg adult would require 35 units of insulin daily; 24 units long acting with the remaining 11 units divided among three meals based upon carbohydrate count of each meal
- (b) Consider twice-daily administration of mixed dose insulin if patient has set routine of meals and activity, needs a simpler regimen, or has economic constraints
  - (i) Amount of regular insulin normally should not exceed 50% of insulin given at any time. Monitoring is done weekly and dosage adjusted based on FPG until glycemic control is achieved. Goal is FPG of 80–130 mg/dL
  - (ii) Do not mix lente or ultralente with regular; zinc in lente precipitates regular, decreasing effective proportion of regular and increasing that of the lente
  - (iii) Do not mix lente with velosulin short acting (Nordisk); phosphate buffer increases concentration of unmodified soluble insulin and diminishes effect of intermediate-acting preparation
  - (iv) Regular insulin should be drawn up first if mixing regular and NPH in same syringe
  - (v) Do not mix glargine with other insulins and do not use syringes that have been used with other insulins to draw up glargine
- (c) Consider more intensive therapy for those with irregular schedule or unstable medical condition, able to adjust insulin doses, and able to monitor and correct hypoglycemia
- (3) Augmentation with insulin is initiated when an individual cannot achieve an A1c equal to or < 7 with diet, exercise, and oral medications
  - (a) Augmentation therapy may begin at a fixed dose of 10 units/day or 0.2 u/kg/day in one long-acting dose or divided between two intermediate acting doses (Henske, Griffith, & Fowler, 2009).
  - (b) If FPG is in range but A1c is still > 7% and postprandial glucose levels are > 180 mg/dL, move to replacement therapy as outlined previously
    - (i) Preprandial plasma glucose goal is less than 140 mg/dL
    - (ii) Adjust one insulin dosage at a time and adjust dosage by no more than 2–5 units every 2–3 days
- (4) Once daily regimen is established, urine and self-monitored plasma-glucose levels are tested 3–4 times a day as indicated by the insulin schedule and severity of the disease
  - (a) Daily dose requirement decreases with progressive renal failure
  - (b) Control is assessed at 3- to 6-month intervals; glycosylated hemoglobin (Hgb), which reflects average glucose levels of the preceding 8–12 weeks, may be helpful
8. Patient education—should begin at time of diagnosis and will extend over several weeks
   a. Cause and general management of diabetes
   b. Importance of diet and weight control
   c. Self-monitoring of blood and urine glucose
   d. Administration of insulin, dosing, action, side effects, and site rotation
   e. Administration of oral hypoglycemic agents, dosing, action, and side effects
   f. Potential alteration in glucose metabolism with acute illness, exercise, and emotional stress
   g. Test for and significance of ketonuria
   h. Recognition and treatment of hypoglycemia
   i. Proper leg and foot care
   j. Sick-day guidelines
   k. Guidelines for economizing with repeated use of needles and splitting glucose test strips
9. Complications
   a. Hypoglycemia
      (1) Causes
          (a) Insulin overdosage
          (b) Omission or delay of meals
          (c) Heavy exercise
          (d) Errors in injection technique
          (e) Renal failure
          (f) Weight loss
          (g) Development of hepatitis, pituitary or adrenal insufficiency, or other conditions that cause hypoglycemia
          (h) Drugs that affect insulin metabolism/action; see **Table 10-3**
      (2) Symptoms
          (a) Weakness
          (b) Sweating
          (c) Shakiness
          (d) Tremors
          (e) Nervousness
          (f) Headache

### TABLE 10-3 Medication Effect on Insulin Metabolism/Action

| Medication | Action |
|---|---|
| Alcohol | Decreased half-life of sulfonylureas in alcoholics, can cause severe hypoglycemia in those on hypoglycemic agents |
| Beta-adrenergic | Inhibit insulin secretion; block most hypoglycemia symptoms; prolong effect of insulin |
| Calcium channel blockers | Inhibit insulin secretion |
| Diazoxide | Inhibits insulin secretion |
| Glucocorticoids | Insulin antagonism |
| Nicotinic acid | Insulin resistance |
| Oral contraceptives | Insulin resistance |
| Phenytoin | Inhibits insulin secretion |
| Sympathomimetics | Insulin antagonism; inhibit insulin secretion |
| Thiazide diuretics | Inhibit insulin secretion |
| MAO inhibitors | Increase effects of antidiabetic agents |
| Salicylates | Increase effects of antidiabetic agents |
| Coumarin | Increase effects of sulfonylureas |
| Phenylbutazone | Increase effects of sulfonylureas |

   (g) Dizziness
   (h) Hunger
   (i) Irritability
   (j) Convulsions, confusion, coma
   (k) Tachycardia, palpitations
  b. Somogyi phenomenon
   (1) Cause—morning rebound hyperglycemia; occurs in response to nocturnal hypoglycemia with excessive insulin administration
   (2) Clues—erratic plasma glucose and urine ketone values; symptoms of nocturnal hypoglycemia (night sweats, nightmares, low serum glucose 2–3 a.m.), weight gain in presence of heavy glycosuria
   (3) Treatment—reduce insulin dose 10–20%
   (4) Distinguish from *dawn phenomenon*, which is early morning fasting hyperglycemia without nocturnal hypoglycemia; thought to be related to circadian rhythm secretion of growth hormone and treated by evening or bedtime dose of insulin
  c. Lipodystrophy
   (1) Atrophy—subcutaneous fat atrophy at insulin injection sites
    (a) Cause—impurities in the insulin, possible autoimmune mechanism
    (b) Treatment—switch to purified insulin, inject directly into atrophic areas
   (2) Hypertrophy—overgrowth of subcutaneous tissue
    (a) Cause—growth-promoting effects of insulin; improper rotation of injection sites
    (b) Treatment—prevent by proper rotation of injection sites
  d. Insulin allergy
   (1) Rare and usually localized
   (2) Treatment—change to human synthetic insulin
   (3) Localized allergies may be treated with antihistamines or corticosteroid; consultation required
  e. Insulin resistance requiring more than 200 units per day
   (1) Rare and even less common with increased use of human insulins
   (2) Cause—overproduction of insulin-binding immunoglobulins
   (3) Treatment—change to less immunogenic pork or human synthetic insulins
   (4) May require glucocorticoid treatment; consultation required
 10. Follow-up
  a. Well-controlled patients—minimum every 3–4 months
  b. Yearly ECG, chest radiograph, creatinine, urinalysis with microprotein analysis, lipid profile, physical examination including fundoscopic, full neurological examination

c. Annual ophthalmological examination by ophthalmologist
d. Skin inspection, feet inspection, fundoscopic, and evaluation of glycemic control by fasting or postprandial plasma glucose measurements at each visit
e. Hemoglobin A1c every 3–6 months
11. Referrals to local support groups and identification of local chapters of the American Diabetes Association for information, support, and publications
12. Routinely screen all adults > 45 years of age or those with a body mass index (BMI) ≥ 26 and the presence of risk factors; if negative, repeat every 3 years

## THYROTOXICOSIS

- Definition—a metabolic state characterized by symptomatic circulating thyroid hormone excess; commonly due to hyperthyroidism, which is a state of excessive secretory activity of the thyroid gland (Graves' disease) or a state of excess circulating thyroid hormone produced by excess exogenous or endogenous thyroid hormone in the presence of a normally functioning gland (subacute thyroiditis, exogenous thyroid hormone administration)

- Etiology/Incidence
  1. Causes
     a. Autoimmune response (Graves' disease accounts for more than 85% of cases)
     b. Subacute thyroiditis—normal gland releases its hormone stores in a burst following glandular insult, e.g., viral inflammation
     c. Toxic multinodular goiter; toxic uninodular goiter (autonomous thyroid adenoma)
     d. Metastatic follicular thyroid carcinoma
     e. Thyrotoxicosis factitia
     f. Thyroid-stimulating hormone (TSH)-secreting pituitary tumor (secondary hyperthyroidism)
     g. Human chorionic gonadotropin (hCG)-secreting tumors (choriocarcinoma, hydatidiform mole)
     h. Testicular embryonal carcinoma
  2. One of the most common endocrine disorders
  3. Highest incidence in women between 20 and 40 years of age

- Signs and Symptoms
  1. Most frequent
     a. Anxiety
     b. Diaphoresis
     c. Fatigue
     d. Hypersensitivity to heat
     e. Nervousness
     f. Palpitations
     g. Weight loss
     h. Insomnia, nightmares
  2. Frequent
     a. Dyspnea
     b. Weakness
     c. Increased appetite
     d. Eye complaints, e.g., difficulty focusing
     e. Swelling of legs
     f. Hyperdefecation without diarrhea, hyperactive bowel sounds
     g. Diarrhea
     h. Oligomenorrhea or amenorrhea
     i. Tremors
     j. Angina
  3. Infrequent
     a. Anorexia
     b. Constipation
     c. Weight gain
     d. Signs of pseudobulbar palsy
  4. Elderly patients may present with few signs or symptoms noted in younger patients (apathetic hyperthyroidism); may present with cardiovascular problems unresponsive to digitalis, quinidine, or diuretics
     a. Atrial fibrillation
     b. Angina
     c. Congestive heart failure

- Differential Diagnosis
  1. Anxiety neurosis, especially in menopause
  2. Other diseases associated with hypermetabolism, e.g., pheochromocytoma and acromegaly
  3. Myasthenia gravis (causes the same ophthalmoplegic signs)
  4. Orbital tumors, which can cause exophthalmos
  5. Psychosis

- Physical Findings
  1. General—thin, muscle wasting may be evident; nervous; quick motions
  2. Vital signs—tachycardia, irregular pulse, widened pulse pressure
  3. Integumentary—skin moist, velvety, may show increased pigmentation or vitiligo; hair thin, fine; spider angiomas and gynecomastia may be evident
  4. Eyes—prominent; appear to "stare"; lid lag; lack of accommodation, chemosis; proptosis (exophthalmos)
  5. Neck—enlarged thyroid gland (goiter) smooth or nodular, symmetric or asymmetric; thyroid bruit or thrill; absence of signs does not rule out hyperthyroidism
  6. Cardiovascular—tachycardia, paroxysmal atrial fibrillation, harsh pulmonary systolic murmur, congestive failure, possible enlargement

7. Neurological—hyperactive reflexes; fine tremors of fingers, tongue; mental changes ranging from mild exhilaration to delirium; in elderly patients, apathy, lethargy, and severe depression may be manifested
8. Lymphatic—lymphadenopathy and splenomegaly may be present

- Diagnostic Tests/Findings (see **Table 10-4** for list of thyroid function tests)
    1. TSH assay best test for thyroid dysfunction—decreased in most forms of thyrotoxicosis; if TSH is elevated in the setting of clinical thyrotoxicosis, consider TSH-producing tumor
    2. Free thyroxine index ($FT_4I$) usually elevated; order if normal and clinical impression is strong for hyperthyroidism
    3. $T_3$, radioimmunoassay ($T_3$, RIA)—elevated with a normal $T_4$ in early hyperthyroidism and $T_3$ toxicosis
    4. $T_4$ level elevated in later stages
    5. TSI present

- Management/Treatment
    1. Refer for hospitalization for suspected "thyroid storm"
        a. High fever
        b. Severe agitation
        c. Confusion
        d. Cardiovascular collapse
        e. Malignant exophthalmus
        f. Difficulty in breathing due to enlarged or tender thyroid gland
    2. Symptomatic and curative treatment
        a. Propranolol 10–60 mg orally every 6 hours to control symptoms
        b. Radioactive iodine ($^{131}I$)
            (1) In United States preferred treatment—refer to interventional radiology
            (2) Therapeutic dose is 80–120 mCi administered in doses of 5–15 mCi based on estimated weight of the thyroid gland
            (3) Most become euthyroid after 6–8 weeks
            (4) Hypothyroidism is frequent and can occur anytime after radioactive iodine therapy
            (5) Contraindicated in pregnancy
        c. Antithyroid drugs—indicated for initial control of thyrotoxicosis especially in pregnant women, those not wanting to take $^{131}I$,

**TABLE 10-4** Thyroid Assessment Tests

| | |
|---|---|
| Thyroxine ($T_4$) | Major hormone secreted by the thyroid gland |
| $T_4$ (RIA-serum) | By radioimmunoassay (RIA); normal adult is 5–12 mg/dL |
| Free Thyroxine Index ($FT_4I$) | Unaffected by thyroxine-binding globulin (TBG) and is a better reflection of the true index hormonal status; serum $T_4$ and $T_3$ resin uptake ($T_3$, RU) used to calculate this index; normal adult is 0.9–2.2 ng/dL |
| $T_3$ Resin Uptake ($T_3RU$) | Indirect measure of $T_4$ levels by assessing $T_4$ binding sites; may be thought of as the reciprocal of the $T_4$ RIA; in hyperthyroidism there is a high $T_3$ resin uptake; in hypothyroidism the $T_3$ is low; normal adult is 25–35% |
| $T_3$ RIA (Serum) | Direct measure of triiodothyronine ($T_3$) thyroid hormone; helpful in diagnosing thyrotoxicosis when $T_4$ is normal; in hypothyroidism $T_3$ often normal; $T_4$ more helpful; normal adult is 80–200 ng/dL (RIA) |
| Antithyroid Peroxidase Antibody (Anti-TPO) (Serum) | Mediate antibody-dependent thyroid cell destruction; when present in a patient with elevated TSH and normal $T_4$, suggests early disease; may be elevated in 10% asymptomatic individuals (nl < 1 IU/mL) |
| Thyroid-Stimulating Immune Globulins (TSI) | Autoantibodies frequently present in Graves' disease; stimulate TSH receptors, accelerating function of the gland independent of the pituitary–thyroid gland feedback loop; normal range < 130% activity, although persons with Graves' disease usually at < 2% |
| Thyroid-Stimulating Hormone (TSH) | Direct measure of TSH secreted from the anterior pituitary in response to thyrotropin-releasing hormone (TRH); normal adult is 2–5.4 mU/mL < 10 mU/mL (RIA); most sensitive indicator of thyroid hormone function |
| TSH Immunoradiometric Assay (IRMA) | Newer assay replacing TSH (RIA); normal adult is 0.5–5 mU/mL; more sensitive to suppressed TSH in hyperthyroidism |
| Radioactive Iodine Uptake (RAIU) | Used primarily to detect hyperthyroidism etiology; radioactive iodine given orally or intravenously; the thyroid is scanned at three different intervals to determine iodine uptake of the thyroid gland; an elevated RAIU indicates hyperthyroidism; normal adult is 2 hour, 1–13%; 6 hour, 2–25%; 24 hour, 15–45% |

or in preparation for surgical removal; effective in patients with small goiters
            (1) Propylthiouracil (PTU)—usual dose 300–400 mg/day in divided doses
                (a) Preferred for use in pregnant women
                (b) During pregnancy, dose kept < 200 mg/day
            (2) Methimazole (MMI)—15–60 mg/day orally in three divided doses
            (3) Side effects
                (a) Dermatitis
                (b) Nausea
                (c) Agranulocytosis (most serious)
                (d) Hypothyroidism, which can cause a TSH-stimulated increase in goiter size
    3. Patient education
        a. Medication is to be taken for about 2 years and not abruptly discontinued
        b. At first sign of infection or fever, drug should be stopped and healthcare professional contacted
        c. Therapeutic effect of medication is not usually evident for about 3 weeks
    4. Surgery
        a. Not typically indicated in Graves' disease
        b. Indicated for children, adolescents, pregnant women unable to tolerate PTU, adults nonresponsive to thiourea treatment who refuse RAI
        c. Usually rendered euthyroid with drugs preoperatively
    5. General considerations
        a. Client education
            (1) Rationale for treatment; dosage and side effects of medications; takes at least 3 weeks before antithyroid medications become effective
            (2) Instructions regarding nutritional needs: high-carbohydrate, high-calorie diet until medication takes effect; avoidance of stimulants such as caffeine
            (3) Symptoms of "thyroid storm"
            (4) Symptoms of hypothyroidism
        b. Follow-up
            (1) Periodic examinations until euthyroid
            (2) All patients who have been treated for hyperthyroidism should be periodically checked for hypothyroidism, which may occur anytime during treatment

# ADULT HYPOTHYROIDISM

- Definition—decreased or deficient thyroid hormone—primary (glandular dysfunction) or secondary (pituitary insufficiency); occurs in all age groups

- Etiology/Incidence
    1. Major classifications
        a. Primary—caused abnormalities of the thyroid gland itself
            (1) Most common cause in adults is autoimmune thyroiditis (Hashimoto's, or chronic lymphocytic)
            (2) Can also be caused by ablation of the gland by surgery, medication, radiation, and goitrogens (thiocyanates, rutabagas, lithium carbonate, amiodarone)
            (3) More common than secondary
        b. Secondary—often related to destructive lesions of the pituitary gland as with chromophobe adenoma or postpartum necrosis (Sheehan's syndrome); frequently associated with signs of adrenal and gonadal disorders
        c. Tertiary—TRH deficiency arising in the hypothalamus; sometimes grouped with secondary
    2. Occurs in all age groups; more prevalent in women and those
        a. With a history of thyroiditis
        b. With previously treated hyperthyroidism (all modalities)
        c. Being treated with lithium or amiodarone
        d. With coexistent autoimmune disorders (e.g., rheumatoid arthritis, lupus, pernicious anemia)

- Signs and Symptoms
    1. Most frequent
        a. Cold intolerance
        b. Coarse skin
        c. Decreased sweating
        d. Dry skin
        e. Lethargy
        f. Swelling of eyelids
    2. Frequent
        a. Anemia (normocytic, normochromic, microcytic, or macrocytic)
        b. Anorexia
        c. Coarse hair
        d. Cold skin
        e. Constipation
        f. Hair loss
        g. Hoarseness or aphonia, thick tongue
        h. Hyperlipidemia including hypercholesterolemia
        i. Leg edema
        j. Menorrhagia
        k. Memory impairment
        l. Swelling of face
        m. Paresthesias
        n. Weight change

- Differential Diagnosis
    1. Rule out coexisting autoimmune disease or secondary hypothyroidism
    2. Nephrotic syndrome
    3. Chronic renal disease

- Physical Findings
    1. Vital signs—bradycardia, mild hypotension, or diastolic hypertension
    2. Edema of hands, face, eyelids
    3. Integumentary—dry, scaly skin with carotenemic tone; brittle nails; alopecia; puffy eyelids; temporal thinning of the eyebrows; generalized hair loss, nonpitting edema
    4. ENT—enlarged tongue, possible hearing decrease, thyroid often enlarged
    5. Cardiovascular—bradycardia, decreased intensity of heart tones, cardiac enlargement (myxedemic heart may be related to pericardial effusion)
    6. Respiratory—pleural effusion
    7. Abdominal—ascites, decreased bowel sounds
    8. Neuromuscular—slow or delayed deep tendon reflexes, cerebellar ataxia, dementia (myxedema madness, manifested with hallucinations, paranoid ideation, and hyperactive delirium), pseudomyotonia, carpal tunnel syndrome

- Diagnostic Tests/Findings (see **Table 10-5**)
    1. TSH elevated in primary hypothyroidism
    2. Free thyroxine index (FTI) or $T_4$; if low, a TSH is helpful in determining etiology
    3. TSH elevated in primary hypothyroidism
    4. If $T_4$ is normal and TSH is elevated, may be mild hypothyroidism
    5. Thyrotropin-releasing hormone (TRH) stimulation done if low TSH with low $T_4$ or low FTI; may indicate secondary hypothyroidism
    6. Complete blood count (CBC)—may demonstrate anemia

- Management/Treatment
    1. Refer for immediate hospitalization any client suspected of developing myxedemic coma—severe hypothyroidism associated with hypothermia, decreased mentation, hypoventilation, respiratory acidosis, relative hypotension, hyponatremia, hypoglycemia
    2. Replacement of hormone deficiency
        a. Average replacement dose of $T_4$ is thyroxine 1.6 mcg/kg/day day in healthy, non-elderly adults
        b. Replacement at 1 mcg/kg/day for those > 50 years of age or with known ischemic heart disease without angina
        c. Dosage begins with ½ projected replacement, increased every 4–6 weeks as tolerated until clinically euthyroid
            (1) 70-kg, 45-year-old female would have projected dose of 70 × 1.6 mcg (112 mcg or 1.12 mg)
            (2) Begin at 50 mcg/day, increase every 4 weeks by 25% until clinically euthyroid
        d. Patients with coexisting adrenal insufficiency, coronary insufficiency, or angina require particular care
        e. Initial effects of replacement not usually perceptible for at least 2 weeks after initiation of therapy and are initially demonstrated by decreased facial edema and increased urination
    3. On follow-up visits, after replacement therapy has been instituted
        a. Laboratory assessment at 8 weeks minimum after dose initiated—TSH of > 4 mU/mL increase dose by 25 mcg/d after appropriate adherence to current therapy ensured
        b. Monitor for symptoms or signs of too vigorous therapy, side effects, and toxic effects of replacement therapy; ask about dyspnea, orthopnea, angina, palpitations, nervousness, insomnia
        c. Be alert to concomitant use of opiates, barbiturates, other central nervous system depressants, digitalis, and insulin; persons with hypothyroidism are particularly sensitive to these agents; as they become euthyroid, dosages may have to be increased
    4. Monitor control of clinical symptoms and periodically monitor serum FTI and TSH; persistently high TSH or low FTI may indicate underreplacement; a high $T_4$ and low TSH with symptoms of hyperthyroidism usually indicates overreplacement
    5. Patient education
        a. Nature and chronicity of the disease and the need for lifelong treatment

**TABLE 10-5** Laboratory Values in Hypothyroidism

| Type | TSH | $FT_4$ | $FT_3$ |
|---|---|---|---|
| Primary | High | Low | Low |
| Subclinical | High | Normal | Normal |
| Secondary (pituitary deficiency) TSH | Low | Low | Low |

TSH = thyroid-stimulating hormone; $T_4$ = thyroxine; $T_3$ = triiodothyronine.

b. Rationale for treatment—dosage, side effects, and toxic effects of treatment
c. Teach signs of hyperthyroidism
d. Management of symptoms of hypothyroidism until abatement with replacement therapy
    (1) Fatigue
    (2) Dry skin
    (3) Constipation (increased fiber, fluids)

## THYROID NODULE

- Definition—discrete enlargements within the thyroid gland

- Etiology unknown, but nodules are common
  1. Palpable in 5–10% of U.S. population
  2. Majority are benign
  3. Risk of nodule malignancy less than 10% in most adults
     a. Men have a higher incidence than women
     b. Papillary and follicular carcinoma are most common types of malignancy
        (1) Papillary tends to spread within the thyroid gland or to cervical lymphatics
            (a) Twice as common in women as men
            (b) Accounts for 80% of thyroid malignancies in adults < 40 years
        (2) Follicular accounts for approximately 20% of all thyroid cancers
            (a) Incidence somewhat higher in older individuals
            (b) Usually slow growing but more aggressive than papillary; can spread rapidly to lymph nodes and to distant sites via the bloodstream, often to lung, bone, brain, or liver
            (c) More aggressive in elderly adults
     c. Medullary and anaplastic carcinoma are rare but tend to metastasize very early; anaplastic carcinoma, because of high invasiveness and early metastasis, results in death in weeks or months regardless of treatment modality
     d. Risk of carcinoma is increased with a history of radiation exposure, particularly during childhood, to the head or neck for acne, tonsils, adenoids; the risk is also increased in those with a family history of thyroid cancer—this is especially true for medullary carcinoma

- Signs and Symptoms
  1. Thyroid mass
  2. Expanding goiter or nodule, which is hard and/or tender
  3. Hoarseness or dysphagia

- Differential Diagnosis—distinguish from nonneoplastic enlargements, e.g., cystic nodules, multinodular goiters

- Physical Findings
  1. Single hard thyroid nodule (or multiple nodules) fixed to overlying tissue
  2. Regional lymphadenopathy

- Diagnostic Tests/Findings
  1. FTI—usually normal; if elevated, chances of malignancy are decreased
  2. RAI scan—nonfunctioning (cold) nodule
  3. Ultrasonography—if cystic, rarely malignant
  4. Thyrocalcitonin—increased in medullary carcinoma
  5. Biopsy (open or needle)—positive cytology if malignant

- Management/Treatment
  1. Treatment may include
     a. Excision of the nodule (complete thyroidectomy in the case of medullary carcinoma) and regional lymph nodes
     b. Ablation of metastasis with large doses of radioactive iodine
     c. Suppression of thyroid function with L-thyroxine
     d. Chemotherapy for anaplastic carcinoma (thyroid suppression and radioactive ablation of metastasis are not effective in medullary thyroid carcinoma)
  2. Client education related to diagnostic tests
  3. Follow-up for detection of metastasis, recurrence, and subsequent treatment is usually on an annual basis

## CUSHING'S SYNDROME (HYPERCORTISOLISM)

- Definition—a constellation of clinical abnormalities due to an excess of corticosteroids

- Etiology/Incidence
  1. Excessive or prolonged administration of glucocorticoids (most common)
  2. Excessive pituitary adrenocorticotropic hormone (ACTH) secretion (Cushing's disease)
  3. Secretion of ACTH by a nonpituitary tumor (ectopic tumor), e.g., carcinoma of the lung or other malignant growths

4. Tumors within the adrenal cortex—adenomas or carcinoma
  5. Cushing's disease and primary adrenal tumors more common in females
  6. Ectopic corticotropin production more common in males

- Signs and Symptoms
  1. Central obesity with slender extremities
  2. Full face
  3. Muscular weakness
  4. Back pain
  5. Mental changes
  6. Thin, fragile skin
  7. Poor wound healing
  8. Acne
  9. Menstrual disorders

- Differential Diagnosis
  1. Hypercortisolism due to alcoholism
  2. Hypercortisolism due to depression

- Physical Findings
  1. Moon face with facial plethora
  2. Hirsutism
  3. Skin—thin and atrophic
  4. Purplish-red striae on abdomen, breasts, or buttocks
  5. Truncal obesity with wasting of limbs
  6. Prominent supraclavicular and dorsal cervical fat pads ("buffalo hump")
  7. Hypertension

- Diagnostic Tests/Findings
  1. Dexamethasone test (most reliable for distinguishing among causes of Cushing's syndrome)
  2. Urinary cortisol—elevated
  3. Plasma cortisol—evening cortisol levels and 24-hour total levels are elevated
  4. MRI, CT, and ultrasonographic imaging for identification of pituitary tumor, nonpituitary ACTH-producing neoplasms
  5. Blood glucose—increased
  6. Hypokalemia, but not hypernatremia

- Management/Treatment
  1. Treatment of choice for Cushing's disease—surgery
  2. Adrenal tumors or hyperplasia—removal
  3. If surgery is contraindicated, radiation and drug therapy (used to control cortisol excess) may be used, which includes ketoconazole 400–500 mg b.i.d.; metyrapone 2 g per day; aminoglutethimide 1 g per day
  4. When surgery and aggressive medical management not options, controlling consequences is indicated
     a. Replace K⁺
     b. Control hypertension
     c. Control hyperglycemia
     d. Aggressive management of wounds and rashes
  5. For Cushing's syndrome due to prolonged administration of steroids
     a. Discontinuation of therapy gradually
     b. Reduction of steroid dose
     c. Changing to an alternate-day schedule

# ADDISON'S DISEASE (PRIMARY ADRENOCORTICAL INSUFFICIENCY)

- Definition—an insidious, usually progressive disease due to destruction of the adrenal cortex
  1. Primary—due to destruction of adrenal cortex
  2. Secondary—lack of corticotropin stimulation

- Etiology/Incidence
  1. Idiopathic autoimmune destruction of adrenal tissue (more than 80%); two to three times more common in females; usually diagnosed between ages 30 and 50 years
  2. Tuberculosis—second most frequent cause (common cause in underdeveloped countries)
  3. Acquired immunodeficiency syndrome (AIDS)—becoming a more frequent cause
  4. Less common—hemorrhage, fungal infections, antineoplastic chemotherapy, abrupt withdrawal of exogenous steroids
  5. Primarily a rare disease

- Signs and Symptoms
  1. Chronic primary adrenocortical insufficiency—develops gradually
     a. Weakness and fatigue, orthostatic hypotension may be early symptoms
     b. Anorexia, weight loss
     c. Tan appearance to the skin
     d. Gastrointestinal symptoms
  2. Acute adrenocortical insufficiency—seen more often in patients without previous diagnosis or those with a diagnosis who are exposed to stress with related increased requirement for glucocorticoids; symptoms of chronic are exaggerated, especially profound hypotension
  3. Most dangerous feature of Addison's disease is hypotension, which may cause shock, especially during stress *and* is nonresponsive to usual treatment; requires glucocorticoid replacement

- Differential Diagnosis
  1. Antidiuretic hormone (ADH) syndrome
  2. Salt-losing nephritis
  3. Hemochromatosis

**172** CHAPTER 10 Endocrine Disorders

- Physical Findings
    1. Hyperpigmentation of skin
    2. Hypotension
    3. Black freckles over forehead, face, neck, and shoulders
    4. Areas of vitiligo
    5. Bluish-black discolorations of the areolae and of the mucous membranes of the lips, mouth, rectum, vagina

- Diagnostic Tests/Findings
    1. Sodium levels—low (< 130 mEq/L; normal 135–145 mEq/L)
    2. Potassium levels—high (> 5 mEq/L; normal 3.5–5 mEq/L)
    3. Blood urea nitrogen (BUN)—elevated
    4. Plasma renin level—increased
    5. ACTH plasma levels—increased
    6. Ratio of serum sodium to potassium (< 30:1)
    7. Low fasting blood glucose (< 50 mg/dL; normal 60–115 mg/dL)
    8. Hematocrit—elevated
    9. White blood cell (WBC) count—low
    10. Eosinophils—increased

- Management/Treatment
    1. In acute crisis referral with hospitalization
    2. Chronic
        a. Lifetime of treatment
        b. Cortisol 15–20 mg orally every a.m.; 5–10 mg 4–6 p.m.
        c. Fludrocortisone acetate 0.05–0.3 mg daily or every other day if insufficient sodium retention with cortisol alone; frequently needed in times of physiological crises, e.g., acute systemic illness, operation
            (1) When fludrocortisone therapy has been initiated, monitor closely for symptoms of sodium and fluid retention
            (2) Discontinue as able when patient recovers from physiological crisis
        d. Monitor weight, blood pressure, and electrolytes
    3. General considerations
        a. Education regarding increasing cortisol during times of stress
        b. Education regarding carrying an identification bracelet or card
        c. Salt additives for excess heat or humidity
        d. Prognosis is excellent with continued substitution therapy

---

### Special Considerations in the Hospitalized Patient

- Diabetic Ketoacidosis
    - Definition—an acute, life-threatening metabolic state characterized by hyperglycemia and ketonemia occurring most commonly in patients with type 1 diabetes mellitus; it can, however, occur in some forms of uncontrolled type 2 diabetes mellitus when severe physiological stressors are present.
    - Etiology/Incidence
        - Undiagnosed and untreated type 1 DM
        - Atypical increased insulin requirements
        - Sepsis
        - Trauma
            - Major surgery
        - Occurs in 5 to 8 per 1,000 persons with diabetes
        - Poor compliance with capillary and urine monitoring increases likelihood
        - More common in insulin-pump users
        - Increased incidence in those on atypical antipsychotics
    - Signs and Symptoms
        - Insidious increase in polyuria and polydypsia
        - Nausea and vomiting
        - Weight loss
        - Decreased perspiration
        - Fatigue
        - Drowsiness
        - Abdominal discomfort
    - Differential Diagnosis
        - Alcoholic ketoacidosis
        - Metabolic acidosis
        - Lactic acidosis
        - Shock
        - Salicylate toxicity
    - Physical Findings
        - Volume contraction
        - Fruity breath
        - Hypotension
        - Tachycardia
        - Orthostasis
        - Hypothermia
        - Abdominal tenderness
        - Altered level of consciousness (frank coma is not typical)
        - Physical findings consistent with predisposing event, e.g., infection
    - Diagnostic Tests/Findings

- Essentials of diagnosis
  - Serum glucose > 250–300 mg/dL
  - Blood pH < 7.3
  - Ketonemia
  - Serum bicarbonate < 15 mEq/dL
- Consequent serum abnormalities
  - Hyperkalemia
  - Hyponatremia
  - Hyperphosphatemia
  - Elevated BUN/creatinine
- Other studies as indicated to evaluate underlying cause, e.g., infection
- Management/Treatment
  - Admit to critical care unit for first 24–48 hours
  - Priorities of treatment are reversal of acidosis and correction of fluid deficit—failure to replace volume adequately is a primary risk factor for poor outcome
    - 0.9% normal saline solution (NSS) 1L/hour for the first 2 hours; then 300–400 mL/hour to infuse total of 4–5 L over an 8-hour period; do not exceed 5 L in 8 hours
    - Change to dextrose-containing solution once serum glucose < 250 mg/dL
    - If presenting serum Na+ is > 150 mEq/L, begin infusion with ½ NSS
    - Regular insulin 0.15μ/kg IV bolus followed by 0.1μ/kg/hour
  - Blood glucose should be measured every 1–2 hours until stable; then every 6 hours; optimal rate of glucose decline is 100 mg/dL/hr
  - Consider K+ replacement; patients may become hypokalemic as acidosis and volume contraction resolves—K+ at 10–30 mEq/hour should be infused as soon as clinical improvement of acidosis is apparent
  - NaHCO$_3$ infusion only if presenting pH is < 7.0
- Hyperosmolar Hyperglycemic State (HHS)
  - Definition—an acute, unstable, metabolic, potentially life-threatening emergency occurring in persons with uncontrolled type 2 diabetes mellitus; it may occur in type 1 DM, and both DKA and HHS have been found to occur simultaneously. It is characterized by severe hyperglycemia, volume contraction, and hyperosmolality in the absence of acidosis.
  - Etiology/Incidence
    - Most often occurs in persons with type 2 DM and underlying illness resulting in decreased fluid intake
    - Stress responses leading to increased catecholamines, cortisol, and glucagon as well as other glucose-mobilizing hormones
    - Patients with underlying congestive heart failure (CHF) and chronic kidney disease (CKD) at higher risk
    - Medications that increase glucose or increase insulin resistance
    - Underhydration
    - Mean onset is in the 7th decade
    - Higher incidence in African Americans, Native Americans, and Latinos (consistent with higher incidence of type 2 DM)
  - Signs and Symptoms
    - Insidious onset of polyuria and polydipsia
    - Generalized weakness
    - Sensory deficits
    - Altered level of consciousness
  - Differential Diagnosis
    - Severe dehydration
    - Diabetes insipidus
    - DKA
  - Physical Findings
    - Physical findings consistent with volume contraction
      - Dry mucous membranes
      - Poor skin turgor
      - Hypotension
      - Tachycardia
      - Findings consistent with underlying type 2 DM
        - Poor wound healing
        - Distal paresthesias
        - Cutaneous rash or fungal infection
        - Onychomycosis
  - Diagnostic Tests/Findings
    - Essentials of diagnosis
      - Serum glucose > 600 mg/dL
      - Serum osmolality > 320 mOsm/kg
      - Absence of acidosis
        - Serum bicarbonate > 15 mEq/dL
        - Blood pH > 7.3
        - Anion gap < 14 mEq/L
    - Hyponatremia in mild cases
    - Hypernatremia as condition progresses and volume loss is severe

*(continues)*

**Special Considerations in the Hospitalized Patient (*continued*)**

- Elevated BUN and creatinine
- Management/Treatment
  - Replace 50% of calculated fluid deficit with 0.9% NSS in the first 12 hours; deficits may exceed 10 L
  - Initial isotonic fluid replacement may be as high as 2 L in the first hour; requires consideration of degree of fluid deficit and the presence of underlying conditions that may be exacerbated by vigorous fluid resuscitation (CHF)
  - Insulin infusion at DKA doses until glucose is < 250 mg/dL
  - K+ replacement when fluid infusion begun; at minimum 5 mEq/L, increase depending on presenting condition
- Diabetes Insipidus (DI)
  - Definition—an endocrine disorder characterized by the passage of large volumes of hypo-osmolar urine and an associated increase in thirst; due to either a deficiency of antidiuretic hormone or a nephrogenic insensitivity to it
  - Etiology/Incidence
    - Central DI
      - Idiopathic
      - Tumors of the brain or pituitary gland
      - Head trauma
      - Head surgery
      - Hereditary DI
      - Hypoxic encephalopathy
      - Metastatic disease
    - Nephrogenic
      - Renal disease
      - Vasopressinase-induced
      - Vasopressin-resistant
      - Hyperglycemia
      - Drug-induced
    - Psychogenic
    - Uncommon condition (3 per 100,000 population) with no gender or ethnic predisposition
  - Signs and Symptoms
    - Intense polydipsia—may ingest up to 20 L daily
    - Polyuria
    - Fatigue
    - Headache
  - Differential Diagnosis
    - Type 1 DM
    - HHS
    - Hypokalemia
    - Hypercalcemia
  - Physical Findings
    - Volume contraction not apparent unless fluid intake restricted
    - Hydronephrosis
    - Bladder distention
    - Flank pain
    - Pelvic fullness
  - Diagnostic Tests/Findings
    - 24-hr urine required to assess volume loss
    - Specific gravity < 1.005
    - Urine osmolality < 200 mOsm/L
    - Water deprivation test
      - All water intake withheld
      - Urine osmolality and body weight measured hourly
      - When two sequential urine osmolalities vary by < 30 mOsm/kg or weight decrease by 3%, 5 units of ADH are administered
      - In the absence of DI, water deprivation should produce a urine osmolality 2–4 × greater than plasma osmolality; this will not occur in DI
      - In the absence of DI, administration of ADH will not produce an increase in urine osmolality of > 9%
        - ADH will produce significant increase in urine osmolality in central DI (problem is ADH deficiency)
        - ADH will not produce significant increase in urine osmolality in nephrogenic DI (problem is ADH resistance)
      - Head imaging if tumor or other structural or traumatic problem suspected
    - Management/Treatment
      - In milder cases fluid can be replaced orally
        - In more severe cases, calculate fluid deficit and replace at 500–750 mL/hour with hypo-osmolar $D_5W$—reduce serum Na+ by 0.5 mEq/L every hour
      - Treat underlying cause as able—transient cases will resolve spontaneously
      - ADH replacement in the form of desmopressin for central DI

- High doses of hydrochlorothiazide (HCTZ), desmopressin, and indomethacin, in a variety of combinations, for nephrogenic DI
- In patients who develop DI after pituitary surgery, monitor closely for DI
- Psychotherapy for psychogenic causes
- Syndrome of Inappropriate Antidiuretic Hormone (SIADH)
  - Definition—an endocrine disorder characterized by inappropriate production or action of antidiuretic hormone (ADH) in the absence of normal physiological triggers, resulting in hypervolemia and hypo-osmolality
  - Etiology/Incidence
    - Central nervous system disorders (CNS)
      - Tumor
      - Head trauma
      - Meningitis
      - Hydrocephalus
      - Cerebrovascular accident
      - Subdural hematoma
      - Acute Psychosis
    - Neoplasms
      - Pulmonary
      - CNS
      - Gastrointestinal
      - Genitourinary
      - Leukemias
    - Pulmonary
      - Abscess
      - Tumors
      - Infection
      - Inflammatory disease
      - Pneumothorax
      - Acute respiratory failure
    - Medications that stimulate or potentiate ADH—list is quite exhaustive; some examples of common triggers include:
      - Antidepressants
      - Antiepileptics
      - Opiates
      - Ecstasy
      - Synthetic ADH (DDAVP)
      - Physiological stress
      - Postoperative state
      - Psychogenic polydipsia
  - Signs and Symptoms
    - Nausea
    - Malaise
    - Headache
    - Lethargy
    - Confusion
    - Muscle cramps
  - Differential Diagnosis
    - Cerebral salt wasting
    - Renal disease
    - Hypervolemic hyponatremia
    - Addison's disease
    - Myxedema coma
  - Physical Findings
    - Vital signs consistent with volume overload—bounding pulse, hypertension, tachycardia
    - Edema
    - Jugular venous distention
    - Mental status changes
    - Neurological findings as hyponatremia progresses
    - Ataxia
    - Seizure
    - Hyporeflexia
    - Asterixis
    - Tremor
    - Dysarthria
  - Diagnostic Tests/Findings
    - Clinical diagnosis characterized by:
      - Serum sodium < 135 mEq/L
      - Serum osmolality < 280 mOsm/kg
      - Absence of heart, renal, hepatic disease
      - Normal thyroid and adrenal function
    - Additional laboratory findings typically include
      - Urine $Na^+$ > 20 mEq/L
      - BUN < 10 mg/dL
      - Serum uric acid < 4 mg/dL
    - Studies as indicated to rule out thyroid, adrenal, renal, hepatic, or cardiac cause of water retention/sodium loss
    - Imaging as indicated if CNS or pulmonary cause suspected
    - Serum ADH typically not contributory and not measured
  - Management/Treatment
    - Fluid restriction in all patients—500 to 1,500 mL/day

(continues)

> **Special Considerations in the Hospitalized Patient** (*continued*)
>
> - Correction of hyponatremia; caution with respect to overcorrection and resultant neurological consequences; raise Na+ 0.5 to 1 mEq/h with no more than 10–20 mEq in the first 24 hours; a variety of calculations have been proposed but none studied extensively; all should serve as guide only to control correction
>   - In less severe cases, loop diuresis and isotonic saline replacement
>   - In severe cases, loop dieresis and hypertonic saline replacement
> - Vasopressin receptor agonists (aquaretics) in severe cases
>   - Facilitate free water excretion
>   - No direct impact on electrolytes
>   - Currently approved forms
>     - Conivaptan—parenteral
>     - Tolvaptan—oral

## QUESTIONS

■ Select the best answer.

### Questions 1 and 2 refer to the following scenario:

Mrs. O. is a 46-year-old female whose hypertension has been controlled with hydrochlorothiazide 50 mg every day for the past 3 years. She is 5'9'' and weighs 220 lbs. Although no other abnormal physical findings were noted, blood work done as part of her routine annual physical examination reveals a fasting blood glucose of 230 mg/dL. Other abnormal laboratory tests included elevated serum cholesterol (250) and triglyceride level (170), a K+ of 3.4, and 4+ glycosuria.

1. You should then:
   a. Discontinue her hydrochlorothiazide
   b. Order a glucose tolerance test
   c. Repeat a fasting glucose
   d. Start insulin therapy

2. Mrs. O. is about how many pounds over her ideal body weight?
   a. 80
   b. 105
   c. 140
   d. 154

3. Persons with type 2 diabetes:
   a. Tend to have peripheral muscle loss
   b. Account for less than 10% of persons with diabetes
   c. Tend to be obese and hypertensive
   d. Have early symptoms similar to persons with type 1 diabetes

4. The pathophysiology of type 2 diabetes frequently includes:
   a. Insulin receptor abnormalities
   b. Islet cell antibody development
   c. Activation of a genetic predisposition
   d. Beta cell insensitivity to insulinogenic stimuli

5. You are managing the primary care needs of a patient with difficult-to-control type 2 diabetes. He is under the care of an endocrinologist and recently started taking pramlintide. Patient education should reinforce the potential for:
   a. Renal dysfunction with contrast dye
   b. Development of hypoglycemia
   c. Significant nausea in the first weeks of therapy
   d. Headache and upper respiratory symptoms

6. Which of the following is not a diagnostic criterion for diabetes mellitus?
   a. HgbA1c> 6.5%
   b. The presence of islet cell antibodies
   c. FPG > 126 mg/dL on two separate occasions
   d. Random plasma glucose (RPG) > 200 mg/dL along with classic symptoms

7. Dietary recommendations for persons with diabetes *do not* include:
   a. Strict carbohydrate restriction
   b. Limiting fats and cholesterol
   c. Limiting protein intake
   d. Eating meals at regular intervals

8. Indications for starting a person with diabetes on oral hypoglycemics include:
   a. Allergy to sulfa drugs
   b. Pregnancy in type 2 diabetes controlled by diet
   c. Diagnosis of type 2 diabetes
   d. Failure to control hyperglycemia with diet in a patient with type 2 diabetes

9. A person with type 2 diabetes has had good control of his blood glucose with oral agents. He is in for a routine 3-month check. He had a complete workup

6 months ago. Which of the following is *least* likely to be done at this visit?

   a. Urinalysis
   b. Foot examination
   c. Fundoscopic examination
   d. ECG

10. Mr. P. is on 30 units of NPH and 5 units of regular insulin each morning and 15 units of NPH each evening to control his type 1 diabetes. His blood glucose levels for the past 3 days have been:

| Fasting | Before Lunch | Before Supper | At h.s. |
|---------|--------------|---------------|---------|
| 200–250 | 95–110 | 110–120 | 95–130 |

   He should be instructed to:
   a. Add 2 units of NPH to his p.m. dose
   b. Add 2 units NPH before breakfast
   c. Add 2 units of regular insulin to his p.m. dose
   d. Do nothing

11. Hemoglobin A1c gives an indication of glucose control over the past:

   a. Week
   b. 4–6 weeks
   c. Month
   d. 60–90 days

12. When treating diabetes, the goal for hemoglobin A1c (normal 4–6%) is:

   a. < 6%
   b. < 7%
   c. < 8%
   d. < 10%

13. Which of the following is an adverse effect of sulfonylureas?

   a. Increased blood pressure
   b. Weight loss
   c. Gastrointestinal distress
   d. Hypoglycemia

14. In addition to controlling glucose levels, metformin may also:

   a. Cause weight loss
   b. Increase total cholesterol levels
   c. Increase triglyceride levels
   d. Be likely to cause hypoglycemia

15. Synthetic human insulin:

   a. Causes more antibody formation
   b. Contains more impurities than purified pork insulin
   c. Is least antigenic of all insulins
   d. Has a more rapid action onset than do pork counterparts

### Questions 16, 17, and 18 refer to the following scenario:

Mr. J. is a 50-year-old male with type 2 diabetes who has been on insulin for the past 6 months. He reports that his fasting blood glucose levels have been running above 200 mg/dL, but they have been great during the rest of the day. His evening dose of NPH insulin has been increased three times in the last 2 weeks with no improvement in the fasting values. Currently, he is on 30 units NPH/4 units regular in the morning and 18 units NPH/4 units regular before supper. This is his most recent glucose pattern:

| Breakfast | Lunch | Supper | h.s. |
|-----------|-------|--------|------|
| 250–280 | 130–144 | 120–132 | 100–120 |

16. If he has fairly good dietary compliance, you should instruct him to:

   a. Increase the evening NPH by 2 more units
   b. Check his blood glucose between 2 and 3 a.m. for the next 2 days
   c. Increase the morning dose of regular insulin by 2 units
   d. Increase the morning dose of NPH insulin by 2 units

17. High fasting glucose after a nocturnal hypoglycemia in a person with diabetes otherwise in good control with insulin would indicate:

   a. Dawn phenomenon
   b. Somogyi phenomenon
   c. Insulin allergy
   d. Lipodystrophy

18. Which action would counteract this problem?

   a. Increase morning dose of NPH
   b. Use human insulin instead of pork insulin
   c. Decrease evening NPH insulin dose
   d. Increase morning dose of regular insulin

19. What is the best option to assess long-term glycemic control in a patient with diabetes who also has sickle cell anemia?

   a. Have the patient keep a log of FPG
   b. Assess serum fructosamine
   c. Subtract 3% from the measured HgbA1c
   d. Measure glycosylated fatty acids

20. Ms. W. is a 34-year-old who is seeking care because of increased irritability, weight loss "despite a great appetite," and diarrhea (not watery but 2–3 stools a day). She feels exhausted but can't seem to sleep and states she "feels like I could jump out of my skin." If excess thyroid hormone is the problem, which of the following might be noted?

    a. Yellowing skin
    b. Fine tremor
    c. Delayed tendon reflex
    d. Sinus bradycardia

21. Graves' disease is caused by:

    a. Viral infection
    b. Use of lithium
    c. An autoimmune response
    d. Excessive ingestion of thyroid hormone

22. In Graves' disease you would expect:

    a. TSH to be decreased
    b. Anti-TP to be increased
    c. TSI to be decreased
    d. $T_4$ to be decreased

23. Upon initial diagnosis of Graves' disease, which medication should be ordered immediately for symptom control?

    a. PTU
    b. Cytomel
    c. $^{131}$I
    d. Propranolol

24. The most serious side effect of both PTU and methimazole is:

    a. Skin rash
    b. Diarrhea
    c. Agranulocytosis
    d. Hepatitis

25. The best guide to adequacy of the dosage of antithyroid medication in thyrotoxicosis is:

    a. Thyroid antibodies
    b. $T_3$ (RIA)
    c. TSH
    d. $T_4$

26. Sally is a 44-year-old who thinks she is beginning menopause because her menstrual periods have become irregular. Her major complaint is a lack of energy and weight gain. Physical examination reveals dry skin, thinning hair, a puffy facial appearance, and an enlarged, nontender thyroid. Her BP is 130/92 mm Hg with a heart rate of 60. These findings are consistent with:

    a. Graves' disease
    b. Hypothyroidism
    c. Plummer's disease
    d. Thyrotoxicosis

27. Which of the following findings would be consistent with a hypothyroid state?

    a. Hyperactive bowel sounds and fine tremor
    b. Oligomenorrhea and constipation
    c. Edema and heat intolerance
    d. Dry skin and weight gain

28. Ms. H. is diagnosed with hypothyroidism and is placed on levothyroxine 0.05 mg per day. After a week she calls to tell you she hasn't seen any improvement and wants to discontinue her medication. Your best response would be to:

    a. Add propranolol to her regimen
    b. Change to desiccated thyroid
    c. Increase her dosage 0.125 mg/day
    d. Encourage her to take this dose for at least another week

29. Ms. L. is a 50-year-old female who has been diagnosed as having primary myxedema. An initial dose of 0.1 mg/day of levothyroxine has been prescribed. Patient education would include which of the following?

    a. Discussion of the chronicity of the disease and the lifelong medication use
    b. That it will take 6 months to a year for her fatigue to disappear
    c. Avoidance of foods causing increased peristalsis
    d. Explanation that after 2 years of therapy this medication may not be needed

30. Your 57-year-old patient has been on prednisone for her rheumatoid arthritis. She has the typical "moon face," carries excess weight in her torso, and is complaining that she bruises easily when she bumps herself. As her primary care provider, the best action would be to:

    a. Discontinue her prednisone immediately
    b. Add an NSAID to her treatment regimen
    c. Convert to an alternate-day schedule
    d. Discontinue prednisone immediately and start on naproxen 250 mg b.i.d.

31. Skin changes in Addison's disease include:
    a. Circumoral pallor
    b. Maculopapular eruptions associated with stress
    c. Hyperpigmentation
    d. Facial plethora and hirsutism

## ■ Answers

| | |
|---|---|
| 1. **c** | 17. **b** |
| 2. **a** | 18. **c** |
| 3. **c** | 19. **b** |
| 4. **a** | 20. **b** |
| 5. **b** | 21. **c** |
| 6. **b** | 22. **a** |
| 7. **a** | 23. **d** |
| 8. **d** | 24. **c** |
| 9. **d** | 25. **c** |
| 10. **a** | 26. **b** |
| 11. **d** | 27. **d** |
| 12. **b** | 28. **d** |
| 13. **d** | 29. **a** |
| 14. **a** | 30. **c** |
| 15. **c** | 31. **c** |
| 16. **b** | |

## BIBLIOGRAPHY

American Diabetic Association. (2013). Standards of diabetes care in 2013. *Diabetes Care, 36*(Suppl. 1), S11–S66.

Berra, K. (2003). Treatment options for patients with "Metabolic Syndrome." *Journal of the American Academy of Nurse Practitioners, 15*(8), 361–370.

Blackwell, J. (2004). Clinical practice guidelines: Evaluation and treatment of hyperthyroidism and hypothyroidism. *Journal of the American Academy of Nurse Practitioners,16,* 422–425.

Dushay, J., & Abrahamson, M. J. (2005). Insulin resistance and type 2 diabetes: A comprehensive review. Retrieved from http://www.medscape.org/viewarticle/501569

Fatourechi, V. (2004). Subclinical hyperthyroidism: When to treat, when to watch? *Consultant, 44*(4), 533–539.

Fitzgerald, P. A. (2014). Endocrine disorders. In S. J. McPhee & M. A. Papadakis (Eds.), *Current medical diagnosis and treatment* (53rd ed.). New York, NY: McGraw-Hill.

Henske, J. A., Griffith, M. L., & Fowler, M. J. (2009). Initiating and titrating insulin in patients with type 2 diabetes mellitus. *Clinical Diabetes, 27*(2), 72–76.

Kirk, L. F., Jr., Hash, R. B., Katner, H. P., & Jones, T. (2000). Cushing's disease: Clinical manifestations and diagnostic evaluation. *American Family Physician, 62,* 1119–1133.

Kutschman, R. F., & Hadley, S. (2004). Diagnosing and treating the metabolic syndrome. *American Journal of Nurse Practitioners, 8*(2), 9–18.

Li, T.-M. (2002). Hypothyroidism in elderly people. *Geriatric Nursing, 23*(2), 88–98.

Liotta, E. A., Elston, D. M., & Brough, A. (2013). Dermatologic aspects of Addison's disease. Retrieved from http://www.emedicine.com/derm/TOPIC761.htm

Mayfield, J. A., & White, R. D. (2004). Insulin therapy for type 2 diabetes: Rescue, augmentation, and replacement of beta-cell function. *American Family Physician, 70*(3), 489–500.

Streetman, D. D., & Khanderia, U. (2004). Diagnosis and treatment of Graves' disease. *American Journal for Nurse Practitioners, 8*(1), 27–40.

Thomas, C. P. (2014). Syndrome of inappropriate antidiuretic hormone secretion treatment and management. Retrieved from http://emedicine.medscape.com/article/246650-treatment#a1156

Umesh, M. (2014). Diabetes mellitus and hypoglycemia. In S. J. McPhee & M. A. Papadakis (Eds.), *Current medical diagnosis and treatment* (53rd ed.). New York, NY: McGraw-Hill.

Whittemore, R., Bak, P. S., Melkus, G. D., & Grey, M. (2003). Promoting lifestyle changes in the prevention and management of type 2 diabetes. *Journal of the American Academy of Nurse Practitioners, 15*(8), 341–350.

# Genitourinary and Gynecological Disorders

*Pamela A. Shuler*

*Mary D. Knudtson*

## ACQUIRED IMMUNODEFICIENCY SYNDROME (AIDS)

- Definition—secondary immunodeficiency syndrome resulting from human immunodeficiency virus (HIV) infection and characterized by opportunistic infections, neurological dysfunction, malignancies, systemic wasting, and a variety of other disorders

- Etiology/Incidence
  1. HIV invades and then multiplies in one or more types of susceptible cells; circulating $CD4^+$ lymphocytes, macrophages, and monocytes are most commonly affected, destroying the host's immune system
  2. Median time from HIV infection to AIDS is 10 years
  3. Estimated 1,106,400 cases in the United States; 21% undiagnosed
  4. Estimated 36,000 people are newly infected in the United States annually
  5. Most diagnoses are made in persons 30–39 years old
  6. HIV is transmitted through direct contact with body fluids (blood, semen, vaginal secretions) and breast milk
  7. Major routes of HIV transmission
     a. Sexual intercourse (homosexual and heterosexual)
     b. Needle sharing (IV drug users)
     c. Reusing needles for medical purposes (e.g., in developing countries)
     d. Transfusions of contaminated blood and blood products
     e. Needle stick, open wound, and mucous membrane exposure to healthcare workers (0.4% incidence according to the Centers for Disease Control and Prevention [CDC])
     f. Injection with previously used unsterilized needle (acupuncture, tattooing, medical injection)
     g. Pregnancy
     h. Breastfeeding
  8. Trends
     a. Approximately 50,000 new infections annually
     b. Two-thirds of new infections occur in men who have sex with men
     c. African Americans and Hispanics are disproportionately represented
     d. One in four new HIV infections occurs in people younger than 20 years
     e. Sexual contact is leading mode of transmission for women who have sex with men

- Signs and Symptoms—CDC classification
  1. Asymptomatic HIV infection (may last > 10 years)—HIV antibody is detectable in at least 95% of people within 3 months of infection
  2. Acute HIV infection
     a. 2–8 weeks after infection 30–40% may have acute viremia symptoms
        (1) High fever, lymphadenopathy, rash, aseptic meningitis, fatigue, myalgias, arthralgias

(2) Usually mistaken for flu or mononucleosis
b. Months to years before AIDS—may have chronic fatigue, weight loss, night sweats, persistent dermatitis, shingles, persistent diarrhea, oral candidiasis, hairy leukoplakia, chronic vaginal candidiasis, tuberculosis, cognitive changes
3. Persistent generalized lymphadenopathy (PGL)
   a. Palpable lymph node enlargement (two sites other than inguinal)
   b. No concurrent illness to explain lymphadenopathy
4. HIV diseases that contribute to progression of AIDS
   a. *Pneumocystis jiroveci* pneumonia, Kaposi's sarcoma, cytomegalovirus, and/or other opportunistic infections/cancers
   b. Encephalopathy
   c. Wasting syndrome (involuntary weight loss greater than 10% of baseline body weight, plus either chronic diarrhea or chronic weakness and documented fever)

- Differential Diagnosis
  1. Cancer
  2. Tuberculosis
  3. Enterocolitis
  4. Endocrine diseases
  5. Primary cytomegalovirus infection
  6. Drug reaction
  7. Epstein-Barr virus (mononucleosis)
  8. Viral hepatitis
  9. Secondary syphilis

- Physical Findings—variable, depending on infection stage

- Diagnostic Tests/Findings
  1. Informed consent with pretest counseling required prior to HIV testing
  2. Posttest counseling also required
  3. Rapid HIV testing
     a. Oral Quick Rapid HIV-1 antibody test
        (1) Oral fluids, serum, or whole blood tested
        (2) Results in 20–60 minutes
        (3) Sensitivity—99.6%, specificity—100%
        (4) Clinical laboratory improvement amendments (CLIA)—waived
     b. Reveal HIV-1 antibody test
        (1) Serum or plasma tested
        (2) More laboratory dependent
        (3) Results in minutes
        (4) Sensitivity—99.8%, specificity—serum 99.1%, plasma 98.6%
        (5) CLIA—moderate complexity
  4. Most commonly used initial blood tests for antibody detection
     a. Enzyme immunoassay (EIA) (screening test)
     b. Western blot or immunofluorescent antibody test—confirmatory blood tests for HIV-specific antibody profile
     c. Some individuals may not generate an antibody response for up to 36 months
  5. Detection/quantification of HIV
     a. HIV-1 p24 antigen used to diagnose infection before antibodies measurable
     b. Qualitative polymerase chain reaction (PCR) circulating cells or plasma—can use in early disease instead of p24
     c. Quantitative viral RNA levels—used to decide when to initiate treatment, as a prognostic indicator, and as a basis for evaluating response to treatment
     d. CD4$^+$ count used to assess magnitude of disease and to monitor effectiveness of treatment
  6. Additional recommended tests if HIV positive
     a. HIV viral load test
     b. Toxoplasma antibody test
     c. Tests for hepatitis A, B, and C viral markers
     d. Purified protein derivative (PPD)
     e. Chest radiograph
     f. Venereal disease research laboratory (VDRL) or rapid plasma regain (RPR)
     g. Complete blood count (CBC)
     h. Fasting blood glucose
     i. Fasting lipid panel
     j. Pap testing in females
     k. Anal pap testing in males
     l. Viral genotype

- Management/Treatment—HIV/AIDS treatment regimens throughout this chapter based on *Guidelines for the Use of Antiretroviral Agents in HIV-1 Infected Adults and Adolescents*, published by the Department of Health and Human Services (DHHS, 2014). Treatment of HIV and AIDS is changing rapidly; recommendations may have changed as a result of new or better treatment options; consult with specialist or expert in AIDS care for latest information
  1. All adults in the United States should be screened
  2. No cure or vaccination for HIV infection at present
  3. New treatment regimens are constantly evolving
  4. Treatment of HIV and opportunistic infections, malignancies, and prophylaxis against opportunistic infections continues to evolve rapidly; basic guidelines include
     a. Therapy for opportunistic infections and malignancies begins with a CD4$^+$ count of 350 cells/$uL$

(1) Conditions include *P. jiroveci* pneumonia, toxoplasmosis, cryptococcus, lymphoma, cytomegalovirus, esophageal candidiasis, herpes simplex and zoster, Kaposi's sarcoma
(2) Medications include antibiotics, antifungals, and corticosteroids

b. Antiretroviral treatment (DHHS, 2014); should be offered at the time of diagnosis unless adherence concerns exist
(1) Recommended treatment—combination drug treatment known as antiretroviral therapy (ART)
(2) Medications
 (a) A variety of combination therapies exist for the treatment-naïve patient and typically include two nucleoside reverse transcriptase inhibitors (NRTI), plus one additional drug from either the non-nucleoside reverse transcriptase inhibitor (NNRTI), protease inhibitor (PI), integrase strand transfer inhibitor (INSTI), or chemokine receptor antagonist (CCR5) class (CDC, 2013)
 (b) Additional combination options are available for patients not responding to initial treatments
 (c) Viral load monitoring—measure viral RNA every 3–4 months, more frequently if
  (i) Noncompliance suspected
  (ii) $CD4^+$ count drops
  (iii) Clinical symptoms appear
  (iv) Drug adjustments are made (measure at 4–8 weeks, then again at 3–4 weeks to document drug effect)

c. Prophylaxis of opportunistic infections
(1) *P. jiroveci* pneumonia (begin when $CD4^+$ count < 350)
 (a) Trimethoprim-sulfamethoxazole (TMP/SMX), 1 double-strength tablet daily or 3 times a week
 (b) Dapsone 100 mg per day or aerosolized pentamidine 300 mg monthly if unable to tolerate TMP/SMX
(2) *Mycobacterium tuberculosis*
 (a) Isoniazid—10 mg/kg/day up to 300 mg plus pyridoxine 50 mg daily for 1 year
 (b) All patients with positive PPD reaction (5 mm of induration or greater) without positive chest radiography should receive prophylactic treatment
(3) Toxoplasmosis—begin when $CD4^+$ count < 100—TMP/SMX 1 double-strength tablet orally 3 times per week or daily
(4) *Mycobacterium avium* complex—begin when $CD4^+$ count < 50
 (a) Clarithromycin 500 mg orally b.i.d., or
 (b) Azithromycin 500 mg orally 3 times a week, or
 (c) Rifabutin 150 mg orally b.i.d.

d. Indications to change treatment regimens
(1) Immunological failure
 (a) $CD4^+$ count falls below baseline
 (b) $CD4^+$ count does not rise > 50 cells after 1 year of therapy
(2) Virologic failure
 (a) Viral load remains > 400 copies after 6 months of therapy or 50 copies after 1 year
 (b) Viral rebound—viral load rises after initial suppression
 (c) Any reproducible threefold increase in viral load after starting therapy
(3) Clinical failure
 (a) Clinical deterioration despite $CD4^+$ or viral load trends
 (b) Occurrence of HIV-related infection
 (c) Intolerance of adverse effects
 (d) Emergence of resistance

e. Recommended immunizations for HIV-infected persons
(1) Pneumococcal vaccination
(2) Annual influenza vaccination
(3) Three-dose schedule of hepatitis B vaccine for those who lack immunity
(4) Tetanus-diphtheria booster
(5) Inactivated polio virus vaccine (IPV)
(6) Measles, mumps, rubella vaccine (no live virus vaccines if $CD4^+$ count < 200 cells/uL)

5. Thorough psychosocial evaluation to include
 a. Signs of severe psychological distress
 b. Behavioral factors related to risk for transmitting HIV
 c. Information concerning partners who should be notified of possible HIV exposure
6. Discuss therapeutic and diagnostic plans
7. Educate regarding prevention, transmission, and treatment of the disease
8. Emphasize importance of behavioral measures to protect and enhance the immune system
 a. No tobacco, street drugs, alcohol use
 b. Nutritious diet
 c. Stress management, imagery
 d. Exercise as tolerated

**184** CHAPTER 11 Genitourinary and Gynecological Disorders

   e. Decrease exposure to infectious agents because HIV virus is spread when immune system is activated
9. Encourage continued "safer sex" practices and/or abstinence
10. Assist patient, as appropriate, in meeting physical, psychological, social, cultural, environmental, and spiritual needs
11. Report AIDS cases to local health department

## GONORRHEA (UNCOMPLICATED GONOCOCCAL INFECTIONS)

- Definition—a sexually transmitted bacterial infection that produces urethritis in men and cervicitis in women

- Etiology/Incidence
  1. Causative organism is *Neisseria gonorrhoeae*, a gram-negative diplococcus
  2. Approximately 300,000 infectious new cases reported annually
  3. Greatest incidence in the 15- to 30-year-old age group
  4. Incubation period usually 3–10 days
  5. Spectrum of infection—cervicitis, urethritis, salpingitis, proctitis, pelvic inflammatory disease (PID), pharyngitis, conjunctivitis, arthritis
  6. A leading cause of female infertility in the United States

- Signs and Symptoms
  1. Female
     a. Often asymptomatic
     b. Dysuria, urinary frequency, urgency with a purulent urethral discharge
     c. Vaginal discharge
     d. Cervicitis
     e. Pelvic pain
     f. Abnormal menstrual bleeding
     g. Pharyngitis
     h. Septic arthritis
     i. Rash—petechial or pustular skin lesions
  2. Male
     a. One-quarter are asymptomatic
     b. Dysuria (urethra most common site in male), frequency
     c. Copious penile discharge (serous/milky to yellow with blood-tinge)
     d. Testicular pain
     e. Pharyngitis
     f. Septic arthritis
     g. Rash—petechial or pustular skin lesions
     h. Proctitis—common in homosexual males

- Differential Diagnosis
  1. Nongonococcal cervicitis, vaginitis, urethritis, or epididymitis
  2. Reiter's syndrome
  3. Pelvic inflammatory disease (PID)
  4. Proctitis (other origin)
  5. Nongonococcal pharyngitis or arthritis

- Physical Findings
  1. Female
     a. Purulent discharge from cervix (primary site in women of reproductive age)
     b. Inflammation of Bartholin's glands
     c. Evidence of PID (untreated infection)
  2. Male
     a. Evidence of urethritis, prostatitis
     b. Evidence of epididymitis (with untreated infection)
     c. Copious purulent discharge

- Diagnostic Tests/Findings
  1. Female tests
     a. Gram stain of endocervical discharge in women shows white blood cells (WBCs) with gram-negative intracellular diplococci; sensitivity only 40–70% in women; greater than 90% in men
     b. Wet prep of purulent cervical discharge may show polymorphonuclear leukocytes (WBC) > 10/HPF
     c. Culture material from endocervix and other suspect sites onto Thayer-Martin or Transgrow media to confirm diagnosis
     d. DNA probe—sensitivity comparable to culture, 2-hour turnaround time, only one specimen needed for chlamydia and *N. gonorrhoeae*
     e. Urine-based ligase chain reaction—highly sensitive and specific in men and women
  2. Male tests
     a. Gram stain of urethral discharge smear shows gram-negative diplococci and WBC
     b. Culture of urethra and other suspect sites
     c. DNA probe
  3. Test for concomitant infection from other STD, including HIV, syphilis, and chlamydia
  4. Test partners

- Management/Treatment
  1. Evaluate and treat all contacts for *N. gonorrhoeae* and chlamydia; evaluate and treat other partners of contacts because patients infected with *N. gonorrhoeae* often are coinfected with chlamydia; dual presumptive therapy should be considered for patients who may not return for test results and for those with signs/symptoms suggestive of a dual diagnosis
  2. Quinolone-resistant *N. gonorrhoeae* is recognized nationally; quinolone options no longer recommended for treatment

3. Recommended treatment regimens for uncomplicated gonococcal infections of the cervix, urethra, and rectum—ceftriaxone 250 mg IM in a single dose PLUS azithromycin 1 g orally in a single dose or doxycycline 100 mg orally twice a day for 7 days if chlamydial infection is not ruled out
4. Alternative regimens for uncomplicated gonococcal infections of the cervix, urethra, and rectum—spectinomycin 2 g IM in a single dose, or ceftizoxime 500 mg IM in a single dose, or cefoxitin 2 g IM in a single dose plus probenecid 1 g orally, or cefotaxime 500 mg IM in a single dose PLUS azithromycin 1 g orally in a single dose or doxycycline 100 mg orally twice a day for 7 days if chlamydial infection is not ruled out
5. Recommended treatment regimens for uncomplicated gonococcal infections of the pharynx—ceftriaxone 250 mg IM in a single dose PLUS azithromycin 1 g orally in a single dose or doxycycline 100 mg orally twice a day for 7 days if chlamydial infection is not ruled out
6. Recommended treatment regimens for uncomplicated gonococcal infections during pregnancy—one of the recommended or alternate cephalosporins should be used, or a single, 2-g dose of spectinomycin IM PLUS erythromycin base 500 mg orally 4 times a day for 7 days, or amoxicillin 500 mg orally 3 times daily for 7 days for presumptive or diagnosed chlamydia during pregnancy; tetracyclines should not be used during pregnancy
7. Test of cure not essential; repeat culture if symptoms persist or recur
8. Discuss therapeutic and diagnostic plans
9. Emphasize importance of complete treatment
10. Avoid sexual intercourse until patient and partner(s) cured
11. Educate regarding prevention, transmission, and treatment of the disease; encourage continued use of condoms
12. Report cases to health department
13. Can cause disseminated infection, acute arthritis, hepatitis, or endocarditis

# GENITAL CHLAMYDIAL INFECTION

- Definition—a sexually transmitted disease that produces urethritis in men and cervicitis in women

- Etiology/Incidence
  1. Causative organism is *Chlamydia trachomatis*
  2. More than 1.2 million new cases occur annually
  3. The most common bacterial sexually transmitted disease in United States
  4. A leading cause of female infertility and ectopic pregnancy in United States
  5. Incubation period 7–21 days
  6. Screening for high-risk individuals recommended—sexually active adolescents and young adults, multiple partners, history of previous or current STD

- Signs and Symptoms
  1. Female
     a. Often asymptomatic
     b. Dysuria
     c. Mucopurulent vaginal discharge/spotting
     d. Lower abdominal/pelvic pain
     e. Dyspareunia
     f. Dysmenorrhea, menstrual irregularity
     g. Infertility
     h. Enlarged, tender inguinal lymph nodes
     i. Friable cervix
  2. Male
     a. Often asymptomatic
     b. Urethral discharge (any color)
     c. Dysuria
     d. Testicular pain/swelling
     e. Enlarged, tender inguinal lymph nodes
     f. Rectal pain, bleeding, and diarrhea

- Differential Diagnosis
  1. Gonococcal cervicitis
  2. Urethritis
  3. Proctitis
  4. PID
  5. Urinary tract infection
  6. Epididymitis
  7. Prostatitis from other infective agent
  8. Vaginitis

- Physical Findings
  1. Female
     a. Mucopurulent urethral and/or cervical discharge
     b. Hypertrophic, eroded, and friable cervix (maybe)
     c. Evidence of PID (advanced infection)
  2. Male
     a. Thin, white urethral discharge; markedly less purulent and copious as gonococcal infection
     b. Evidence of prostatitis
     c. Evidence of epididymitis (untreated infection)

- Diagnostic Tests/Findings
  1. Female
     a. Wet prep or gram stain shows WBC > 10/HPF
     b. Most common tests—EIA and direct fluorescence assay (DFA) *or* lipase chain reaction (LCR) for confirmation

c. Other tests include tissue culture, DNA hybridization, and PCR
2. Male
   a. Gram stain or wet prep shows WBC > 10/HPF
   b. Same indirect antigen-detection tests
3. Test for concomitant infection from other STD in patient (HIV, gonorrhea, syphilis, trichomoniasis)
4. Test partners

- Management/Treatment
  1. Evaluate and treat all contacts and partners of contacts
  2. Recommended treatment regimens for uncomplicated chlamydial infections—azithromycin 1 g orally in a single dose (preferred), or doxycycline 100 mg orally twice a day for 7 days
  3. Alternative regimens for uncomplicated chlamydial infections—erythromycin base 500 mg orally 4 times a day for 7 days, or erythromycin ethylsuccinate 800 mg orally 4 times a day for 7 days, or ofloxacin 300 mg orally twice a day for 7 days, or levofloxacin 500 mg orally for 7 days
  4. Recommended treatment regimens for uncomplicated chlamydial infections during pregnancy—erythromycin base 500 mg orally 4 times a day for 7 days, or amoxicillin 500 mg orally 3 times daily for 7 days
  5. Alternative treatment regimens for uncomplicated chlamydial infections during pregnancy—erythromycin base 250 mg orally 4 times a day for 14 days, or erythromycin ethylsuccinate 800 mg orally 4 times a day for 7 days, or erythromycin ethylsuccinate 400 mg orally 4 times a day for 14 days, or azithromycin 1 g orally, single dose
  6. Test-of-cure not recommended UNLESS patient was treated with erythromycin, is pregnant, has persistent symptoms, or reinfection suspected (wait > 3 weeks after treatment for repeat testing preferably by culture)
  7. Discuss therapeutic and diagnostic plans
  8. Emphasize importance of complete treatment
  9. Avoid sexual intercourse until patient and partner(s) complete treatment
  10. Educate regarding prevention, transmission, and treatment of the disease; encourage continued use of condoms
  11. Report cases to health department

## SYPHILIS

- Definition—complex infectious disease that can affect almost any organ or tissue in the body and mimics many diseases

- Etiology/Incidence
  1. Causative organism is *Treponema pallidum*, a spirochete
  2. Transmission primarily occurs through minor skin or mucosal lesions during sexual encounters; genital and extragenital areas may be inoculated
  3. Can be transmitted via placenta (after 10th week) from mother to fetus (congenital rate—1 in 10,000 pregnancies)
  4. Incidence has declined since 1990s; 49,903 cases were reported in the United States in 2012
  5. Risk of contraction—30–50% (partner-primary syphilis)

- Signs and Symptoms
  1. Primary
     a. Painless chancre
     b. Regional lymphadenopathy
  2. Secondary
     a. Skin rash—especially palmar, plantar, and oral mucosa
     b. Malaise, anorexia
     c. Alopecia
     d. Arthralgias/myalgias/flu-like symptoms
     e. Other symptoms depending on affected organs
     f. Generalized lymphadenopathy
     g. Low-grade fever
     h. Condylomata lata
  3. Latent
     a. May be asymptomatic
     b. Integumentary, ocular, cardiovascular, gastrointestinal, respiratory, or neurological manifestations may be present
  4. Neurosyphilis
     a. May occur during any stage of syphilis
     b. Optic, auditory, cranial nerve, and/or meningeal symptoms are most common

- Differential Diagnosis
  1. Primary
     a. Herpes genitalis
     b. Chancroid
     c. Neoplasm
     d. Lymphogranuloma venereum (LGV)
     e. Granuloma inguinale
  2. Secondary
     a. Conditions associated with rash or other presenting symptoms, e.g., flu, mononucleosis, pityriasis rosea, drug eruptions
     b. Infectious hepatitis
  3. Latent
     a. Neoplasms of skin, liver, lung, stomach, or brain
     b. Other forms
        (1) Meningitis

(2) Cardiovascular disorders
(3) Central nervous system (CNS) disorders
(4) Arthritis
(5) Primary neurological lesions
- Physical Findings
  1. Neurological signs may be present at any stage
  2. Primary
     a. Indurated ulcer (chancre) on
        (1) Genitals
        (2) Mouth
        (3) Rectum
        (4) Nipple
     b. Regional lymphadenopathy
  3. Secondary
     a. Low-grade fever
     b. Highly variable skin rash (including palms and soles)
     c. Mucous patches
     d. Evidence or manifestations of condyloma latum
     e. Generalized lymphadenopathy
     f. Evidence of meningitis, iritis, hepatitis, glomerulonephritis
  4. Latent
     a. May have no clinical signs of infection
     b. Granulomatous lesions (gummas)—skin, mucous membranes, bone
     c. Leukoplakia
     d. Evidence of periostitis, osteitis, or arthritis
     e. Gummatous infiltrates in larynx, trachea, pulmonary parenchyma, stomach, and/or liver
     f. Diminished coronary circulation
     g. Acute myocardial infarction
     h. Cardiac insufficiency
     i. Aortic aneurysm
     j. Meningitis
     k. Hemiparesis
     l. Hemiplegia
     m. Tabes dorsalis
     n. General paresis
- Diagnostic Tests/Findings
  1. Early syphilis—primary, secondary, or latent syphilis of less than 1 year's duration
     a. Definitive methods
        (1) Darkfield microscopy
        (2) Direct fluorescent antibody tests of lesion exudate or tissue
     b. Presumptive methods (neither test alone is sufficient for diagnosis)
        (1) Treponemal serologic tests
           (a) Fluorescent treponemal antibody absorption (FTA-ABS) test
           (b) Microhemagglutination assay for antibody to *T. pallidum* (MHA-TP)
           (c) Tests/titers should be reported as positive or negative and used to confirm nontreponemal tests
           (d) FTA-ABS or MHA-TP confirmation tests positive in 85–95% of primary and in 100% of secondary cases
        (2) Nontreponemal serologic tests
           (a) Venereal Disease Research Laboratory (VDRL)
        (3) Rapid plasma reagin (RPR)
  2. Latent syphilis of more than 1 year's duration and cardiovascular syphilis
     a. VDRL or RPR test (+ in 75% of cases)
     b. FTA-ABS or MHA-TP confirmation test (+ in 98% of cases)
     c. Lumbar puncture with tests on cerebrospinal fluid (CSF)
  3. Neurosyphilis (occurs at any stage)
     a. Treponemal and nontreponemal serologic test results dependent upon stage of disease
     b. CSF examinations as above
  4. Test for concomitant infection from other STD in patient and contacts
     a. HIV
     b. Gonorrhea
     c. Chlamydia
  5. Test partners

- Management/Treatment
  1. Pregnant patients with any stage of syphilis should be treated with penicillin after inpatient desensitization
  2. Alternative antibiotic regimens are available for nonpregnant patients at any stage except neurosyphilis
  3. Early syphilis and persons exposed within last 90 days
     a. Treat all partners
     b. First choice—benzathine penicillin G, 2.4 million units IM once
     c. Penicillin allergy—doxycycline 100 mg orally b.i.d. for 2 weeks or tetracycline 500 mg orally q.i.d. for 2 weeks
  4. Late latent cases and cardiovascular syphilis (normal CSF examination)
     a. First choice—benzathine penicillin G, 2.4 million units IM weekly for 3 weeks
     b. Penicillin allergy—doxycycline 100 mg orally b.i.d. for 4 weeks or tetracycline 500 mg orally q.i.d. for 4 weeks
  5. Neurosyphilis
     a. First choice—18–24 million units aqueous crystalline penicillin G daily, administered as 3 to 4 million units IV every 4 hours for 10–14 days

b. Alternate regimen if compliance ensured—2.4 million units procaine penicillin IM daily, plus probenecid 500 mg orally q.i.d., both for 10–14 days
6. Posttreatment follow-up
   a. Primary and secondary baseline RPR or VDRL at time of treatment and repeated every 3 months; titer should fall fourfold in 3 months, eightfold in 6 months, and become negative within 2 years (MHA-TP and FTA-ABS will be positive for lifetime)
   b. Latent—RPR or VDRL repeated at 6-month and 12-month intervals; titer should fall fourfold in 12–24 months
   c. Neurosyphilis—CSF examination every 6 months until normal
7. Discuss therapeutic and diagnostic plans
8. Emphasize importance of complete treatment
9. Avoid sexual intercourse until patient and partner(s) cured
10. Educate regarding prevention, transmission, and treatment of the disease; encourage continued use of condoms
11. Report cases to health department
12. All patients with syphilis should be tested for HIV infection

## HERPES GENITALIS

- Definition—a viral STD that produces recurrent, painful genital lesions and has no cure

- Etiology/Incidence
  1. Caused by herpes simplex virus (HSV) types 1 (5–15%) and 2 (85–95%)
  2. Initial (primary) and recurrent infections affect approximately 40 million people annually
  3. Duration of initial infection—10–14 days; recurrent 7–10 days; viral shedding (without clinical symptoms) occurs during latency (interval between outbreaks)
  4. Virus resides in presacral ganglia during latency
  5. Can lead to neuralgia, meningitis, ascending myelitis, urethral strictures, and lymphatic suppuration
  6. Infection during pregnancy can lead to spontaneous abortion or fetal morbidity/mortality; risk for transmission to neonate appears highest among women with first episode near time of delivery
  7. Incubation period 2–21 days after exposure

- Signs and Symptoms
  1. First clinical episode occurs in all persons within 6 weeks of contracting infection
     a. Fever/chills
     b. Malaise
     c. Headache
     d. Dysuria
     e. Vaginal discharge, abnormal bleeding
     f. Dyspareunia
     g. Lymph nodes tender, enlarged, firm
     h. Painful genital vesicles that appear in groups on an erythematous base, then rupture and become painful ulcers before resolution—mean duration 12 days
     i. Prodrome frequently absent
  2. Recurrent episodes
     a. Characterized by a prodrome of tingling, burning, or other neuropathic symptoms for 1 or more days
     b. Grouped vesicles that rupture into less painful ulcers; mean duration 4.5 days
     c. Severity of outbreak typically less than initial presentation unless immune compromise is present

- Differential Diagnosis
  1. Syphilis
  2. Lymphogranuloma venereum
  3. Gonorrhea
  4. Chlamydia
  5. Chancroid
  6. Vaginitis
  7. Herpes zoster
  8. Condyloma latum
  9. Erythema multiforme
  10. Neoplasm (especially cervical)

- Physical Findings
  1. Fever—first episode
  2. Single or multiple vesicles surrounded by inflammation/edema on external genitalia, penis, scrotum, anus, vagina, or cervix (75%); vesicles spontaneously rupture and form painful, erythematous ulcers, scab over, and heal
  3. Cervix may appear diffusely inflamed, edematous with large punched-out ulcers or a granulomatous-appearing tumor-like mass covered with gray exudate
  4. Profuse, watery vaginal discharge often present and may be only sign
  5. Regional lymphadenopathy may be present

- Diagnostic Tests/Findings
  1. Tzanck stain—identification of multinucleated giant cells with intranuclear inclusions in a cytologic smear
  2. Identification of HSV virus(es) from tissue (vulvar, vaginal, cervical) cultures, antigen test, DNA probe, or PCR assay
  3. Serologic tests for HSV types 1 and 2 antibodies are also available

4. IgM and IgG markers distinguish recent from remote infection
5. Test for concomitant infection of other STD in patient and contacts
   a. HIV
   b. Syphilis
   c. Condylomata acuminata
   d. Gonorrhea
   e. Chlamydia
   f. Chancroid

- Management/Treatment
  1. Symptomatic treatment—drying and antipruritic agents and topical anesthetic agents
  2. Chemotherapeutic agents—acyclovir (available in topical, oral, and intravenous formulation), famciclovir, or valacyclovir
     a. Topical therapy—minimal benefit except may be useful for immunocompromised patients, use is discouraged
     b. Oral therapy
        (1) First clinical episode of genital herpes
            (a) Acyclovir 400 mg orally 3 times a day for 7–10 days, or
            (b) Acyclovir 200 mg orally 5 times a day for 7–10 days, or
            (c) Famciclovir 250 mg orally 3 times a day for 7–10 days, or
            (d) Valacyclovir 1 g orally twice a day for 7–10 days
        (2) Episodic recurrent genital herpes
            (a) Acyclovir 400 mg orally 3 times a day for 5 days, or
            (b) Acyclovir 200 mg orally 5 times a day for 5 days, or
            (c) Acyclovir 800 mg orally twice a day for 5 days, or
            (d) Famciclovir 125 mg orally twice a day for 5 days, or
            (e) Valacyclovir 500 mg orally twice a day for 3–5 days, or
            (f) Valacyclovir 1 g orally once a day for 5 days
            (g) One-day regimens of famciclovir and valacyclovir available if taken at the beginning of prodrome before vesicles erupt
        (3) Suppressive therapy for recurrent genital herpes
            (a) Acyclovir 400 mg orally twice a day, or
            (b) Famciclovir 250 mg orally twice a day, or
            (c) Valacyclovir 500 mg orally once a day, or
            (d) Valacyclovir 1 g orally once a day
     c. Intravenous therapy
        (1) Used in severe disease and when complications necessitate hospitalization
        (2) Acyclovir 5–10 mg/kg IV every 8 hours for 2–7 days followed by oral antiviral therapy to complete at least 10 days total therapy
     d. Acyclovir is eliminated by the kidneys; hydration is particularly important
     e. Safety of systemic treatment has not been established during pregnancy
  3. Avoid sexual intercourse when lesions present; encourage continued use of condoms
  4. Educate regarding prevention, transmission, and treatment of the disease and dangers during pregnancy
  5. Up to 80% may have viral shedding during asymptomatic periods

# GENITAL WARTS (CONDYLOMATA ACUMINATA)

- Definition—sexually transmitted warty growths appearing on any part of the genitalia

- Etiology/Incidence
  1. More than 100 types of human papillomavirus (HPV) cause genital warts; visible genital warts usually are caused by types 6 or 11; types 16, 18, 31, 33, 35 are predominately detected in high-grade neoplastic lesions and cervical cancer
  2. HPV increases risk of penile, vulvar, and cervical cancers
  3. Greatest incidence in the 15- to 25-year-old age group; correlated with multiple sex partners, early coitus, and lack of contraceptive barrier methods
  4. Approximately 6 million new cases each year
  5. Approximately 20 million people currently infected in the United States
  6. The most common symptomatic viral STD in the United States; highly contagious

- Signs and Symptoms
  1. Painless, pruritic, or burning warts on external genitalia (male and female)
  2. Possibly—dyspareunia, dysuria, bleeding

- Differential Diagnosis
  1. Condyloma latum
  2. Neoplasm
  3. Granuloma inguinale
  4. Moles
  5. Molluscum contagiosum

- Physical Findings
  1. Single or multiple soft, fleshy, papillary, or sessile, painless keratinized growths (may

be multilobulated papules and quite large) around anus, vulvovaginal area, penis, urethra, perineum, or oral cavity
  2. In women, similar lesions may appear in vagina/on cervix; vaginal discharge from coexisting infection(s) may be present; men may have lesions in urethra
  3. May have no signs because flat warts are visible only by colposcopy
- Diagnostic Tests/Findings
  1. Tissue sample (biopsy) for detection of viral DNA is available, but expense limits clinical utility
  2. Biopsies may be taken to rule out dysplasia and carcinoma
  3. Pap smear may indicate HPV infection on cervix; see section on dysplasia later in this chapter
  4. Test for concomitant infection of other STD
     a. HIV
     b. Gonorrhea
     c. Syphilis—RPR or VDRL to rule out condyloma latum
     d. Chlamydia
- Management/Treatment
  1. Prevention
     a. Condoms may lower risk; however, HPV can be shed into areas not covered by condoms
     b. HPV vaccination
        (1) Gardasil indicated for females and males aged 9–26
           (a) Prevents four HPV types
              (i) Types 16 and 18, which cause 70% of cervical cancers
              (ii) Types 6 and 11, which cause 90% of genital warts
              (iii) No effect on HPV-related disease
           (b) May be given to sexually active girls/women and those who already have HPV infection because most not infected with all four types
           (c) Should not be given in pregnancy
           (d) Should not be given in the setting of moderate or severe illness
           (e) Given as a series of 3 IM injections at baseline, 2 months, and 6 months
        (2) Cervarix indicated for females aged 10–25
           (a) Prevents two HPV types
              (i) Types 16 and 18, which cause 70% of cervical cancers
              (ii) No effect on HPV-related disease
           (b) May be given to sexually active girls/women and those who already have HPV infection because most not infected with all four types
           (c) Should not be given in pregnancy
           (d) Should not be given in the setting of moderate or severe illness
           (e) Given as a series of 3 IM injections at baseline, 2 months, and 6 months
  2. New treatment regimens are evolving to ameliorate symptoms; no current methods are curative
     a. Small vulvar and perianal warts
        (1) Self-treatment with podofilox 0.5% solution or gel—apply with cotton tip applicator b.i.d. for 3 days followed by no treatment for 4 days; cycle can be repeated 4 times (caution with podophyllin use concerning size of treatment area)
        (2) 80–90% solution of trichloroacetic acid (TCA) or tincture of podophyllin weekly for 6 weeks (patient must wash off podophyllin in 4 hours); protect surrounding skin with petroleum jelly
        (3) TCA is preferred because it is more effective, not absorbed, and can be used during pregnancy and on penis; treatment may be slightly more painful than podophyllin; immediate application of sodium bicarbonate paste following treatment will decrease pain
        (4) Self-treatment with imiquimod 5% cream applied at bedtime 3 times a week for 16 weeks; wash off 6–10 hours after application
        (5) Surgical removal with tangential scissor or shave excision, curettage, or electrosurgery
        (6) Intralesional interferon
        (7) Cryotherapy with liquid nitrogen
     b. Large warts (> 2 cm), vulvar/vaginal warts
        (1) $CO_2$ laser
        (2) Electrodesiccation, electrocautery, cryocautery, Leep, intralesional interferon
  3. NO MORE THAN ⅓ OF LESION ENCIRCLING AN ORIFICE SHOULD BE TREATED AT SINGLE VISIT
  4. Cervical warts—see section on dysplasia later in this chapter
  5. Discuss therapeutic and diagnostic plans

6. Educate regarding prevention, transmission, and treatment of the disease; encourage continued use of condoms
7. Emphasize importance of follow-up, particularly if Pap abnormal
8. Discuss possible chronicity
   a. Treatment may not be successful
   b. High recurrence rate due to dormant and asymptomatic viral shedding
   c. Individuals who smoke have more difficulty with recurrence
   d. Smoking is HPV cofactor for cervical cancer

## PELVIC INFLAMMATORY DISEASE (PID)

- Definition—infection of the upper genital tract, including the endometrium, oviducts, ovaries, uterine wall/serosa, broad ligaments, and pelvic peritoneum

- Etiology/Incidence
  1. A disease of polymicrobial infection caused by a variety of aerobic and anaerobic bacteria including *N. gonorrhoeae*, *C. trachomatis*, group B streptococcus, *Escherichia coli*, bacteroides, *Mycoplasma hominis*, and *Ureaplasma urealyticum*
  2. Clinical PID is usually a polymicrobial infection
  3. More than 1 million episodes occur annually
  4. Most prevalent serious infection for women 16–25 years of age
  5. After initial infection, women more susceptible to reinfection, ectopic pregnancy, and infertility
  6. Oral contraceptives and barrier methods with spermicide provide significant protection
  7. Depot-medroxyprogesterone acetate and Norplant cause changes in cervical mucosa, which provide some protection from PID
  8. Annual costs of PID and its sequelae are $4.2 billion

- Signs and Symptoms
  1. Symptoms may be mild, atypical, subtle, or absent
  2. Fever/chills
  3. Nausea/vomiting
  4. Dysuria
  5. Vaginal discharge
  6. Dysmenorrhea
  7. Abnormal menstrual bleeding
  8. Lower abdominal/pelvic pain (usually < 1 week duration)
  9. Dyspareunia
  10. Infertility

- Differential Diagnosis
  1. Appendicitis
  2. Ectopic pregnancy
  3. Septic abortion
  4. Hemorrhagic or ruptured ovarian cysts or tumors
  5. Twisted ovarian cyst
  6. Degeneration of a myoma
  7. Enteritis

- Physical Findings and Diagnostic Tests/Findings (clinical criteria for diagnosing PID)
  1. Minimum criteria—empiric treatment required if both are present
     a. Uterine/adnexal tenderness
     b. Cervical wall motion tenderness
  2. Additional criteria to enhance specificity of diagnosis
     a. Laboratory documentation of cervical infection with *C. trachomatis* or *N. gonorrhoeae*
     b. Oral temperature > 38.3° C or 101° F
     c. Abnormal cervical or vaginal mucopurulent discharge
     d. White blood cells on saline microscopy of vaginal secretions
     e. Elevated erythrocyte sedimentation rate and/or C-reactive protein
  3. Definitive criteria for diagnosis—warranted in select cases
     a. Histopathological evidence of endometritis on endometrial biopsy
     b. Tubo-ovarian abscess on sonography or other radiological tests
     c. Laparoscopic abnormalities consistent with PID

- Management/Treatment
  1. Resolution of symptoms and preservation of tubal function are the primary goals in management of PID; ideally, all patients are hospitalized; however, for economic and practical reasons, many are treated as outpatients
  2. Hospitalization is highly recommended if
     a. Diagnosis is uncertain and surgical emergencies (i.e., appendicitis) cannot be excluded
     b. Tubo-ovarian abscess is suspected
     c. Patient is pregnant
     d. Severe illness, e.g., nausea and vomiting, precludes outpatient treatment
     e. Patient unable to follow or tolerate outpatient regimen
     f. Patient has failed to clinically respond to outpatient treatment
  3. Outpatient treatment

a. Recommended treatment for PID—ceftriaxone 250 mg IM in a single dose plus azithromycin 1 g in a single dose (preferred) or doxycycline 100 mg orally twice a day for 14 days WITH or WITHOUT metronidazole 500 mg orally twice a day for 14 days
b. Alternative treatments—cefoxitin 2 g IM in a single dose and probenecid 1 g orally administered concurrently in a single dose, PLUS azithromycin 1 g in a single dose (preferred) or doxycycline 100 mg orally twice a day for 14 days WITH or WITHOUT metronidazole 500 mg orally twice a day for 14 days
c. Alternative treatment—other parenteral third-generation cephalosporin PLUS azithromycin 1 g in a single dose or doxycycline 100 mg orally twice a day for 14 days WITH or WITHOUT metronidazole 500 mg orally twice a day for 14 days
4. Follow-up appointment in 72 hours; should be substantially improved; if not, hospitalization usually required
5. Some clinicians advocate test-of-cure 4–6 weeks posttreatment
6. Test and treat partners
7. Discuss therapeutic and diagnostic plans
8. Emphasize importance of complete treatment
9. Avoid sexual intercourse until patient and partner(s) cured
10. Education regarding prevention, transmission, and treatment of the disease; encourage continued use of condoms
11. Discuss fertility issues as appropriate

## VULVOVAGINITIS

- Definition—inflammation and infection of the vulva/vagina

- Etiology/Incidence
  1. Commonly caused by *Trichomonas vaginalis* (a motile protozoan), bacterial vaginosis (a polymicrobial bacterial vaginal infection), or *Candida albicans* (a fungi or yeast)
  2. *Trichomonas*—transmitted through intercourse, can infect the lower urinary tract in men and women
  3. Bacterial vaginosis (BV)—the most frequently diagnosed symptomatic vaginitis in the United States; unclear whether BV results from sexually transmitted pathogen, but incidence is higher in those who are sexually active; should be treated in pregnant women because the infection has been associated with premature rupture of membranes, preterm labor, and preterm birth
  4. Vulvovaginal candidiasis (VVC)—occurs in close to 40–75% of women; is not considered to be an STD; is predisposed by pregnancy, diabetes, use of broad-spectrum antibiotics or corticosteroids; heat, moisture, and occlusive clothing also increase risk; VVC has been divided into two categories
     a. Uncomplicated VVC—sporadic or infrequent vulvovaginal candidiasis or mild-to-moderate vulvovaginal candidiasis is likely to be *C. albicans* in nonimmunocompromised women
     b. Complicated VVC—recurrent vulvovaginal candidiasis (four or more episodes of symptomatic VVC in 1 year) or severe vulvovaginal candidiasis or nonalbicans candidiasis, or women with uncontrolled diabetes, debilitation, or immunosuppression in those who are pregnant
  5. Several types of vaginitis may coexist

- Signs and Symptoms
  1. Trichomoniasis
     a. Malodorous yellow-green discharge with pruritus
     b. Dyspareunia
     c. Dysuria (male partners may also have dysuria)
  2. Bacterial vaginosis
     a. Malodorous, white ("fishy") discharge
     b. Spotting
     c. 50% of patients are asymptomatic
  3. Candida vaginitis
     a. Thick, "cottage cheese" discharge with pruritus
     b. Erythema of vagina and vulva

- Differential Diagnosis
  1. Chlamydia
  2. Gonorrhea
  3. Herpes genitalis
  4. Condylomata acuminata
  5. Allergy, contact dermatitis
  6. Atrophic vaginitis

- Physical Findings
  1. Trichomoniasis
     a. Diffuse vaginal erythema
     b. Intensely inflamed lesions on cervix and vaginal mucosa—"strawberry patches"
     c. Discharge
        (1) Ranges from white/watery to green, thick, and frothy
        (2) Vaginal pH—higher than 4.5
  2. Bacterial vaginosis
     a. Watery, grayish, or white homogenous discharge, fishy odor

b. Discharge slightly adherent to vaginal walls
3. Candida vaginitis
    a. White, "cottage-cheese" discharge
    b. Marked vulvovaginal erythema/edema with intense pruritus

- Diagnostic Tests/Findings
    1. Wet prep microscopic examination of vaginal secretions viewed on low or high power
        a. Trichomoniasis—discharge mixed with saline will show motile *Trichomonas* on microscopic examination
        b. Bacterial vaginosis—discharge mixed with saline will show clue cells on microscopic examination; amine-like odor present when discharge alkalinized with 10–20% potassium hydroxide (KOH) "whiff test"; vaginal pH of 4–5 or more
        c. Candida vaginitis—discharge mixed with 10% KOH will show branched and budding pseudohyphae on microscopic examination
    2. Test for concomitant infection from other STD
        a. HIV
        b. Syphilis
        c. Condylomata acuminata
        d. Gonorrhea
        e. Chlamydia

- Management/Treatment
    1. Trichomoniasis
        a. Recommended treatment—metronidazole 2 g orally as a single dose, alternative treatment metronidazole 500 mg b.i.d. for 7 days; treat partner
        b. Treatment during pregnancy—2 g of metronidazole in single dose
        c. Caution patient to avoid alcohol during metronidazole therapy due to possible disulfiram-like reaction
    2. Bacterial vaginosis
        a. Recommended treatment
            (1) Clindamycin cream 2%, 1 full applicator 5 g intravaginally at bedtime for 7 days
            (2) Metronidazole 500 mg orally b.i.d. for 7 days, or
            (3) Metronidazole gel 0.75%, 1 full applicator (5 g) intravaginally q.d. or b.i.d. for 5 days
        b. Alternative treatment
            (1) Clindamycin 300 mg orally b.i.d. for 7 days (safe during pregnancy)
            (2) Metronidazole 2 g orally in a single dose
            (3) Clindamycin ovules 100 g intravaginally at bedtime for 3 days
        c. Treatment during pregnancy
            (1) Metronidazole 250 mg orally 3 times a day for 7 days
            (2) Clindamycin 300 mg orally twice a day for 7 days
    3. Vulvovaginal candidiasis
        a. Recommended regimens for uncomplicated VVC
            (1) Intravaginal agents—variety of intravaginal antifungal agents available over the counter in single dose, 3-, 5-, 7-, or 14-day regimens
            (2) Oral agent—fluconazole 150-mg oral tablet, 1 tablet in single dose
            (3) Return for follow-up if symptoms recur within 2 months—need to consider underlying cause of recurrent susceptibility to fungal infection
            (4) Intravaginal creams and suppositories are oil-based and may weaken latex condoms and diaphragms
        b. Recommended regimens for complicated VVC
            (1) Recurrent VVC—7–14 days of topical azole therapy or a 150-mg oral dose of fluconazole repeated 3 days later
                (a) Maintenance regimens include clotrimazole (500-mg dose vaginal suppositories once weekly), or ketoconazole (100-mg dose once daily), or fluconazole (100- to 150-mg dose once weekly), or itraconazole (400-mg dose once monthly or 100-mg dose once daily)
                (b) Maintenance regimens usually continue for 6 months
                (c) Patients receiving long-term treatment with ketoconazole should be monitored for hepatic toxicity
            (2) Severe VVC (i.e., extensive vulvar erythema, edema, excoriation, and fissure formation)—7–14 days of topical azole or 150 mg of fluconazole in two sequential doses (second dose 72 hours after initial dose) are recommended
            (3) Nonalbicans VVC—7–14 days of treatment with a nonfluconazole azole drug are recommended
                (i) For recurrence—600 mg of boric acid in a gelatin capsule are recommended, administered vaginally once daily for 2 weeks; referral to a specialist is advised
            (4) Pregnancy—only topical azole therapies, applied vaginally for 7 days

4. Discuss therapeutic and diagnostic plans
5. Avoid sexual intercourse until patient and partner(s) cured
6. Education regarding prevention, transmission, and treatment of the disease; encourage continued use of condoms
7. Emphasize importance of treating BV, trichomoniasis, and infections during pregnancy
8. Education regarding dangers of douching and incidence of infection
9. Education regarding PID; association with bacterial vaginosis

## LOWER URINARY TRACT INFECTION (LUTI; CYSTITIS: ACUTE, UNCOMPLICATED)

- Definition—inflammation and infection of the urinary bladder; urethra may be involved

- Etiology/Incidence
  1. Most common causative organisms—*E. coli* (women) and *Proteus* species (men)
  2. More common in women than in men; urological evaluation should be considered for men with UTI
  3. 30–40% of women will experience at least one UTI
  4. Contributing factors in women
     a. Sexual intercourse; diaphragm use
     b. Pregnancy
     c. Diabetes
     d. Catheterization
     e. Instrumentation
     f. Retaining urine in bladder despite urge to void
  5. Contributing factors in men
     a. Residual urine (prostatic enlargement)
     b. Neuropathic bladder
     c. Calculi
     d. Prostatitis
     e. Catheterization
     f. Instrumentation

- Signs and Symptoms
  1. Dysuria, frequency, urgency
  2. Lower abdominal discomfort
  3. Suprapubic discomfort
  4. Foul-smelling urine

- Differential Diagnosis
  1. Vaginitis (females)
  2. Prostatitis (males)
  3. Gonorrhea
  4. Chlamydia infection
  5. Renal calculi
  6. Pyelonephritis
  7. Epididymitis

- Physical Findings
  1. Urinary meatus may be erythematous/edematous
  2. Negative costovertebral angle tenderness
  3. Negative pelvic or prostate examination; women may experience discomfort when bladder palpated during pelvic examination
  4. May have suprapubic tenderness on palpation

- Diagnostic Tests/Findings
  1. Pyuria—> 10 WBC/HPF
  2. Complete urinalysis (clean catch) with culture and sensitivity testing
     a. Bacteria count of more than 100,000 organisms per milliliter in fresh "clean catch" midstream specimen is reliable indicator of active urinary tract infection; women with acute cystitis may have more than $10^3$ but less than $10^5$ per mL in midstream urine cultures
     b. Leukocyte esterase dipstick test—positive
     c. Urine dipstick positive for protein, blood, nitrites suggestive of UTI

- Management/Treatment for Women (men need urological referral)
  1. Single-dose regimens—fosfomycin tromethamine 3-g single dose
  2. Three-day regimen examples (uncomplicated lower tract infection, e.g., women < 65 years old who are not pregnant)
     a. TMP/SMX DS tablet b.i.d.
     b. Fluoroquinolones in cases of TMP/SMX resistance or allergy
        (1) Ciprofloxacin 250 mg b.i.d.
        (2) Norfloxacin 400 mg b.i.d.
        (3) Ofloxacin 200 mg b.i.d.
        (4) Levofloxacin 250 mg daily
  3. 7- to 10-day regimen examples (for complicated infection, e.g., men, women > 65 years of age)
     a. TMP/SMX 1 DS tablet b.i.d.
     b. Nitrofurantoin 100 mg q.i.d.
     c. Fluoroquinolones in cases of TMP/SMX resistance
        (1) Norfloxacin 400 mg b.i.d.
        (2) Ciprofloxacin 250–500 mg b.i.d.
        (3) Levofloxacin 250 mg daily
  4. Treatment during pregnancy—nitrofurantoin 100 mg b.i.d. for 7–10 days or amoxicillin 500 mg orally t.i.d. for 7–14 days; cephalosporin 500 mg q.i.d. for 7–14 days
  5. Consider adding phenazopyridine hydrochloride 200 mg orally t.i.d. for 2 days for discomfort associated with urinary tract irritation (caution patient of orange/red tinge to urine)

6. Consider possibility of urethritis from chlamydia if failure of short-course therapy in sexually active women
7. Increase water and decrease carbonated drink intake
8. Encourage frequent voids; do not hold urine in bladder
9. Patient education regarding perineal hygiene
10. Repeat urinalysis with culture and sensitivity after medication regimen completed if still symptomatic
11. Discuss therapeutic and diagnostic plans
12. Advise return appointment if symptoms increase or no improvement
13. Emphasize importance of complete treatment

## ACUTE PYELONEPHRITIS (UPPER UTI)

- Definition—an acute bacterial infection of the upper urinary tract (kidney and renal pelvis); usually results from an ascending infection

- Etiology/Incidence
  1. *E. coli* (gram negative) accounts for 80% of infections; *Staphylococcus saprophyticus* and *Streptococcus faecalis* (gram positive) account for 5–10%
  2. If urological abnormalities or calculi present, the following organisms may cause infection— *Enterobacter, Proteus, Klebsiella, Serratia,* and *Pseudomonas*
  3. Majority of infections occur in young women; rare occurrence in men younger than age 50 years
  4. Most commonly occurs in patients who are pregnant or have disruptive urinary flow, neurogenic bladder dysfunction, or vesicoureteral reflux
  5. May follow incomplete treatment of lower urinary tract infection

- Signs and Symptoms—usually develop rapidly over a few hours
  1. Shaking chills
  2. Malaise, generalized muscle tenderness
  3. Nausea, vomiting, and diarrhea
  4. Flank/back pain (unilateral or bilateral)
  5. Abdominal pain
  6. Dysuria, frequency, or urgency (may be absent)

- Differential Diagnosis
  1. Cystitis
  2. Prostatitis
  3. Musculoskeletal back pain
  4. Appendicitis
  5. Diverticulitis
  6. Pelvic inflammatory disease
  7. Ectopic pregnancy

- Physical Findings
  1. Fever, tachycardia
  2. Costovertebral angle pain (unilateral or bilateral) upon percussion
  3. Peritoneal signs are usually absent
  4. Patient may appear very ill

- Diagnostic Tests/Findings
  1. Microscopic urinalysis
     a. 5–10 WBC/HPF
     b. Occasional erythrocytes
     c. White cell casts may be present
     d. Mild proteinuria
  2. Urine culture—> 100,000 bacteria per mL of urine; sensitivity testing should be done
  3. Gram stain of uncentrifuged urine—one bacterium per oil-immersion correlates with 100,000 bacteria per mL of urine or more
  4. CBC—leukocytosis with left shift
  5. Elevated erythrocyte sedimentation rate (ESR)
  6. Blood urea nitrogen (BUN) and creatinine usually normal
  7. Electrolytes may be abnormal if dehydrated

- Management/Treatment
  1. Outpatient therapy—if compliant/reliable with immediate access to healthcare services, if condition worsens, and if not elderly or pregnant
     a. Antibiotics may include fluoroquinolones for 7-day regimen as treatment of choice; alternative regimens include TMP/SMX, first-generation cephalosporins, or amoxicillin/clavulanate, for 14-day course
     b. Resistance to amoxicillin is 30%; therefore, should not be used as sole therapy
     c. Follow-up within 24 hours
     d. Hydration measures
  2. Inpatient therapy
     a. Patients who are pregnant, have underlying illness, have decreased renal reserve, very toxic (high fever, hypotensive, etc.), or unable to tolerate oral therapy should be hospitalized for parenteral antibiotics
     b. IV antimicrobial therapy is based on culture and sensitivity report
     c. IV hydration is also required
  3. Repeat urine culture 2 weeks after completed course of antibiotics
  4. Discuss therapeutic and diagnostic plans
  5. Emphasize importance of complete treatment and follow-up appointments
  6. Instructions regarding no sexual intercourse until treatment completed

7. Education regarding emergency signs and symptoms if managed as outpatient
8. Second episode of acute pyelonephritis requires urological consultation or workup

## ACUTE BACTERIAL PROSTATITIS

- Definition—inflammation/infection of the prostate gland

- Etiology/Incidence
  1. *E. coli* or other gram-negative bacteria are common causative agents
  2. Occasionally acute urinary retention develops, requiring urgent hospitalization; suprapubic drainage may be necessary; URINARY CATHETERIZATION SHOULD BE AVOIDED
  3. Absence of zinc in prostatic fluid can predispose patient to infection
  4. Young adult men may be more prone to nonbacterial prostatitis or prostatosis
     a. WBC are present in expressed prostatic secretions, but no organisms are cultured
     b. Causative agents include mycoplasma, ureaplasma, gonorrhea, and chlamydia—sexually transmitted organisms more likely in men < 35 years of age

- Signs and Symptoms
  1. Fever/chills, malaise, myalgias
  2. Low back pain
  3. Dysuria, urgency, nocturia, frequency
  4. Perineal pain increased with defecation

- Differential Diagnosis
  1. Acute/chronic bacterial cystitis (urinary retention)
  2. Chronic prostatitis
  3. Nonbacterial prostatitis
  4. Prostatodynia
  5. Prostatic or seminal vesicle abscesses
  6. Benign prostatic hypertrophy
  7. Prostatic cancer
  8. Epididymitis
  9. Acute diverticulitis

- Physical Findings
  1. Fever
  2. Prostate—edematous, firm or "boggy," warm and tender; AVOID VIGOROUS MASSAGE, CAN LEAD TO BACTEREMIA

- Diagnostic Tests/Findings
  1. Urine cultures—positive
  2. Prostatic secretions—expressed prostatic secretions (EPS), WBC > 20 cells/HPF is abnormal
  3. Diagnosis is best made by performing simultaneous quantitative bacterial cultures of urethral urine, bladder urine, and EPS, the three-glass test
  4. Patient often treated based only on physical findings and urine culture

- Management/Treatment
  1. Patients who appear septic and/or have urinary retention should be hospitalized
  2. Outpatient treatment
     a. First choice if age > 35 years is TMP/SMX double-strength tablet b.i.d. for 4–6 weeks; if age < 35 years azithromycin 1 g orally in a single dose or doxycycline 100 mg orally b.i.d. for 10 days plus ceftriaxone 250 mg IM 1 time or ofloxacin 400 mg once then 300 mg b.i.d. for 10 days
     b. Alternative choices are carbenicillin 2 tablets orally q.i.d. for 2–4 weeks or ciprofloxacin 500 mg orally b.i.d. for 2–4 weeks
  3. Bed rest
  4. Sitz bath t.i.d. for 30 minutes
  5. Follow-up appointment 48–72 hours
  6. Discuss therapeutic and diagnostic plans
  7. Avoid sexual intercourse until acute phase resolved; encourage continued use of condoms if multiple partners
  8. Education regarding signs/symptoms of urinary retention and epididymitis
  9. Emphasize importance of follow-up appointments

## CHRONIC BACTERIAL PROSTATITIS

- Definition—chronic inflammation/infection of prostate gland

- Etiology/Incidence
  1. Causative organisms are *E. coli*; *Enterobacter* organisms, *Proteus* species, *C. trachomatis*—sexually transmitted organisms more likely in men < 35 years of age
  2. Often associated with urethritis or infection of lower urinary tract
  3. One of the most common causes of recurrent urinary tract infection in men

- Signs and Symptoms
  1. Symptoms similar to, but milder than, acute bacterial prostatitis
  2. Hallmark of disease is relapsing UTI due to same pathogen found in prostatic secretions
  3. Urinary frequency, dysuria, decreased flow, hesitancy, dribbling
  4. Vague lower abdominal pain
  5. Lumbar and perineal pain

6. Fever and urethral discharge uncommon
7. May experience swelling and severe tenderness of scrotum

- Differential Diagnosis—same as acute bacterial prostatitis

- Physical Findings
  1. May involve scrotal contents, producing intense local discomfort, swelling, erythema, and severe tenderness to palpation
  2. Prostate may be tender, irregularly indurated, or boggy

- Diagnostic Tests/Findings—diagnosis made by examination of EPS and quantitative bacterial cultures
  1. EPS—abnormal if greater than 10 WBC/HPF
  2. More than 1 or 2 lipid-laden macrophages/HPF—abnormal
  3. EPS culture—positive

- Management/Treatment
  1. Often difficult to treat
  2. Usual antibiotics—TMP/SMX, doxycycline, ciprofloxacin, levofloxacin, norfloxacin for 12 weeks
  3. Sitz baths, prostatic massage
  4. Regular ejaculation through intercourse and/or masturbation
  5. Avoid over-the-counter decongestants if urinary outlet symptoms

## EPIDIDYMITIS

- Definition—an acute intrascrotal infection

- Etiology/Incidence
  1. Caused by infection from bladder urine, the prostate, or an ascending urethral infection
  2. Common affliction of men 35 years and younger; chlamydia usual causative organism for this population (*N. gonorrhoeae* far less common)
  3. Infection in men > 35 years usually arises from bladder bacteriuria secondary to coliform organisms or following instrumentation, catheterization, or surgery (prostatectomy)
  4. "Sterile" epididymitis associated with vigorous physical activity is caused by vasal reflux of sterile urine, which leads to a chemical inflammation of the epididymis
  5. Epididymitis in boys may indicate underlying congenital anatomic abnormalities (i.e., ectopic ureter, posterior urethral valve)
  6. Condition is usually unilateral
  7. Epididymitis may be complicated by development of testicular necrosis, testicular atrophy, or infertility

- Signs and Symptoms
  1. Painful, scrotal swelling (pain may radiate up the spermatic cord into the lower abdomen)
  2. Sensation of scrotal heaviness
  3. Symptoms of prostatitis or UTI may be present
  4. Systemic symptoms may develop—fever, chills, and malaise

- Differential Diagnosis
  1. Mumps
  2. Testicular torsion
  3. Testicular abscess
  4. Tumor of testicle with or without hemorrhage
  5. Hydrocele
  6. Trauma
  7. Infarction

- Physical Findings
  1. Enlarged, tender indurated epididymis
  2. Urethral discharge may be present
  3. Massaging prostate may exacerbate epididymitis
  4. Pain relieved with scrotal elevation (Prehn's sign)
  5. Cremasteric reflex present

- Diagnostic Tests/Findings
  1. Men
     a. STD testing (chlamydia, gonorrhea, and syphilis)
     b. Culture and gram-stained smear of uncentrifuged urine
     c. Scrotal ultrasonography if condition initially severe or if fever continues while on antibiotics (rule out abscess)
     d. CBC—may show increased white blood cell count with left shift
     e. Pyuria
  2. Boys—require more extensive workup; refer for consult
     a. Intravenous urography
     b. Cystourethroscopy
     c. Voiding cystourethrography
     d. Scrotal ultrasonography (with or without Doppler imaging)
     e. Radionuclide scanning
     f. Surgical exploration may be required

- Management/Treatment
  1. Physician referral or consult required if
     a. Patient is a child
     b. Systemic symptoms of infection (leukocytosis, fever) present in adults; patient should be hospitalized for parenteral antibiotics
     c. Possible torsion of testes
  2. Outpatient therapy

a. Antibiotic therapy based on patient's age and symptoms
   (1) Adult < 35 years of age—first choice is ceftriaxone 250 mg IM in a single dose plus azithromycin 1 g orally in a single dose or doxycycline 100 mg orally b.i.d.; alternative choice for men 17 years of age or older if no gonococcal or chlamydial infection is ofloxacin 200–400 mg orally b.i.d. for 10 days or levofloxacin 500 mg orally once daily for 10 days
   (2) Adult > 35 years of age—TMP/SMX 1 double-strength tablet orally b.i.d. or ciprofloxacin 250–500 mg orally b.i.d. for 10 days; or levofloxacin 250–500 mg daily for 10 days; treat for 4 weeks if underlying prostatitis present
b. Scrotal elevation, support, and bed rest
c. Analgesics—nonsteroidal anti-inflammatory agents
d. Ice (early), heat (late)
e. Spermatic cord block with lidocaine may be used

3. Follow up within 48 hours if symptoms persist or worsen
4. If STD present or suspected, instruct patient to refer sex partners for evaluation and treatment
5. Discuss therapeutic and diagnostic plans
6. Emphasize importance of complete treatment
7. Avoid sexual intercourse until course of antibiotics completed
8. Inform patient that swelling and discomfort may persist for weeks or months after eradication of infecting organism; epididymis may remain enlarged or indurated indefinitely
9. Educate regarding prevention, transmission, and treatment of sexually transmitted disease (if causative agent); encourage continued use of condoms
10. Encourage patient to discuss concerns and/or fears

# BENIGN PROSTATIC HYPERPLASIA (BPH)

- Definition—progressive, benign hyperplasia of prostate gland tissue

- Etiology/Incidence
  1. Cause is uncertain
  2. Approximately 50% of men have BPH by age 60; incidence increases to 90% by age 85
  3. The most common cause of bladder outlet obstruction in males > 50 years
  4. Symptoms are attributed to mechanical obstruction of the urethra by the enlarged prostate gland

- Signs and Symptoms
  1. May be asymptomatic
  2. Frequency, urgency, urge incontinence
  3. Nocturia, dysuria
  4. Weak urinary stream, dribbling, hesitancy
  5. Sensation of full bladder immediately after voiding
  6. Retention
  7. Urinary tract infection may be first indicator of BPH-induced urinary retention

- Differential Diagnosis
  1. Urethral stricture
  2. Prostate or bladder cancer
  3. Neurogenic bladder
  4. Bladder calculus
  5. Acute or chronic prostatitis
  6. Bladder neck contracture
  7. Medications that affect micturition

- Physical Findings
  1. Abdomen—may have distended bladder secondary to retention
  2. Prostate (patient should void prior to examination)
     a. Nontender with asymmetrical or symmetrical enlargement; gross enlargement atypical
     b. Consistency is smooth and rubbery (consistency of a pencil eraser)
     c. Distinct nodules (spheroids) may be present—differentiation between BPH nodules and cancerous ones is based on induration or firmness of gland; may require biopsy
     d. Blunting of the central sulcus

- Diagnostic Tests/Findings
  1. Urinalysis—typically normal; may be secondary indices of infection
  2. Urinary flow rate—voided volume and peak urinary flow rate (uroflowmetry) tests prostatic obstruction
  3. Abdominal ultrasound—rules out associated upper tract pathology
  4. Serum creatinine and BUN—normal
  5. Prostate-specific antigen (PSA) levels should be normal

- Management/Treatment
  1. Observation
  2. Urology consult required for mechanical or surgical treatments
  3. Pharmacological—drugs selected that reduce bulk and/or tone of gland
     a. Alpha-adrenergic antagonists
        (1) Terazosin—1 mg orally at bedtime, increase up to 10 mg at bedtime

(2) Prazosin—1 mg orally b.i.d. to t.i.d.; increase up to 6–15 mg per day
(3) Doxazosin—1 mg orally every day up to 16 mg if required
(4) Tamsulosin—0.4 mg orally daily; alpha antagonist activity specific to prostate
b. 5-alpha reductase inhibitors
(1) Finasteride—5 mg orally daily
(a) Pregnancy category X
(b) Must not be handled by pregnant women or those trying to become pregnant
(2) Dutasteride—0.5 mg orally daily
(a) Same precautions for pregnant women as finasteride
(b) Patients should not donate blood until > 6 months after last dose
c. Dutasteride/tamsulosin combination (Jalyn)
(1) Fixed dose combination of alpha blocker and 5-alpha reductase inhibitors
(2) Same precautions as each medication individually
4. Mechanical—balloon dilation of prostatic urethra
5. Surgery—indications
a. Acute urinary retention (urgent urology referral)
b. Gross hematuria
c. Epididymitis (especially if recurrent)
d. Recurrent urinary tract infections
e. Renal failure from obstruction
f. Intolerable chronic symptoms
6. Discuss therapeutic and diagnostic plans
7. Educate regarding signs/symptoms of urinary retention, renal failure, and epididymitis
8. Emphasize importance of follow-up appointments
9. Avoid caffeine and alcohol to decrease bladder irritation
10. Avoid decongestants, antihistamines, tricyclic antidepressants, anticholinergics

# PROSTATE CANCER

- Definition—a malignant neoplasm of the prostate gland

- Etiology/Incidence
  1. Etiology is unknown; environmental factors may be involved; adenocarcinoma is most common type
  2. Most common malignancy in American men and second most common cause of cancer deaths in men older than 65 years
  3. The relative survival rates have improved over the past 30 years (as a result of increased awareness and early detection, rather than improved therapy)
  4. May be associated with high-fat diet
  5. Risk factors—family history, age, African American

- Signs and Symptoms
  1. Many patients are asymptomatic
  2. Symptoms may mimic BPH with frequency, dribbling, nocturia, hesitancy
  3. Occasionally bone pain from metastases (advanced stage)
  4. Occasionally symptoms of uremia due to urethral obstructions (advanced stage)

- Differential Diagnosis
  1. BPH, urethral stricture
  2. Bladder cancer
  3. Neurogenic bladder
  4. Bladder calculus
  5. Acute/chronic prostatitis
  6. Bladder neck contracture
  7. Medications that affect micturition

- Physical Findings
  1. May present with lymphadenopathy, signs of uremia, or urinary retention with distended bladder
  2. More common physical findings are confined to prostate—on rectal examination prostate feels harder than normal and normal boundaries of gland may be obscured; nodules may be present
  3. Prostate may have asymmetric enlargement

- Diagnostic Tests/Findings (performed by consultant physician)
  1. Transperineal or transrectal needle biopsy of prostate—diagnostic accuracy rate > 90%
  2. PSA levels between 4 and 10 ng/mL may indicate BPH, levels > 10 ng/mL are suggestive of carcinoma; false negatives occur
  3. Transrectal ultrasound can aid in identification of solid nodules and is used to guide biopsy
  4. Other tests such as bone scans may be conducted

- Management/Treatment
  1. Consult/referral required
  2. Treatment predicated largely on stage of tumor; accurate staging is therefore essential
  3. Methods of treatment include surgery, radiation, hormonal therapy
  4. Assistance as appropriate in meeting physical, psychological, social, cultural, environmental, and spiritual needs
  5. Emphasize importance of follow-up appointments

## FIBROCYSTIC BREAST CHANGES

- Definition—benign breast condition characterized by increased growth of fibrous tissue, proliferation of the ductal epithelial lining, and/or formation of cysts

- Etiology/Incidence
  1. Cause is unknown, estrogen dependency is suspected; condition occurs clinically in 50% and histologically in 90% of women
  2. Three types of fibrocystic changes have been identified
     a. Nonproliferative lesions—most common type; no increased risk of breast cancer
     b. Proliferative lesions without atypia—minimal increased risk of breast cancer
     c. Cellular atypia—fivefold increased risk of breast cancer
  3. May be related to dietary intake of methylxanthines, e.g., coffee, chocolate (inconclusive)

- Signs and Symptoms (more pronounced premenstrually)
  1. Cyclic breast tenderness, engorgement, increased density, increased nodularity, enlargement of cystic lump(s)
  2. Nipple discharge may be present
  3. Symptoms of discomfort decrease after menopause

- Differential Diagnosis
  1. Fibroadenosis/fibroadenoma
  2. Fat necrosis
  3. Carcinoma (especially in women > 40 years)
  4. Breast cysts

- Physical Findings
  1. Skin and contour usually normal
  2. Mass or thickened area present
     a. Location—upper outer quadrant or any area
     b. Size—varies
     c. Shape—round, oval, or nodular
     d. Mobility—mobile
     e. Consistency—soft to firm (depends on tension of fluid within cysts)
     f. Number—solitary or multiple (may give impression of "beads on a string")
     g. Nipple—clear/serous discharge may be present (rare)
     h. Signs and symptoms may fluctuate with the menstrual cycle

- Diagnostic Tests/Findings
  1. Fine needle aspiration (FNA)—fluid should return if cyst
  2. Excisional biopsy (most definitive test)—no cancer cells
  3. Mammography—negative (for women > 35 years)
  4. Ultrasound—distinguishes cyst vs. solid mass

- Management/Treatment
  1. Warm compresses applied t.i.d.; supportive brassiere
  2. Low-salt diet; diuretics may also be given premenstrually
  3. Elimination of dietary methylxanthines (coffee, tea, colas, chocolate) (inconclusive) and tobacco use
  4. Vitamin E—400–600 international units orally daily
  5. Vitamin $B_6$—50–100 mg daily
  6. Evening primrose oil 1,000 mg/day (Katz & Dotters, 2012)
  7. Hormonal and antihormonal therapy are controversial; the following agents may be used in severe cases
     a. Oral contraceptives—low estrogen with relatively high progesterone
     b. Danazol
     c. Bromocriptine
     d. Tamoxifen
  8. Surgical excision is controversial
  9. Discussion of diagnostic and therapeutic plans
  10. Reassurance of low risk for malignancy
  11. Instruction and demonstration of breast self-examination
  12. Encouragement to report any new mass that does not resolve following menstruation
  13. At follow-up, assess for progression of condition and/or concurrent malignancy

## BREAST CANCER

- Definition—a malignant neoplasm of the breast

- Etiology/Incidence
  1. Estimated that one in nine women in the United States will develop breast cancer if they live to be 90 years old
  2. Frequency increases steadily after age 35
  3. Whites have higher incidence than nonwhites in United States
  4. Approximately 182,000 new cases occur annually
  5. Most common cause of cancer in women and second most common cause of cancer death in women
  6. Risk factors include
     a. Increasing age
     b. Postmenopausal long-term estrogen therapy—conflicting data

c. Nulliparity
   d. Late first pregnancy (over age 30)
   e. Early menarche and late menopause (after age 55)
   f. Cellular atypia
   g. Previous endometrial cancer
   h. Alcohol intake
   i. High-fat diet (polyunsaturated)
   j. Obesity
7. Patients with higher risk
   a. Positive family history (premenopausal more significant)
   b. Family history suggestive of an inherited predisposition to breast cancer
   c. Confirmation of an inherited mutation ($BRCA_1$ or $BRCA_2$) on a breast cancer susceptibility gene
   d. Prior personal history of breast cancer
   e. Fibrocystic changes associated with cellular atypia

- Signs and Symptoms
  1. Often asymptomatic
  2. Single, firm, nontender, painless mass is usual presenting sign
  3. Later manifestations
     a. Skin erythema, dimpling, ulceration
     b. Breast pain
     c. Nipple retraction, eczema, or ulceration
     d. Nipple discharge

- Differential Diagnosis
  1. Fibrocystic breast changes
  2. Fibroadenoma
  3. Intraductal papilloma
  4. Lipoma
  5. Fat necrosis
  6. Mastitis
  7. Dermatitis (Paget's disease)

- Physical Findings
  1. Most common manifestation is single, firm, nontender, ill-defined lump in breast; associated findings may include
     a. Diffuse nodularity
     b. Skin dimpling
     c. Nipple retraction, discharge (usually bloody)
     d. Lymphadenopathy
     e. Ulcerated/fungating mass (rare)
     f. Palpable supraclavicular and/or axillary lymph nodes
  2. Inflammatory cancer—skin erythema/edema, pain
  3. Paget's disease
     a. Associated with about 5% of mammary carcinomas
     b. Nipple erosion, crusting, bloody discharge
     c. Eczema-like change in skin

- Diagnostic Tests/Findings
  1. Mammography—mass or calcifications indicated; may be negative because 10% of palpable masses are missed on mammogram
  2. Ultrasound—distinguishes cyst vs. solid mass
  3. FNA cytology—fluid vs. solid mass, 10% false negative
  4. Large-needle (core needle) biopsy—histological examination reveals cancer cells (problems with sampling occur)
  5. Excisional biopsy—most reliable diagnostic test where staging of the tumor is done
  6. Determination of hormone receptor tumor cells
  7. Various tests may be conducted if metastasis is suspected including bone and organ scans

- Management/Treatment
  1. Secondary prevention
     a. Clinical breast examination every 3 years to age 40
     b. Clinical breast examination annually over age 40
     c. Mammography annually beginning at age 40 or 10 years before the age of diagnosis in women with first-degree family history
  2. Tertiary prevention
     a. Referral to an oncology team is required
     b. Dependent on tumor stage, presence of hormone receptors, and patient's symptoms/preferences
     c. May include surgery, chemotherapy, radiation therapy, and/or hormonal therapy
  3. Discussion of diagnostic and therapeutic plans
  4. Encouragement to express concerns and fears
  5. Education to patient and family members, especially daughters
  6. Encouragement to report new mass or changes
  7. Assistance, as appropriate, in meeting physical, psychological, sexual, social, cultural, environmental, and spiritual needs
  8. Emphasis on importance of maintaining follow-up with specialists and primary care providers

# DYSFUNCTIONAL UTERINE BLEEDING (DUB)

- Definition—excessive, abnormal uterine bleeding that occurs at irregular intervals, with no demonstrable organic cause

- Etiology/Incidence

1. Usually results from irregular sloughing of endometrium during anovulatory cycles (90% of cases); but occasionally occurs with poor quality ovulatory cycles
2. Most frequently due to abnormalities of endocrine function
3. Estrogen withdrawal or estrogen breakthrough bleeding
4. Progesterone breakthrough bleeding—continuous low-dose contraceptives
5. Heaviest bleeding due to high sustained levels of estrogen and seen with
    a. Polycystic ovarian disease
    b. Obesity
    c. Immaturity of the hypothalamic-pituitary-ovarian axis (postmenarchal teenagers)
    d. Late ovulations (perimenopausal women)
    e. Unopposed estrogen replacement therapy
6. Not related to oral contraceptive use

- Signs and Symptoms
   1. A carefully obtained history and character of bleeding pattern is critical to assist in ruling out other conditions
   2. Bleeding is usually characterized by one or more of the following
       a. Persistent or intermittent uterine bleeding
       b. Episodes of extremely heavy bleeding
       c. Oligomenorrhea
   3. DUB bleeding patterns
       a. Intermenstrual bleeding—variable amounts of bleeding that occur between regular menstrual periods
       b. Menometrorrhagia—prolonged, frequent, excessive uterine bleeding that occurs at irregular intervals
       c. Menorrhagia (hypermenorrhea)—prolonged (> 7 days) and excessive (> 80 mL) uterine bleeding occurring at regular intervals
       d. Metrorrhagia—uterine bleeding between normal cycle
       e. Polymenorrhea—frequent, irregular bleeding < 18-day intervals
       f. Oligomenorrhea—infrequent, irregular uterine bleeding that occurs at intervals > 40 days

- Differential Diagnosis
   1. *Inappropriate* to assume that abnormal uterine bleeding is endocrine in origin; other conditions must be ruled out according to reproductive age
   2. Adolescents
       a. Vaginal trauma secondary to athletics or early sexual exposure
       b. Hypothalamic-pituitary dysfunction secondary to exercise
       c. Pregnancy
       d. Genital infection
       e. Oral contraceptive use/misuse
       f. Blood dyscrasias
   3. Women in reproductive years
       a. Previously noted causes
       b. Endocrine-related anovulatory abnormal uterine bleeding, common with exercise
       c. Organic pathology
          (1) Uterine fibroids
          (2) Endometrial polyps
          (3) Chronic systemic illness, e.g., liver cirrhosis, renal failure
       d. Neoplasia
       e. Secondary to stress
       f. Excessive weight change
   4. Perimenopausal women
       a. Previously listed causes
       b. Follicular dysfunction (predominant cause)
   5. Postmenopausal women
       a. Previously noted causes
       b. Hormone replacement therapy
       c. Cancer

- Physical Findings
   1. A thorough general and pelvic examination should be performed to assist in ruling out conditions included in the differential diagnosis; source of bleeding must be determined
   2. For DUB, the examination may be essentially negative, or an adnexal mass may indicate polycystic ovaries or other pathology

- Diagnostic Tests/Findings
   1. Of secondary importance and usually only substantiates a diagnosis already determined by history and physical examination findings
   2. Three most important initial tests
       a. Pregnancy test (quantitative beta hCG)
       b. Prolactin determination (hyperprolactinemia may initially present as ovulatory dysfunction or anovulation and abnormal uterine bleeding)—may be elevated after breast examination
       c. Thyroid-stimulating hormone (TSH)
   3. Additional initial tests should include
       a. Follicle-stimulating hormone (FSH) and luteinizing hormone (LH)
       b. Complete blood count, blood smear, platelet count
       c. Cervical Pap smear
       d. STD screening tests
   4. Additional tests may be done to rule out other conditions as indicated by the history and physical examination, such as
       a. Coagulation profile
       b. Serum iron studies if anemic

c. Pelvic ultrasound
   5. Tests more important in older women
      a. Endometrial biopsy
      b. D&C

- Management/Treatment
  1. Should be considered according to amount of blood loss and with an age-related perspective
  2. Physician consultation may be required
  3. Arrest of heavy, acute, or prolonged bleeding may require intravenous conjugated estrogens followed by combined oral contraceptives or medroxyprogesterone acetate to prevent recurrence
  4. Induction of ovulation is reserved for those desiring pregnancy (use of clomiphene citrate)
  5. Iron supplementation if indicated
  6. Patient should maintain a basal body temperature chart and record symptoms during cycles
  7. Provide instruction regarding basal body temperature monitoring
  8. Discuss therapeutic and diagnostic plans
  9. Review emergency instructions for acute, heavy bleeding
  10. Review nutritional requirements and encourage intake of iron-rich foods
  11. Encourage expression of concerns and fears
  12. Emphasize importance of maintaining follow-up

## DYSPLASIA: ABNORMAL PAPANICOLAOU (PAP) SMEAR MANAGEMENT

- Definition—*squamous intraepithelial lesions* (SIL) refers to precancerous cellular development of the cervix (includes mild, moderate, and severe dysplasia) and carcinoma in situ (CIS) of the cervix

- Etiology/Incidence
  1. Etiology is most likely related to a sexually transmitted factor; human papillomavirus (HPV) is suspected to be an initiator of malignant transformation
  2. Suspected HPV cofactors include cigarette smoking and folate deficiency
  3. Major risk factors for cervical cancer
     a. Sexual intercourse prior to age 18
     b. More than three sexual partners in a lifetime
     c. Intercourse with a male who has had multiple sexual partners
     d. Smoking or history of smoking
     e. Presence or history of HPV (types 16, 18, 31, 33, 35) more commonly associated with high-grade lesions—see section on genital warts (condylomata acuminata) earlier in this chapter
     f. Intercourse with man who has HPV
  4. SIL may persist, spontaneously regress, or advance to invasive disease
  5. Globally, carcinoma of the cervix is a leading cause of death; in the United States it ranks as the third most common gynecological malignancy (behind endometrial and ovarian cancers)

- Cervical Cancer Screening
  1. The Papanicolaou (Pap) smear has reduced disease-related mortality in the United States by 50% in the past 40 years
  2. Screening has also increased detection of pre-invasive cervical neoplasms, including dysplasia and CIS
  3. 30% of Pap smears may have false-negative results
  4. Risk of invasive cervical cancer significantly increases when screening exceeds 3-year intervals
  5. Recommended screening criteria (American Cancer Society [ACS], 2014)
     a. Initiate at age 21 and perform every 3 years until age 29; no HPV screening is recommended for this age group
     b. Perform Pap smears with HPV screening every 5 years until age 65
     c. After age 65 routine screening should be discontinued if findings are normal on three or more consecutive Pap smears and no abnormal/positive cytology tests occurred within the last 10 years
     d. Routine Pap smear screening in women who have had a total hysterectomy for benign disease is NOT recommended

- Pap smear interpretation—the Bethesda Classification System is most commonly used
  1. Specimen type—indicate conventional smear (Pap smear) vs. liquid-based preparation vs. other
  2. Specimen adequacy
     a. Satisfactory for evaluation—(describe presence or absence of endocervical/transformation zone component and any other quality indicators, e.g., partially obscuring blood, inflammation)
     b. Unsatisfactory for evaluation (specify reason)
        (1) Specimen rejected/not processed (specify reason)
        (2) Specimen processed and examined, but unsatisfactory for evaluation of epithelial abnormality because of (specify reason)
  3. Interpretation/Result

a. Negative for intraepithelial lesion or malignancy—(when there is no cellular evidence of neoplasia); the presence of organisms or other nonneoplastic findings should be noted
    (1) Organisms
        (a) *T. vaginalis*
        (b) Fungal organisms morphologically consistent with *Candida* species
        (c) Shift in flora suggestive of bacterial vaginosis
        (d) Bacteria morphologically consistent with *Actinomyces* species
        (e) Cellular changes consistent with herpes simplex virus
    (2) Other non-neoplastic findings (optional to report; list not inclusive)
        (a) Reactive cellular changes associated with
            (i) Inflammation (includes typical repair)
            (ii) Radiation
            (iii) Intrauterine contraceptive device (IUD)
        (b) Glandular cells status posthysterectomy
        (c) Atrophy
b. Endometrial cells (in a woman > 40 years of age)—specify if negative for squamous intraepithelial lesion
c. Epithelial cell abnormalities
    (1) Squamous cell
        (a) Atypical squamous cells
            (i) Of undetermined significance (ASC-US)
            (ii) Cannot exclude HSIL (ASC-H)
        (b) Low-grade squamous intraepithelial lesion (LSIL) encompassing: HPV/mild dysplasia/CIN 1
        (c) High-grade squamous intraepithelial lesion (HSIL) encompassing: moderate and severe dysplasia, CIS; CIN 2 and CIN 3
            (i) With features suspicious for invasion (if invasion is suspected)
        (d) Squamous cell carcinoma
    (2) Glandular cell
        (a) Atypical
            (i) Endocervical cells, not otherwise specified (NOS) or specify in comments
            (ii) Endometrial cells, NOS or specify in comments
            (iii) Glandular cells, NOS or specify in comments
        (b) Atypical
            (i) Endocervical cells, favor neoplastic
            (ii) Glandular cells, favor neoplastic
        (c) Endocervical adenocarcinoma in situ
        (d) Adenocarcinoma
            (i) Endocervical
            (ii) Endometrial
            (iii) Extrauterine
            (iv) NOS
        (e) Other malignant neoplasms (specify)
4. Ancillary testing
5. Automated review

- Management of Pap smear results
    1. Within normal limits—maintain normal screening practices as indicated according to cervical cancer risk factors and age
    2. Infection
        a. Treat based on agent causing inflammation
        b. Repeat Pap smear in 1 year
    3. Reactive or reparative changes
        a. Treat if infectious agent present
        b. May be related to contraceptive mechanical devices (IUD), atrophic changes, chemotherapy, and/or radiotherapy, etc.
        c. Repeat Pap in 4–6 months
    4. Atypical squamous cells of undetermined significance (ASC-US)
        a. 10–40% risk of SIL and 5–10% of these are HSIL
        b. Repeat Pap smear every 4–6 months, three times
        c. Colposcopy and cervical biopsies with endocervical curettage (ECC) if HSIL develops or HIV positive
        d. If peri- or postmenopausal, treat with vaginal estrogen cream prior to repeat Pap or colposcopy (even if patient is on hormone therapy [HT])
    5. Low- and high-grade SIL
        a. Colposcopy and cervical biopsies with ECC
        b. Low-grade lesions may be monitored with Pap smears every 6 months for 2 years if ECC is negative
        c. Common treatments include cryotherapy, large loop excision of transformation zone (LLETZ), laser vaporization
        d. Referral to physician specialist if carcinoma in situ present
    6. Squamous cell carcinoma, adenocarcinoma, and other epithelial or nonepithelial malignant neoplasm—refer to physician specialist

7. Hormonal evaluation—treat atrophic changes if present
8. Discuss therapeutic and diagnostic plans along with common complications of treatment
9. Emphasize importance of regular screening
10. Review patient's individual risk factors as appropriate
11. Educate regarding recommended management and treatment as appropriate
12. Encourage patient to discuss concerns and/or fears

## AMENORRHEA

- Definitions
    1. Primary amenorrhea—absence of normal spontaneous menstrual period by age 16
    2. Secondary amenorrhea—cessation of menses after a variable period of normal function, usually 3–6 consecutive cycles

- Etiology/Incidence—potential underlying conditions
    1. Primary amenorrhea
        a. Hypergonadotropic hypogonadism
        b. Turner syndrome (gonadal dysgenesis)
        c. Severe malnutrition
        d. Pituitary tumors
        e. Head trauma
        f. Encephalitis
        g. Uterine malformations, congenital absence of uterus
        h. Imperforate hymen, cervical stenosis
        i. Androgen insensitivity
        j. Polycystic ovaries
    2. Secondary amenorrhea
        a. Pregnancy (most common cause)
        b. Oral contraceptives
        c. Menopause
        d. Emotional stress
        e. Malnutrition
        f. Excessive exercise
        g. Lactation
        h. Hyperprolactinemia (pituitary tumor)
        i. Anorexia/obesity
        j. Drug use
        k. Polycystic ovaries, anovulation
        l. Hypothalamic suppression
        m. Hyper- and hypothyroidism
        n. Addison's disease
        o. Cervical stenosis

- Signs and Symptoms
    1. Primary amenorrhea
        a. Absence of menarche
        b. Failure to develop pubic hair and other secondary sex characteristics may or may not occur
        c. Abnormal growth and development may be present
        d. Normal breast development may or may not occur
        e. Patient symptoms are dependent on the etiology of the amenorrheic condition
    2. Secondary amenorrhea
        a. Absence of menses at expected time intervals
        b. Previous regular menses

- Differential Diagnosis
    1. First rule out pregnancy
    2. All the potential underlying conditions listed under etiology should be considered in the differential diagnosis
    3. A thorough and complete history/physical examination, with supplemental diagnostic/laboratory testing will assist in ruling out unrelated etiologies

- Physical Findings
    1. A thorough general and pelvic examination should be performed, partially directed by the history
    2. Findings will be related to the underlying etiology
    3. The examination may be essentially negative if the amenorrhea is secondary to such conditions as oral contraceptive use or unreported emotional stress

- Diagnostic Tests/Findings
    1. Primary amenorrhea—refer to endocrinologist if suspected
    2. Secondary amenorrhea
        a. Pregnancy test (quantitative beta hCG)—initial test
        b. Prolactin (if negative pregnancy test), FSH, LH
            (1) Elevated prolactin—rule out micro- and macroadenomas with CT scan of sella turcica
            (2) Physician consult may be required if prolactin, FSH, or LH elevated
        c. Progestin challenge test
        d. TSH
            (1) Elevated TSH—hypothyroid
            (2) Normal TSH—rule out pituitary adenoma
        e. Cervical Pap smear
        f. STD screening tests
        g. Urinalysis
    3. Additional tests may be done to rule out other conditions as indicated by the history and physical examination

- Management/Treatment
  1. Dependent on underlying etiology
  2. Specialty consult is often required
  3. Discuss therapeutic and diagnostic plans
  4. Encourage expression of concerns and fears
  5. Emphasize importance of maintaining follow-up

# DYSMENORRHEA

- Definition—crampy pain that occurs prior to or during menses, often with a constellation of other symptoms
  1. Primary—usually begins in women younger than 20 years; related to menses with no other organic cause
  2. Secondary—usually occurs after age 20 in women with pelvic pathology or IUD use

- Etiology/Incidence
  1. Primary—probably the result of excessive uterine prostaglandin production; usually appears shortly after onset of ovulatory cycles; affects approximately 50% or more of all menstruating females
  2. Secondary—usually occurs in the presence of organic disease, e.g., endometriosis, pelvic adhesions, adenomyosis, cervical stenosis, uterine fibroids, chronic pelvic infection, or with the use of an IUD

- Signs and Symptoms
  1. Primary
     a. Pain usually crampy in nature, may radiate to back, thighs, and lower abdomen
     b. May also have other symptoms, e.g., nausea, vomiting, diarrhea, headache, fatigue
     c. Usually begins at onset of menstruation or several hours before; duration is usually 48–72 hours
  2. Secondary
     a. Signs and symptoms associated with organic disease listed under Etiology/Incidence
     b. Pain occurs at any point in cycle
     c. Associated symptoms may include dyspareunia, infertility, and abnormal bleeding

- Differential Diagnosis
  1. Differentiation between primary and secondary dysmenorrhea
  2. Rule out secondary pathological conditions as noted under Etiology/Incidence

- Physical Findings
  1. Primary—usually no significant physical findings; uterine corpus may be tender during menstruation; no pelvic masses or uterine fixation
  2. Secondary—findings associated with organic disease

- Diagnostic Tests/Findings
  1. Primary—usually none, but if diagnosis unclear, CBC, erythrocyte sedimentation rate, and genital culture for pathogens
  2. Secondary—tests related to suspected organic pathology; may include pelvic ultrasound, hysterosalpingogram, laparoscopy, hysteroscopy, or dilatation and curettage

- Management/Treatment
  1. Primary
     a. Prostaglandin synthetase inhibitors (PGSI), e.g., naproxen, indomethacin, mefenamic acid, ibuprofen
     b. Oral contraceptives for sexually active individuals
     c. Moderate exercise on a regular basis
     d. Diet high in whole grains, beans, vegetables, fruit
     e. Elimination of or decreased salt, sugar, caffeine
     f. Alternative therapies that have been shown to be more effective than placebo are omega-3 fatty acids, thiamine ($B_1$), magnesium supplements, and vitamin E
  2. Secondary—treatment related to organic pathology

# PREMENSTRUAL SYNDROME (PMS)

- Definition—a group of somatic and affective symptoms occurring during the luteal phase of the menstrual cycle, decreasing shortly after onset of menstruation

- Etiology/Incidence
  1. Exact cause unknown
  2. Postulated etiologic factors include insufficient progesterone, fluid retention, nutritional problems, glucose metabolism disorders, vitamin deficiencies, ovarian infections, altered serotonin, endorphin levels, elevated prolactin levels
  3. Peak prevalence in the thirties with a decline noted in the forties
  4. Incidence ranges from 5–95%; generally agreed about 40% of women are significantly affected at one time or another; only 2–3% of women of childbearing age suffer severe symptoms
  5. Premenstrual dysphoria may be considered a severe subtype of PMS
  6. Most women experience some physical and emotional changes before onset of menstrual flow

- Signs and Symptoms
  1. Bloated feeling, feeling of weight increase
  2. Breast pain or tenderness
  3. Skin disorders
  4. Hot flashes
  5. Headache
  6. Pelvic pain
  7. Change in bowel habits
  8. Irritability, aggression, tension, anxiety, depression, crying, lethargy
  9. Insomnia, fatigue
  10. Change in appetite, thirst
  11. Change in libido
  12. Loss of concentration
  13. Poor coordination, clumsiness, accidents

- Differential Diagnosis
  1. Depression
  2. Anxiety disorders
  3. Marital discord
  4. Substance abuse
  5. Thyroid disease
  6. Impaired glucose tolerance or diabetes
  7. Early menopause
  8. Dysmenorrhea
  9. Endometriosis
  10. Anemia
  11. Polycystic ovaries

- Physical Findings
  1. Because etiology is still unknown, diagnosis is made by history
  2. Complete history and physical examination should be conducted to rule out any medical problems that could be influencing symptomatology

- Diagnostic Tests/Findings
  1. Thyroid profile
  2. Fasting blood sugar, HgbA1c
  3. FSH, LH (if early menopause suspected)
  4. CBC with differential
  5. Complete metabolic panel

- Management/Treatment
  1. Exercise 3–4 times per week, especially during luteal phase
  2. Appropriate diet with reasonable amounts of protein (from fish and poultry rather than red meats), vegetables, and fruit
  3. Elimination of tobacco, alcohol, caffeine
  4. Pyridoxine, multiple vitamins
  5. Diuretics, if fluid retention predominates
  6. Progesterone is controversial; in several studies no more effective than placebo
  7. Prostaglandin inhibitors, e.g., mefenamic acid, naproxen sodium
  8. Oral contraceptives
  9. Danazol
  10. Bromocriptine for mastalgia
  11. PMS support group referral
  12. Selective serotonin reuptake inhibitors (SSRIs) for severe cases

## Special Considerations in the Hospitalized Patient

Although common GU/GYN disorders do not typically warrant hospitalization in the otherwise healthy patient, in certain circumstances infectious disease of the genitourinary tract may disseminate to involve multiple-system sepsis. Always consider that in the elderly patient infection mobilizes quickly and is a leading cause of delirium, which requires hospitalization for diagnosis and initial management

- Acute Pyelonephritis
  - Sepsis can occur in certain at-risk patients and may prompt hospitalization at the time of diagnosis or in the event that the patient does not demonstrate some improvement within 24 hours of initiating therapy; hospitalization should also always be considered if follow-up of outpatient management cannot be ensured. Consider hospitalization in patients with
    - Underlying diabetes mellitus
    - HIV/AIDS with a CD4+ count < 350 cells
    - Cancer chemotherapy
    - Immunosuppressive therapy
    - Renal disease
    - Pregnancy
    - Renal anatomic abnormality
    - Age > 60 years
    - Persistent vomiting
  - Treatment options for hospitalized patients with acute pyelonephritis should include
    - Aggressive rehydration
    - Intravenous antibiotics for 7–14 days
      - Indicated for all—fluoroquinolone and aminoglycoside
      - May include—ampicillin or third-generation cephalosporin
    - If no improvement in 48 hours
      - Repeat blood and urine cultures
      - Renal imaging
      - Consider surgical evaluation

(*continues*)

> **Special Considerations in the Hospitalized Patient (*continued*)**
>
> - Pelvic Inflammatory Disease
>   - When to hospitalize
>     - Pregnancy
>     - No clinical response to outpatient therapy within 72 hours
>     - Cannot tolerate outpatient regimen or follow-up cannot be ensured
>     - Severe systemic illness, e.g., vomiting or high fever
>     - Tubo-ovarian abscess
>   - Treatment options for hospitalized patients—should be continued until 24 hours after the patient has experienced significant improvement
>     - Cefotetan 2 g IV q.12.hours or cefoxitin 2 g IV q.6.hours and
>     - Doxycycline 100 mg p.o. q.12.hours
>     - Alternative regimen
>       - Clindamycin 900 mg q.8.hours and
>       - Gentamicin with a loading dose followed by maintenance dependent on peak and trough
>     - After discharge an oral regimen should be continued for 14 days
>     - Surgical consult for tubo-ovarian abscess

## QUESTIONS

■ **Select the best answer.**

1. Which of the following statements regarding HIV/AIDS is correct?

   a. The greatest increase in cases is in those 15–24 years old
   b. Close to 4 million people in the United States are infected
   c. 21% of cases are undiagnosed
   d. The Western blot is a screening test

2. During the acute phase of HIV infection (first 2–8 weeks), which of the following symptoms may be present?

   a. Rash
   b. Shingles
   c. Oral candida
   d. Pulmonary symptoms

3. Which of the following is not considered in a new HIV treatment program?

   a. NRTIs
   b. Protease inhibitors
   c. Nutritious diet and stress management
   d. Fusion inhibitors

4. Secondary prevention of AIDS includes:

   a. Condom use
   b. Virologic monitoring every 3–6 months
   c. Educating about safe sex practices
   d. ELISA assessment of men who have sex with men

5. Which of the following is a diagnostic test for gonorrhea?

   a. Western blot assay
   b. VDRL
   c. Wet prep with WBC
   d. Culture of endocervix on Thayer-Martin media

6. Which of the following is not a correct statement regarding *Neisseria gonorrhoeae*?

   a. One of the leading causes of infertility among U.S. females
   b. The majority of male patients are asymptomatic
   c. PID is a possible complication
   d. In most cases it is confined to the genitourinary tract

7. You are evaluating a male patient who is concerned because he has developed a profound purulent penile discharge. He admits to unprotected casual sex. His symptom is most consistent with:

   a. Chlamydia
   b. Epididymitis
   c. Gonorrhea
   d. Prostatitis

8. The most common serious gonococcal complication that occurs in women is:

   a. PID
   b. Cervicitis
   c. Arthritis
   d. Conjunctivitis

9. Patients with gonorrhea should also be treated for:

   a. Chlamydia
   b. Syphilis
   c. *Trichomonas*
   d. Herpes

10. The causative organism of chlamydia is:
    a. *Chlamydia coli*
    b. *Chlamydia megalovirus*
    c. *Chlamydia trachomatis*
    d. *Chlamydia hominos*

11. A 20-year-old female presents to your clinic with dysuria, dyspareunia, and mucopurulent discharge. She reports that her boyfriend was recently treated for nongonococcal urethritis. What STD has she most likely been exposed to?
    a. Gonorrhea
    b. HPV
    c. Chlamydia
    d. *Trichomonas*

12. Which of the following represents the best description of chlamydia in women?
    a. It is the third most common bacterial STD
    b. It is frequently asymptomatic
    c. It is characterized by "strawberry spots" on the cervix
    d. Coinfection with HPV is common

13. Which of the following is true with respect to syphilis?
    a. It can affect every body system
    b. More than 350,000 cases are diagnosed annually
    c. Treatment with fluoroquinolones is no longer recommended because of resistance
    d. It is frequently asymptomatic in the early stages

14. Which of the following is not a characteristic of secondary syphilis?
    a. Skin rash
    b. Arthralgias
    c. Chancre
    d. Malaise

15. The treatment of choice for a 32-year-old male with early syphilis who is allergic to penicillin is:
    a. Ciprofloxacin
    b. Doxycycline
    c. Erythromycin
    d. Amoxicillin/clavulanate

16. During laboratory assessment, syphilis is characterized by:
    a. A fishy odor with KOH testing
    b. > 20 clue cells/HPF
    c. The presence of multinucleated cells
    d. Treponemes on darkfield microscopy

17. Which of the following is a confirmatory test for syphilis?
    a. VDRL
    b. FTA-Abs
    c. STS
    d. RPR

18. A 24-year-old female seen in your clinic has been diagnosed with urethral strictures. What STD is probably included in her past history?
    a. Chlamydia
    b. Herpes genitalis
    c. Syphilis
    d. HPV

19. Which of the following statements regarding herpes genitalis is not true?
    a. Causative agent is a virus
    b. Genital lesions are painless
    c. Infection during pregnancy can lead to spontaneous abortion
    d. Treatment focuses on relieving symptoms

20. The most common symptomatic viral STD in the United States is:
    a. Gonorrhea
    b. Chlamydia
    c. Genital warts (HPV)
    d. Herpes genitalis

21. Which of the following statements regarding genital warts is incorrect?
    a. More than 40 types of HPV cause genital warts
    b. They increase risk of developing cervical, penile, and vulvar cancer
    c. There is a vaccine available
    d. RPR aids in diagnosing cervical lesions

22. PID is typically characterized by cervical wall motion tenderness, adnexal tenderness, and:
    a. Hypotension
    b. Grouped vesicles on an erythematous base
    c. Solitary papules, macules, or pustules
    d. Lower abdominal discomfort

23. Which of the following is the best treatment regimen for PID?
    a. Ciprofloxacin 500 mg p.o. b.i.d. for 10 days with or without metronidazole
    b. Augmentin 875 mg p.o. b.i.d. for 14 days with azithromycin 1 g, single dose

c. TMP/SMX DS tab p.o. b.i.d. for 14 days
d. Ceftriaxone 250 mg IM with doxycycline 100 mg b.i.d. for 14 days

24. Which of the following is not considered an STD?
   a. Chlamydia
   b. Trichomoniasis
   c. Bacterial vaginitis
   d. Epididymitis

25. A 22-year-old female seen in your clinic has the following signs and symptoms—malodorous, greenish discharge, perineal itching, red macular cervical lesions, and a vaginal pH of 5–7. What type of vulvovaginitis does she probably have?
   a. Candidiasis
   b. Gardnerella
   c. Bacterial vaginosis
   d. Trichomoniasis

26. Which of the following is not related to bacterial vaginosis?
   a. Multiple bacterial causative agents
   b. "Curdy" white discharge
   c. Positive "whiff test"
   d. Metronidazole is a treatment of choice

27. A classic description of the discharge associated with candida vaginitis is:
   a. "Cottage-cheese"
   b. "Fishy" odor
   c. Green, frothy
   d. Nonpruritic

28. One of the most common causative organisms of UTI in women is:
   a. *Klebsiella*
   b. Beta-hemolytic streptococci
   c. *Chlamydia*
   d. *E. coli*

29. Patient education for the patient with urinary tract infection should include all of the following except:
   a. Reminders to empty the bladder frequently
   b. Counseling that the course of antibiotic therapy must be completed
   c. Instruction to increase intake of grapefruit juice
   d. Information about proper perineal hygiene

30. Which of the following is not a characteristic sign or symptom associated with a UTI?
   a. Fever
   b. Pyuria
   c. Urgency
   d. Negative CVA tenderness

31. Which of the following activities is contraindicated in a patient with suspected acute bacterial prostatitis?
   a. Ejaculation
   b. Urinary catheterization
   c. Prostate examination
   d. Masturbation

32. The drug of choice for a 40-year-old monogamous male with prostatitis is:
   a. Metronidazole
   b. Doxycycline
   c. TMP/SMX
   d. Carbenicillin

33. Assessment of BPH may typically include all of the following except:
   a. Symmetrical enlargement
   b. A prostate the consistency of firm rubber
   c. Obliteration of the central sulcus
   d. Fever

34. Which of the following is a true statement about prostate cancer?
   a. It may be present with hard nodules
   b. A PSA of > 10 ng/dL is diagnostic
   c. It is the third leading cause of cancer in men
   d. Men of western European descent are at greatest risk

35. What is the most common physical finding associated with prostate cancer?
   a. Boggy prostate
   b. Tender prostate
   c. Enlarged, smooth prostate
   d. Hard, nodular prostate

36. When counseling a patient with suspected prostate cancer, the NP should advise the patient that:
   a. He will need a needle biopsy of the prostate for diagnosis
   b. Incontinence is a likely consequence of most treatment options

c. He should refrain from sexual activity until the diagnosis is confirmed
d. He may need to take alpha-adrenergic antagonists as an adjunct to treatment

37. The type of fibrocystic breast change that has been associated with malignancy is:
    a. Proliferative changes without atypia
    b. Nonproliferative changes
    c. Cellular atypia
    d. Dysplasia

38. Which physical change is not consistent with fibrocystic breast disease?
    a. Strand of pearls to palpation
    b. A tender lump
    c. Enlarged skin pores
    d. Symptoms that are exacerbated during the menstrual cycle

39. A 30-year-old woman is diagnosed with fibrocystic breast changes. All of the following components may be included in the treatment plan *except*:
    a. Yearly mammograms starting now
    b. Low-salt diet
    c. Limited consumption of caffeine
    d. Oral contraceptives

40. All of the following are risk factors for breast cancer except:
    a. First-degree family history
    b. Late onset of menarche
    c. Increasing age
    d. Obesity

41. Primary prevention of breast cancer includes:
    a. Mammography beginning at age 40
    b. Clinical breast exam every 3 years until age 40
    c. Self-breast exam monthly
    d. Weight loss for obese women

42. Which description is most characteristic of breast cancer?
    a. Single, firm, nontender, ill-defined breast lump
    b. Multiple, firm, nontender, ill-defined breast lumps
    c. Single, firm, tender, circumscribed breast lump
    d. Single, rubbery, nontender, circumscribed breast lump

43. Which of the following is not true with respect to breast cancer?
    a. 10% of palpable masses are missed on mammography
    b. Core needle biopsy is the most reliable diagnostic test
    c. Paget's disease affects the nipple
    d. Inflammatory breast cancer may be painful

44. Dysfunctional uterine bleeding is most often caused by:
    a. Polycystic ovaries
    b. Low estrogen levels
    c. An endocrine abnormality
    d. Low body fat content

45. *Menorrhagia* refers to:
    a. Uterine bleeding that occurs at regular intervals < 21 days apart
    b. Prolonged and excessive uterine bleeding occurring at regular intervals
    c. Infrequent uterine bleeding that occurs at intervals > 40 days apart
    d. Uterine bleeding that occurs at irregular but frequent intervals

46. Differential diagnosis of dysfunctional uterine bleeding for a perimenopausal woman includes all of the following *except*:
    a. Neoplasia
    b. Blood dyscrasias
    c. Pregnancy
    d. Vaginal trauma

47. The diagnostic evaluation of primary amenorrhea should include:
    a. Assessment for Turner syndrome
    b. Serum prolactin
    c. Abdominal ultrasound
    d. Endometrial biopsy

48. The most common cause of secondary amenorrhea is:
    a. Oral contraceptives
    b. Polycystic ovaries
    c. Pregnancy
    d. Anovulation

49. What is the first test that should be ordered in a woman who presents with secondary amenorrhea?
    a. Thyroid profile
    b. Prolactin
    c. Pregnancy test
    d. Progestin challenge

50. Who among the following is not a candidate for Gardasil vaccination?
    a. A 14-year-old female who has had HPV diagnosed on Pap screening
    b. A 27-year-old woman who has never been sexually active
    c. An 11-year-old female who has a family history of cervical cancer
    d. A 24-year-old woman who has had a low-grade SIL

## ■ Answers

| | | | |
|---|---|---|---|
| 1. | c | 26. | b |
| 2. | a | 27. | a |
| 3. | d | 28. | d |
| 4. | d | 29. | c |
| 5. | d | 30. | a |
| 6. | b | 31. | b |
| 7. | c | 32. | c |
| 8. | a | 33. | d |
| 9. | a | 34. | a |
| 10. | c | 35. | d |
| 11. | c | 36. | a |
| 12. | b | 37. | c |
| 13. | a | 38. | c |
| 14. | c | 39. | a |
| 15. | b | 40. | b |
| 16. | d | 41. | d |
| 17. | b | 42. | a |
| 18. | b | 43. | b |
| 19. | b | 44. | c |
| 20. | c | 45. | b |
| 21. | d | 46. | d |
| 22. | d | 47. | a |
| 23. | d | 48. | c |
| 24. | c | 49. | c |
| 25. | d | 50. | b |

## BIBLIOGRAPHY

American Cancer Society (ACS). (2014). *American Cancer Society guidelines for the early detection of cancer.* Retrieved from http://www.cancer.org/healthy/findcancerearly/cancerscreeningguidelines/american-cancer-society-guidelines-for-the-early-detection-of-cancer

American College of Obstetricians and Gynecologists. (2006). ACOG Practice Bulletin: Clinical management guidelines for obstetrician-gynecologists, number 72, May 2006. Vaginitis. *Obstetrics & Gynecology 107*(5), 1195–1206.

Branson, B. M. (2003). *Rapid HIV testing: 2003 update.* Atlanta, GA: Centers for Disease Control and Prevention.

Brusch, J. L., Bavaro, M. F., Cunha, B. A., & Tessier, J. M. (2007). *Cystitis in females.* Retrieved from http://www.emedicine.com/med/TOPIC2835.htm

Centers for Disease Control and Prevention. (2008). HPV vaccine information for clinicians. Retrieved from http://www.cdc.gov/std/HPV/STDFact-HPV-vaccine-hcp.htm

Centers for Disease Control and Prevention. (2012). *Sexually transmitted disease surveillance.* Atlanta, GA: Author.

Centers for Disease Control and Prevention. (2013). HIV prevalence estimates—United States, 2006. *Morbidity and Mortality Weekly Report, 57*(39), 1073–1076.

Danforth, D. N., Scott, J. R., & Gibbs, R. S. (Eds.). (2008). *Danforth's obstetrics and gynecology* (10th ed.). Philadelphia, PA: Lippincott Williams & Wilkins.

Department of Health and Human Services (DHHS), Panel on Antiretroviral Guidelines for Adults and Adolescents. (2014). *Guidelines for the use of antiretroviral agents in HIV-1-infected adults and adolescents.* Retrieved from http://aidsinfo.nih.gov/contentfiles/lvguidelines/adultandadolescentgl.pdf

Harris, J. R., Lippman, M. E., & Morrow, M. (Eds.). (2004). *Diseases of the breast.* Philadelphia, PA: Lippincott Williams & Wilkins.

Katz, V. L., & Dotters, D. (2012). Breast diseases: Diagnosis and treatment of benign and malignant disease. In G. M. Lentz, R. A. Lobo, D. M. Gershenson, & V. L. Katz (Eds.), *Comprehensive gynecology* (6th ed.). Philadelphia, PA: Elsevier Mosby.

McClain, R., & Gray, M. L. (2002). A prostate cancer primer. *Clinical Advisor, 5*(3), 37–38, 41, 44–47, 49.

McPhee, S. J., Papadakis, M. A., & Rabow, M.W. (Eds.). (2014). *Current medical diagnosis and treatment* (53rd ed.). New York, NY: McGraw-Hill.

Rakel, R. E., & Bope, E. T. (Eds.). (2004). *Conn's current therapy 2004.* Philadelphia, PA: Saunders, The Curtis Center.

Solomon, D., Davey, D., Korman, R., Moriarty, A., O'Connor, D., Prey, M., . . . Young, N. (2002). The 2001 Bethesda System: Terminology for reporting results of cervical cytology. *Journal of the American Medical Association, 16*(287), 2114.

U.S. Preventive Services Task Force. (2014). *The guide to clinical preventive services: Recommendations of the United States Preventive Services Task Force.* Retrieved from http://www.ahrq.gov/professionals/clinicians-providers/guidelines-recommendations/guide/index.html

Wein, A. J., Kavoussi, L. R., Novick, A. C., Partin, A. W., & Peters, C. A. (Eds.). (2011). *Campbell's urology* (10th ed.). Philadelphia, PA: Saunders.

# Musculoskeletal and Associated Immunological Disorders

*Madeline Turkeltaub*

## OSTEOARTHRITIS (OA)

- Definition—a noninflammatory, degenerative disorder of movable joints characterized by an imbalance between synthesis and degradation of articular cartilage, leading to classic cartilaginous and joint destruction. Subsequent formation of osteophytes, bony cysts, and hypertrophy may occur.

- Etiology/Incidence
  1. Idiopathic
     a. Occurs without obvious cause
     b. Familial tendency
     c. Obesity—exacerbates stress on weight-bearing joints
  2. Secondary osteoarthritis—results from underlying abnormality
     a. Trauma
     b. Congenital
     c. Metabolic/endocrine/neuropathic
     d. Other underlying medical causes
  3. Overall affects 26.9 million adults
  4. Higher incidence in females, especially after age 50

- Signs and Symptoms
  1. Pain
     a. Worsens throughout the day; patient feels best upon awakening and discomfort progresses
     b. Aggravated by activity and relieved with rest; may become persistent as disease progresses
  2. Joints affected become edematous, but not hot or red
  3. Limitation of movement in affected joint
  4. Joints most frequently involved
     a. Weight bearing—hips, knees, lower back
     b. Distal interphalangeal joints (DIP), proximal interphalangeal joints (PIP)
     c. Neck, metatarsophalangeal (MTP)

- Differential Diagnosis
  1. Rheumatic disease
  2. Pseudogout
  3. Reiter's syndrome
  4. Arthritis of chronic ulcerative colitis
  5. Fibromyalgia
  6. Multiple myeloma

- Physical Findings
  1. Hands
     a. Heberden's nodes—enlargement of DIP joints
     b. Bouchard's nodes—enlargement of PIP joints
  2. Joints
     a. Localized tenderness
     b. Crepitus on movement
     c. Bony consistency to enlargement
     d. Decreased range of motion (ROM)
     e. No gross deformity
  3. Neurological—pain due to pressure on nerves by affected joints
  4. Knee—instability
  5. Hips—reduced internal rotation, pain may be referred to knee

**214 CHAPTER 12** Musculoskeletal and Associated Immunological Disorders

- Diagnostic Tests/Findings
    1. Radiograph—cardinal radiological features
        a. Unequal loss of joint space
        b. Osteophytes
        c. Juxta-articular sclerosis
        d. Subchondral bone
        e. Sharpened articular bone
    2. Synovial fluid aspirate is usually normal
    3. Serological markers of inflammation within normal limits

- Management/Treatment
    1. Preserving function and decreasing pain are goals of treatment
    2. Treating biomechanical factors
        a. Weight loss in obese patients
        b. Correct uneven leg length with heel wedge
        c. Use canes on opposite side or crutches to decrease weight bearing on affected joint
        d. Quadriceps setting for knee involvement
        e. Cervical collar for cervical spine pain
        f. Isometric exercises for abdominal muscles decreases lumbosacral spine pain
        g. Orthotic shoe modification
    3. Local measures
        a. Ice to improve range of motion and exercise performance
        b. Moist heat to decrease muscle spasm and relieve morning stiffness
        c. Temporary rest such as removable splint to decrease motion
    4. Medications
        a. Acetaminophen 500 mg to 1 g t.i.d. or q.i.d.
            (1) Caution with high doses over extended periods
            (2) May cause significant GI upset and liver toxicity
        b. Nonsteroidal anti-inflammatory drugs (NSAIDs), e.g., ibuprofen 400–800 mg t.i.d.; indomethacin 50–200 mg/day up to 1 g q.i.d.
            (1) COX-2 inhibitors for selected patients with history of or high risk for GI bleeding, e.g., Celebrex (celecoxib) 100–200 mg/day
            (2) Consider risk of GI toxicity and cardiovascular events with all COX inhibitors
            (3) Consider $H_2$ blocker or proton pump inhibitor (PPI) when using NSAID
            (4) Instruction on side effects of NSAID, including
                (a) Gastrointestinal intolerance
                (b) Fluid retention
                (c) Platelet abnormalities
                (d) Hepatic and renal dysfunction
        c. NSAIDs may be added to acetaminophen when acetaminophen alone is inadequate
        d. Topical therapies such as lidocaine patches and capsaicin may contribute to pain control
        e. Adjuvant medications such as antiepileptics and antidepressants for neuropathic component
        f. Opioids when other measures are inadequate
        g. Intra-articular injections of hyaluronic acid, e.g., Hyalgan, Synvisc
        h. Intra-articular steroid injection 2–3 times yearly as alternate option
    5. Surgery—refer to orthopedics for procedures, such as fusion or joint replacement when other options fail
    6. Educate regarding body mechanics, muscle strengthening, range-of-motion exercises, and weight-reduction strategies

## RHEUMATOID ARTHRITIS (RA)

- Definition—chronic multisystem disease resulting in symmetrical joint inflammation, loss of normal synovial joint anatomy and mobility, pain, increased risk for a variety of systemic diseases including coronary artery disease and cancer, and shortened life expectancy

- Etiology/Incidence
    1. Cause unknown—may have autoimmune component
    2. Other diseases of joints, such as gout and OA may predispose to RA
    3. Affects approximately 1% of the adult population
    4. 30% of patients have mild disease with remissions and little deformity
    5. 10% have a single period of active disease with only occasional exacerbations
    6. About one-half of patients have progressive disease
    7. Two to three times more common in women
    8. Peak age of onset 40–60 years

- Signs and Symptoms
    1. Morning stiffness lasting several hours
    2. Pain—joint pain and/or stiffness develops insidiously over several weeks to months in three or more joints symmetrically
    3. Fatigue, malaise, weakness, low-grade fever
    4. Proximal interphalangeal (PIP) and metacarpophalangeal (MCP) joints are the most commonly affected; distal interphalangeal (DIP) joints not affected in RA
    5. The first ROM loss is full extension
    6. Patient may report decrease in ability to perform specific functions such as

a. Turn on faucets
b. Hold a hairbrush or toothbrush
c. Open jars
d. Hold cups or drinking glasses

- Differential Diagnosis
    1. Ankylosing spondylitis
    2. Rheumatic fever
    3. Systemic lupus erythematosus
    4. Arthritis of inflammatory intestinal disease
    5. Psoriatic arthritis
    6. Reiter's syndrome
    7. Lyme disease

- Physical Findings
    1. Soft-tissue swelling
        a. Most frequently in MCP joints, wrists, and PIP joints
        b. Usually symmetrical
        c. Positive squeeze test precedes radiographic or laboratory evidence of disease—vigorous squeeze of metacarpals produces significant pain
    2. Tenderness and pain on passive motion
    3. Warmth at site of inflamed joint
    4. Limited ROM at joint
    5. Permanent deformity in chronic disease
        a. Flexion contractures
        b. Subluxation
        c. Ulnar deviation of fingers at MCP joints or deformities of fingers (swan neck, boutonniere)
    6. Synovial cysts can be visualized and palpated; Baker's cysts (synovial cysts of popliteal space) are common
    7. Extra-articular manifestations
        a. Ocular manifestations
        b. Skin and/or muscle atrophy
        c. Splenomegaly
        d. Lymph node enlargement

- Diagnostic Tests/Findings
    1. Anticyclic citrullinated peptide antibodies (anti-CCP)
        a. Higher specificity for RA than rheumatoid factor
        b. Similar or higher sensitivity than rheumatoid factor; present in 40% of people with negative rheumatoid factor
        c. Higher predictive value than rheumatoid factor
        d. Not all patients anti-CCP positive
    2. Rheumatoid factor can be isolated in 70–80% of patients at some course in disease
        a. Less than 50% patients positive in first 6 months of disease
        b. Not specific to RA
        c. High titer early suggests poor prognosis
        d. Titers not useful to follow—once positive, no need to check again
    3. Erythrocyte sedimentation rate may be elevated; not particularly helpful or useful in diagnosis or prognosis
    4. Antinuclear antibodies are present in 20% of patients
    5. Radiograph findings
        a. Early changes are often limited to periarticular osteoporosis and soft-tissue swelling, joint effusion; radiograph not helpful in diagnosing early disease
        b. Primary value is to assess degree of joint destruction
    6. Joint fluid shows inflammatory changes
    7. Complete blood count (CBC)—mild to moderate normocytic anemia

- Management/Treatment
    1. The primary goal of treatment is to arrest or delay disease progression with disease-modifying antirheumatic drugs (DMARDs)
    2. Additional goals include
        a. Pain relief
        b. Prevention of deformity
        c. Decrease rate of extra-articular manifestations; patients with RA have
            (1) Cardiovascular disease risk 10 years earlier
            (2) Increased incidence of pulmonary disease
            (3) Increased gastrointestinal (GI) bleeding
            (4) Twice the risk for certain cancers
            (5) Six to nine times higher incidence of serious infection
    3. Patients with suspected rheumatoid arthritis should be immediately started on disease-modifying antirheumatic drugs (DMARDs)—methotrexate preferred, supplemented with folate 1 mg daily or 7 mg once weekly
    4. Other management strategies include
        a. Tumor necrosis factor (TNF) inhibitors
            (1) Etanercept, infliximab, adalimumab
            (2) Very effective in modifying/treating RA
            (3) Concern over serious risk of infections
            (4) Patients must be well screened and monitored closely for infection
        b. Antimalarials, e.g., hydroxychloroquine sulfate
        c. Gold salts—intramuscular or orally
        d. Corticosteroids (not more than 10 mg of prednisone or equivalent per day) on short-term basis to relieve disabling symptoms; may be used at start of therapy as a bridge to DMARDs

e. Intra-articular corticosteroids if medications do not relieve symptoms
f. Education
g. Rest
h. Physical therapy
i. Nonsteroidal anti-inflammatory agents
j. Cold and heat therapies
5. Education
   a. Abstinence from alcohol while taking methotrexate
   b. Methotrexate is contraindicated in pregnancy (category X) and in those with impaired renal function

## SYSTEMIC LUPUS ERYTHEMATOSUS (SLE)

- Definition—a multisystem, inflammatory autoimmune disorder that affects primarily women of childbearing age. The disease course is highly variable and uncertain. Many of its clinical manifestations are secondary to trapping of antigen–antibody complexes in capillaries of visceral structures or to autoantibody-mediated destruction of host cells. The clinical course is marked by spontaneous remission and relapses. It can range from a mild episodic disorder to a rapidly fulminating fatal illness. A variety of pharmacological agents have been implicated as causing a lupus-like syndrome.

- Etiology/Incidence
  1. Autoantibody development to nuclear antigens
  2. Drug-induced: procainamide, hydralazine, isoniazid, chlorpromazine, quinidine, methyldopa
  3. Sex hormones may contribute to development
  4. Higher incidence in women
  5. Occurs four times more often in African Americans
  6. Family history increases risk

- Signs and Symptoms
  1. Fever
  2. Anorexia
  3. Malaise
  4. Weight loss
  5. Fingertip lesions
  6. Raynaud's phenomenon in 20% of patients
  7. Joint symptoms
  8. Photosensitivity
  9. Vasculitis
  10. Nephritis
  11. Ocular manifestations
  12. Serositis
  13. Abdominal pain, ileus, peritonitis

- Differential Diagnosis
  1. Parvovirus
  2. Viral infection
  3. Polyarthritis
  4. Vasculitis
  5. Pleuritic chest pain
  6. Pericarditis
  7. Pancytopenia
  8. Photosensitivity

- Physical Findings
  1. Butterfly rash on face
  2. Periungal erythema
  3. Splinter hemorrhages
  4. Alopecia
  5. Discoid rash
  6. Oral ulcers
  7. Systolic murmur in 70% of patients

- Diagnostic Tests/Findings
  1. ANA (antinuclear antibodies) positive in 95% of patients—used as screening, but not diagnostic without clinical findings
  2. Anti-dsDNA
  3. Anti-Sm
  4. Anti-SSA (Ro) or Anti-SSB 9 (La)
  5. Anticardiolipin
  6. Lupus anticoagulant
  7. Direct Coombs test
  8. Anti-histone
  9. CBC
  10. Comprehensive metabolic panel (CMP)
  11. Urinalysis with microscopy
  12. Erythrocyte sedimentation rate (ESR) or C-reactive protein (CRP)
  13. Diagnostic acronym for SLE: SOAP BRAIN MD
      a. Serositis
      b. Oral ulcers
      c. Arthritis
      d. Photosensitivity
      e. Blood disorders—thrombocytopenia, leucopenia
      f. Renal involvement
      g. Antinuclear antibodies
      h. Immunological phenomena
      i. Neurological disorder
      j. Malar rash
      k. Discoid rash

- Management/Treatment
  1. Mild symptoms—bedrest, midafternoon naps, avoidance of fatigue
  2. Sun protection
  3. Topical corticosteroids for skin lesions
  4. NSAID for arthritis, arthralgias, serositis, fever
  5. Hydroxychloroquine 200–400 mg daily for joint symptoms not responsive to NSAIDs, photosensitivity, alopecia

6. Glucocorticoids for life-threatening manifestations—60–100 mg prednisone in divided doses
7. Pulse therapy for progressive renal failure
8. Immunosuppressant drugs for steroid-resistant cases
9. Coumadin (warfarin) for INR > 3 in patients with antiphospholipid antibodies

## GIANT CELL ARTERITIS

- Definition—a systemic panarteritis affecting medium-sized and large arteries in patients > 50 years of age; commonly known as temporal arteritis because it often affects the temporal artery. This condition accounts for 15% of all cases of fever of unknown origin in patients > 65 years of age and may result in blindness.

- Etiology/Incidence
  1. Autoimmune inflammation of the endothelial surface of the arteries
  2. Higher incidence in persons of northern European descent
  3. Age is most important risk factor; most common in patients > 50 years of age
  4. Higher incidence in the northern United States
  5. More common in Caucasians
  6. More common in women by almost a 4:1 ratio

- Signs and Symptoms
  1. Headache/scalp tenderness
  2. Visual symptoms
  3. Jaw claudication
  4. Throat pain
  5. Rigors and chills
  6. Transient diplopia
  7. Visual loss

- Differential Diagnosis
  1. Polymyalgia rheumatica (may coexist)
  2. Granulomatosis with polyangiitis (Wegener's granulomatosis)
  3. Dental disease
  4. Migraine
  5. Stroke
  6. Arteriosclerotic vascular disease
  7. Systemic infection
  8. Neoplasms

- Physical Findings
  1. Fever—often > 102.5° F
  2. Nodular temporal artery
  3. Pulseless temporal artery
  4. Nystagmus
  5. Ptosis
  6. Pupil abnormalities
  7. Fundoscopic abnormalities, e.g., central retinal artery occlusion

- Diagnostic Tests/Findings
  1. Erythrocyte sedimentation rate (ESR) or C-reactive protein (CRP) typically elevated
  2. Normal white blood cell count
  3. Temporal artery biopsy
  4. American College of Rheumatology (ACR) diagnostic criteria
     a. Age > 50
     b. New-onset localized headache
     c. Temporal artery tenderness to palpation
     d. ESR ≥ 50 mm/hour
     e. Positive arterial biopsy

- Management/Treatment
  1. Prednisone 60 mg/day for 1–2 months before beginning taper
  2. ESR may be used as a guide to begin taper
  3. Patients should be instructed in symptom recognition; condition tends to recur

## GOUT

- Definition—gout is a metabolic disease associated with abnormal accumulation of urates in the body and characterized by recurring acute arthritis; classic gouty attack is podagra, involving the big toe

- Etiology/Incidence
  1. Due to deposition of crystals of monosodium urate (MSU)
  2. Related to either excess production or decreased excretion of uric acid
  3. Decreased uric acid excretion is present in 90% of patients
  4. 90% of patients with primary gout are men older than 30 years
  5. The onset in women is usually at menopause plus 20–30 years
  6. Rapid fluctuation of serum urate levels may be precipitated by alcohol and food excess; surgery, infection, diuretics, or uricosuric drugs
  7. Gout is the most common cause of monoarticular joint inflammation

- Signs and Symptoms
  1. Acute onset, frequently monoarticular, affecting the first metatarsophalangeal joint, called podagra
  2. Tophi due to accumulation of urate crystals may be found in ears, hands, feet
  3. Remissions and exacerbations; exacerbations may occur years apart
  4. Involved joint is swollen, tender, warm, red; pain may wake patient from sleep and interfere with activities of daily living (ADLs)
  5. Temperature elevation to 39° C (102.2° F)
  6. May become chronic with progressive loss and disability

- Differential Diagnosis
  1. Diagnosis may be confirmed based on dramatic response to NSAID or colchicine
  2. Acute stage may be confused with cellulitis or septic joint, e.g., gonorrhea, staphylococcal infection
  3. Pseudogout presents with similar symptoms but normal serum uric acid
  4. Chronic gout may mimic rheumatoid arthritis
  5. Chronic lead intoxication may result in attacks of gout
  6. See also section on rheumatoid arthritis earlier in this chapter

- Physical Findings
  1. Limited, painful ROM in affected joint
  2. Elevated temperature during acute attack
  3. Palpation of tophi in areas indicated previously
  4. Affected area hot to touch

- Diagnostic Tests/Findings
  1. Synovial fluid aspirate contains monosodium urate crystals
  2. In later stages of disease, radiograph may show punched-out areas in bone
  3. Erythrocyte sedimentation rate elevated
  4. White cell count elevated
  5. Uric acid elevated
  6. Hyperuricemia—serum urate > 7.5 mg/dL

- Management/Treatment
  1. Acute attack should be treated first, hyperuricemia later
  2. NSAID—indomethacin, 50 mg every 8 hours, continued until symptoms resolve
  3. Colchicine
     a. Most effective during first 24–48 hours
     b. Dose—0.5–0.6 mg orally, every hour, until pain relieved or GI symptoms occur or maximum dose of 6 mg
  4. Corticosteroids—used for patients who cannot tolerate NSAID
  5. Analgesics—codeine or meperidine may be indicated; acetylsalicylic acid (ASA) is *contraindicated*
  6. Bed rest—for 24 hours after acute attack subsides
  7. Discontinue thiazide diuretics if in use
  8. Diet to maintain daily output of 2,000 cc of urine; avoid obesity and prevent dehydration; low-purine diet has little effect on blood levels
  9. Support is needed during remissions for patient to maintain medical regimen, including
     a. Diet instruction
     b. Prophylactic medication
        (1) Xanthine oxidase inhibitors—begin 40 mg daily, may increase to 80 mg daily if no effect within 2 weeks; liver function abnormalities most common adverse effect
        (2) Allopurinol—100 mg/day for 1 week initially, then 200–300 mg daily; observe for rash associated with hypersensitivity
  10. Comfort may be obtained with cold or hot compresses and elevation of affected area during acute attack

## OSTEOPOROSIS

- Definition—demineralization of bone, resulting in decrease in bone mass with an otherwise normal structural matrix

- Etiology/Incidence
  1. Most common metabolic bone disease in the United States
  2. Clinically evident in middle years and beyond
  3. Type I—affects women more frequently than men, especially postmenopausal women
  4. Type II—in men and women older than 75 years
  5. Caucasians have highest incidence, then Asians, then African Americans
  6. Most frequently associated with
     a. Lack of estrogen (postmenopausal or postoophorectomy)
     b. Lack of activity (immobilization)
     c. Malabsorption (postgastrectomy, lactase deficiency)
     d. Vitamin D deficiency
     e. Low calcium intake
  7. Family history of osteoporosis
  8. Sedentary lifestyle
  9. Smoking (more than one pack per day)
  10. Excessive alcohol intake
  11. Small body frame
  12. Secondary causes—drug related, endocrine, gastrointestinal, neoplastic, renal, rheumatological disorders
  13. Affects 25 million women and more than 5 million men in the United States

- Signs and Symptoms
  1. Loss of height
  2. Kyphosis
  3. Backache
  4. Spontaneous fracture or collapse of vertebrae

- Differential Diagnosis
  1. Adrenal cortical excess
  2. Hyperthyroidism
  3. Metabolic bone disease, such as hyperparathyroidism and osteomalacia

4. Multiple myeloma
5. Metastatic bone disease

- Physical Findings
  1. There may be no specific physical findings, unless a fracture is present; FRACTURE IS THE CARDINAL FINDING OF OSTEOPOROSIS
  2. Loss of height is most common
  3. Kyphosis ("dowager's hump") is evident with vertebral compression fractures

- Diagnostic Tests/Findings
  1. Serum calcium, phosphorus, and alkaline phosphatase are within normal limits
  2. Standard radiography is not a reliable indicator because more than 25–30% of bone loss must occur for detection with this method
  3. Lateral radiograph of spine might show
     a. Anterior wedging of thoracic vertebral bodies
     b. Widening intervertebral bodies
     c. New or old fractures of vertebrae
  4. Dual-energy x-ray absorptiometry (DEXA)—more sensitive to bone loss
     a. Results reported as standard deviation in the general population (T-score)
     b. T-score above −1 is normal
     c. T-score between −2.5 and −1 is osteopenia
     d. T-score below −2.5 is osteoporosis
  5. Additional laboratory tests may be ordered for older patients, including
     a. Albumin (to allow interpretation of serum calcium)
     b. Serum and urine protein electrophoresis (differentiate multiple myeloma)
     c. BUN and creatinine (to rule out chronic renal disease)
  6. Record accurate serial height measurements

- Management/Treatment—treatment of established osteoporosis must take into consideration severity of disease, age, and coexisting medical problems; prevention is key factor
  1. Prevention and treatment of osteoporosis include
     a. Balanced diet—protein not to exceed 20% of total calories; diet counseling to include dietary sources high in calcium and low in fat
     b. Exercise
        (1) Prevention
           (a) Weight-bearing, at least 30 minutes 3–4 times per week
           (b) Encourage lifestyle changes related to importance of exercise
           (c) Strength training, e.g., lifting weights, swimming
        (2) Moderate walking for those with diagnosed osteoporosis, depending on severity
        (3) Active or passive ROM exercises for bedridden patients
     c. Estrogen therapy in postmenopausal women or postoophorectomy—decreases rate of bone resorption
        (1) Indicated for prevention
        (2) Consider other medications unless also using estrogen to treat vasomotor symptoms or vulva/vaginal atrophy
        (3) Use short term—5 years
        (4) Progestin required for women with intact uterus
     d. Bisphosphonates—inhibit osteoclast-mediated bone resorption
        (1) Indicated for treatment of osteopenia and osteoporosis
        (2) A variety of weekly, monthly, and annual oral and infusion options available
        (3) Oral forms taken with 8 ounces of water at least one-half hour prior to eating
     e. Salmon calcitonin—decreases bone resorption
        (1) Indicated for treatment only
        (2) Alleviates bone pain
     f. Selective estrogen receptor modulators (SERMs)—agonist and antagonist effects on estrogen receptors
        (1) Indicated for prevention and treatment
        (2) Raloxifene
        (3) Estrogen-like effect on bone
        (4) Estrogen-like effect on lipid levels
        (5) Estrogen antagonist effect on breast and endometrial tissue
     g. Adequate calcium intake
        (1) Ages 13–18—1,300 mg/day (adolescents)
        (2) Ages 19–50—1,000 mg/day (adults and pregnant women)
        (3) Ages 51–70 years
           (a) Men 1,000 mg/day
           (b) Women 1,200 mg/day
        (4) Adults 71+ years—1,200 mg/day
     h. Calcium may be obtained through dietary sources or through calcium supplements; calcium carbonate—least expensive; calcium citrate—absorbed easily; calcium phosphate—decreased chance of constipation
     i. 400–600 IU vitamin D daily
  2. Elderly patients must be protected from falls—educate family regarding safe environment
  3. Alcohol and smoking should be avoided

4. Judicious use of glucocorticoids
5. Regular follow-up with mammogram and pelvic examination for women on hormone therapy (HT)
6. Educate teens and young women regarding adequate calcium intake and dangers of excessive exercise
7. Treatment for acute back pain includes
   a. Rest
   b. Analgesia
   c. External support
   d. Heat
   e. Stool softeners

## LOW BACK PAIN (LBP)

- Definition—acute, chronic, or recurrent pain occurring in the lumbosacral spine region and associated musculoskeletal areas; in the absence of contributory history and physical exam findings, most LBP is a consequence of lumbosacral strain or radiculopathy

- Etiology/Incidence
  1. Most acute back pain is caused by muscle strain and spasm of the paraspinal muscle groups
  2. Low back pain from trauma or mechanical causes is most common between 30 and 40 years of age
  3. 80% of the population will experience low back pain (LBP) sometime during their lifetime
  4. LBP is a self-limited condition
     a. 40% remit in 1 week
     b. 60–80% in 3 weeks
     c. 90% in 2 months
  5. Risk factors include
     a. Obesity
     b. Poor body mechanics
     c. Physical deconditioning

- Signs and Symptoms
  1. Lumbosacral strain
     a. Discomfort confined to the lower back region; may radiate to the anterior superior iliac crest, but no farther
     b. Symptoms exacerbated by activity/movement
     c. Tenderness reproducible with palpation of paraspinal muscles
  2. Lumbar radiculopathy
     a. Pain radiates beyond the back and hip depending on the nerve path affected
     b. Discomfort described as electric, burning, numbness, and other manifestations of neuropathic involvement
     c. Symptoms exacerbated by maneuvers that increase intra-abdominal pressure, e.g., straining for a bowel movement, Valsalva maneuver

- Differential Diagnosis
  1. Congenital disorders, e.g., asymmetry
  2. Tumors involving nerve roots or meninges
  3. Trauma
     a. Lumbar strain
     b. Compression fracture
  4. Spondylosis and spondylolisthesis
  5. Metabolic disorders, e.g., osteoporosis
  6. Arthritis of the spine
  7. Degenerative diseases
  8. Herniated nucleus pulposus
  9. Infections
  10. Mechanical causes, e.g., weak abdominal muscles, pelvic tumors, prostate disease
  11. Cauda equina syndrome
  12. Psychogenic

- Physical Findings
  1. Lumbosacral strain
     a. Physical findings typically normal
     b. Possible decreased ROM to lumbosacral spine as a function of pain
     c. No neurological findings
     d. Normal straight leg raise
  2. Lumbar radiculopathy
     a. Abnormal straight leg raise
     b. Other neurological abnormalities depending on area affected
        (1) Altered deep tendon reflexes
        (2) Great toe dorsiflexion
        (3) Sensory impairment
        (4) Foot eversion
        (5) Atrophy of calf muscle
        (6) Flexing thigh on pelvis (femoral stretch test)—associated with $L_3$ problems
        (7) $L_{3-4}$ disc
            (a) Pain in lower back, hip, anterior leg to great toe
            (b) Numbness in anteromedial thigh and knee
            (c) Weakness in quadriceps leading to atrophy
            (d) Diminished patellar reflex
        (8) $L_{4-5}$ disc
            (a) Pain over sacroiliac joint, hip, lateral thigh
            (b) Numbness of lateral leg, web of great toe
            (c) Weakness on dorsiflexion, difficulty walking on heels
            (d) Reflexes usually unchanged

(9) $L_5$–$S_1$ disc
- (a) Pain over sacroiliac joint, hip, back of thigh, and leg to heel
- (b) Numbness in back of calf and lateral foot to small toe
- (c) Difficulty walking on toes
- (d) Atrophy of gastrocnemius
- (e) Diminished or absent Achilles tendon reflex

3. Complete physical examination to rule out nonmusculoskeletal etiology—urgent findings that require immediate referral
   a. Bilateral leg weakness
   b. Saddle anesthesia
   c. Pain unrelieved by rest
   d. Pain worsens at night

- Diagnostic Tests/Findings
  1. None indicated in the presence of an otherwise normal history and physical examination; conservative management of a clinical diagnosis is indicated
  2. If conservative management is not effective in 4–6 weeks or referral to specialty service is being considered, an MRI is indicated
  3. Standard radiography—anterior-posterior (AP), lateral and oblique only if bony structure abnormalities, fracture, metastasis, or other abnormal conditions need to be ruled out

- Management/Treatment—key elements include
  1. Bed rest not indicated—limit select activities that increase pain
  2. Analgesia
     a. Salicylates or acetaminophen
     b. Nonsteroidal anti-inflammatory drugs
     c. Occasionally, opiates may be required
  3. Muscle relaxants
     a. Limit use to 1–2 weeks
     b. Avoid in older patients
  4. With radiculopathy
     a. 5-day steroid dose pack at first visit if pain severe
     b. Schedule second visit 1 week after first visit, if no improvement, consider referral to specialist for epidural steroid injection (ESI)
  5. Patient education
     a. Good body mechanics
     b. Diet—weight loss if indicated
     c. Appropriate exercise
     d. Sleeping posture
  6. Traction
  7. Back and abdominal exercises for prevention and recurrences; contraindicated during acute episode; walking better than jogging
  8. Back massage
  9. Many times there is a psychosocial overlay—a psychosocial assessment should be conducted for
     a. Stress
     b. Depression
     c. Domestic violence
     d. Inadequate coping ability
     e. Marriage/family problems
  10. Early return to work with limited activity
  11. Stress management

# BURSITIS

- Definition—inflammation of the synovial membrane lining of a bursal sac; more than 150 bursae throughout the body

- Etiology/Incidence
  1. Infection in a joint space
  2. Inflammation as part of a systemic process, such as RA or gout
  3. Occurs most commonly in middle and old age, following trauma or unaccustomed repetitive use of the part
  4. Most common locations
     a. Subdeltoid
     b. Olecranon
     c. Ischial
     d. Prepatellar

- Signs and Symptoms
  1. Abrupt onset of pain that increases on motion (superficial)
  2. Local tenderness
  3. Fluctuant edema
  4. Erythema may be present
  5. Regional tenderness and limited motion (deep bursitis)

- Differential Diagnosis
  1. RA
  2. Gout or pseudogout
  3. Septic arthritis

- Physical Findings
  1. Restriction of movement
  2. Tenderness over rotator cuff
  3. Swelling and redness (prepatellar/olecranon)

- Diagnostic Tests/Findings
  1. None indicated in chronic, stable, painless disease
  2. Aspirate fluid with 18-gauge needle and request laboratory analysis
     a. Culture
     b. White blood cell (WBC) count—elevation is associated with bacterial infection

c. Red blood cell (RBC) count—associated with trauma
d. Glucose—decreased with bacterial infection
e. Crystals—associated with microcrystalline bursitis
f. Mucin clot—poor clot associated with bacterial infection

- Management/Treatment
  1. If bursitis is traumatic
     a. Splint part
     b. Apply heat 30 minutes t.i.d. or q.i.d.
     c. ASA or NSAID—naproxen 250 mg b.i.d. or t.i.d.
  2. If symptoms recur and fluid reaccumulates, inject long-acting corticosteroids into bursa
  3. If septic bursitis
     a. Incision and drainage
     b. Parenteral antibiotics
  4. Education regarding care of injured part
     a. Ice for first 24 hours
     b. After swelling is stabilized, warm, moist heat several times daily

# EPICONDYLITIS (TENNIS ELBOW)

- Definition—an overuse syndrome resulting in inflammation in the region of the lateral epicondyle of the humerus at the origin of the common extensor muscles

- Etiology/Incidence
  1. Repetitive stress on the tendons
  2. Specific pathogenesis of tennis elbow is not known
  3. Occurs most frequently in the dominant extremity during midlife (may be athletic or work related)

- Signs and Symptoms
  1. Pain exacerbated by constant motion of the forearm and twisting motions, aggravated by hand and wrist movements
  2. Gradual onset of dull pain along lateral aspect of elbow
  3. Point tenderness over the epicondyle
  4. Limited motion

- Differential Diagnosis
  1. RA
  2. Localized intra-articular pathology
  3. Radial tunnel syndrome
  4. Trauma
  5. Septic joint

- Physical Findings
  1. Burning or aching pain with grasping or lifting
  2. Point tenderness present at or just distal to lateral epicondyle

- Diagnostic Tests/Findings—radiographs usually normal or show small calcium deposits

- Management/Treatment
  1. Pain relief
     a. Mild analgesics
     b. Rest
     c. Ice to tendon
  2. Counterforce brace; wrist splint
  3. Peri-tendon cortisone injection
  4. For continued pain
     a. Immobilize for 6–8 weeks in a long arm cast with 90° elbow flexion
     b. Physical therapy to restore strength and motion when cast is removed
  5. Reinforce an exercise program to condition muscle groups in the forearm and wrist
  6. If associated with a sport, evaluate whether improper technique was responsible for injury
  7. If nonoperative management fails, surgical intervention recommended

# CARPAL TUNNEL SYNDROME

- Definition—median nerve compression of wrist beneath transverse carpal ligament

- Etiology/Incidence
  1. Related to repeated forceful wrist flexion
  2. More common in women
  3. Frequently involves dominant hand
  4. May be associated with
     a. Pregnancy (likely to resolve within 6 weeks after delivery)
     b. Endoneural edema in diabetes mellitus
     c. Thyroid disease
     d. Occupational activities

- Signs and Symptoms
  1. Burning, tingling, numbness sensation along distribution of median nerve
  2. Pain exacerbated with dorsiflexion of wrist
  3. Night pain that interferes with sleep
  4. Clumsiness in performing fine hand movements
  5. May be unilateral or bilateral

- Differential Diagnosis
  1. Compression syndromes of median nerve
  2. Mononeuritis multiplex
  3. Cervical radiculopathy
  4. Tendonitis

- Physical Findings
  1. Decreased two-point discrimination on affected side
  2. Positive Tinel's sign—sensation of electric shock on percussion of volar aspect of wrist
  3. Positive Phalen's sign—pain and/or paresthesia when hands are held in forced flexion for 30–60 seconds
  4. Decreased sensation and muscle atrophy of thenar eminence

- Diagnostic Tests/Findings
  1. Electromyography—assists in documenting motor involvement
  2. Segmental sensory and motor conduction testing
  3. Abnormal monofilament test—used to determine sensation
  4. Radiography not routinely indicated but appropriate when there is history of trauma

- Management/Treatment
  1. Elevate extremity
  2. Splint hand and forearm
  3. Injection of corticosteroids into carpal tunnel if bursitis is involved
  4. Refer to surgeon for surgical intervention
  5. Notification of healthcare provider if symptoms increase
     a. Numbness and tingling persist
     b. Sensation in fingers decreases
  6. Take NSAID with food and report any gastric distress
  7. Consideration of occupational changes if appropriate

# KNEE PAIN

- Definition—knee pain is due to mechanical, inflammatory, and/or degenerative problems

- Etiology/Incidence
  1. Trauma
  2. Most frequently an exercise-related condition
  3. Tears of medial meniscus 10 times more common than lateral meniscus
  4. Increasingly overweight population has resulted in an increased prevalence of osteoarthritis of the knee

- Signs and Symptoms
  1. Locking—most frequently indicative of meniscal tear or loose bodies
  2. "Giving way" or "buckling"—related to patella dislocation or ligamentous instability or anterior cruciate tear
  3. Effusions around knee—associated with hemarthrosis and anterior cruciate ligament; fluid under patella noted on ballottement
  4. Crepitus

- Differential Diagnosis
  1. Single painful knee with minimal edema
     a. Dislocated patella
     b. Degenerative joint disease (DJD)
     c. Prepatellar bursitis
  2. Single edematous knee
     a. Baker's cyst
     b. Torn ligaments
     c. Loose bodies
     d. Meniscal tears

- Physical Findings—the physical examination is confirmatory, following a careful history
  1. McMurray's test—a palpable or audible click when knee is raised slowly with foot externally rotated; examiner's hand rests on joint line; positive = medial meniscal injuries
  2. Anterior drawer test—positive = anterior cruciate ligament (ACL) tear; posterior drawer test—positive = posterior cruciate ligament (PCL) tear
  3. Lachman test—(anterior drawer test for ACL tear) most sensitive and easy to perform test on a swollen, painful knee; place knee in 20–30° flexion, grasp leg with one hand with anterior force to proximal tibia (to stress ACL) while opposite hand stabilizes thigh; graded 11 to 31 grade of displacement
  4. Pain on resisted knee extension
  5. Apley's grind test—flex knee to 90° with patient prone; put pressure on heel with one hand while rotating the lower leg internally and externally; pain or click = positive = medial or lateral collateral ligament damage

- Diagnostic Tests/Findings
  1. Radiographs of knees—AP and lateral to rule out fracture, arthritis
  2. MRI to assess tendon and ligament disease if unresponsive to conservative therapies or physical examination inconsistent with symptoms

- Management/Treatment
  1. Rest, cold pack, immobilization for acute sprain/strain, fractures
  2. NSAID for pain management
  3. ROM of knee, if possible, to prevent stiffness
  4. Hinged knee brace for grades I, II, III collateral ligament sprains
  5. Cruciate ligament sprains may require surgical repair, physical therapy

6. Meniscal tears require arthroscopic repair
7. Review ROM and muscle-strengthening exercises

## ANKLE SPRAIN

- Definition—stretched, partially torn, or completely ruptured ligaments; usually a consequence of forced inversion or eversion—ankle sprain is most common sports-related injury

- Etiology/Incidence
  1. Lateral ankle sprains most frequent sports-related injury
  2. Between 5 million and 10 million ankle sprains occur annually
  3. Most commonly involved structures include the anterior talofibular and fibulocalcaneal ligaments
  4. 10% of ankle sprains are injuries to the medial ligament as a result of pronation and eversion of the ankle

- Signs and Symptoms
  1. Sprains are classified on a grading system of 1–3; signs and symptoms are associated with each grade as follows
     a. Grade 1—related to a stretched ligament; mild or minimal sprain
        (1) Mild localized tenderness
        (2) Normal ROM
        (3) No functional disability
     b. Grade 2—characterized by incomplete or partial rupture of ligament fibers
        (1) Moderate to severe pain with weight bearing; difficulty walking
        (2) Abnormal ROM
        (3) Swelling and local ecchymosis
        (4) Pain immediately after injury
     c. Grade 3—complete disruption of ligament
        (1) Ambulation is impossible
        (2) Resists any motion of the foot
        (3) Marked pain, edema, hemorrhage
        (4) Egg-shaped swelling within 2 hours of injury

- Differential Diagnosis
  1. Avulsion fractures of the malleoli or tarsal bones
  2. Epiphyseal fractures in young patients
  3. Fracture of the calcaneus
  4. Fracture of the fifth metatarsal base
  5. Injury to the bifurcate ligament

- Physical Findings—drawer sign determines anterior talofibular rupture—tibia is stabilized with one hand with foot in neutral and plantar-flexed position, force applied to heel with other hand, positive if anterior displacement of talus occurs

- Diagnostic Tests/Findings
  1. Radiograph if fracture suspected
  2. Arthrography—determines site and extent of ligamentous injury
  3. MRI

- Management/Treatment—treatment depends upon the degree of injury
  1. General treatment
     a. Rest
     b. Ice—15–20 minutes every 1–2 hours for 72 hours, then begin contrast baths
     c. Compression
     d. Elevation
     e. Nonweightbearing
     f. NSAID for 10–14 days
     g. Begin ROM when asymptomatic
     h. Reevaluate grades 1 and 2 sprains in 7–10 days
     i. Refer grade 3 sprains for casting
  2. Rehabilitation may begin on the first day after injury and is individualized
     a. ROM
     b. Achilles tendon stretching
     c. Isometrics
     d. Manual resistance exercises
     e. Build up ankle strength after healing to prevent subsequent injury

## MUSCLE STRAIN

- Definition—overuse of muscle tendons, resulting in inflammation, often associated with repetitive motion; does not include disruption of tissue

- Etiology/Incidence—strains occur during mild stress by overusing muscle groups not usually used

- Signs and Symptoms—pain after overuse or injury

- Differential Diagnosis
  1. Sprain
  2. Fracture

- Physical Findings
  1. Pain on ROM
  2. Edema
  3. Ecchymosis
  4. Pain of muscle strain resolves after 1–2 days

- Diagnostic Tests/Findings—usually none indicated unless symptoms persist or to rule out suspected fracture

- Management/Treatment
  1. Rest of affected part with assistive devices, if needed
  2. Ice t.i.d. for 20 minutes
  3. Compression
  4. Elevation
  5. Analgesics
  6. NSAID
  7. Education efforts focus on prevention
  8. Increase awareness of repetitive motion
  9. Identify possible changes that will decrease stress on the extremity
  10. Emphasize warm-up and stretching before any activity—occupational or sports related

### Special Considerations in the Hospitalized Patient

Most musculoskeletal disorders do not typically warrant hospitalization in the otherwise healthy patient unless a surgical intervention is required. Conversely, in certain circumstances systemic lupus erythematosus may deteriorate to the point that hospitalization is required.

- Systemic lupus erythematosus
  - SLE may present with a clinical course that is rapidly deteriorating and/or that produces profound organ system involvement. Consider hospitalization in patients with
    - Rapidly progressive glomerulonephritis
    - Pulmonary hemorrhage
    - Transverse myelitis
    - Fever
    - Severe neurological involvement
    - Systemic vasculitis
    - Severe infection when the patient is on immunosuppressive therapy
  - Treatment options for hospitalized patients include
    - High-dose systemic pulse steroid therapy with methylprednisolone 0.5 to 1 gm IV over 1 hour daily for 3 days
    - Immunosuppressives, e.g., cyclophosphamide
    - Rheumatology and other consultants depending on organ systems affected
    - Plasma exchange or intravenous immunoglobulin (IVIG) in cases of diffuse alveolar hemorrhage may be indicated

## QUESTIONS

### Select the best answer.

1. Mr. Johnson, age 55, has developed a slight limp and pain in his right knee, which is worse with weight bearing. Which other findings would be most consistent with osteoarthritis?
   a. Soft-tissue swelling on radiograph
   b. A BMI of 34
   c. A positive McMurray's test
   d. A positive serum CCP

2. Which of the following injectable therapies is used in the treatment of osteoarthritis?
   a. Methotrexate
   b. Enbrel
   c. Hyaluronic acid
   d. Anti-citrullinated antibody

3. On physical examination, enlargement of an 83-year-old patient's distal interphalangeal joints is noted. Enlargement of these joints is known as:
   a. Heberden's nodes
   b. Bouchard's nodes
   c. Tinel's sign
   d. Tenosynovitis

4. Most frequently, synovial fluid aspirate to diagnose gout reveals:
   a. WBCs
   b. RBCs
   c. Urate crystals
   d. High protein content

5. Osteoarthritis is often associated with:
   a. Systemic symptoms of disease
   b. Restricted joint motion
   c. Elevated temperature
   d. Inflammation of the proximal interphalangeal joints

6. Which of the following is not a radiological feature of osteoarthritis?
   a. Unequal loss of joint space
   b. Subchondral bone
   c. Osteophytes
   d. Osteoporosis

7. What is the primary goal of therapy for rheumatoid arthritis?
   a. Control pain
   b. Modify disease progression
   c. Reduce incidence of serious infection
   d. Maintain function with ADLs

8. Rheumatoid arthritis is often associated with:
   a. Systemic symptoms
   b. Weight-bearing joints
   c. Obesity
   d. High-purine diet

9. Nonsteroidal anti-inflammatory medications are frequently used in the treatment of musculoskeletal conditions. It is important to remind a patient to:
   a. Take antacids 1 hour after taking NSAID
   b. Exercise at least ½ hour after taking medication
   c. Take the medication at least once a day
   d. Take NSAID with food

10. The onset of rheumatoid arthritis is most frequent:
    a. During 20s and 30s
    b. During 60s and 70s
    c. During 30s and 40s
    d. During 40s and 50s

11. Mrs. Franklin has been complaining of sore hands upon awakening, difficulty opening jars, and trouble holding her hairbrush. The most useful diagnostic study would be:
    a. Serum RF
    b. Anti-CCP
    c. Radiographic assessment
    d. ESR

12. Which joints are most commonly affected by rheumatoid arthritis?
    a. Proximal interphalangeal and metacarpophalangeal joints
    b. Distal interphalangeal joints
    c. Spinous processes
    d. Elbow and shoulder

13. When diagnosing rheumatoid arthritis, which of the following would not be considered a potential differential diagnosis?
    a. Reiter's syndrome
    b. Multiple sclerosis
    c. Rheumatic fever
    d. Ankylosing spondylitis

14. Primary prevention of osteoarthritis includes:
    a. Physical therapy
    b. Synvisc injections
    c. NSAIDs with $H_2RA$ medications
    d. Weight reduction in obese patients

15. Methotrexate is included in which category of medication used to treat rheumatoid arthritis?
    a. Antimalarials
    b. Corticosteroids
    c. Nonsteroidal anti-inflammatory agents
    d. Disease-modifying antirheumatic drugs

16. Podagra is an example of:
    a. Pseudogout
    b. Gout
    c. Osteosarcoma
    d. Septic arthritis

17. Patients with rheumatoid arthritis who are on TNF inhibitors should be especially watchful for the development of:
    a. Symptoms of infection
    b. Cognitive impairment
    c. Extreme fatigue
    d. Loss of pigmentation

18. Mr. Adams, age 55, has a history of chronic exposure to lead. He presents with pain and swelling of his left foot. These facts are both associated with:
    a. Rheumatoid arthritis
    b. Gout
    c. Fracture
    d. Osteoarthritis

19. What is the most common metabolic bone disease in the United States?
    a. Rickets
    b. Scurvy
    c. Osteomyelitis
    d. Osteoporosis

20. A patient with a T-score of 1.5 has:
    a. Osteomalacia
    b. A normal bone density
    c. Osteopenia
    d. Osteoporosis

21. When a patient with gout experiences mild pain, the medication indicated is:

    a. ASA
    b. NSAID
    c. Allopurinol
    d. Probenecid

22. Mr. Jones, age 27, is complaining of acute-onset lower back pain after helping to move a refrigerator. His pain is on the right and shoots down the back of his thigh. The intervertebral space most likely affected is:

    a. $L_4$–$L_5$
    b. $L_5$–$S_1$
    c. $L_3$–$L_4$
    d. $T_{10}$–$L_1$

23. Mr. Jones, the patient from the previous question, returns one week later. His pain is on the right and shoots down the back of his thigh. Mr. Jones's pain persists for 1 week. He has been treated with activity limitation and NSAID with minimal relief. His symptoms are worsening, and you are considering specialty consultation. What is the first diagnostic test to be ordered?

    a. MRI
    b. Anteroposterior and lateral radiograph of the spine
    c. CT scan
    d. Spinal tap

24. A scan for a patient with back pain would be indicated if:

    a. Spinal nerve entrapment is suspected
    b. The history and physical exam do not suggest a cause
    c. The pain radiates to one or both legs
    d. The patient is pregnant

25. Aspirate from a joint space affected by bursitis may be indicative of a bacterial infection when:

    a. WBC is decreased
    b. Glucose is decreased
    c. RBC is increased
    d. Glucose is increased

26. Tennis elbow is a type of:

    a. Tenosynovitis
    b. Rheumatic disease
    c. Epicondylitis
    d. Osteoarthritis

27. The treatment of choice for chronic, stable bursitis is:

    a. Aspiration of fluid
    b. No intervention
    c. NSAIDs
    d. Antibiotic therapy targeting gram-positive organisms

28. Positive Tinel's and Phalen's signs are associated with:

    a. Carpal tunnel syndrome
    b. Torn medial meniscus
    c. Baker's cyst
    d. Epicondylitis

29. "Loose bodies" in the knee would result in the following symptom:

    a. Inflammation
    b. "Click" on extension
    c. "Locking"
    d. Instability

30. Mrs. Abbott, age 32, "turned" her ankle when stepping off a curb. She immediately experienced pain on weight bearing and had limited range of motion on examination. What is the most likely diagnosis?

    a. Muscle strain
    b. Grade 2 ankle sprain
    c. Fractured calcaneus
    d. Grade 3 ankle sprain

## ■ Answers

| 1. **b**  | 16. **b** |
|-----------|-----------|
| 2. **c**  | 17. **a** |
| 3. **a**  | 18. **b** |
| 4. **c**  | 19. **d** |
| 5. **b**  | 20. **c** |
| 6. **d**  | 21. **b** |
| 7. **b**  | 22. **b** |
| 8. **a**  | 23. **a** |
| 9. **d**  | 24. **a** |
| 10. **d** | 25. **b** |
| 11. **b** | 26. **c** |
| 12. **a** | 27. **b** |
| 13. **b** | 28. **a** |
| 14. **d** | 29. **c** |
| 15. **d** | 30. **b** |

# BIBLIOGRAPHY

American College of Rheumatology. (2012). Update of the 2008 guidelines of the American College of Rheumatology recommendations for the use of disease-modifying antirheumatic drugs and biologic agents in the treatment of rheumatoid arthritis. *Arthritis Care and Research, 64*(5), 625–639.

Anders, M., Turner, L., & Wallace, L. S. (2007). Use of decision rules for osteoporosis prevention and treatment: Implications for nurse practitioners. *Journal of the American Academy of Nurse Practitioners, 19*(6), 299–305.

Anderson, B. C. (2006). *Office orthopedics for primary care* (3rd ed.). Philadelphia, PA: Saunders.

Brigham and Women's Hospital. (2003). *Lower extremity musculoskeletal disorders: A guide to diagnosis and treatment.* Boston, MA: Author.

Daniels, J. M., Zook, E. G., & Lynch, J. M. (2004). Hand and wrist injuries: Part I. Nonemergent evaluation. *American Family Physician, 69*(8), 1941–1948.

Follin, S. L., & Hansen, L. B. (2003). Current approaches to the prevention and treatment of postmenopausal osteoporosis. *American Journal of Health-System Pharmacy, 60*(9), 883–901.

Holm, G. B. (2004). Office management of back and neck pain. *Advance for Nurse Practitioners, 12*(7), 38–42.

Klareskog, L., Catrina, A. I., & Paget, S. (2009). Rheumatoid arthritis. *Lancet, 373,* 659–672.

McPhee, S., & Papadakis, M. (Eds.). (2014). *Current medical diagnosis and treatment* (53rd ed.). New York, NY: McGraw-Hill.

Newsome, G. (2002). Guidelines for the management of rheumatoid arthritis: 2002 update. *Journal of the American Academy of Nurse Practitioners, 14,* 432–437.

Peterson, E. L. (2007). Fibromyalgia—management of a misunderstood disorder. *Journal of the American Academy of Nurse Practitioners, 19*(7), 341–348.

# Neurological Disorders

*Sally K. Miller*

## HEADACHE

- Definition—very common complaint; may be the diagnosis itself (primary headache) as in tension, migraine, or cluster, or the symptom of an underlying disorder (influenza, giant cell arteritis, structural lesion, intracranial or dural bleed); because there are many types of headaches, all with varying degrees of severity, proper assessment of headache and associated symptoms is critical.

- Etiology/Incidence
  1. Primary (headache is the diagnosis)
     a. Tension
     b. Migraine
        (1) Classic (occurs with aura)
        (2) Common (no aura)
        (3) Frequently associated with characteristic nausea, vomiting, photophobia, and/or phonophobia
     c. Cluster headaches
        (1) Frequently associated with characteristic ipsilateral conjunctivitis, rhinitis, or other histamine-mediated symptoms
  2. Secondary (due to an underlying process—typically accompanied by associated systemic symptoms, and typically progressive or variable in character)
     a. Toxic
        (1) Viral infection
        (2) Medication induced
     b. Subdural hematoma
     c. Subarachnoid hemorrhage—medical emergency requiring immediate hospitalization
     d. Meningeal irritation
     e. Giant cell arteritis
     f. Structural lesion—infrequently presents as headache, but must be considered
     g. Referred pain from eyes, ears, sinuses, teeth
     h. Visual strain
     i. Narrow angle glaucoma
     j. Hypertensive headache
     k. Post-traumatic headache
     l. Cough headache
     m. Depression

- Components of Headache Evaluation
  1. Chronology is most important item—headache of recent onset that becomes progressively more frequent and/or severe is more ominous than extremely intense headache that has presented in same fashion over a period of time
  2. Location, duration, and quality—should be evaluated because they will provide clues to the underlying cause
  3. Associated activity—exertion, sleep, tension, relaxation
  4. Timing of menstrual cycle in women
  5. Presence of associated symptoms such as neurological symptoms, systemic symptoms of illness (rhinitis, pharyngitis), symptoms of anxiety or depression (sleep disturbance, inability to concentrate)
  6. Presence of triggers—things that seem to be associated with headache onset such as certain foods, stress, alcohol, weather changes

7. Age and character of onset—headaches of very abrupt onset (apoplectic) are much more ominous, as are those that occur < 5 or > 50 years of age

## TENSION HEADACHES

- Definition—headache associated with prolonged contraction of muscles of the head

- Etiology/Incidence
  1. Physical or emotional stress
  2. Circumstances producing physical tension, prolonged muscle contraction

- Signs and Symptoms
  1. Associated complaints of poor concentration and other vague, nonspecific symptoms
  2. Usually lasts for several hours
  3. Usually described as generalized and bilateral—may be most intense about the neck or back of head
  4. Described as vise-like or tight in quality
  5. Occur frequently during or following stressful circumstances
  6. No associated focal neurological symptoms
  7. No aura

- Differential Diagnosis
  1. Evaluation of social history very important in differentiating tension headache
     a. Work history
     b. Family circumstances
     c. Recent life changes—birth, death, marriage, divorce
  2. Other syndromes producing similar headache patterns
     a. Common migraine
     b. Toxic headache
     c. Hypertensive headache
     d. Referred pain from other structures in the head
     e. Meningeal irritation

- Physical Findings
  1. Often no physical findings
  2. May find cervical muscle pain/tenderness to palpation
  3. Other findings depending on severity
     a. Tremor
     b. Disinterest in appearance

- Diagnostic Tests/Findings
  1. Headache diary is particularly helpful in identifying triggers for primary headache syndromes
  2. Radiographic imaging of head as appropriate to rule out organic disorder
  3. Other diagnostic evaluation as indicated in the presence of systemic symptoms to rule out secondary causes

- Management/Treatment
  1. Definitive management of tension headache involves determining and modifying source of tension
  2. Over-the-counter analgesics for paincontrol—should be taken as soon as headache begins
     a. Acetaminophen 650–1,000 mg q.i.d.
     b. Aspirin 650–1,000 mg q.i.d.
     c. Ibuprofen 400 mg q.i.d.
     d. Other NSAIDs as preferred by the patient; caution regarding gastrointestinal (GI) toxicity with prolonged use
  3. Relaxation or stress-reducing techniques
     a. Biofeedback
     b. Massage
     c. Hot baths
  4. Explore underlying cause of stress/anxiety
  5. When initial measures fail, a trial of antimigraine agents is appropriate

## MIGRAINE HEADACHE

- Definition—an extremely painful headache syndrome that is disabling during acute attack; commonly divided into two categories
  1. Classic migraine occurring after an aura—aura precedes pain and may include visual disturbances; auditory, visual, or olfactory hallucinations; or other neurological symptoms
  2. Common migraine—not associated with an aura

- Etiology/Incidence
  1. Categorized as a neurovascular disorder
     a. Dilation and excessive pulsation of intracranial pathways stimulate trigeminal pain pathways
     b. Excess release of vasoactive peptides exacerbates pain
  2. Variety of triggers—a headache diary should be kept by the patient to identify them
     a. Emotional or physical stress
     b. Lack of or excess sleep
     c. Missed meals
     d. Specific foods
     e. Alcoholic beverages
     f. Menstruation
     g. Changes in weather
     h. Nitrate-containing foods
     i. Hormonal contraception

3. Onset usually in adolescence or early adult years
4. Often family history of migraine
5. Females more often affected than males are

- Signs and Symptoms
  1. Episodic unilateral, lateralized, throbbing headache
  2. Builds up gradually and lasts several hours or longer
  3. Focal neurological disturbances may precede or accompany migraines
  4. Visual disturbances frequently occur
     a. Visual field defects
     b. Luminous visual hallucinations (stars, sparks, zigzag of lights)
  5. Aphasia, numbness, tingling, clumsiness, or weakness
  6. Nausea and vomiting
  7. Photophobia
  8. Phonophobia

- Differential Diagnosis
  1. Subarachnoid hemorrhage
  2. Cluster headaches
  3. Hypertensive headache
  4. Cerebrovascular accident
  5. Space-occupying lesion
  6. Giant cell arteritis
  7. Post-traumatic headache

- Physical Findings
  1. Physical examination usually normal
  2. Patient appears acutely ill during migraine
  3. Thorough neurological examination
     a. Focal deficits may accompany migraine but are usually mild and self-limiting
     b. Focal deficits may indicate tumor

- Diagnostic Tests/Findings
  1. None available specific to migraine
  2. Patients with new onset migraine require baseline studies to rule out organic cause; abnormalities may indicate organic cause of pain
     a. Blood chemistries
     b. Complete blood count
     c. Syphilis screening
     d. Erythrocyte sedimentation rate
     e. Radiographic imaging of the head
     f. Other studies indicated by history and physical examination

- Management/Treatment—prophylactic
  1. Avoidance of trigger factors very important
  2. Relaxation and stress management techniques described in management of tension headache
  3. Prophylactic pharmacological therapy if attacks occur more than 2–3 times per month
     a. Aspirin 650–1,950 mg daily; other nonsteroidal anti-inflammatory drugs (NSAIDs) may be useful
     b. Propranolol 10–20 mg b.i.d. starting dose, gradually increase to effective dose of 80–120 mg daily—contraindicated in reactive airway disease, heart block, and severe depression
     c. Clonidine 0.2–0.6 mg daily
     d. Amitriptyline 10–150 mg daily
        (1) Other tricyclic antidepressants helpful
        (2) Must be taken for 2–4 weeks before improvement seen
        (3) Contraindicated in cardiac dysrhythmia, narrow angle glaucoma, and urinary difficulties
     e. Selective serotonin reuptake inhibitors (SSRIs)
        (1) Better choice for geriatric patients and those with cardiac disorders
        (2) Fluoxetine, sertraline, paroxetine, and venlafaxine are common choices
           (a) Start low dose every day at 7:00 a.m., build to therapeutic dose in 7–10 days
           (b) Contraindicated in severe depression
     f. Calcium channel blockers widely used, but not as effective
        (1) Verapamil 40 mg t.i.d., increased to 80 mg t.i.d. over 2–3 weeks; maximum dose 160 mg t.i.d.
        (2) Contraindicated in congestive heart failure, heart block, hypotension

- Management/Treatment—acute attack
  1. Rest in dark, quiet room
  2. Serotonin (5-HT) agonists are mainstay of acute pharmacotherapy
     a. Multiple options available within the class
        (1) Sumatriptan available by injection, nasal spray, and orally
        (2) Zolmitriptan available orally and by disintegrating tablet
        (3) Rizatriptan available orally and by disintegrating tablet
        (4) Others include naratriptan, almotriptan
     b. Contraindicated in coronary artery disease, Prinzmetal's angina, basilar and hemiplegic migraine, uncontrolled hypertension, history of anaphylaxis, and recent ergotamine use
     c. May cause chest tightness
  3. Simple analgesics (aspirin) taken immediately upon onset may provide some relief
  4. Nonsteroidal agents

a. Naproxen 250 mg, repeat in 1–4 hours as needed
b. Ketorolac 10 mg, repeat in 1–4 hours as needed
5. Butalbital-containing medications
   a. Aspirin, caffeine, butalbital combination
   b. Acetaminophen, caffeine, butalbital combination
6. Opiates—may be effective, but should be used with caution
   a. Butorphanol 1 mg every 4 hours
   b. Meperidine 75–100 mg with hydroxyzine 50 mg IM every 4 hours
7. Ergot alkaloids orally or as suppository—contraindicated in pregnancy, uncontrolled hypertension, peripheral vascular disease, coronary artery disease, liver and kidney disease, and concomitant use of sumatriptan
8. Migranal 2 mg intranasal spray
9. Medicate for nausea as indicated
10. Acetaminophen, aspirin, and caffeine preparation (oral)

## CLUSTER HEADACHES

- Definition—among the most painful of all pain-inducing conditions

- Etiology/Incidence
  1. Intrinsic histamine-mediated dilation of external carotid artery
  2. Decreased oxygen saturation due to intrinsic hypothalamic abnormality stimulates brainstem, causing pain
  3. Episodic (90%); chronic (10%)
  4. Cycles occur the same time each year—most often during fall and spring
  5. Males more often affected than females are, although that trend is decreasing; published male:female ratio ranges from 8:1 to 1.9 with narrowing in recent years
  6. Most common in middle age, but affects all age groups
  7. May be precipitated by alcohol ingestion

- Signs and Symptoms
  1. Severe unilateral, orbital, supraorbital, and/or temporal pain occurring in clusters of days or weeks with pain-free period in between
  2. Pain lasts 15 minutes to 2 hours
  3. Attacks occur 1–8 times daily
  4. May rock, pace, or put fist against the painful eye

- Differential Diagnosis
  1. Migraine headache
  2. Narrow angle glaucoma
  3. Structural lesions

- Physical Findings
  1. May be none
  2. Conjunctival injection
  3. Ipsilateral nasal congestion
  4. Rhinorrhea
  5. Forehead or facial sweating
  6. Miosis
  7. Ptosis
  8. Eyelid edema

- Diagnostic Tests/Findings
  1. None diagnostic of cluster headache
  2. As indicated to rule out organic disorders
     a. CT scan of the head
     b. MRI of the head
     c. Complete blood count (CBC)
     d. Serum chemistries
     e. Erythrocyte sedimentation rate (ESR)
     f. Electroencephalogram (EEG)

- Management/Treatment—prophylaxis
  1. Ergotamine tartrate 2 mg every day, 0.5–1 mg per rectum, or 0.25 mg SQ t.i.d. 5 days weekly
  2. Prednisone 20–40 mg daily or q.o.d. for 2 weeks, then taper
  3. Verapamil 240–480 mg every day
  4. Methysergide 4–6 mg every day
  5. Lithium 300–600 mg every day

- Management/Treatment—acute attack
  1. As described for acute migraine
  2. Inhalation of 100% oxygen—typically only effective in case of cluster headache

## TRANSIENT ISCHEMIC ATTACK (TIA)

- Definition—interruption in the cerebral vascular flow, causing ischemia and resultant temporary focal neurological deficits; two types of TIA—carotid and vertebrobasilar; treatments are same for either type, but presenting signs and symptoms differ; by definition attacks are transient, typically lasting < 1 hour, but in all cases < 24 hours

- Etiology/Incidence
  1. Embolization is an important cause
     a. Cardiac dysrhythmia
     b. Rheumatic heart disease
     c. Mitral valve disease
     d. Ulcerated plaque on a major artery
     e. Infective endocarditis
     f. Mural thrombus following myocardial infarction
  2. Fibromuscular dysplasia
  3. Inflammatory disorders
     a. Giant cell arteritis
     b. Systemic lupus erythematosus

4. Hypotension in clients with extracranial artery stenosis
5. Hematological disorders
   a. Polycythemia
   b. Sickle cell disease
   c. Severe anemia
6. Risk factors for vascular disease are often present
   a. Diabetes mellitus
   b. Tobacco use
   c. Hypertension
   d. Elevated serum cholesterol
7. Patients with acquired immunodeficiency syndrome (AIDS) at increased risk
8. 30,000–150,000 occur annually (may be underreported)

- Signs and Symptoms (carotid TIA)
  1. Weakness of the contralateral arm, leg, or face, singly or in combination
  2. Numbness or paresthesia of the contralateral side may occur alone or in combination with motor deficits
  3. Homonymous hemianopsia
  4. Ipsilateral monocular vision loss
  5. Symptoms usually disappear within 1 hour and must resolve completely within 24 hours for a diagnosis of TIA
  6. Any of the preceding symptoms may occur singly or in combination with other symptoms

- Signs and Symptoms (vertebrobasilar TIA)
  1. Unilateral or bilateral weakness
  2. Vertigo
  3. Ataxia
  4. Diplopia
  5. Dysarthria
  6. Perioral numbness
  7. Drop attacks may occur as a result of bilateral leg weakness
  8. Dysphasia
  9. Hearing loss
  10. Symptoms may occur singly or in any combination

- Differential Diagnosis
  1. Focal seizures
  2. Classic migraine
  3. Hypoglycemia
  4. Cerebral vascular attack
  5. Vitamin $B_{12}$ deficiency
  6. Drug toxicities
  7. Electrolyte imbalance

- Physical Findings
  1. Physical findings present only during event
  2. Hyperactive deep tendon reflexes
  3. Slowness of movement
  4. Flaccid weakness with pyramidal distribution
  5. May identify sensory impairment
  6. May see atherosclerotic changes on funduscopic examination
  7. Carotid artery bruit
  8. Cardiac examination may suggest source
     a. Murmur
     b. Dysrhythmia
  9. Physical findings absent if patient examined after resolution of symptoms

- Diagnostic Tests/Findings
  1. Clinical and laboratory evaluation must include assessment of risk factors for vascular disease
     a. Complete blood count
     b. Serum glucose
     c. Serum cholesterol
     d. Syphilis screening
     e. Electrocardiogram
     f. Chest radiograph
  2. Echocardiography if cardiac emboli suspected
  3. Evaluate for hypertension
  4. Holter monitor if transient disturbance in cardiac rhythm suspected
  5. CT scan of the head to rule out small hemorrhage, infarct, or tumor
  6. Ultrasound to evaluate cerebral circulation and major vessels to head
  7. Arteriography is definitive study of vasculature—should be considered if patient is good operative risk, CT scan is normal, and no apparent source of cardiac emboli present

- Management/Treatment
  1. Medical management aimed toward preventing further attacks because 30% of patients with cerebrovascular accident have history of TIA
     a. Cessation of tobacco use
     b. Control of underlying medical conditions with emphasis to thromboembolic disease
        (1) Hyperlipidemia
        (2) Diabetes mellitus
        (3) Hypertension
        (4) Arteritis
        (5) Hematological disorders
     c. Immediate anticoagulation when cardiac emboli is strong possibility
     d. Aspirin 325 mg daily when cardiac emboli not strong possibility or when risks of anticoagulation are significant
     e. Platelet inhibitors in those intolerant of aspirin
  2. Carotid thromboendarterectomy considered when
     a. Arteriography reveals a surgically accessible stenosis > 70%

## 234 CHAPTER 13 Neurological Disorders

    b. Relatively little atherosclerosis elsewhere
    c. Patient is a good surgical candidate

## SEIZURE DISORDER

- Definition
  1. A disorder characterized by transient disturbance of cerebral function due to an abnormal paroxysmal neuronal hyperexcitability and discharge in the brain
  2. Two main classifications of seizure
     a. Partial seizures
        (1) Simple partial seizure
        (2) Complex partial seizure
        (3) Secondarily generalized tonic-clonic seizures
     b. Generalized seizures
        (1) Absence (petit mal) seizure
        (2) Tonic seizure
        (3) Clonic seizure
        (4) Myoclonic seizure
        (5) Atonic seizure
        (6) Tonic-clonic (grand mal) seizure
  3. Partial seizures result from an activation of part of one hemisphere (unilaterally)
  4. Generalized seizures result from a generalized activation of the brain (bilateral)

- Etiology/Incidence
  1. Congenital abnormalities and perinatal injuries may result in seizures presenting in infancy and early childhood
  2. Metabolic disorders
     a. Hypocalcemia
     b. Hypoglycemia
     c. Hyponatremia
     d. Pyridoxine deficiency
     e. Renal failure
     f. Acidosis
     g. Alcohol withdrawal
  3. Infectious diseases
     a. Bacterial meningitis
     b. Herpes encephalitis
     c. Neurosyphilis
  4. Trauma an important cause in young adults
  5. Tumors and other space-occupying lesions
  6. Vascular disease, an increasingly frequent cause in the older population—most common cause when seizure onset is after age 60
  7. May be due to unknown cause
  8. Overall affects approximately 0.5% of the population in the United States

- Signs and Symptoms—simple partial seizure
  1. No loss of consciousness
  2. Lasts approximately 1 minute
  3. Focal motor symptoms (convulsive jerking)
  4. Speech arrest or vocalizations
  5. Jacksonian march
  6. Special sensory symptoms
     a. Light flashes
     b. Buzzing
  7. Paresthesias
  8. Autonomic symptoms
     a. Flushing
     b. Diaphoresis
     c. Pupillary dilation
  9. Dysmnesic symptoms (déjà vu)

- Signs and Symptoms—complex partial seizures—any symptoms of simple partial seizure accompanied by a period of impaired consciousness before, during, or after episode

- Signs and Symptoms—absence (petit mal) seizures
  1. Impairment of consciousness
  2. Mild tonic, clonic, or atonic components
  3. Occasional autonomic components
     a. Flushing
     b. Diaphoresis
     c. Enuresis
  4. Onset and termination very brief, lasting seconds—individual may break off in midsentence for a few seconds
  5. Almost always begin in childhood
  6. Frequently cease by age 20, occasionally replaced by other forms of generalized seizure

- Signs and Symptoms—myoclonic seizures
  1. Single or multiple myoclonic jerks
  2. No loss of consciousness

- Signs and Symptoms—tonic-clonic (grand mal) seizures
  1. Sudden loss of consciousness
  2. Patient becomes rigid, falls to the ground
  3. Respiration is arrested
  4. Clonic phase follows tonic phase—jerking of body musculature lasting 2–3 minutes followed by stage of flaccid coma
  5. Urinary and/or fecal incontinence may occur
  6. Lips or tongue may be bitten
  7. After one tonic-clonic cycle, patient may
     a. Recover consciousness
     b. Fall into deep sleep (postictal state)—headache, disorientation, soreness, nausea, and drowsiness common upon awakening
     c. Experience more attacks after recovering consciousness (serial seizures)
     d. Experience more attacks without recovering consciousness (status epilepticus)
     e. Display postepileptic automatism

(1) Behave in an abnormal fashion in immediate postictal period
(2) Have no subsequent memory of events

- Differential Diagnosis—partial seizures
  1. Transient ischemic attacks
  2. Rage attacks
  3. Panic attacks

- Differential Diagnosis—generalized seizures
  1. Syncope
  2. Cardiac dysrhythmia
  3. Brain stem ischemia
  4. Pseudoseizures

- Physical Findings
  1. May be none
  2. May show evidence of underlying disorder
     a. Trauma
     b. Focal neurological deficits (brain lesion)
     c. Hyperactive reflexes
  3. Muscle soreness following grand mal seizure
  4. Tongue trauma

- Diagnostic Tests/Findings
  1. As indicated to investigate underlying cause and as indicated by history and age of patient
  2. Initial evaluation in patients older than 10 years of age should include the following tests in order to investigate cause and provide a baseline for subsequent monitoring of long-term treatment
     a. Complete blood count
     b. Serum glucose
     c. Liver function tests
     d. Renal function tests
     e. Serologic test for syphilis
     f. Head imaging
  3. EEG for paroxysmal abnormalities containing spikes or sharp waves
     a. May help classify disorder
     b. Support clinical diagnosis of seizure
     c. Evaluate candidates for surgical treatment by localizing epileptogenic source
  4. CT scan or MRI to rule out lesion or neoplasm when
     a. Focal neurological signs and symptoms present
     b. EEG findings suggestive of focal disturbance
     c. Onset after age 30
     d. Seizure disorder is progressive
  5. Chest radiograph to rule out primary or secondary neoplasms
  6. Lumbar puncture (LP)—rule out infectious process

- Management/Treatment—acute seizures
  1. Diazepam 5–10 mg slow IV
  2. Lorazepam 4 mg slow IV

- Management/Treatment—preventive
  1. May need to be reported to Department of Motor Vehicles
  2. Treat underlying problem as appropriate
     a. Infectious process
     b. Metabolic disturbance
  3. Pharmacological choice depends on type of seizure
  4. Pharmacological options for generalized tonic-clonic or partial seizures
     a. Levetiracetam 1,000–3,000 mg daily in divided doses—does not require serum level monitoring
     b. Phenytoin 200–400 mg daily or in divided doses
        (1) Maintain serum level 10–20 mg/mL
        (2) Contraindicated in patients with sino-atrial or atrioventricular block
     c. Carbamazepine 600–1,200 mg in 2 divided doses daily
        (1) Maintain serum level 4–12 mg/mL
        (2) Contraindicated in patients with known hypersensitivity to tricyclic antidepressants, patients with past or present bone marrow depression, and patients on monoamine oxidase inhibitors
     d. Valproic acid 1,500–2,000 mg in 3 divided doses daily
        (1) Maintain serum level 50–100 mg/mL
        (2) Contraindicated in patients with known hepatic disease
  5. Pharmacological choices for petit mal seizures
     a. Ethosuximide 1,000–1,500 mg in 2 divided doses daily
        (1) Maintain serum level 40–100 mg/mL
        (2) Use with extreme caution in patients with hepatic or renal disease
     b. Valproic acid at doses indicated for tonic-clonic seizure
     c. Clonazepam 0.05–0.2 mg/kg in 2 divided doses daily
        (1) Maintain serum level 20–80 ng/mL
        (2) Contraindicated in patients with known hypersensitivity to benzodiazepines, hepatic disease, chronic respiratory disorders, and untreated glaucoma
  6. Pharmacological choice for myoclonic seizures
     a. Valproic acid at doses indicated for tonic-clonic seizure
     b. Clonazepam at doses indicated for petit mal seizure

7. Newer antiseizure medications for adjunctive therapy of partial or secondary generalized seizures
   a. Gabapentin 900–1,800 mg daily in divided doses
   b. Lamotrigine 100–500 mg daily in divided doses
   c. Topiramate 200–400 mg daily in divided doses
8. Patients should be advised to avoid dangerous situations
9. When first drug choice does not provide control, add second drug until therapeutic levels obtained, and then first drug gradually withdrawn
10. Prophylactic medication not generally indicated based on one seizure unless further attacks occur or investigation identifies untreatable pathology
11. Withdrawal of medication should be considered only when patient has been free of seizure activity for at least 4 years
    a. Dose reduction over a period of weeks/months
    b. Reinstitution of same drug(s) if seizure recurs

# PARKINSON'S DISEASE

- Definition—degenerative central nervous system disorder characterized by any combination of tremor, rigidity, bradykinesia, or progressive postural instability

- Etiology/Incidence
  1. Degeneration of the dopaminergic nigrostriatal system leads to dopamine depletion and consequently a dopamine/acetylcholine imbalance
  2. Most commonly idiopathic, but causes may include
     a. Exposure to toxins
        (1) Manganese dust
        (2) Carbon disulfide
        (3) Carbon monoxide
     b. Postencephalitic parkinsonism
  3. Onset usually between 45 and 65 years of age
  4. Approximately equal gender distribution
  5. Occurs in all ethnic groups

- Signs and Symptoms
  1. Any combination of
     a. Tremor
     b. Rigidity
     c. Bradykinesia
     d. Progressive postural instability
  2. Wooden facies
  3. Impaired swallowing
  4. Decreased automatic movement
  5. Seborrhea of scalp and face

- Differential Diagnosis
  1. Side effects of high-potency neuroleptics
  2. Brain tumor
  3. Depression
  4. Benign essential tremor
  5. Dementia
  6. Huntington's disease
  7. Creutzfeldt–Jakob disease

- Physical Findings
  1. Relatively immobile face with wide palpebral fissures
  2. Infrequent blinking
  3. Seborrhea
  4. Myerson's response—repetitive tapping over bridge of nose produces sustained blinking response
  5. Drooling
  6. Bradykinesia
  7. Slow cycle tremor—most conspicuous at rest
  8. No muscle weakness
  9. No alteration in deep tendon reflexes or plantar response
  10. Slow shuffling steps; loss of automatic arm swing

- Diagnostic Tests/Findings
  1. None specific to Parkinson's disease
  2. As indicated to rule out toxins
  3. As indicated to rule out differential diagnoses

- Management/Treatment
  1. Levodopa/carbidopa 25/100 or sustained release form 50/200 t.i.d.
     a. Initial drug of choice in more progressive disease
     b. Improves all clinical features, but does not halt progression
     c. Contraindicated in
        (1) Narrow angle glaucoma
        (2) Psychotic illness
        (3) Patients taking monoamine oxidase A inhibitors
     d. Use caution with malignant melanoma or active ulcer disease
     e. Generally loses effectiveness after several years of treatment; generally, 5 years therapeutic efficacy anticipated
  2. Dopamine agonists—stimulate dopamine receptors in brain; may be used as monotherapy early in disease or in combination with levodopa/carbidopa
     a. Ropinirole 0.25–3 mg t.i.d.—adverse effects include orthostatic hypotension, syncope, hallucinations

  b. Pramipexole 1.5–6 mg daily—adverse effects include orthostatic hypotension, hallucinations, somnolence, nausea, vomiting
  c. Bromocriptine 1.25 mg b.i.d. titrate to symptom improvement—contraindicated in
   (1) History of mental illness
   (2) Recent myocardial infarction
   (3) Peripheral vascular disease
   (4) Bleeding ulcers
  d. May delay need to initiate levodopa, subsequently prolonging the therapeutic life span of pharmacotherapy
  e. Adverse effects similar to those of levodopa but typically more pronounced
  f. May be preferred initial treatment for younger patients
 3. Catechol-o-methyltransferase (COMT) inhibitors
  a. Used as an adjunct to levodopa/carbidopa for those with unsatisfactory clinical response
  b. All agents in this class have black box warning; require close monitoring for hepatic toxicity
  c. Tolcapone 100–200 mg t.i.d.
  d. Entacapone 200 mg with each dose levodopa/carbidopa to maximum 1,600 mg daily
  e. Because of risk of hepatocellular injury, tolcapone should be discontinued in 3 weeks if no clinical response noted
 4. Selegiline 5 mg b.i.d. with breakfast and lunch with levodopa
  a. Clinical responses not consistent
  b. Evidence that it arrests the progression of disease requires it be considered for patients with early disease or mild forms
 5. Anticholinergics to alleviate tremor and rigidity
  a. Benztropine mesylate 1–6 mg daily
  b. Trihexyphenidyl 6–20 mg daily
  c. Biperiden 2–12 mg daily
  d. Poorly tolerated by elderly; side effects include
   (1) Urinary retention
   (2) Increased intraocular pressure
   (3) Dysrhythmia
   (4) Constipation
  e. Contraindicated in
   (1) Narrow angle glaucoma
   (2) Prostatic hypertrophy
   (3) Obstructive gastrointestinal disease
 6. Amantadine 100 mg b.i.d.
  a. Mode of action unclear
  b. Improves clinical features in mild disease
  c. Side effects include confusion, depression, restlessness, hypotension, and cardiac abnormalities
 7. Clozapine 6.25 mg; titrate to 25–100 mg for confusion, psychosis, and dyskinesias; monitor CBC
 8. Physical therapy and speech therapy may be helpful
 9. Surgical thalamotomy or pallidotomy a consideration for those with severe disease and medication intolerance

# MULTIPLE SCLEROSIS (MS)

- Definition
  1. Pathological focal areas of demyelination with reactive gliosis scattered in white matter of brain and in optic nerve; single lesions cannot explain clinical findings
  2. Months or years may pass between initial symptom appearance and recurrence or exacerbation, but eventually progressive disability usually results (relapsing, remitting)
  3. Less commonly, symptoms worsen steadily from onset and disability occurs early (primary progressive)

- Etiology/Incidence
  1. Cause unknown
  2. May be familial incidence
  3. Association with HLA-DR2 antigen suggests genetic predisposition
  4. Immunological basis suspected
  5. Greatest incidence in young adults—onset usually < 55 years of age
  6. More common in persons of western European descent who live in temperate climates through adolescence
  7. Certain factors may trigger exacerbation
     a. Pregnancy and postpartum period
     b. Infection
     c. Trauma
  8. 300,000 cases in the United States
  9. Female to male ratio 2.5:1
  10. Family history with first-degree relative increases risk by 15%

- Signs and Symptoms
  1. Weakness, numbness, tingling, or unsteadiness in a limb
  2. Spastic paraparesis
  3. Diplopia
  4. Disequilibrium
  5. Urinary urgency or hesitancy
  6. Vertigo
  7. Sphincter disturbance

- Differential Diagnosis
  1. Anxiety
  2. Brain tumor

3. Spinal cord lesion
4. Neurosyphilis
5. Systemic lupus erythematosus
6. Metastatic carcinoma

- Physical Findings
    1. Optic atrophy
    2. Nystagmus
    3. Ataxia
    4. Dysarthria
    5. Muscle weakness
    6. Decreased vibratory sense
    7. Hyperactive deep tendon reflexes
    8. Positive Babinski with clonus
    9. Sensory deficits in some or all limbs

- Diagnostic Tests/Findings
    1. Definitive diagnosis cannot be based on laboratory findings alone
    2. Diagnostic tests as indicated to rule out other causes of symptoms
        a. Serum vitamin $B_{12}$
        b. Syphilis screening
        c. Serum antinuclear antibody (ANA)
    3. Mild lymphocytosis
    4. Cerebrospinal fluid abnormalities
        a. Slightly elevated protein
        b. Elevated IgG
        c. Discrete bands of IgG called oligoclonal bands—presence of oligoclonal bands not specific but supportive
    5. MRI preferred to CT scan
        a. Demonstrates multiplicity of lesions
        b. Rule out surgically treatable lesions
        c. Visualize foramen magnum to rule out Arnold-Chiari malformation
        d. Neurophysiological assessment of electrocerebral responses to evaluate subclinical involvement of cerebral pathways

- Management/Treatment
    1. No definitive method of arresting disease process, but areas of investigation include
        a. Immunosuppressive therapy
        b. Plasmapheresis
        c. Beta interferon used in relapsing-remitting form of disease
        d. Cop 1 (a random polymer-stimulating myelin basic protein) may be helpful to patients with relapsing-remitting form
    2. Methylprednisolone 1 g intravenously for 3 days followed by prednisone 80 mg daily for 1 week, then tapered for 2–3 weeks
        a. May hasten recovery from acute exacerbation
        b. Does not improve the extent of recovery
        c. Does not slow progression of disease
    3. Treatment of urinary retention
        a. Various pharmacological options to stimulate urination
        b. Intermittent self-catheterization
        c. Indwelling Foley catheter last option
    4. Diazepam and carbamazepine may relieve paresthesias
    5. Medications to relieve fatigue
        a. Antidepressants
        b. Amantadine
        c. Modafinil
    6. Rest/activity balance
    7. Treatment of constipation
        a. High-fiber diet
        b. Stool softeners/laxatives as indicated
    8. Emotional support, patient education
        a. Sexual dysfunction may be a problem
        b. Other social/intimacy issues
            (1) Questions regarding marriage
            (2) Questions regarding having children
    9. Avoidance of triggers

# DEMENTIA

- Definition—a cognitive disorder that involves deterioration in mental, behavioral, and emotional function; typically includes gradual regression and loss of intellectual functioning, such as thinking, remembering, and reasoning, of sufficient severity to interfere with daily functioning. Definitive diagnostic features include
    1. Cognitive impairment
    2. Change in personality
    3. Mood swings
    4. Erratic behavior
    5. Significant short-term memory impairment
    6. Impairment in abstract thinking
    7. Aphasia, apraxia, agnosia

- Etiology/Incidence
    1. Alzheimer's disease (AD)
        a. Affects 4.5 million Americans; 10% of people ages 65 and older; the prevalence doubles every 10 years thereafter; half the population 85 years and older may have AD
        b. Most common type of dementia; 16% of women and 6% of men who survive to an average life expectancy will develop Alzheimer's disease
        c. Gradual onset
        d. Senile plaques and neurofibrillary tangles seen on autopsy

e. Proven risk factors are age and a positive family history; especially for early onset prior to age 65
2. Vascular dementia (VaD)
   a. Onset may be sudden; deterioration is more stepwise, less insidious as with AD
   b. Generalized symptoms of disorientation, confusion, behavior change
   c. Depression more common in VaD
   d. VaD coexists in 15–20% of AD
   e. Risk factors include high blood pressure, vascular disease, diabetes, or previous stroke
3. Parkinson's disease (PD)
   a. Lack of dopamine, which controls muscle activity
   b. Symptoms include tremors, stiffness, and slow speech
   c. Late in the course, some individuals develop dementia
4. Other related disorders include Huntington's disease, Creutzfeldt–Jakob disease, Pick's disease, Lewy body dementia, and normal pressure hydrocephalus
5. Rare causes of dementia include alcohol, drugs, nutritional and metabolic disorders, and tumor

- Signs and Symptoms
  1. Cognitive dysfunction common to all types—short-term memory decrease, performing on mental status examination consistent with dementia
  2. Symptoms are insidious, persistent, progressive, and not reversible
  3. Other symptoms depend on type
     a. Alzheimer's dementia—progresses over many years and may deteriorate to include
        (1) Visuospatial abnormalities
        (2) Paranoia
        (3) Wandering
        (4) Hallucinations and delusion
        (5) Loss of control of bodily functions
     b. Vascular dementia
        (1) Depression
        (2) Incremental "stepwise" deterioration
        (3) Personality changes

- Differential Diagnosis
  1. Delirium
  2. Mild cognitive impairment
  3. Organic disease
  4. Repetitive head injury
  5. Psychiatric disease
  6. Depression

- Physical Findings
  1. May be normal
  2. Other symptoms of vascular disease in vascular dementia

- Diagnostic Tests/Findings
  1. Mental status examination to evaluate cognitive dysfunction
  2. CBC
  3. Comprehensive metabolic panel (CMP)
  4. Thyroid-stimulating hormone (TSH)
  5. Vitamin $B_{12}$
  6. Rapid plasma regain (RPR)
  7. HIV testing
  8. Head imaging
  9. Other tests as indicated by history to evaluate cause

- Management/Treatment
  1. Good preventive health practices may affect the risk of developing dementia
  2. Use of lists to assist with memory impairment
  3. Correct vision and hearing deficits
  4. Use of day hospital and outpatient day care centers
  5. Make few environmental changes to avoid confusion
  6. Pharmacological treatment has demonstrated improved short-term memory, delayed long-term care placement, and maintenance of function
     a. Combination therapy with acetylcholinesterase inhibitors and NMDA inhibitors is standard of care; should be instituted in mild-moderate Alzheimer's disease
        (1) Acetylcholinesterase inhibitors
        (2) NMDA inhibitors
     b. Both classes of drug ultimately attempt to preserve/protect acetylcholine-producing neurons in the midbrain
  7. Dietary recommendations focus on neuroprotection and the effect of dietary fat composition on the risk of AD; some evidence suggests that elevated blood cholesterol is related to the development of AD; some studies report dietary intake of fish, nuts, seeds, and eggs may protect against AD; although it is generally advised that individuals should limit intake of foods high in saturated and transunsaturated fats such as red meat, butter, ice cream, commercially baked products, and partially hydrogenated oils, there is no direct evidence that this will improve risk for dementing disorders

## Special Considerations in the Hospitalized Patient

- Acute iodiopathic polyneuropathy (Guillain-Barré syndrome)
  - A progressive process characterized by demyelination of the ascending peripheral nerves resulting in ascending paralysis; cause is unclear but is observed more commonly in those recovering from exacerbation of acute illness; may have an immunological component
    - Symptoms begin in the lower extremities
    - Ascend symmetrically; may involve respiratory muscles
    - Autonomic manifestations may occur
      - Tachycardia or bradycardia
      - Hypotension or hypertension
      - Flushing
    - May last weeks or months
    - Some patients require life support, e.g., mechanical ventilation
- Treatment
  - Mainstay of care is supportive therapy; all cases resolve spontaneously, although time course can vary from weeks to > 1 year
  - Prednisone is ineffective and actually prolongs recovery time
  - Plasmapheresis
  - Meningitis
    - An infectious/inflammatory process of the pia mater and arachnoid mater; may be septic (bacterial, infectious), aseptic (viral), or chronic (due to a variety of infectious or noninfectious causes)
    - Signs and symptoms presentation includes profound headache, stiff neck, and fever in 85% of patients—additional symptoms such as confusion, photophobia may occur as well as symptoms dependent on specific type; bacterial and viral characterized by acute onset, whereas chronic is more insidious and overall symptoms are less severe
    - Bacterial—symptoms most profound, patients typically clearly septic
    - Viral—symptoms still very uncomfortable, but not as profound as bacterial
    - Chronic—meningitis symptoms less intense, other symptoms of underlying cause will likely be present (infectious, autoimmune, neoplastic)
  - Diagnostic evaluation
    - All patients should have a CBC at minimum to help differentiate among types of meningitis
    - Serum glucose (to compare to cerebrospinal fluid glucose) (see **Table 13-1** for a comparison of characteristics of cerebrospinal fluid in purulent versus aseptic meningitis)
    - Serum electrolytes
    - Other studies as indicated to rule in causes of chronic meningitis; toxicology screen, cancer markers
    - Lumbar puncture is diagnostic but should be delayed until after head imaging if clinical signs or symptoms suggest a space-occupying lesion
      - Papilledema
      - Coma
      - Focal neurological deficits
      - Seizures
- Treatment
  - All patients need aggressive pain and fever management
  - Purulent meningitis requires high-dose parenteral antibiotics for the patient and oral antibiotics for contacts
  - Dexamethasone is used in some cases; some evidence it can reduce residual damage/deficits
  - Management of specific symptoms as appropriate, e.g., seizures, shock
- Ischemic cerebrovascular accident
  - A thrombotic or embolic event of the cerebral vasculature resulting in a sudden loss of circulation and resultant neurological symptoms; incidence of subclinical stroke increased in migraine sufferers. Signs and symptoms include
    - Abrupt onset of symptoms—screening tools include the Cincinnati Stroke Scale, which assesses three items: (1) ability to smile, (2) ability to extend arms parallel to the floor and rapidly rotate hands, and (3) ability to say, "no ifs, ands, or buts"
    - Hemisensory deficits
    - Diplopia or visual field deficits
    - Dysarthria
    - Ataxia
    - Aphasia
    - Change in level of consciousness

- Patients must be triaged to assess suitability for fibrinolytic therapy; stroke mimics should be ruled out, and the time of symptom onset (last time the patient was seen symptom free) should be clearly established. Physical examination should include
  - Cranial nerve assessment
  - Mental status examination
  - Gait
  - Sensory and motor function
- Diagnostic evaluation
  - Noncontrast CT scan to confirm diagnosis
  - Coagulation studies
  - Cardiac biomarkers
  - Other diagnostic evaluation to rule out other etiologies depending on age and history of the patient
- Treatment options include
  - Complete all indicated evaluation within 60 minutes
  - Begin thrombolytic therapy if appropriate within 60 minutes of emergency department (ED) arrival (see **Table 13-2**)
  - If patient is not a candidate for thrombolytics, supportive care for stroke in evolution includes
    - Ruling out underlying cause
    - Initiating blood pressure control if BP exceeds 220/120 mm Hg
    - Supplying symptomatic and supportive care
    - Controlling risk factors

**TABLE 13-1** Spinal Fluid Characteristics in Purulent versus Aseptic Meningitis

|  | Cell Count | Glucose | Protein | Opening Pressure |
|---|---|---|---|---|
| **Purulent** | 200–20,000 PMN/μL | < 45 cells/μL | > 50 cells/μL | Markedly high |
| **Aseptic** | 100–1,000 lymphocytes/μL | Normal | > 50 cells/μL, but < than purulent | Normal/slightly elevated |

Note: Cerebrospinal fluid features in chronic meningitis vary based on underlying cause but in general are more consistent with aseptic meningitis. PMN = polymorphonuclear leukocytes.

**TABLE 13-2** Characteristics of Patients Who Are Suitable Candidates for Recombinant Tissue Plasminogen Activator (rtPA)

Diagnosis of ischemic stroke causing measurable neurological deficit
The neurological signs should not be clearing spontaneously
The neurological signs should not be minor and isolated
Caution should be exercised in treating a patient with major deficits
The symptoms of stroke should not be suggestive of subarachnoid hemorrhage
Onset of symptoms < 4.5 hours before beginning treatment
No head trauma or prior stroke in previous 3 months
No myocardial infarction in the previous 3 months
No gastrointestinal or urinary tract hemorrhage in previous 21 days
No major surgery in the previous 14 days
No arterial puncture at a noncompressible site in the previous 7 days
No history of previous intracranial hemorrhage
Blood pressure not elevated (systolic < 185 mm Hg and diastolic < 110 mm Hg)
No evidence of active bleeding or acute trauma (fracture) on examination
Not taking an oral anticoagulant or, if anticoagulant being taken, INR 1.7
If receiving heparin in previous 48 hours, aPTT must be in normal range
Platelet count 100,000 mm$^3$
Blood glucose concentration 50 mg/dL (2.7 mmol/L)
No seizure with postictal residual neurological impairments
CT does not show a multilobar infarction (hypodensity > ⅓ cerebral hemisphere)
The patient or family members understand the potential risks and benefits from treatment

INR = international normalized ratio; aPTT = activated partial thromboplastin time.

## CHAPTER 13  Neurological Disorders

**TABLE 13-3** Spinal Cord Syndromes

|  | Autonomic Dysreflexia | Brown–Sequard Syndrome | Central Cord Syndrome |
|---|---|---|---|
| Location | Injury above T6 | Spinal cord | Cervical spinal cord |
| Cause | Traumatic injury | Penetrating trauma | Hyperextension injury |
| Symptoms | Exaggerated autonomic responses to a stimulus; diaphoresis and flushing above the injury, chills and vasoconstriction below the injury; hypertension; bradycardia; headache; nausea | Ipsilateral motor disturbance and proprioception; contralateral loss of pain and temperature appreciation | Upper and lower extremity weakness (more deficits in upper) with varying degrees of sensory loss; impaired pain, temperature, light touch, and position sense below level of injury |
| Treatment | Remove stimulus; manage autonomic manifestations | Immobilization, transfer to trauma, steroids | ICU monitor for 24 hours, monitor for autonomic dysreflexia, hypertension |

## QUESTIONS

■ **Select the best answer.**

1. All of the following are considered primary headache syndromes *except*
   a. Hypertension
   b. Common migraine
   c. Classic migraine
   d. Tension

2. Which of the following causes of headache is a medical emergency?
   a. Toxic headache
   b. Classic migraine
   c. Subarachnoid hemorrhage
   d. Subdural hematoma

3. A systematic and thorough assessment of the headache is important in making the appropriate diagnosis. Which of the following components of headache assessment is the most important?
   a. Presence of associated symptoms
   b. Chronology of headache
   c. Presence of triggers
   d. Age of onset

4. Your patient describes a headache that is quite painful and vise-like in quality. The pain is generalized about the head and lasts for several hours at a time. There does not appear to be an aura, and the patient does not report any symptoms suggestive of focal neurological deficits. Based on your knowledge of headache evaluation, you know that the most likely diagnosis is:
   a. Cluster headache
   b. Common migraine
   c. Tension headache
   d. Hypertensive headache

5. Migraine and cluster headaches are both extremely painful headache syndromes that may be difficult to differentiate. Based on known epidemiological patterns, who is most likely to suffer from migraines?
   a. A 45-year-old male with history of excess alcohol use
   b. A 35-year-old female with history of excess alcohol use
   c. A 19-year-old female with family history of migraine
   d. A 24-year-old male with family history of migraine

6. Excess release of vasoactive peptides is proposed as possible etiological factor in:
   a. Migraine headache
   b. Seizure disorder
   c. Parkinson's disease
   d. Multiple sclerosis

7. Which of the following is not typically a trigger of migraine headache?
   a. Menstruation
   b. Excess sleep
   c. Changes in weather
   d. Loud noise

8. 5-HT agonists are considered primary therapy for acute migraine headache. Which of the following is a contraindication to their administration?
   a. A history of serotonin syndrome
   b. Current treatment with beta-adrenergic antagonists

c. Current treatment with calcium channel antagonists
d. A history of angina

9. Cluster headaches are different from other headache syndromes in that they are sometimes responsive to therapy with:
   a. NSAIDs
   b. Inhaled oxygen
   c. 5-HT agonists
   d. Clonidine

10. Propranolol is a pharmacological agent used in the prophylactic management of migraine, but there are several contraindications to its use. In which of the following patients is propranolol not contraindicated?
    a. A 40-year-old man with asthma
    b. A 39-year-old woman with Graves' disease
    c. A 32-year-old woman with type 1 heart block
    d. A 24-year-old man with severe depression

11. Amitriptyline is an antidepressant medication that can be useful in the prophylactic management of migraine headache. Which of the following statements is true regarding amitriptyline therapy for migraine prophylaxis?
    a. It is the only antidepressant that is useful in migraine prophylaxis
    b. Improvement is usually seen in 2–4 weeks
    c. It is contraindicated in severe depression
    d. It has fewer side effects than paroxetine does

12. Possible organic causes of cluster headache include:
    a. Histamine release
    b. Constriction and rebound dilation of arteries
    c. Physical tension of muscle tissue
    d. Chronic alcohol ingestion

13. Many headache-inducing conditions are difficult to diagnose because there are no associated physical exam findings. Ptosis, eyelid edema, conjunctival injection, and ipsilateral nasal congestion are findings associated with:
    a. Classic migraine
    b. Toxic headache
    c. Narrow angle glaucoma
    d. Cluster headache

14. Tapered corticosteroids are a recommended prophylactic regimen in the treatment of:
    a. Cluster headache
    b. Tension headache
    c. Migraine headache
    d. Subdural hematoma

15. Which of the following is a diagnostic criterion for transient ischemic attack?
    a. Numbness or paresthesia with motor deficits
    b. Symptoms resolve in < 24 hours
    c. Symptoms include homonymous hemianopsia
    d. Lacunar infarct on CT scan

16. Medical management of transient ischemic attack (TIA) is aimed toward preventing further attacks and subsequent cerebrovascular accident (CVA). When atrial fibrillation is discovered during the clinical examination, therapy of TIA should include:
    a. Aspirin
    b. Coumadin
    c. Ticlopidine
    d. Verapamil

17. When are platelet aggregate inhibitors preferred in the management of TIA?
    a. When the patient is intolerant of aspirin
    b. When cardiac emboli is suspected
    c. When heparin has been administered for 5–7 days
    d. When the patient is dysrhythmic

18. What is the most common cause of seizure disorder in the elderly population?
    a. Congenital abnormalities
    b. Renal failure
    c. Neurosyphilis
    d. Vascular disease

19. What is the primary difference between a simple partial seizure and complex partial seizure?
    a. There are no EEG changes
    b. Simple partial seizures do not require chronic medication therapy
    c. There is no loss of consciousness
    d. There is no postictal state

20. Which type of seizure is almost exclusively found in children and young adults?
    a. Myoclonic
    b. Simple partial
    c. Absence
    d. Tonic-clonic

21. Postepileptic automatism is characterized by:
    a. More tonic-clonic attacks with periods of consciousness in between
    b. Headache, disorientation, and nausea

c. More tonic-clonic attacks without periods of consciousness in between
d. Abnormal behavior in the immediate post-ictal period

22. The most important information in seizure assessment is usually provided by:
    a. An eyewitness
    b. EEG
    c. CT scan
    d. MRI

23. Which form of seizure disorder does not require antiepileptic drug (AED) therapy?
    a. Simple partial
    b. Complex partial
    c. Absence
    d. Alcohol withdrawal

24. An EEG is helpful in the evaluation of seizure disorder for several reasons. Which of the following is *not* accomplished with an EEG?
    a. Classification of the disorder
    b. Etiology of the disorder
    c. Localization of the epileptogenic source
    d. Support of clinical diagnosis

25. What is the drug of choice for acute seizure management?
    a. Phenytoin
    b. Clonazepam
    c. Lorazepam
    d. Valproic acid

26. Several antiepileptic drugs are characterized by:
    a. A tendency to promote tolerance requiring progressively higher doses
    b. A narrow range of effectiveness to safety requiring periodic assessment of serum levels
    c. The potential risk for clotting abnormalities and subsequent bleeding disorders
    d. Potentially dangerous interactions with benzodiazepines, which are required for acute seizure suppression

27. When is it appropriate to withdraw seizure medication?
    a. When the patient is pregnant
    b. When the patient has been seizure free for 4 years
    c. When the patient is an alcoholic
    d. When the patient has untreatable pathology

28. What is the most common etiology of parkinsonism?
    a. Postencephalitic
    b. Manganese dust
    c. Exposure to toxins
    d. Idiopathic

29. Immobile face with wide palpebral fissures is a common physical finding in the patient with:
    a. Absence seizure
    b. Depression
    c. Multiple sclerosis
    d. Parkinson's disease

30. When are dopamine agonists preferred for initial management of Parkinson's disease?
    a. In the younger patient
    b. In a patient no longer responsive to levodopa
    c. When liver function abnormalities prohibit use of COMT inhibitors
    d. When there is comorbid schizophrenia

31. Which of the following is true regarding the use of corticosteroids in treating multiple sclerosis?
    a. It hastens recovery from exacerbation
    b. It improves the extent of recovery
    c. It slows progression of the disease
    d. It relieves paresthesias

32. One of the primary differences in clinical presentation of Alzheimer's dementia and vascular dementia is that:
    a. The symptoms of Alzheimer's dementia present before the sixth decade
    b. Depression is a common feature in early Alzheimer's disease
    c. Vascular dementia responds better to environmental interventions
    d. The symptoms of vascular dementia present incrementally

33. Which of the following is not a true statement with respect to drug management of Alzheimer's dementia?
    a. Vitamin E has shown promising results in terms of slowing progression of neuronal degeneration
    b. Combination therapy with AChE inhibitors and NMDA receptor inhibitors is the standard of care
    c. Pharmacological therapy can delay institutionalization
    d. Transdermal options are now available

34. Mrs. G. is an 86-year-old female who lives alone. She has been functionally independent until 2 days ago when her daughter found her to be disheveled, incontinent of urine, and "talking nonsense." When evaluating Mrs. G. to rule out causes of delirium, the nurse practitioner knows that which of the following is not typically a cause?

    a. Infection
    b. Polypharmacy
    c. Hyponatremia
    d. Depression

35. Some forms of Alzheimer's dementia have a clear genetic, familial component. A distinct feature of familial disease is that it:

    a. Is more rapidly progressive
    b. Presents before the age of 50
    c. Does not respond to traditional pharmacological therapy
    d. Affects men disproportionately

## ■ Answers

| | |
|---|---|
| 1. a | 19. c |
| 2. c | 20. c |
| 3. b | 21. d |
| 4. c | 22. a |
| 5. c | 23. d |
| 6. a | 24. b |
| 7. d | 25. c |
| 8. d | 26. b |
| 9. b | 27. b |
| 10. b | 28. d |
| 11. b | 29. d |
| 12. a | 30. a |
| 13. d | 31. a |
| 14. a | 32. d |
| 15. b | 33. a |
| 16. b | 34. a |
| 17. a | 35. b |
| 18. d | |

## BIBLIOGRAPHY

Aminoff, M. J., & Kerchner, G. A. (2012). Nervous system. In S. J. McPhee & M. A. Papadakis (Eds.), *Current medical diagnosis and treatment* (51st ed., pp. 936–1009). New York, NY: McGraw-Hill.

Fenstermacher, K., & Hudson, B. (2003). *Practice guidelines for family nurse practitioners* (3rd ed.). Philadelphia, PA: Saunders.

French, J. A., Kanner, A. M., Bautista, J., Abou-Khalil, B., Browne, T., Harden, C. L., . . . Glauser, T. A. (2004). Efficacy and tolerability of the new antiepileptic drugs I: Treatment of new onset epilepsy: Report of the Therapeutics and Technology Assessment Subcommittee and Quality Standards Subcommittee of the American Academy of Neurology and the AES. *Neurology, 62*(8), 1252–1260.

Goolsby, M. J. (2003). Migraine headaches. *Journal of the American Academy of Nurse Practitioners, 15*(12), 536–538.

Jauch, E. C., & Stettler, B. (2014). Ischemic stroke. Retrieved from http://emedicine.medscape.com/article/1916852-overview

Ko, D. Y. (2009). Epilepsy and seizures treatment and management. Retrieved from http://emedicine.medscape.com/article/1184846-treatment

Luzzio, C. (2006). Multiple sclerosis. Retrieved from http://www.emedicine.com/neuro/TOPIC228.htm

Scott, B. L., & Stacy, M. A. (2009). The management of Parkinson's disease in the primary care setting. *Clinician Reviews, 19*(6 Suppl.), 3–11.

# Psychosocial Disorders

*Sister Maria Salerno*

## DEPRESSION (MAJOR)

- Definition—a complex clinical syndrome consisting of physical, affective, and cognitive symptoms that range from mild to severe; it is attributable to a variety of organic, environmental, and developmental causes and is diagnosed according to diagnostic criteria presented in the *Diagnostic and Statistical Manual of Mental Disorders, Fifth Edition* (*DSM–V*). Depression may present as depressed mood or in the form of physical complaints for which no organic cause is identified. Most forms of depression are accompanied by a sense of worthlessness, which aids in differentiating from a normal grief or situational reaction—common subtypes of depression include
    1. Adjustment disorder with depressed mood
        a. Occurring within 3 months of an identifiable stressor
        b. Depressed mood and impairment of function or symptoms in excess of those normally expected
        c. Symptoms ease as stressor passes
        d. Often self-limiting but can lead to major depression
    2. Major depression (MD)
        a. Five of nine symptoms are present continuously during the same 2-week period; the five must include (1) or (2) below along with at least four of the remaining
            (1) Presence of depressed mood
            (2) Anhedonia (loss of interest or pleasure in most all activities most of the day)
            (3) Increased or decreased appetite or significant weight loss or gain—more than 5% of body weight in a month
            (4) Sleep disturbance—hypersomnia or insomnia
            (5) Psychomotor agitation or retardation
            (6) Fatigue or loss of energy
            (7) Feelings of worthlessness or inappropriate guilt or low self-esteem
            (8) Decreased ability to think, concentrate, or make decisions
            (9) Recurrent thoughts of death, suicidal ideation without an attempt or specific plan
        b. The symptoms represent a change from previous functioning and are severe and disabling
        c. The onset is variable and may be superimposed on dysthymia
    3. Dysthymia—chronic depression characterized by symptoms for 2 or more years
        a. Milder than MD
            (1) Depressed mood
            (2) At least two other symptoms
            (3) Loss of self-esteem prominent
        b. Poor coping skills
        c. Often associated with chronic drug use
        d. No clear onset
    4. Depressive disorder not otherwise specified (NOS)
        a. Depressed mood and two to four moderate to severe symptoms
        b. Does not meet criteria for MD or dysthymia
        c. Includes several subcategories

(1) Atypical depression—characterized by
    (a) Hypersomnia
    (b) Hyperphagia
    (c) Lethargy
    (d) Rejection sensitivity
(2) Seasonal affective disorder
    (a) Disturbance of circadian rhythm
    (b) Related to light spectrum exposure
    (c) Carbohydrate craving, lethargy, hyperphagia, and hypersomnia are characteristic
(3) Premenstrual dysphoric disorder—symptoms occur year-round during the late luteal phase of the cycle and resolve when menses begins
    (a) More disabling than premenstrual syndrome
    (a) Cardinal feature is irritability; a variety of additional symptoms produce emotional and physical disability
(4) Prenatal depression and postpartum depression
    (a) 10–15% accompanied by obsessive concerns about ability to care for infant or fear of doing harm to the infant
    (b) Usually occurs 2 months to 1 year postpartum
    (c) Occurs in approximately 20% of the population
    (d) Is *not* postpartum psychosis—no recognized danger to infant; if safety concerns exist, they are for the mother

5. Bipolar disorder—recurrent episodes of depression interspersed with bouts of mania
   a. Heredity a strong factor
   b. Tricyclic antidepressants (TCA) often precipitate a manic response called "hypomania"
   c. Early onset, usually before age 30
   d. Incidence in African Americans and whites similar
   e. Incidence is similar in males and females
6. Organic mood syndrome—major depressive episode associated with a general medical condition or medications
   a. Substance abuse (alcoholism is a common cause)
   b. Endocrinopathy, e.g., hypothyroidism, Cushing's disease, Addison's disease
   c. Neurological disorders—left-sided stroke, parkinsonism
   d. Pancreatic cancer
   e. Common causative medications include
      (1) Reserpine
      (2) Corticosteroids
      (3) Beta-adrenergic antagonists
      (4) Centrally acting antiadrenergic agonists
      (5) Interferons
      (6) Opiates
      (7) Benzodiazepines

- Etiology/Incidence
  1. Psychosocial and/or biochemical causes for depression have been theorized
     a. Psychosocial
        (1) Psychoanalytical
            (a) Anger turned inward
            (b) Regression to a less mature stage of functioning
        (2) Environmental
            (a) Stressful life events
            (b) Changes or inadequacies in social support
        (3) Psychodynamic
            (a) Personality development
                (i) Passive/dependent
                (ii) Obsessive-compulsive
            (b) Effects of past relationships and developmental tasks on coping styles, particularly use of defense mechanisms
                (i) Denial
                (ii) Suppression
                (iii) Sublimation
        (4) Cognitive
            (a) Self-reinforcing habit of unrealistic negative ideas
            (b) Recent or past style of thinking and relating
            (c) Learned helplessness
     b. Biochemical
        (1) Catecholamine
            (a) Poorly functioning neurotransmitter
            (b) Primarily dopamine, norepinephrine, epinephrine, and serotonin
        (2) Endocrine
            (a) Cortisol
            (b) Thyroid-releasing hormone
  2. Incidence
     a. Depressive illness most common mental health problem seen in general practice
     b. Estimated 30% of the general population suffer from depressive illness, yet fewer than a third will receive treatment
     c. Twice as many women as men with major depression worldwide
     d. Lifetime risk for developing depressive illness
        (1) 20% for females
        (2) 10% for males
     e. Major depression can occur in any age group

Depression (Major)

(1) Adolescents and the elderly at higher risk
(2) Peak incidence 55–65 years old
(3) Other risk factors
   (a) Family history of depressive illness, chemical dependency, substance abuse, or major medical illness
   (b) Prior depressive episode or suicide attempt
   (c) Recent childbirth (postpartum)
   (d) Unanticipated or prolonged stress
   (e) Lack of social support
f. Bipolar disorder occurs equally among the genders
g. Race is not a factor; prevalence is equal among ethnic groups
h. Major depression has a 50–85% recurrence rate within 3–9 years
i. 15% of patients with depression successfully commit suicide
j. Only one-half of patients with depression receive treatment

- Signs and Symptoms
  1. None specific
     a. Aggravation of any physical pathology
     b. Pains of undetermined etiology in a variety of anatomical sites
  2. Mnemonic device to recall major symptoms—IN SAD CAGES
     a. *IN*terest—loss of interest or pleasure in just about any activity
     b. *S*leep disturbances
        (1) Hypersomnia or insomnia
        (2) Early morning awakenings with painful ruminations
     c. *A*ppetite and/or weight change
     d. *D*epressed mood
        (1) Tends to be most pervasive symptom
        (2) May manifest as crying spells
     e. *C*oncentration poor; indecisiveness, inability to act, procrastination
     f. *A*ctivity—agitation or retardation
     g. *G*uilt, low self-esteem
     h. *E*nergy loss, fatigue
     i. *S*uicidal ideation, thoughts of death, suicide attempts

- Differential Diagnosis
  1. Because depression may be a manifestation of many illnesses, the differential diagnosis must include a thorough search for factors or organic diseases that may be responsible for symptom manifestation, including
     a. Infections, inflammation
     b. Neurological neoplasms, stroke, trauma
     c. Endocrine disorders
     d. Nutritional deficiencies
     e. Electrolyte disturbances
  2. Differentiate major depression from other mental disorders, e.g., schizophrenia, dementia, adjustment disorder with depressed mood
  3. Currently, the trend is to address the signs and symptoms of major depression; if criteria presented previously are met, the diagnosis is made regardless of comorbidity; when contributing organic conditions are optimally managed, antidepressants may be discontinued under supervision

- Physical Findings
  1. General—may show lack of personal grooming and hygiene, inattention to dress, slouched posture, slowed speech and movements, long pauses in response to questions, tearfulness; weight may be less than or more than ideal for body size, may appear dehydrated
  2. Mental status—poor concentration, decreased memory, indecision, pessimism

- Diagnostic Tests/Findings
  1. Initial tests
     a. Complete blood count (CBC)—normal
     b. Chemical profile, including liver function—normal
     c. Urinalysis and urine toxicology screen—normal
     d. Thyroid function—normal
     e. Venereal disease research laboratory (VDRL)—normal
     f. Vitamin $B_{12}$ level—normal
     g. EKG—normal
     h. Chest radiograph—normal
     i. In first or second episode
        (1) CT scan or MRI of the brain—normal
        (2) HIV screen—normal
  2. Depression screening instruments—scores indicative of depression
     a. Beck Depression Inventory
     b. Yesavage Geriatric Depression Scale
     c. Zung Self-Rating Depression Scale
     d. Patient Health Questionnaire (PHQ) 9
  3. Special tests (primarily used in psychiatric and research settings)
     a. Thyroid-stimulating hormone (TSH) response to thyroid-releasing hormone (TRH) may be decreased
     b. Dexamethasone suppression test (DST) used to distinguish between major and minor depression
     c. EEG sleep profile—may show reduction in REM sleep
     d. Platelet monoamine oxidase (MAO) activity—increased

e. Biogenic amines (norepinephrine, serotonin)—increased levels
f. Dementia screening test in at-risk populations

- Management/Treatment
  1. General considerations
     a. Assess degree of problem related to daily functioning
     b. Refer those with evidence of
        (1) Hallucinations, delusions
        (2) Loss of contact with reality
        (3) Suicidal thoughts, wishes, tendencies (see section on suicide later in this chapter)
  2. Mild depression (no clear criteria but general functional status tends to be high)
     a. Cognitive behavioral intervention (CBI) is the mainstay of therapy for mild depression and should be a component of all depression management
     b. Structured monitoring with weekly appointments with phone contact for backup
     c. Use therapeutic communication skills to
        (1) Encourage verbalization, clarification of feelings and fears, as well as relationship of feelings to specific events if known
        (2) Assess and discuss losses that have occurred and their meaning
        (3) Help correct cognitive errors in thinking
     d. Use crisis or social skills models to teach and promote more effective coping strategies
        (1) Help patient recognize need for and identify alternative coping methods
        (2) Encourage interaction with other people
        (3) Encourage planned, regular physical activity
        (4) Teach relaxation techniques
        (5) Provide patient with anticipatory guidance regarding feelings and usual course of the problem, e.g., gradual improvement and abatement of symptoms
     e. Provide consistency and caring, avoiding a judgmental or blaming attitude
     f. Reinforce positive behaviors
     g. Avoid actions or response that could be interpreted as punishment
     h. Selective serotonin reuptake inhibitors (SSRIs) are the drug of choice when pharmacotherapy required for mild depression
        (1) Ensure an adequate trial of both time and dose—primary care providers often underdose and abort therapy before allowing adequate time (at least 6 weeks at appropriate dose for any improvement, 3 months for therapeutic control)
        (2) Consider implications of half-life and cytochrome P450 drug interactions when choosing an agent
  3. Moderate to severe depression
     a. Consultation with psychiatry regarding patients who may
        (1) Be a potential danger to self or others; be unable to meet basic needs; exhibit suicidal ideation or behavior
        (2) Have impaired cognition or judgment
        (3) Need skilled observation for diagnosis, assessment, or monitoring of therapy
        (4) Have inadequate social supports for outpatient treatment
     b. Medication is typically required at the start of therapy; all forms of depression treatment should include cognitive behavioral interventions as well
        (1) SSRI is the initial drug of choice for patients with functional depression
           (a) Initial choice based on predominant symptom (hypersomnia, depressed mood, agitation, etc.), potential for drug interaction, and half life
           (b) Fluoxetine should be avoided in the elderly because of its prolonged half-life as compared to other SSRI options
           (c) Fluoxetine and paroxetine are most central nervous system (CNS) activating and sedating, respectively; also have the greatest potential for cytochrome P450–mediated drug interaction
           (d) Excellent safety profile—no cardiovascular effects, may have undesirable adverse sexual effects, weight gain, and nausea
        (2) Serotonin–norepinephrine reuptake inhibitors (SNRI) indicated for those not fully functional at the time of presentation as well as patients with SSRI-resistant depression or comorbid neuropathic pain
           (a) Consider risk of hypertension in higher doses
           (b) Generally safe, but be alert to hypertension in higher doses

resulting from the norepinephrine reuptake inhibitor effects
- (3) Tricyclic antidepressant (TCA) drugs very effective, but adverse effect profile prohibitive; not used routinely by primary care providers
  - (a) Potentially cardiotoxic with impact on conduction system
  - (b) Powerful anticholinergic properties
  - (c) Among the most efficacious drugs for endogenous depression
  - (d) Patients who require TCAs for depression management should be comanaged with psychiatry
- (4) Only 65% have complete remission with any one drug
- (5) Choice based on predominant symptoms, side effects, cost, and complexity of dosing—affect compliance
- (6) Most will demonstrate some response within 4–6 weeks of beginning treatment
- (7) Cannot assess therapeutic efficacy before 3 months of treatment
- (8) Continue medication full 6–12 months after complete remission of symptoms
- (9) When drugs are discontinued, taper over 6–8 weeks
- (10) Long-term prophylaxis—full treatment dosage for those with recurrent episodes (at least three)
- (11) Some controversy regarding efficacy in minor depression, dysthymia, and adjustment disorder
  c. Electroconvulsive therapy (ECT)
  - (1) More rapid improvement than with pharmacological agents
  - (2) Indicated for severely depressed or suicidal persons for whom pharmacological agents are contraindicated or ineffective
  - (3) Benzodiazepines used prior to the procedure
  - (4) Confusion, headache, temporary amnesia lasting 1–2 weeks are common side effects in about 40%; may be clinically apparent up to 1 month
  - (5) Avoided in persons with brain tumor, recent (3 months) myocardial infarction (MI), cerebrovascular accident (CVA), or perforated viscus repair
  d. Other options include exercise and light therapy
4. Patient education
   a. Disease course, expected outcomes, and usual treatment modalities
   b. Purpose, dosage, side effects of medication
      (1) Improvement in symptoms not evident for 3–4 weeks
      (2) Importance of adhering to prescribed pharmacological regimen; avoid abrupt discontinuation of medications
      (3) Caution against concomitant use of over-the-counter preparations
      (4) Interactions with food or other medications
5. Secondary prevention
   a. Screening those populations who have the means for treatment is recommended
   b. Asking the patient one of two questions is considered a highly sensitive screening tool
      (1) Over the last 2 weeks have you felt depressed?
      (2) Over the last 2 weeks have you felt disinterested in your activities of living?
6. Persons with major depression should be followed at least weekly for first 6–8 weeks, preferably by a mental health professional for medication adjustment and brief psychotherapeutic support
7. Persons known to be on antidepressants or receiving care for depression, who are being seen for other reasons, should be routinely checked for
   a. Suicidal feelings, plans, intentions, risks
   b. Tremor, blurred vision, dry mouth, tachycardia, postural hypotension

## SUICIDE

- Definition
  1. The intentional taking of one's own life
  2. Usually described as
     a. Attempted—unsuccessful conscious attempt to take one's own life
     b. Threatened—verbal or physical indication of intent for self-destruction
     c. Ideation—thoughts or behaviors indicating conscious intent for self-destruction; ominous when it includes the development of a viable plan

- Etiology/Incidence
  1. Often a manifestation or complication of depressive illness or anxiety states
  2. Approximately 2–9% of depressed patients commit suicide
  3. Tenth leading cause of death in United States; third leading cause of death in teenagers

4. Risk factors include
   a. Sudden crisis or loss
   b. Destructive coping mechanisms
   c. Few or no significant others
   d. Poor social or personal resources
   e. Past suicide attempts or family history of suicide
   f. Previous psychotic problems
   g. Unstable lifestyle
   h. Specific plan
   i. Substance abuse
   j. Recent initiation of pharmacotherapy for depression
5. Eight of 10 persons who state an intent to commit suicide do so; risk for depressed patients is greatest during the first month of treatment when the individual begins to feel better and has more energy
6. In the United States women attempt suicide more often, but men are three times as likely to succeed; in elderly, suicide among males outnumbers that among women at a rate of 4:1
   a. Female rates peak at age 55
   b. Male rates peak at age 75
7. Caucasian males older than 75 years have the highest incidence of successful suicide
8. In adolescents increased risk has been associated with
   a. Extreme parental control or permissiveness
   b. Loss of communication with parents and teachers
   c. Hostility and difficulty in school or with the law
   d. Lack of social supports (peers, social, work, and school)

- Signs and Symptoms
  1. Feelings of worthlessness and/or helplessness
  2. Preoccupation with a dead relative or friend
  3. Excessive denial, indignation, or anger in response to being questioned about suicide
  4. Verbalization or rehearsal of a realistic plan
  5. Sudden mood elevation in a depressed patient often accompanied by more energy and calmer, more placid manner
  6. Giving possessions away
  7. Setting affairs in order
  8. Making a will
  9. Presence of hallucinations or delusions
  10. Intuition on the part of the health professional
  11. In adolescents these may be more prominent
      a. Taking excessive risks
      b. Self-destructive behaviors, e.g., drug abuse, accident proneness
      c. Negative self-concept
      d. Expression of wish to die
      e. Withdrawal from family and people
      f. Increased interest and companionship with animal/pets
  12. All depressed patients need to be asked about suicide. If patients do not volunteer information, ask directly about thoughts of taking their own life. Also ask direct questions to elicit information about a plan, its lethality, and any mental or actual rehearsals of the plan. Risk is highest if planned in 24 hours; low or moderate if planned for a later time
      a. Presence of five or more risk factors constitutes high risk
      b. Mnemonic device to recall risk factors—SAD PERSONS
         (1) *S*ex
         (2) *A*ge
         (3) *D*epression
         (4) *P*revious attempt
         (5) *E*thanol abuse
         (6) *R*ational thinking diminished
         (7) *S*ocial support loss or absence
         (8) *O*rganized plan
         (9) *N*o spouse
         (10) *S*ick

- Differential Diagnosis
  1. Depression with melancholic features
  2. Depression with seasonal pattern (seasonal affective disorder)
  3. Nonfatal self-inflicted injury
  4. Organic disease

- Physical Findings
  1. No specific physical findings; however, those of depression may be evident
     a. General appearance—unkempt, slumped or stooped posture, slow speech pattern, lack of expression or dejected look, or agitation, hostility, tremulousness
     b. Mental status—disorientation, poor concentration, agitation, hallucinations, or delusions
  2. Old scars or evidence of injury from past attempts or high-risk behaviors

- Diagnostic Tests/Findings—there are no specific laboratory tests. See Diagnostic Tests/Findings in "Depression" section earlier in this chapter

- Management/Treatment
  1. Treatment usually includes hospitalization with psychotherapy, antidepressant medications, and/or ECT; see Management/Treatment in "Depression" section earlier in this chapter

2. If a patient is deemed suicidal or if there is concern about the patient's potential for suicide, do not leave the patient alone, but obtain immediate psychiatric consultation
3. There is no evidence that suicide screening reduces mortality

## ANXIETY

- Definition
  1. A condition characterized by a combination of psychological symptoms, e.g., excess worry, tension, or coping mechanisms, and somatic symptoms arising from the autonomic nervous system or specific organ system
  2. Major categories
     a. Generalized anxiety disorder—unrealistic or excessive anxiety and worry about life circumstance
     b. Panic disorders—unfounded morbid dread of seemingly harmless object or situation often leads to agoraphobia
     c. Obsessive-compulsive disorder (OCD)—repetitive thoughts (obsession) that a person is unable to control and/or urge to perform an act that cannot be resisted without great difficulty (compulsion) and that interferes with functional abilities
     d. Post-traumatic stress disorder (PTSD)—delayed (at least 6 months) anxiety after a severe trauma often perceived as a threat to physical integrity or self-concept; intrusive thoughts, flashbacks, and nightmares form the symptomatic triad
     e. Other categories include adjustment disorder with anxious mood, simple and social phobias, and dissociative disorders

- Etiology/Incidence
  1. Various theories related to etiology include
     a. Psychodynamic
        (1) Freudian—conflict between id and superego; ego not strong enough to resolve the conflict
        (2) Sullivanian—fear of disapproval from mother figure; conditional love leads to fragile ego, lack of self-confidence, lack of self-esteem, fear of failure
        (3) Dollar and Miller—learned response to innate drive to avoid pain; anxiety the result of two competing drives or goals
     b. Biological
        (1) Genetic influence with high family incidence
        (2) Autonomic nervous system response—fight-or-flight mechanism
        (3) Biological abnormalities of neurotransmitter receptors in the central nervous system, particularly gamma aminobutyric acid (GABA) receptors
     c. Family dynamics
        (1) Individual with dysfunctional behavior is representative of family system problems
        (2) Carrier of problems resulting from disrupted interrelationships
  2. Incidence
     a. Anxiety disorders occur in 10–15% of patients seen in healthcare settings
        (1) Only 1 in 4 diagnosed and treated
        (2) 3% of Americans will experience an anxiety disorder in their lifetime
        (3) Slight preponderance in women
        (4) Lower incidence in the elderly
        (5) Often associated with depression in the elderly
     b. Panic disorders
        (1) Occur more frequently in women than in men
        (2) Onset usually in late teens or early adulthood
        (3) More common in those who have had an early traumatic event, e.g., the death of a parent
     c. Obsessive-compulsive disorder
        (1) Most often seen in adolescence and early adulthood
        (2) Males and females affected equally
        (3) More frequent in upper middle class and in persons with higher levels of intellectual functioning

- Signs and Symptoms
  1. Generalized anxiety and panic attacks
     a. A feeling of tightness in the throat
     b. Difficulty breathing; feelings of suffocation
     c. Palpitations
     d. Chest tightness or pain
     e. Tachypnea, tachycardia
     f. Gastric distress or discomfort
     g. Nausea
     h. Diarrhea
     i. Feeling of weakness in lower limbs
     j. Tingling, numbness of extremities
     k. Feeling of light-headedness
     l. Dryness of the mouth
     m. Feeling of something caught in the throat
     n. Cold, sweaty hands
     o. Feelings of loss of control; irritability; impatience
     p. Motor tension—shakiness, jitteriness, trembling, restlessness
     q. Anxiety insomnia, difficulty falling asleep

r. Symptoms of panic generally develop suddenly and have been related to mitral valve prolapse
    2. OCD
        a. Recurrent, persistent thoughts, ideas, or images experienced as intrusive
        b. Repetitious, purposeful, intentional behaviors that are distressing, time consuming, or interfere with functioning
    3. PTSD
        a. Intrusive thoughts, flashbacks, nightmares related to the traumatic event
        b. Poor impulse control, unpredictability, and/or aggressiveness
        c. Avoidance symptoms
            (1) Avoids reminders of event
            (2) Memory difficulty
            (3) Detachment and restricted affect
        d. Hyperarousal symptoms
            (1) Hypervigilance
            (2) Insomnia
            (3) Irritability, poor concentration
- Differential Diagnosis
    1. Drug abuse, withdrawal, or intoxication
    2. Thyrotoxicosis
    3. Hypoglycemia
    4. Acute hypoxia
    5. Myocardial infarction
    6. Pheochromocytoma
    7. Seizure disorder
    8. Side effects of chemical agents or medications, e.g., caffeine, nicotine, beta-adrenergic agonists
- Physical Findings
    1. Between attacks may all be within normal limits
    2. During an attack
        a. General appearance—looks worried, frightened, restless
        b. Vital signs—tachycardia, increased respirations, elevated blood pressure (BP)
        c. Integumentary—pallor, flushed face, cold, clammy hands
        d. Gastrointestinal—possible loss of bowel or bladder control
        e. Mental status—hypervigilance, easy distractibility, poor concentration
        f. Motor tension—tremulous
- Diagnostic Tests/Findings
    1. Serum drug analysis—negative
    2. Thyroid function tests—normal
    3. Serum glucose—normal
    4. ECG—normal
    5. Diagnostic criteria for each type of anxiety disorder found in *DSM-V*
- Management/Treatment
    1. Depends on careful workup and identified anxiety subtype
    2. Cognitive behavioral therapy more effective for generalized anxiety than for panic attacks
        a. Assess usual coping mechanisms, lifestyle, social supports
        b. Establish a trusting, warm, empathetic, respectful relationship
        c. Assist patient to identify and describe emotional and physical feelings and to identify the relationship between them
        d. Identify patient behaviors that cause anxiety in the healthcare provider
        e. Use supportive confrontation as needed
        f. Keep focus of responsibility on the patient
        g. Encourage use of and teach or refer for relaxation techniques, biofeedback, and meditation
    3. Antianxiety medications
        a. For chronic anxiety management
            (1) SSRIs are drug of choice for most anxiety syndromes
            (2) Doses may need to be higher than those for depression
            (3) Consider those that are most sedating, e.g., paroxetine, citalopram
            (4) SNRIs may be considered for those unresponsive to SSRIs, those with chronic neuropathic pain, or those in whom symptoms are more severe at time of diagnosis
        b. For acute anxiety management
            (1) Benzodiazepines drug of choice for acute, short-term management
                (a) Not intended for long-term use
                (b) May result in fatal withdrawal syndrome if discontinued abruptly after extended use
            (2) Benzodiazepines may provide short-term symptom control until SSRI reaches therapeutic efficacy
            (3) Most have behavioral profile similar to alcohol
            (4) All have hypnotic properties
            (5) Antihistamines for those with chronic obstructive pulmonary disorder (COPD) or potential for abuse of benzodiazepines
        c. Beta-adrenergic blockers, e.g., propranolol more effective in reducing marked autonomic symptoms (tachycardia, palpations, breathlessness)
        d. Tricyclics and MAO inhibitors good for panic attacks, but not for generalized anxiety; safety profile limits their utility as first-line agents

e. Buspirone only anxiolytic not classified as a tranquilizer
   (1) Not linked to dependence or depressant effects
   (2) Does not impair motor skills
   (3) Does not potentiate alcohol effects
f. Optimal duration of treatment not well established
4. Patient education
   a. Disease course, expected outcome
      (1) Reassurance that anxiety rarely evolves into a more serious disorder
      (2) Reassurance that symptoms can be alleviated with appropriate therapy
      (3) Condition is temporary and with appropriate therapy and time, anxiety may be alleviated
      (4) Dosage, side effects, expected action of pharmacological agents
   b. Chart attacks—date, time, situation, level of anxiety or symptoms on a scale of 0 to 10

## ALCOHOLISM

- Definition
  1. Recurrent use of alcohol to the extent it significantly interferes with the individual's physical, social, and/or emotional life
  2. Characterized by preoccupation with the drug, loss of control over its use, physical dependence, and tolerance

- Etiology/Incidence
  1. Multifactorial and poorly understood; several etiologic theories have been developed
     a. Psychological
        (1) Retarded ego, weak superego
        (2) Fixed in lower level of psychosocial development
           (a) Dependent personality with poor impulse control
           (b) Low frustration tolerance
           (c) Low self-esteem
        (3) No evidence to support distinct personality predisposition
     b. Biological
        (1) Physiological changes in enzymes, genes, brain chemistry, hormones cause the disorder
        (2) May be familial, inherited, or acquired
  2. About 1 in 12 persons have serious problems related to alcohol use
     a. Children of alcoholics are four times as likely to develop alcoholism as children of nonalcoholics
     b. Three times as many men as women are alcoholics, and they are more likely to develop the problem early in life
     c. Highest prevalence of drinking problems in 18- to 29-year-olds
  3. Risk factors include
     a. Use of alcohol or other psychoactive substance
     b. Family history of alcohol abuse
     c. Being a young, single male
     d. Heavy drinking—five or more drinks in one sitting or getting drunk once a week
     e. Family or social background that accepts or promotes intoxication
     f. Ready accessibility
     g. Comorbid psychiatric disease or disorder
     h. Cultural or environmental conditioning

- Signs and Symptoms
  1. Definite (level I)
     a. Blackouts
     b. Alcoholic hepatitis
     c. Withdrawal symptoms—hallucinations; fine tremors of face, tongue, and hands; disorientation; seizures
     d. Memory loss, confabulation
     e. Nystagmus
     f. Prior exhibition of signs and symptoms of levels II and III
  2. Probable (level II)
     a. Previous diagnosis of
        (1) Cirrhosis
        (2) Pancreatitis without cholelithiasis
     b. Loss of control over alcohol intake, increased alcohol tolerance
     c. Numbness of hands and feet
     d. Increased incidence of infection
     e. Weight loss
     f. Forgetfulness
     g. Trauma from accidents or altercations—cigarette burns, healed fractures
     h. Hypothermic injuries
     i. Attempted suicide
     j. Symptoms of associated diseases; see **Table 14-1**

**TABLE 14-1 Conditions Commonly Associated with Substance Abuse**

| |
|---|
| 1. Frequent upper respiratory infection |
| 2. Slowly healing skin ulcers |
| 3. Recurrent vaginal infections |
| 4. Hepatitis |
| 5. Sexually transmitted disease |
| 6. Mononucleosis |
| 7. Malnutrition |
| 8. HIV infection |
| 9. Pancreatitis |
| 10. Tuberculosis |

3. Possible (level III)
   a. Blurred or dim vision
   b. Nocturnal diuresis
   c. Anxiety or depression
   d. Impotence
   e. Symptoms of associated diseases; see Table 14-1
   f. History of chronic gastritis, anemia, clotting disorders, marital discord, or loss of significant relationships (job, family, friends)
   g. Preoccupation with alcohol; thinking about it when not drinking

- Differential Diagnosis
  1. Other substance abuse disorders
  2. Anxiety disorder
  3. Other psychiatric disorder
  4. Central nervous system disease

- Physical Findings
  1. Definite (level I)
     a. General appearance—fearful, anxious, stuporous, hyperactive, or incoherent
     b. Vital signs—mild fever, tachycardia, increased or labile blood pressure
     c. Integumentary—flushed face and/or palms, spider nevi, angiomas on face, numerous scars, ecchymotic areas; generalized tissue edema, and dry, dull hair
     d. Head, ear, eye, nose, throat (HEENT)—pupil constriction, nystagmus, parotid adenopathy, inflamed buccal cavity, alcoholic odor to breath, fissures at corners of mouth
     e. Cardiovascular—tachycardia; dysrhythmias; weak, irregular peripheral pulses
     f. Abdomen—gastric distention, ascites, enlarged liver, tenderness
     g. Musculoskeletal—muscle wasting, healed or new fractures
     h. Neurological—memory loss, confabulation, hallucinations, disorientation, fine motor tremors, unsteady ataxic gait, gaps in word-finding, conversation
  2. Probable (level II) and possible (level III)
     a. General appearance—no major abnormalities
     b. Vital signs—normal or possible tachycardia, hypertension, and cardiac dysrhythmias
     c. Integumentary—unexplained ecchymosis
     d. HEENT—parotid adenopathy, angiomas
     e. Abdomen—hepatomegaly, tenderness
     f. Neurological—hyperreflexia; unsteady walk, ataxia (Wernicke–Korsakoff syndrome)

- Diagnostic Tests/Findings
  1. Use of CAGE screening test—≥ 2 yes answers indicates alcoholism
     a. Four questions related to drinking patterns
        (1) *Cut*—Ever felt you ought to cut down on your drinking?
        (2) *Annoyed*—Have people annoyed you by criticizing your drinking?
        (3) *Guilt*—Ever felt bad or guilty about your drinking?
        (4) *Eye-opener*—Ever had an eye-opener to steady nerves in the a.m.?
  2. Blood alcohol/drug levels—may or may not be severely elevated depending on amount and time of consumption
     a. 300 mg/100 mL at anytime = definite diagnosis
     b. 100 mg/mL on routine exam = definite diagnosis
     c. 150 mg/mL without evidence of intoxication = alcohol tolerance
  3. CBC—increased or depressed white count; macrocytosis with or without anemia; decreased platelets
  4. Blood glucose—hyper- or hypoglycemia
  5. Electrolytes—hypokalemia and hypomagnesemia
  6. Liver function—all may be increased
     a. Gamma glutamyl transferase (GGT)—> 30 units/L suggests recent episode of heavy drinking, not sensitive to chronicity
     b. Alanine aminotransferase (ALT) elevated to 3 times normal
     c. Aspartate aminotransferase (AST) elevated to 3 times normal with a level above that of ALT
     d. Elevated lactate dehydrogenase (LDH)
  7. Total bilirubin and amylase—increased
  8. Hypertriglyceridemia without elevations in other cholesterol indices
  9. Prothrombin time—prolonged in severe disease
  10. Urinalysis—infection, ketones
  11. Nutritional—albumin and total protein decreased, folic acid low
  12. Chest radiograph—enlarged heart, right lower lobe pneumonia
  13. ECG—dysrhythmias, cardiac myopathies, ischemic heart disease

- Management/Treatment
  1. Consider need for detoxification—will need acute pharmacological management in acute withdrawal phase
     a. Benzodiazepines for seizure suppression
     b. Blood pressure management; significant hypertension possible
     c. May need management of psychosis

2. Confront patient with diagnosis "alcoholism"
3. Do not use nebulous statements, e.g., "We think you might have a drinking problem" or "You need to cut down on your drinking"
4. Tell the patient it is a disease and treatable
5. Describe treatment options; many treatment programs will not accept pregnant women
6. Make appropriate referral for treatment and follow-up
   a. Alcoholics Anonymous (most successful)
   b. Behavioral approaches
7. Provide family members with information on alcoholism and encourage involvement in Al-Anon (for families of alcoholics) and/or Ala-Teen and Ala-Tots (for teenagers and young children of alcoholics)
8. General considerations
   a. Alcoholic women have a higher incidence of suicide attempts than both alcoholic men and the female population as a whole; see "Suicide" section earlier in this chapter
   b. Females, even with less alcohol consumption, are more likely to develop liver disease than males are
   c. Alcohol use by pregnant women is the leading cause of mental retardation
   d. Women's drinking and drug problems are often viewed as less serious than men's and are more frequently misdiagnosed
   e. If seeing a patient who was referred for treatment of alcoholism, reinforce participation in treatment and use of any agreed upon treatment aids
   f. Avoid compounding the problems or hindering recovery by prescribing sedatives or other depressants (cross-tolerance)

## PSYCHOACTIVE SUBSTANCE ABUSE

- Definition
  1. Misuse of any substance capable of producing altered state of consciousness and/or euphoria
  2. Addiction or compulsive use includes
     a. Psychological craving
     b. Physiological dependence (withdrawal symptoms with discontinuance)
     c. Tolerance (need for larger and larger doses to produce desired effect)
- Etiology/Incidence
  1. As with alcohol abuse, several theories have been developed to explain the cause of substance abuse, which include
     a. Psychological
        (1) Failure to complete developmental tasks
        (2) Underdeveloped ego
        (3) Dependent personality
        (4) Poor impulse control
        (5) Ego breakdown with subsequent drug use as a coping mechanism
     b. Biological hereditary/genetic factors
        (1) Neurotransmitter deficiency
        (2) Enzyme deficiency
     c. Family dynamics
        (1) Dysfunctional family system
        (2) Absent parent
        (3) Tyrannical or weak, ineffective parent
        (4) Negative role models
        (5) Drugs used for stress relief
        (6) Cultural perceptions of drug abuse
  2. Incidence
     a. 26% of females and 24% of males between the ages of 12 and 17 years have used an illicit drug
     b. More than 1 million women are on legal psychoactive drugs
     c. 66% of psychoactive drugs are prescribed for women
     d. Most commonly used substances alone or in combination
        (1) Depressants—benzodiazepines, barbiturates, opiates, morphine, heroin, alcohol, sedatives, hypnotics, and minor tranquilizers
            (a) Most widely used and abused drugs
            (b) Often prescribed for anxiety, depression, or sleep disorders
        (2) Stimulants (amphetamines, cocaine, caffeine, tobacco)
            (a) Most commonly abused stimulants other than caffeine and nicotine are amphetamine and cocaine
            (b) Twice as many males as females use stimulants, primarily in the 21- to 44-year age range
        (3) Hallucinogens (lysergic acid diethylamide, LSD; myristicin, nutmeg; dimethyltryptamine, DMT; psilocybin, magic mushroom; phencyclidine, PCP or angel dust; mescaline, peyote; cannabis, hashish and marijuana; and chemically related substances)
     e. Solvents/gases
        (1) Used to reproduce effects of depressants, stimulants, hallucinogenics
        (2) Produce inebriation similar to volatile anesthetics
        (3) Examples include gasoline, paint thinners, correction fluid
- Signs and Symptoms
  1. Depressants
     a. Nausea/vomiting

b. Myalgia, deep bone or muscle pain (methadone abusers)
c. Rhinorrhea, sneezing, excessive lacrimation
d. Headache
e. Miosis
f. Euphoria
g. Apathy, dysphoria, depression
h. Drowsiness, psychomotor retardation, slurred speech
i. Impaired attention, memory, social judgment (disinhibition)
j. Ataxia, tremors, lack of coordination
k. Mood swings, aggression, combativeness; loss of impulse control
l. Auditory hallucinations, paranoia
m. Bradycardia/respiratory depression
n. Fever, perspiration (with withdrawal)
o. Altered level of consciousness
2. Stimulants
a. Restlessness, irritability, anxiety, confusion, aggression
b. Tachycardia, cardiac dysrhythmia, chest pain (cocaine), increased blood pressure
c. Elation, grandiosity
d. Perspiration or chills
e. Hyper- or hypothermia
f. Abdominal pain, nausea/vomiting, diarrhea, frequent urination
g. Insomnia
h. Paranoia, hallucinations (visual and tactile with cocaine)
i. Dilated pupils
3. Hallucinogenics
a. Dilated pupils, vertical and horizontal nystagmus
b. Flushed skin
c. Increased pulse and BP
d. Marked anxiety; panic paranoia, hypomania
e. Hallucinations, visual and sensory distortions
f. Rapid, severe mood changes, hostility, aggression, violence
g. Depression, suicidal thoughts
h. Grandiosity, euphoria
i. Tremors
j. Flashbacks
k. Insensitivity to pain
4. Solvents/gases (inhaled)
a. Euphoria
b. Slurred speech
c. Hallucinations/confusion
d. Unconsciousness
e. Cardiopulmonary depression or failure

- Differential Diagnosis
1. Poly abuse is common and may present with intoxication, overdose, and/or in various stages of withdrawal
2. Rule out other disorders that may account for presenting signs and symptoms, for example
a. Seizure disorders
b. Hypo- or hyperthyroidism, thyroid storm
c. Hyper- or hypoglycemia
d. Schizophrenia, mania
e. Head injury

- Physical Findings—in addition to drug-specific signs, some general physical findings might include
1. General appearance—unkempt, poor hygiene
2. Vital signs—temperature elevation, increased or decreased BP, tachycardia, tachypnea
3. Integumentary—bruises, burns, needle marks, infections, cellulitis, ulcerations, abscesses
4. HEENT—changes in pupil size, reaction to light, and extraocular movements; poor oral hygiene, puncture wounds under the tongue, pharyngitis, inflammation and/or erosion of the nasal mucosa
5. Abdomen—tenderness, organomegaly
6. Cardiovascular—dysrhythmia
7. Neuromuscular—incoordination; decreased pain perception (PCP); alterations and distortions in consciousness, attention, sensory perceptions

- Diagnostic Tests/Findings
1. CBC—leukocytosis; anemia
2. Urine and drug screens—positive for abused substance(s)
3. If associated diseases are present, other alterations will be noted, e.g., abnormal liver enzymes, thyroid function tests, or glucose levels; positive HIV test

- Management/Treatment
1. Depressant abuse
a. Identify drugs taken, when taken, and route of administration if possible
b. Assess level of consciousness
c. Evaluate for evidence of head trauma
d. Refer to emergency care or drug detoxification unit if acute overdose or intoxication is noted
e. Immediate management includes providing a quiet, lighted room and do not leave patient alone
f. Monitor vital signs
2. Stimulant abuse
a. In cases of intoxication, overdose, or withdrawal, refer to emergency care
b. Immediate management includes providing a quiet area with reduced stimuli and high staff profile; aggressive behavior is associated with amphetamine use

c. Monitor cardiac rate and rhythm; ventricular arrhythmia and/or cardiac arrest may occur with toxic levels of cocaine
   d. Persons experiencing stimulant withdrawal may be suicidal as a result of profound CNS rebound depression; use suicide precautions until patient is transferred to emergency department or detoxification unit
   e. For nonemergency cases refer to drug rehabilitation unit
3. Hallucinogenic abuse
   a. Hallucinogenics do not have a withdrawal syndrome and do not require detoxification as such
   b. Refer patients with psychotic symptoms to the psychiatric unit
   c. Protect patient and others from injury
      (1) Darkened, quiet, nonthreatening environment to decrease the likelihood of confusion, fear, and violent behavior
      (2) Speak in a soft, nonthreatening voice
         (a) If LSD has been taken, provide reassurance verbally and by touch and orient the individual ("talking down")
         (b) If PCP intoxication is present, do not attempt "talking down" because it will increase the patient's agitation and tendency for violent behavior
      (3) Suspiciousness and paranoia, visual and auditory hallucinations, and agitation make suicide or accidental injury a likely possibility; take precautions early
      (4) If frightened and hallucinating, avoid the use of physical restraints; however, use of restraints with PCP users may be necessary for the safety of self and others; PCP is an anesthetic and alters thinking; persons on PCP are a danger to themselves as well as to others
4. General considerations
   a. Primary role is diagnosis and referral
   b. Consult with specialty care regarding medication use
      (1) Period of drug-free observation usually recommended
      (2) Haloperidol may be given to control psychotic and assaultive behaviors
      (3) Diazepam is used to reduce muscle spasm and restlessness
      (4) Phenothiazine neuroleptics should be avoided in patients on PCP because of the possibility of potentiating the anticholinergic effects of PCP
      (5) Vitamin C tablets (ascorbic acid) or cranberry juice may be used to acidify the urine and promote excretion of PCP
   c. Many treatment programs will not accept pregnant women
   d. Many treatment programs do not provide child care or other alternatives for women, which can be a significant barrier to help
   e. Alcoholics Anonymous, Al-Anon will also accept other substance abusers; family members should be given information on Al-Anon and Ala-Teen even if patient refuses treatment
   f. Narcotics Anonymous (substance abusers) and Nar-Anon (families of substance abusers) groups are available in some areas

## DELIRIUM (ACUTE CONFUSION)

- Definition—a transient global disorder of attention, with clouding of consciousness and cognitive impairment; considered a symptom of underlying abnormality rather than a disease entity

- Etiology/Incidence
  1. Usually the result of systemic problems, e.g., infection, medications, hypoxia, dehydration, or electrolyte imbalance—examples include
     a. Intoxication—alcohol, analgesics, bromides, sedatives, psychedelics
     b. Withdrawal from alcohol, sedatives, hypnotics, or corticosteroids
     c. Infections—urinary, respiratory, meningitis, encephalitis, septicemia, syphilis—most common cause of delirium in the elderly population
     d. Endocrine disorders—diabetes, hyper- or hypothyroidism, Addison's disease, Cushing's syndrome
     e. Nutritional deficiencies especially of vitamins $B_1$, $B_6$, $B_{12}$
     f. Medications—anticholinergics, antidepressants, digoxin, $H_2$ blockers, overdose of recreational drugs
     g. May be related to sensory deprivation or overload
     h. Sleep deprivation
     i. Psychological stress
  2. Can occur in any age group, but the elderly are particularly vulnerable
  3. Estimated that 40–80% of elderly patients hospitalized for acute physical illness exhibit delirium at time of admission or soon after
  4. Prolongs hospital length of stay by an average of 6 days

- Signs and Symptoms
  1. Symptom onset is acute and global
  2. Cognitive impairment

a. Inability to focus attention/short attention span
b. Impaired recent memory and recall
c. Problems in perceptual processing
d. Disorientation
e. Impaired judgment
3. Emotional lability
4. Impaired impulse control
5. Anxiety/irritability
6. Mild to moderate depression
7. Visual and auditory hallucinations
8. Confabulation
9. Fluctuating mental status; worse in the evening, "sundowning," more common in those with preexisting dementia
10. Psychomotor restlessness with insomnia
11. Tachycardia, dilated pupils, sweating

- Differential Diagnosis
  1. Dementia
  2. Pseudodementia
  3. Amnestic syndrome
  4. Substance-induced hallucinosis
  5. Schizophrenia
  6. Other psychoses

- Physical Findings—vary according to the underlying cause
  1. General appearance—may be restless, hyper- or hypovigilant; dazed expression
  2. Tachycardia, elevated blood pressure, increased temperature, tachypnea
  3. Focal neurological symptoms may be present
  4. Additional symptoms depending on underlying cause
     a. Fever
     b. Poor skin turgor
     c. Pale skin and mucosa
     d. Muscle twitch; hyperactive deep tendon reflexes (DTR)
     e. Seizure
     f. Cyanosis of nail beds or extremities

- Diagnostic Tests/Findings
  1. Thorough history and physical examination with mental status and neurological examination—may reveal clues to etiology
  2. Basic laboratory workup may include
     a. CBC with differential, chemical screen, blood gas analysis
     b. Electrocardiogram
     c. Chest radiograph
     d. Urinalysis and urine toxicology screen
  3. Special tests as needed
     a. EEG—tends to show general slowing in delirium
     b. CT scan or MRI of the brain—expect to be normal
     c. Blood levels for medications

- Management/Treatment
  1. Diagnostic consult with physician
  2. Identify suspected cause
  3. Remove or modify etiology when possible, e.g., treat infections with antimicrobials, discontinue or simplify medication regimens
  4. Nonpharmacological interventions
     a. Provide adequate nutrition, hydration, oxygenation
     b. Institute environmental controls to control stimuli levels
     c. Provide reassurance and institute safety measures
     d. Institute reorientation measures; provide patient and family with sensitive reassurance
  5. Pharmacological intervention
     a. Judicious use of sedation to promote rest, reduce anxiety, decrease agitation and restlessness
     b. No ideal drug
     c. Short-acting anxiolytics without active metabolites
        (1) Oxazepam 10–50 mg/day
        (2) Lorazepam 0.5–2 mg/day
        (3) Alprazolam 0.5–4 mg/day
     d. For immediate calming of acute agitation—haloperidol 0.5 mg IV combined with 0.5–1 mg lorazepam, repeated in 30 minutes
        (1) Repeat every hour until calming achieved
        (2) Once delirium cycle is broken, sedation may be continued particularly in evening and night hours
  6. General considerations
     a. Anticipate delirium when risk factors are present
        (1) Being > 80 years of age
        (2) Having visual or hearing impairments
        (3) Pain
        (4) Multiple medications
        (5) Urine elimination problems
        (6) Fracture injury
        (7) Multiple chronic diseases
        (8) Previous history of acute confusion
        (9) Immobilized
        (10) Low scores on mental status examinations
        (11) Being hospitalized or experiencing a change in environment
        (12) Drug or alcohol withdrawal

b. Prevention strategies
   (1) Avoid polypharmacy
   (2) Monitor medication intake and monitor for side effects, interactions, toxicity
   (3) Maintain adequate hydration and oxygenation
   (4) Maintain adequate nutrition
   (5) Assess for adequate pain control
   (6) Control environmental stimuli to avoid sensory deprivation or overload
   (7) Provide assistive devices to supplement sensory alterations, e.g., glasses, hearing aids, controlled lighting

## QUESTIONS

■ **Select the best answer.**

1. Which of the following is one of the two conditions required for a diagnosis of major depression?
   a. Contemplating a plan for suicide
   b. Unplanned weight loss > 10% body weight
   c. Unresponsive to cognitive-behavioral therapy
   d. Loss of interest or pleasure in activities

2. Which is true of major depression?
   a. Majority of patients will have a reoccurrence
   b. It may be a normal grief reaction
   c. It is often self-limiting
   d. Strongly associated with chronic drug use

3. What class of drug represents the first choice for the management of both depression and chronic anxiety?
   a. SNRI
   b. TCA
   c. SSRI
   d. MAO-B inhibitors

4. Post-traumatic stress disorder is marked by which triad of findings?
   a. Intrusive thoughts, nightmares, flashbacks
   b. Tendency to globalize, psychomotor retardation, hypersomnia
   c. Weight loss, feelings of helplessness, irritability
   d. Indifference, decreased concentration, hyperphagia

5. Contraindications to TCA therapy do not include:
   a. Coronary artery disease controlled with beta-adrenergic blockade
   b. Unmedicated hypertension
   c. Chest tightness that may represent acute anxiety
   d. An eating disorder characterized by a BMI < 19

6. Therapy for depression should always include:
   a. A trial of SSRIs
   b. Short-term benzodiazepines when anxiety component present
   c. Cognitive-behavioral intervention
   d. Quantification of symptoms with a depression rating scale

7. Premenstrual dysphoric disorder (PMDD):
   a. Is disabling in some way
   b. Is an exacerbation of PMS
   c. Improves in the luteal phase
   d. Is not recognized by *DSM-V* as a distinct diagnosis

8. Which population has the highest rate of completed suicides?
   a. Single Caucasian men > 75 years old
   b. Latina girls ages 15–19 years
   c. Persons of all ages with a history of substance abuse
   d. Persons who were recently treated for depression with pharmacological therapy

9. Who among the following is the most appropriate candidate for benzodiazepine initial therapy for anxiety?
   a. A 65-year-old male whose wife just died of colon cancer
   b. A 29-year-old female who is unable to work because of her excessive anxiety
   c. A 33-year-old female who has been in recovery from alcoholism for 1 year and is having anxiety related to a new relationship
   d. A 49-year-old male who is having flashbacks from a severe motorcycle accident

### Questions 10–13 refer to the following scenario.

A 17-year-old male student comes into the student health service complaining of weight loss, fatigue, and anorexia. He states that the symptoms began about a month ago after he broke up with his girlfriend. He has difficulty sleeping and says he wakes up thinking about her. He says that since she left him he just doesn't enjoy going out anymore and has been spending most of his free time in his room. His affect is flat, and he shows little expression as he relates his problem. The physical examination is within normal limits.

10. You suspect depression to be his problem. Your next step would be to:
    a. Prescribe an anti-anxiety medication
    b. Find out how he has coped with losses in the past
    c. Explain that this is a temporary situation and will probably clear up in another couple of weeks
    d. Ask him directly about feelings or thoughts of harming himself

11. Which factors in the available data might lead you to suspect that he might be suicidal?
    a. Weight loss, fatigue, anorexia
    b. Insomnia, loss of pleasure, social withdrawal
    c. Gender, emotional loss, signs of depression
    d. Intrusive thoughts, flat affect, with normal physical exam

12. Upon further questioning, he admits to suicidal ideation. Knowing which of the following would be most helpful in assessing his suicide risk?
    a. Whether there have been any suicides in his family
    b. If he rooms alone or has a roommate
    c. If his family lives nearby
    d. If he has a viable plan for suicide in the next 24 hours

13. This patient has a roommate, but his family lives in another state. He denies substance abuse or definite plan or time for suicide. What would be the least useful action at this point?
    a. Consult with a physician regarding psychotherapy and antidepressants
    b. Assess him with a structured suicide screening tool
    c. Contract with him to not harm or kill himself until he talks with you at a defined point in the near future
    d. Consult with psychiatry to evaluate need for hospitalization

**Questions 14 and 15 refer to the following scenario.**

A 38-year-old married male comes to the clinic asking for an AIDS test. He has been awakening at night with sweating and his heart pounding. He has read in *Time* magazine that night sweats were a sign of AIDS, and a few years ago he had to have a transfusion after a car accident. He would also like to have a radiograph of his throat because he feels like there's something stuck in it and wonders if it might be cancer. At times he feels like he's losing control. He denies IV drug use or high-risk sexual activities. He denies marital or work problems. In fact, he just got a promotion 2 weeks ago, and he and his wife have bought a new home.

14. What other information would be most helpful to you in your diagnosis?
    a. The duration of symptoms
    b. The presence of nightmares
    c. A family history of major mental health problems
    d. Past medical history significant for mitral valve prolapse

15. If he denies nightmares, has had symptoms for about 2 weeks, and the physical findings are normal, you should:
    a. Order a barium swallow
    b. Refer to a gastroenterologist
    c. Consider a post-traumatic stress syndrome as the probable diagnosis
    d. Consider situational anxiety as the probable diagnosis

16. Benzodiazepines are used in anxiety disorders. They are:
    a. Contraindicated in narrow angle glaucoma
    b. Not helpful for short-term use in situational anxiety
    c. Usually physiologically addicting
    d. As effective as beta blockers for control of palpitations

17. The most common mental health problem seen in general practice is:
    a. Anxiety
    b. Depression
    c. Alcoholism
    d. Schizophrenia

18. Which of the following symptoms is least characteristic of anxiety?
    a. Sleep disorder
    b. Decreased concentration
    c. Irritability
    d. Indifference

19. All of the following organic conditions may produce anxiety-like symptoms *except*:
    a. Thyrotoxicosis
    b. Hyperglycemia
    c. Hormone-releasing tumor
    d. Prolapsed mitral valve

20. A potential consequence of prescribing antidepressants in undiagnosed bipolar disorder is:

    a. Precipitating a manic episode
    b. Desensitizing the patient to serotonin reuptake inhibition
    c. Producing physiological dependence
    d. Contributing to serotonin syndrome

21. Mrs. J. is a 65-year-old widow who completed a series of ECT treatments 1 week ago with positive results. Both she and her daughter are concerned that she continues to experience significant memory loss. It is most appropriate to tell Mrs. J. that:

    a. She may need to take memory-enhancing agents for 4–6 months
    b. This is an unfortunate but common adverse effect of ECT
    c. The loss is temporary and full memory will return
    d. Memory will improve as her mood stabilizes

22. Mr. P. is a 45-year-old divorced male who presents for a physical exam required by his employer. During the interview he reveals previous hospitalization for pancreatitis and long-term self-medication for gastritis. His physical exam is normal except for slight tenderness in the RUQ. A CBC reveals macrocytic, megaloblastic anemia. Which diagnostic test would be most helpful at this point?

    a. ECG and electrolytes
    b. Liver function, vitamin $B_{12}$ and folic acid levels, and triglycerides
    c. Chest radiograph and ultrasound of the gallbladder
    d. Blood albumin levels and bone marrow studies

23. Ms. Z., a 35-year-old female, comes into the clinic demanding to be seen immediately. She is agitated and complaining loudly of police brutality. She states that she was unjustly jailed overnight because of a misunderstanding and that she was shackled for more than 3 hours causing bruises on her wrists and ankles. Upon further elaboration she states the police altered a blood test and said her blood alcohol level was 300. This information alone indicates:

    a. Paranoid ideation
    b. Alcoholism
    c. Need for legal services referral
    d. The patient may have a drinking problem

24. Noncompliance with medication is a concern in outpatient treatment of patients with mental health problems. Which of the following would be least helpful in promoting medication regimen compliance?

    a. Patient involvement in treatment decision making
    b. Providing the patient with information about expected action and side effects of the medications
    c. Arranging follow-up visits with whatever staff are available
    d. Maintaining telephone communication with the patient to monitor effects and response to medication

25. One of the most effective treatments for alcoholism is:

    a. Psychoanalysis
    b. Active participation in AA
    c. Aversion therapy with Antabuse (disulfiram)
    d. Active participation in Al-Anon

26. Ms. C. is brought by her friends to the emergency department after a party. She is stuporous, seems confused, and has pinpoint pupils. These signs are consistent with:

    a. PCP intoxication
    b. Heroin use
    c. LSD
    d. Amphetamine withdrawal

27. A 23-year-old male comes to the clinic to obtain treatment for a cut on his arm he received in a street fight. His face is badly bruised from a previous fight. He is unkempt and shows evidence of poor personal hygiene. He has a history of alcohol abuse. At present he is tachycardic and has an elevated blood pressure. His pupils are dilated and he is slightly diaphoretic. He complains of chest pain. These signs are consistent with:

    a. Acute alcohol intoxication
    b. Chronic heroin use
    c. Recent use of hallucinogenics
    d. Recent use of cocaine

28. A young adult male is brought into the emergency department by the police. He is highly agitated, hostile, verbally abusive, and threatening. He has several lacerations and bruises he sustained in a fight at a local club where he "tore the place apart." You should:

    a. Suspect police brutality
    b. Suspect heroin use

c. Try to talk the patient down and keep him oriented
d. Be prepared to administer a chemical restraint

29. Which of the following is *not* associated with physiological dependence?
    a. Heroin
    b. Phenobarbital
    c. LSD
    d. Amphetamines

30. A cocaine overdose may typically present with all of the following symptoms *except*:
    a. Extreme anxiety
    b. Bleeding
    c. Angina or MI
    d. Stupor

31. Your first action in a suspected cocaine overdose should be to:
    a. Administer antipsychotics
    b. Prepare for cardiopulmonary support
    c. Prepare for mechanical restraint
    d. Administer reversal agents

32. To enhance the excretion of PCP from the body give:
    a. Haloperidol
    b. Ascorbic acid
    c. Valium
    d. A phenothiazine

33. Withdrawal from opiates is often characterized by:
    a. Palpitations and anginal chest pain
    b. Abdominal cramping and diarrhea
    c. Tonic-clonic seizures and delirium
    d. Progressive, deteriorating consciousness

34. CNS rebound is seen in withdrawal of:
    a. CNS depressants
    b. Stimulants
    c. Hallucinogenics
    d. Alcohol

35. Aggressive behavior can be seen with abuse of which of the following?
    a. Amphetamines
    b. Depressants
    c. Hallucinogenics
    d. Any psychoactive substance

## ■ Answers

| 1. d  | 19. b |
| 2. a  | 20. a |
| 3. c  | 21. c |
| 4. a  | 22. b |
| 5. d  | 23. c |
| 6. c  | 24. c |
| 7. a  | 25. b |
| 8. a  | 26. b |
| 9. b  | 27. d |
| 10. d | 28. d |
| 11. c | 29. c |
| 12. d | 30. d |
| 13. b | 31. b |
| 14. a | 32. b |
| 15. d | 33. b |
| 16. a | 34. a |
| 17. b | 35. d |
| 18. d |       |

## BIBLIOGRAPHY

American Psychiatric Association. (2013). *Diagnostic and statistical manual of mental disorders* (5th ed.). Arlington, VA: American Psychiatric Publishing.

Brown, M. N., Lapane, K. L., & Luisi, A. F. (2002). The management of depression in older nursing home residents. *Journal of the American Geriatric Society, 50*(1), 69–76.

Brown, R. L., Leonard T., Saunders, L. A., & Papasouliotis, O. (2001). Two-item conjoint screen for alcohol and other drug problems. *Journal of the American Board of Family Practice, 14*(2), 95–106.

Burke, W. J., Schultz, S. K., & Smith, M. (2004). Management of anxiety in late life. *Annals of Long-Term Care, 12*(8), 28–33.

Centers for Disease Control and Prevention. (2005). Web-based Injury Statistics Query and Reporting System (WISQARS). Retrieved from http://www.cdc.gov/ncipc/wisqars/default.htm

Chychula, N. M., & Sciamanna, C. (2002). Help substance abusers attain and sustain abstinence. *Nurse Practitioner, 27*(11), 30–47.

Davis, B. D. (2004). Assessing adults with mental disorders in primary care. *Nurse Practitioner, 29*(5), 19–29.

Eisendrath, S. J., & Lichtmacher, J. E. (2012). Psychiatric disorders. In S. J. McPhee & M. A. Papadakis (Eds.), *Current medical diagnosis and treatment* (51st ed., pp. 1010–1064). New York, NY: Lange Medical Publishing/McGraw-Hill.

Enoch, M. A., & Goldman, D. (2002). Problem drinking and alcoholism: Diagnosis and treatment. *American Family Physician, 65*, 441–448.

Gerhardt, A. M. (2004). Identifying the drug seeker: The advanced practice nurse's role in managing prescription drug abuse. *Journal of the American Academy of Nurse Practitioners, 16*(6), 239–243.

Hollander, E., & Wong, C. M. (2000). *Contemporary diagnosis and management of common psychiatric disorders* (2nd ed.). Newtown, PA: Handbooks in Health Care.

Kosten, T. R., & O'Connor, P. G. (2003). Management of drug and alcohol withdrawal. *New England Journal of Medicine, 348*, 1786–1795.

Longo, L. P., & Johnson, B. (2000). Addiction: Part I. Benzodiazepines—side effects, abuse risk, and alternatives. *American Family Physician, 6*(7), 2121–2128.

Lyon, D. E., Chase, L. S., & Farrell, S. P. (2002). Using an interview guide to assess suicidal ideation. *Nurse Practitioner, 27*(8), 26–31.

Pokorny, A. D., Miller, B. A., & Kaplan, H. B. (1972). The brief MAST: A shortened version of the Michigan Alcoholism Screening Test. *American Journal of Psychiatry, 129*, 342–345.

Sekula, L. K., DeSantis, J., & Gianetti, V. (2003). Considerations in the management of the patient with comorbid depression and anxiety. *Journal of the American Academy of Nurse Practitioners, 15*(1), 23–33.

Sobczak, J. A. (2009). Managing high-acuity depressed adults in primary care. *Journal of the American Academy of Nurse Practitioners, 21*(7), 362–370.

# Advanced Practice, Role Development, Current Trends, and Health Policy

*Leanne C. Busby and Mary A. Baroni*

## INTRODUCTION

Advanced practice registered nurses (APRNs) must remain informed regarding role development, current issues and trends related to their practice, as well as changes in healthcare policy, as each has an impact on the evolving practice environment. Although current information is presented, the reader is encouraged to contact local and state regulatory bodies for variations in practice requirements.

## ADVANCED PRACTICE NURSING

- Definition of Advanced Practice Registered Nurse (APRN)
  1. National Council of State Boards of Nursing (NCSBN)—an APRN is an individual who has "(a) completed a graduate-level educational program, (b) passed a national certification examination that matches the educational preparation, (c) acquired advanced clinical skills and knowledge, (d) practice built upon the competencies of an RN, (e) been educationally prepared to assume responsibility and accountability, (f) clinical experience of sufficient breadth and depth to reflect the intended license, and (g) obtained a license to practice as an APRN in one of the four roles" (National Council of State Boards of Nursing [NCSBN], 2008). Practice as an advanced practice registered nurse means an expanded scope of nursing, with or without compensation or personal profit, and includes but is not limited to

     a. Assessing patients, synthesizing and analyzing data, and understanding and applying nursing principles at an advanced level
     b. Analyzing multiple sources of data, identifying alternative possibilities as to the nature of a healthcare problem, and selecting appropriate treatment
     c. Making independent decisions in solving complex patient care problems
     d. Developing a plan that establishes diagnoses, sets goals to meet identified healthcare needs, and prescribes a regimen of health care
     e. Performing acts of diagnosing, prescribing, administering, and dispensing therapeutic measures, including legend drugs and controlled substances, within the advanced practice registered nurse's focus of practice
     f. Managing patients' physical and psychosocial health–illness status
     g. Providing for the maintenance of safe and effective nursing care rendered directly or indirectly
     h. Promoting a safe and therapeutic environment
     i. Providing expert guidance and teaching
     j. Participating in patient and health systems management
     k. Advocating for patients and communities by attaining and maintaining what is in the best interest of the patient or group

The authors would like to thank Patricia Burkhardt, DrPH, CNM, for her contributions to this chapter.

l. Evaluating responses to interventions, the effectiveness of the plan of care, and the health regimen
m. Communicating and working effectively with patients, families, and other members of the healthcare team
n. Utilizing research skills and acquiring and applying critical new knowledge and technologies to practice domain
o. Teaching the theory and practice of advanced practice nursing (NCSBN, 2008)
2. Advanced practice registered nurses (APRNs) are educationally prepared to provide care to patients across the health wellness–illness continuum; the emphasis and how implemented within each of the four APRN roles vary. The four APRN roles are identified as (a) certified registered nurse anesthetists, (b) certified nurse-midwives, (c) certified nurse practitioners, and (d) and clinical nurse specialists (NCSBN, 2008)

## ROLE DEVELOPMENT

- The first nurse practitioner (NP) program established in 1964 prepared pediatric nurse practitioners (PNPs) through the collaborative efforts of Loretta C. Ford, EdD, RN, and Henry K. Silver, MD, at the University of Colorado
  1. PNP role development provided a model for other emerging NP specialties
  2. Original support of PNP role as "physician extender" to improve access concerns due to shortage of primary care providers (PCPs)
  3. Most early PNP education occurred within certificate and/or continuing education programs; e.g., Colorado program included 4 months didactic study followed by 18 months clinical practicum training
  4. Early research focused on quality of care, cost-effectiveness, productivity, clinical decision-making skills, and role satisfaction of the PNP
  5. National Association of Pediatric Nurse Practitioners (NAPNAP) organized in 1973 to establish PNP practice guidelines
  6. Early resistance to NP role as too much of a "medical model" from mainstream graduate nursing education that focused on "nursing model" of clinical nurse specialist (CNS) role development
  7. From 1980 to 1989 more physicians resulted in less need for NPs
  8. From 1990 to 1998 increased emphasis on primary care resulted in decreased need for specialty care; NP seen as viable, cost-effective member of healthcare delivery team

- Majority of NP programs currently at the master's-degree level within mainstream nursing education with increasing numbers moving toward the Doctor of Nursing Practice (DNP) program
  1. By 1989, 85% federally funded NP programs were graduate level
  2. Distinction between NP and CNS roles in practice has blurred
  3. Blended NP/CNS programs focusing on advanced practice nursing (APN) emerged within graduate nursing education
  4. Advantages/disadvantages of blended NP/CNS role remain controversial
  5. Most current programs require 2 years of full-time or 3–4 years of part-time graduate study
  6. In October 2004 the American Association of Colleges of Nursing (AACN) endorsed the *Position Statement on the Practice Doctorate in Nursing*
  7. As of January 2012, 141 colleges and universities in the United States offered DNP programs; another 100 schools were in the planning stages

- Curriculum Guidelines and Content
  1. Association of Faculties of Pediatric Nurse Practitioner and Associate Programs (AFPNP/AP)—first published terminal competencies in 1981; later updated in 1996
  2. National Organization of Nurse Practitioner Faculties (NONPF)—published curriculum guidelines and standards for NP education in 1990; later updated in 1995 and again in 2000 as *Domains and Competencies of Nurse Practitioner Practice*
  3. Core graduate nursing content includes nursing theory and research, organizational/leadership theory, ethical/legal issues, multicultural care, economics, community-based care, managed care, and healthcare delivery systems
  4. Advanced practice core content includes advanced health assessment, pharmacology, physiology, advanced pathophysiology or other related sciences depending on the APRN specialty, clinical decision-making process, advanced nursing interventions/therapeutics, health promotion/disease prevention, community-based practice, role differentiation, and interpersonal and family theory
  5. APRN specialty content includes information that is unique to type of APRN role, information that is unique to healthcare needs of respective specialty population, information that supports standards and competencies established by professional

specialty organizations, clinical decision making applied to specialty practice, and faculty supervised clinical practice experience
6. NONPF competencies now available in specialty-specific form to include acute care nurse practitioner, psychiatric mental health nurse practitioner, and primary care in specialty areas, e.g., adult, family, gerontology, women's health, and pediatrics

- Conceptual Models for Advanced Practice Nursing
  1. Benner's model of expert practice (1984)
  2. Calkin's model of advanced nursing practice (1984)
  3. Shuler's model of NP practice (1993a, 1993b, 1998)
     a. Holistic patient needs
     b. NP–patient interaction
     c. Self-care
     d. Health prevention
     e. Health promotion
     f. Wellness

## ADVANCED PRACTICE TRENDS AND ISSUES

- Components of Advanced Practice Registered Nursing Role
  1. Coordinator of care
  2. Patient advocate
  3. Accountable for patient outcomes and cost-effectiveness
  4. Direct caregiver
  5. Educator
  6. Administrator
  7. Researcher
  8. Consultant
  9. Case manager
  10. Change agent
  11. Leader
  12. Policymaker

- Standards and Scope of Practice
  1. Standards of practice
     a. Described by American Nurses Association (American Nurses Association [ANA], 2004) as authoritative statements by which to measure quality of practice, service, or education
     b. Establish minimum levels of acceptable performance
     c. Provide consumer with means to measure quality of care received (Hawkins & Thibodeau, 2002)
     d. Both generic and specific specialty standards exist
     e. Specialty groups have also developed standards, including the American Association of Critical-Care Nurses
     f. Can be used to provide legal expectations of practice, but were not designed to define standards of practice for clinical or legal purposes
  2. Scope of practice
     a. Based on what is legally allowable in each state under the state's nurse practice act
     b. Provides guidelines vs. specific mandates for nursing practice
     c. Is not mandated
     d. Varies widely from state to state (Hawkins & Thibodeau, 2002) and over time
     e. Often based on legal requirements within state and national standards
  3. *AACN Scope and Standards for Acute Care Nurse Practitioner Practice*
     a. Published by the American Association of Critical-Care Nurses in 2012 consistent with the APRN Consensus Model (American Association of Critical-Care Nurses, 2012)
     b. Defines scope of practice, standards of care, and standards of professional performance
     c. Scope of practice
        (1) Recognizes that scope of practice is regulated by state law
        (2) Articulates definition, role, practice population, environment, educational preparation, clinical practicums, regulation, and ethical issues for the acute care nurse practitioner
     d. Standards of care
        (1) Advanced assessment
        (2) Differential diagnosis
        (3) Outcomes identification
        (4) Plan of care
        (5) Implementation of treatment
        (6) Evaluation
     e. Standards of professional performance
        (1) Professional practice
        (2) Education
        (3) Collaboration
        (4) Ethics
        (5) Systems thinking
        (6) Resource utilization
        (7) Leadership
        (8) Collegiality
        (9) Quality of practice
        (10) Clinical inquiry
  4. Nurse practice acts
     a. Authorize boards of nursing in each state to establish statutory authority for licensure of registered nurse (RN)

b. Authority includes use of title, authorization for scope of practice, and disciplinary grounds (Bosna, 1997)
c. Evolve from statutory law, which after interpretation becomes regulatory language
d. NCSBN website—(https://www.ncsbn.org) has full-text state practice acts for most states

5. Clinical practice guidelines or protocols
   a. Definition—"systematically developed statements to assist practitioner and patient about appropriate care for specific clinical outcomes" (Institute of Medicine [IOM], 1990)
   b. Need/requirements for guidelines/protocol development
      (1) Variable requirements depending on individual state nurse practice act and standards of practice
      (2) Protocol requirements may be met with recognized reference books and published clinical guidelines
   c. Examples of practice guidelines for preventive care
      (1) Guidelines for Adolescent Preventive Services (GAPS) (American Medical Association [AMA])
      (2) Guide to Clinical Preventive Services (U.S. Preventive Services Task Force [USPSTF])
   d. Examples of practice guidelines for illness management
      (1) Asthma (National Institutes of Health [NIH], American Academy of Pediatrics [AAP])
      (2) Hearing screening (NIH, AAP)
      (3) HIV—Agency for Healthcare Research and Quality (AHRQ), formerly Agency for Health Care Policy and Research (AHCPR)
      (4) Otitis media with effusion (AHRQ)
      (5) Pain (AHRQ)
      (6) Sickle cell disease (AHRQ)
      (7) Hypertension (Eighth Report of the Joint National Committee on Prevention, Detection, Evaluation, and Treatment of High Blood Pressure [JNC VIII])
      (8) Diabetes (American Diabetes Association [ADA])
      (9) Dyslipidemia (Adult Treatment Panel III [ATP-III]) and American Heart Association/American College of Cardiology Guideline on the Treatment of Blood Cholesterol to Reduce Atherosclerotic Cardiovascular Risk in Adults

- Regulation of Advanced Nursing Practice
  1. Credentialing—regulatory mechanism(s) to ensure accountability for competent practice
     a. Mandates accountability/responsibility for competent practice
     b. Validation of required education, licensure, and certification
     c. Necessary to assure public of safe health care provided by qualified individuals
     d. Necessary to ensure compliance with federal and state laws related to nursing practice
     e. Acknowledges APRN advanced scope of practice
     f. Should provide appropriate avenues for public or individual practice complaints
     g. Allows profession to be accountable to public and its members by enforcing professional standards for practice (Hickey, Ouimette, & Venegoni, 2000)
     h. Tension between certification bodies, state boards of nursing, and nursing education accrediting organizations regarding role and responsibility for credentialing intensified in the 1990s with the proliferation of NP programs
     i. National task force on quality nurse practitioner education convened in 1995 with broad-based representation
        (1) National Organization of Nurse Practitioner Faculties (NONPF)
        (2) American Academy of Nurse Practitioners (AANP)
        (3) American Association of Colleges of Nursing (AACN)
        (4) American Nurses Credentialing Center (ANCC)
        (5) National Association of Neonatal Nurses (NANN)
        (6) National Association of Nurse Practitioners in Women's Health (NPWH) (formerly the National Association of Nurse Practitioners in Reproductive Health)
        (7) National Association of Pediatric Nurse Practitioners (NAPNAP)
        (8) National Certification Board for Pediatric Nurse Practitioners and Nurses (NCBPNP/N)—Pediatric Nursing Certification Board (PNCB) as of 2003
        (9) National Certification Corporation (NCC)
        (10) National League for Nursing (NLN)
        (11) National League for Nursing Accrediting Commission (NLNAC)
     j. Nurse practitioner credentialing remains within the domain of nongovernmental professional agencies with oversight of accreditation standards by the National Commission for Certifying Agencies

(NCCA), http://www.credentialingexcellence.org/p/cm/ld/fid=86
- k. NP credentialing currently available through NCCA-recognized certifying agencies
  - (1) American Nurses Credentialing Center (ANCC) 600 Maryland Avenue, SW Suite 100 West Washington, DC 20024-2572 (1-800-284-2378)
    - (a) Adult-gerontological primary nurse practitioner
    - (b) Family nurse practitioner
    - (c) Adult gerontological acute care nurse practitioner
    - (d) Women's health nurse practitioner
    - (e) Pediatric nurse practitioner
    - (f) Gerontological nurse practitioner
    - (g) Psychiatric mental health nurse practitioner
    - (h) Major revisions to transition in 2013 and 2014 as a result of the blending of adult/gerontological primary care nurse practitioner and acute care/gerontological nurse practitioner certification as required by the Consensus Model for Advanced Practice Registered Nurse (APRN) practice
  - (2) American Academy of Nurse Practitioners (AANP) Certification Administration P.O. Box 12926 Austin, TX 78711 (1-512-442-4262)
    - (a) Family nurse practitioner
    - (b) Adult nurse practitioner
    - (c) Adult-gerontology primary nurse practitioner
  - (3) American Association of Critical Care Nurses 101 Columbia Aliso Viejo, CA 92656-4109 (1-949-362-2050)
    - (a) Acute care nurse practitioner-adult gerontology
2. Certification
   - a. Definition—process by which nongovernmental agency or association confirms that an individual licensed professional has met certain predetermined standards as specified by that profession for specialty practice
   - b. Purpose—to assure the public that an individual has mastered a body of knowledge and acquired skills in a particular specialty
   - c. Required for licensure in most states, and reimbursement available by most insurers
3. Prescriptive authority
   - a. Some level of prescriptive authority for NP and certified nurse-midwives (CNM) since mid-1970s
   - b. As of 2009, all states have approved and/or implemented some degree of prescriptive authority
   - c. Required pharmacology education within graduate program and continuing education to maintain authority—specific requirements vary by state
   - d. Scope of prescriptive authority varies by state; full scope includes ability to obtain federal Drug Enforcement Administration (DEA) registration number
4. Multistate Nurse Licensure Compact
   - a. Since 1998, 24 states have passed legislation to recognize nursing RN licensure among participating states
   - b. In 2000, Wisconsin became the first state to include advanced practice nurses within legislation on multistate compacts
   - c. NCSBN and NP stakeholders developed a position paper in 2000 to guide multistate recognition of APRN licenses/authority to practice
5. Clinical privileges
   - a. Possibility of hospital staff membership opened to nonphysician providers by Joint Commission on Accreditation of Healthcare Organizations (JCAHO; now The Joint Commission) in 1983
   - b. Current issue for APRN practice

- Practice Issues
  1. Collaborative practice
     - a. Definition—ANA's (2003) *Nursing's Social Policy Statement* describes collaboration as "true partnership" in which all players have and value power, recognize and accept separate and combined areas of responsibility and activity, and share common goals
     - b. Purpose—to enhance quality of care and improve patient outcomes through ongoing continuity and coordination of care (Hickey et al., 2000)
     - c. Interdisciplinary teams—examples of collaborative practice
  2. Case management
     - a. Definition—"case management is a collaborative process of assessment, planning, facilitation, and advocacy for options and services to meet an individual's health needs through communication and available resources to promote quality cost-effective outcomes" (Case Management Society of America, 2010)
     - b. Purpose—to provide the means by which persons and firms offering services or products within or to the case management field may voluntarily coordinate

their efforts to advance the practice in all respects
- c. Components of role
  - (1) Planning care for cost-effectiveness and optimal outcomes
  - (2) Procuring and coordinating care
  - (3) Monitoring and evaluating outcomes
  - (4) Performing physical assessments
  - (5) Selecting laboratory and other tests
  - (6) Prescribing medications
  - (7) Requires that provider have strong communication skills and clinical expertise
  - (8) Provides care along continuum, decreases fragmentation of services, enhances patient and family quality of life, and contains costs
- d. Key features associated with case management models
  - (1) Standardize appropriate use of resources aimed at identified outcomes within appropriate time frames
  - (2) Promote collaborative practice among disciplines
  - (3) Promote coordinated continuity of care over course of illness
  - (4) Promote job satisfaction for providers
  - (5) Promote patient and provider satisfaction with care delivery while minimizing cost to institution (Hickey et al., 2000)
- e. Populations appropriate for case management
  - (1) Those for whom course of treatment is costly and unpredictable
  - (2) Those who experience frequent or chronic readmission to hospital
  - (3) Those involved with multiple providers or multiple disciplines

3. Quality improvement (QI)
   a. Definition—a formal approach to the analysis of performance and systematic efforts to improve performance
   b. Alternative terms—total quality management (TQM), continuous quality improvement (CQI); differs from quality assurance (QA) in being continuous rather than episodic process
   c. Systematic, organized structures, processes, and expected outcomes focus on defining excellence and ensuring accountability for quality of care
   d. Provides framework for ongoing evaluation of practice through identification of norms, criteria, and standards that measure program effectiveness and minimize liability
   e. QI mechanisms and strategies
      (1) Peer review
         (a) Recognizes and rewards nursing practice
         (b) Leads to higher standards of practice
         (c) Discourages practice beyond scope of legal authority
         (d) Improves quality of care (Cherry & Jacob, 2002)
         (e) Provides for accountability and responsibility
      (2) Other methods of evaluation
         (a) Audit—retrospective measurement of quality
         (b) Interviews and questionnaires
         (c) Patient satisfaction surveys or interviews

4. Risk management
   a. Systems and activities designed to recognize and intervene to decrease risk of injury to patients and subsequent claims against healthcare providers; based on assumption that many injuries to patients are preventable
   b. Evaluates sources of legal liability in practice such as
      (1) Patients
      (2) Procedures
      (3) Quality of record keeping
   c. Areas of liability/risk
      (1) Practitioner–patient relationship
      (2) Communication and informed consent
      (3) Clinical expertise
      (4) Self-evaluation by professionals of need to stay current
      (5) Documentation
      (6) Consultation and referral
      (7) Policies, procedures, and protocols
      (8) Supervision of others
   d. Includes educational activities that decrease risk in identified areas

5. Malpractice
   a. Professional misconduct, unreasonable lack of skill; infidelity in professional or fiduciary duties; illegal, immoral conduct resulting in patient harm
   b. Alleged professional failure to render services with degree of care, diligence, and precaution that another member of same profession in similar circumstances would render to prevent patient injury
   c. Malpractice insurance
      (1) Does not protect APRN from charges of practicing medicine without a license if APRN is practicing outside legal scope of practice for that state
      (2) National Practitioner Data Bank collects information on adverse actions

against healthcare practitioners, including nurses
- (3) Types of coverage
  - (a) Occurrence coverage—covers malpractice event that occurred during policy period, regardless of date of discovery or when claim filed
  - (b) Claims made coverage—covers only claims filed during policy coverage period, regardless of when event occurred
  - (c) Tail coverage—covers malpractice event from the time that a claims-made policy ends through the statute of limitations in the practitioner's state
6. Negligence—failure of individual to do what a reasonable person would do that results in injury to another
7. Reimbursement—whether working independently, sharing a joint practice with a physician, or practicing within a hospital or managed care system, APRNs must be reimbursed appropriately. Standards that determine private pay insurance mechanisms are often modeled after federal policies such as Medicaid and Medicare. However, even when the federal government establishes mandates that encourage direct payment of nonphysician healthcare providers, barriers to reimbursement are often encountered in state-level rules and regulations (Hamric, Spross, & Hanson, 2000)
    a. Medicaid
      (1) Authorized in 1965 as Title XIX of Social Security Act
      (2) Federal/state matching program with federal oversight
      (3) Financed through federal and state taxes, with between 50% and 83% of total Medicaid costs covered by federal government
      (4) Does not cover all people below federal poverty level, but state Medicaid programs are required by the federal government to cover certain categories such as
        (a) Recipients of Aid to Families with Dependent Children (AFDC)—states set own eligibility requirements for AFDC
        (b) People older than 65 years, blind persons, or people who are totally disabled who are eligible for cash assistance under federal Supplemental Security Income (SSI) program
        (c) Pregnant women (for pregnancy-related services only) and children younger than 6 years with family incomes up to 133% of federal poverty level
        (d) Children born after September 1983 in families whose income is at or below federal poverty level
      (5) States can choose to cover "medically needy"
      (6) Coverage required for certain services
        (a) Hospital and physician services
        (b) Laboratory and radiographic services
        (c) Nursing home and home healthcare services
        (d) Prenatal and preventive services
        (e) Medically necessary transportation
      (7) States can add services to list and can place certain limitations on federally mandated services
      (8) Although Medicaid recipients cannot be billed for services, states can impose nominal copayments or deductibles for certain services (Bodenheimer, 2002)
    b. Medicare
      (1) Federally mandated program established in 1965, provides health insurance for aged and disabled individuals
      (2) Eligibility covers hospital service, physician services, and other medical services
      (3) Income level does not affect eligibility
      (4) Medicare Part A
        (a) Those 65 years of age and older who are eligible for Social Security are automatically enrolled, whether or not they are retired—persons are eligible for Social Security when they (or their spouses) have paid into Social Security system through employment for 40 quarters or more
        (b) Those who have paid into system for fewer than 40 quarters can enroll in Medicare Part A by paying monthly premium
        (c) Those who are younger than age 65 and who are totally and permanently disabled may enroll in Medicare Part A after receiving Social Security disability benefits for 24 months
        (d) Those with chronic renal disease requiring dialysis or transplant may also be eligible for Part A without a 2-year waiting period

(e) Services covered include some hospitalization costs; some skilled nursing facility costs, although custodial care is not covered; home health care—100% for skilled care; 80% of approved amount for medical equipment; and hospice care—100% for most services
(f) Payment for hospitalization is based on projected costs of caring for patient with given problem—each Medicare patient admitted to a hospital is classified according to a diagnosis-related group (DRG); the hospital is then paid a predetermined amount for each patient admitted with the given DRG; if hospital costs are above payment rate, the hospital must absorb loss; if costs are below payment rate, hospital allowed to keep a percentage of excess
(g) APRN not paid directly for services delivered in a hospital
(5) Medicare Part B—Supplementary Medical Insurance (SMI)
(a) Monthly premium is charged
(b) Some low-income people are eligible to have monthly premium paid by Medicaid
(c) Financed by general federal revenues and by Part B monthly premiums
(d) Covers all medically necessary services—80% of an approved amount after annual deductible; includes physician services; physical, occupational, and speech therapy; medical equipment and diagnostic tests and some preventive care such as Pap tests, mammograms; hepatitis B, pneumococcal, and influenza vaccines can be included in medical expenses
(6) Medicare Part C—Medicare Advantage Plans
(a) Like traditional preferred provider organization (PPO) or health maintenance organization (HMO) plans
(b) The plan pays all Part A and Part B costs
(c) May offer additional coverages, e.g., vision, hearing, dental, and wellness
(d) Most offer prescription coverage
(7) Medicare Part D—Prescription Drug Coverage
(a) Plan allows senior citizens to receive prescription drugs at reduced out-of-pocket costs for a monthly fee
(b) Allows some brand and generic drugs that are commonly prescribed to seniors to be covered; drugs have to fall into "commonly prescribed" categories
(c) Plan requires that first $250 per year be paid by the patient
(i) Patient pays 25% of drug costs from $251 to $2,250 in 1 year
(ii) Patient pays for cost of $2,251 to $5,100 in 1 year
(iii) Any costs > $5,100 paid completely by the plan
c. APRN—Medicaid/Medicare coverage
(1) Omnibus Budget Reconciliation Act (OBRA) 1989—mandated Medicaid reimbursement for certified pediatric and family nurse practitioners began July 1, 1990; providers required to practice within the scope of state law and do not have to be under supervision or associated with a physician or other provider
(a) Level of payment determined by states—reimbursement rates range from 70% to 100% of fee-for-service physician Medicaid rate
(b) States can elect to pass laws allowing them to extend Medicaid payment to other types of NPs not identified in federal statutes
(2) Legislation (2005) has expanded direct Medicare reimbursement for APRNs in all geographic locations
(a) APRN reimbursement at 85% of physician fee schedule when billing independently using APRN billing number; direct physician supervision not required
(b) When APRN is employed by physician, the physician practice may receive 100% of customary physician charge, according to "incident to" rules (Buppert, 2012)
(c) APRN must be RN currently licensed to practice in the state in which services are rendered; must meet requirements for NP practice in state in which services are rendered; must be currently certified as a primary care

NP; must have successfully completed a formal advanced practice educational program of at least 1 academic year that includes at least 4 months of classroom instruction and awards a degree, diploma, or certificate OR must have successfully completed a formal advanced practice educational program and have been performing in that expanded role for at least 12 months during the 18-month period immediately preceding February 8, 1978, the effective date for the provision of services of NPs as reflected in the conditions for certification for rural health clinics
      (d) NP covered services are limited to services an NP is legally authorized to perform under the state law in which the NP practices, and the NP must meet training, education, and experience requirements prescribed by the Federal Secretary of Health and Human Services
   (3) NP services covered under Part B if service would be considered physician's services if furnished by medical doctor (MD) or doctor of osteopathy (DO); if NP is legally authorized to perform services in the state in which the services are performed; if services are performed in collaboration with MD/DO (collaboration specified as a process whereby NP works with physician to deliver health care within scope of NP expertise with medical direction and appropriate supervision as provided for in jointly developed guidelines or other mechanisms defined by federal regulations and law of the state in which services are performed); and if services are otherwise precluded from coverage because of one of the statutory exclusions
   (4) "Incident to" refers to services provided as an integral, yet incidental, part of the physician's personal, professional services in the course of diagnosis or treatment of injury or illness—these services must occur under direct personal supervision of a physician, and the APRN must be an employee of the physician group; services must occur during the course of treatment in which the physician performs an initial service and subsequent services in a manner that reflects the physician's active participation and management of the course of treatment—direct personal supervision does not mean that the physician must be in the same room as the APRN; however, the physician must be present in the office suite and available for assistance and direction while the APRN provides patient care (Buppert, 2012)
   (5) When APRN performs "incident to" service in physician's office, billing must be submitted to Medicare by employing physician, under the physician's name, provider number, and Current Procedural Terminology (CPT) code—payment is made at full physician rate and is paid to physician or physician practice
   (6) When APRN provides service in skilled nursing facility, or nursing facility located in urban area as defined by law, Medicare payment can be obtained—Medicare reimbursement is also available for APRN services in skilled nursing facilities (SNFs) in nonrural areas on a reasonable-charge basis; this amount may not exceed physician fee schedule amount for service, and payment is made to the APRN's employer
   (7) Centers for Medicare and Medicaid Services (CMS)
      (a) Formerly Health Care Financing & Administration (HCFA)
      (b) Oversight of several federal programs including Medicare, Medicaid, State Children's Health Insurance Program (SCHIP), Health Insurance Portability and Accountability Act (HIPAA), and clinical laboratory improvement amendments (CLIA)
      (c) Website: http://www.cms.hhs.gov
   d. Other third-party payers
      (1) Private insurer reimbursement is contract specific per state insurance commission
      (2) Triple Option Benefit Care Program (TRICARE), formerly Civilian Health and Medical Program of the Uniformed Services (CHAMPUS)
         (a) Federal health plan for military personnel, including surviving dependents, families, and retirees
         (b) APRN reimbursement for services

(3) Federal Employee Health Benefits Program (FEHBP)
    (a) One of largest employer-sponsored group health insurance programs
    (b) APRN recognized as designated healthcare provider
e. Methods of payment for advanced practice nurses
  (1) Fee-for-service model
    (a) Unit of payment by visit or procedure
    (b) Can occur with utilization review in which case payer has right to authorize or deny payment of expensive medical interventions such as hospital admission, extra hospital days, and surgery
  (2) Episodic model
    (a) One sum is paid for all services delivered during a given illness
    (b) DRG fee payment
  (3) Capitation model, PPO, and HMO are covered in section on managed care later in this chapter

- Professional Organizations
  1. Purpose and benefits
     a. Establish practice standards
     b. Collective voice to promote nursing and quality of care
     c. Monitor and influence policy and legislative initiatives
     d. Position papers on practice issues
     e. Disseminate information
  2. Examples
     a. American Nurses Association (ANA)
     b. National Conference of Gerontological Nurse Practitioners (NCGNP)
     c. National Organization of Nurse Practitioner Faculties (NONPF)
     d. American Association of Nurse Practitioners (AANP)
     e. Nurse Practitioner Associates for Continuing Education (NPACE)

- Research in Advanced Practice
  1. Major trend is outcome studies
  2. Sources of federal funding
     a. Agency for Healthcare Research and Quality (AHRQ)
        (1) Formerly the Agency for Health Care Policy and Research (AHCPR)
        (2) Website: http://www.ahcpr.gov/
     b. National Institutes of Health (NIH)
        (1) Includes the National Institute for Nursing Research (NINR)
        (2) Website: http://www.nih.gov/
     c. Maternal and Child Health Bureau (MCHB)
        (1) Functions within Health Resources and Services Administration (HRSA)
        (2) Website: http://www.mchb.hrsa.gov/
  3. Sources of research findings
     a. Conferences
     b. Scholarly publications
     c. Distribution of summaries of research studies (Hawkins & Thibodeau, 2002)
  4. Use of research in practice setting
     a. Develop research-based clinical pathways
     b. Track clinical outcomes and variances
     c. Demonstrate quality and cost-effectiveness of care
     d. Give structure to demonstration projects
     e. Persuade lawmakers of NP value and contributions in today's healthcare system
     f. Improve quality and patient outcomes
  5. Benefit of research for patients
     a. Provides thorough understanding of patient situation
     b. Provides more accurate assessment of situations
     c. Increases effectiveness of interventions
     d. Increases provider sensitivity to patient situations
     e. Assists providers to more accurately determine need for and effectiveness of interventions
  6. Barriers to research utilization
     a. Time and cost of conducting research studies
     b. Resistance to change in work setting
     c. Lack of rewards for using research findings
     d. Lack of understanding or uncertainty regarding research outcomes
  7. Strategies to overcome barriers to research utilization
     a. Creation of organizational culture that values and uses research
     b. Creation of environment where questions are encouraged, critical thinking is appreciated, and nursing care is evaluated
     c. Support for research through time allocation and financial commitment

# HEALTH POLICY

- Policy Influences
  1. *Healthy People 2020*
     a. Released in 2010 by U.S. Department of Health and Human Services (DHHS)
     b. Builds on initiatives set in *Healthy People 2010*
     c. Purpose—designed to achieve four overarching goals

(1) Attain high-quality, longer lives free of preventable disease, disability, injury, and premature death
(2) Achieve health equity, eliminate disparities, and improve health of all groups
(3) Create social and physical environments that promote good health for all
(4) Promote quality of life, healthy development, and healthy behaviors across all life stages

2. Prevention guidelines—*Guide to Clinical Preventive Services* (U.S. Preventive Services Task Force, 2014) presents national clinical preventive services guidelines for practice and educational settings
   a. Age and gender specific
   b. Suggests targeted examinations, immunizations, and health counseling that should be part of periodic health visits

3. Nursing's Agenda for Health Care Reform – initially published in 1991, revised in 2008 as ANA's Health System Reform Agenda)
   a. Supports creation of a healthcare system that ensures access, quality, and services at affordable costs
   b. Supports ongoing primary care
   c. Calls for basic core of essential health services to be available to all, and for restructured healthcare system focusing on consumers and their health and healthcare delivery in familiar, convenient sites
   d. Proposes shift from focus on illness and cure to orientation on wellness and caring
   e. Supports provisions for long-term care and insurance reforms to ensure improved access to coverage
   f. Calls for establishment of public/private sector review of resource allocations, cost-reduction plans, and fair and consistent reimbursement for all providers

- Utilization of Health Policy
  1. Shifting trend toward primary care and early preventive measures; supports need for APRN
  2. Four major factors influencing healthcare delivery services
     a. Payers—individual healthcare consumers, businesses that pay for health insurance for employees, and government through public programs and entitlement programs such as Medicare and Medicaid
     b. Insurers—take money from payers, assume risks, and pay providers
     c. Providers—include hospitals, physicians, nurses, APRNs, physician assistants, pharmacies, home health agencies, and long-term care facilities
     d. Suppliers—pharmaceutical and medical supply industries
  3. Legislative strategies and political involvement
     a. Professional organizations monitor policy issues and keep membership informed—e.g., NAPNAP legislative newsletter
     b. Local networks of APRN develop practice guidelines and advocate for policies to enhance practice

- Types of Healthcare Delivery Systems
  1. Primary health care
     a. Definition—"primary care is the provision of integrated, accessible healthcare services by clinicians who are accountable for addressing a large majority of personal healthcare needs, developing a sustained partnership with patients, and practicing in the context of family and community"
     b. Activities and/or functions define boundaries of primary care, such as curing or alleviating common illnesses and disabilities
     c. Entry point to a system that includes access to secondary and tertiary care
     d. Attributes include care that is accessible, comprehensive, coordinated, continuous, and accountable
     e. Strategy for organizing healthcare system as a whole; gives priority and allocates resources to community-based rather than hospital-based care
     f. Categories of primary PCP and nature of care
        (1) Medical specialties—family medicine, general internal medicine, general pediatrics, obstetrics and gynecology
        (2) Other experts have included NP and physician assistants (PAs) as PCPs
     g. Many definitions stress self-responsibility for health
  2. Managed care
     a. Defined as any arrangement for health care in which an organization, such as an HMO, another type of doctor–hospital network, or an insurance company, acts as intermediary between the person seeking care and the physician, according to the *American Heritage Medical Dictionary*
        (1) Network connects consumers, sponsors, providers, and third-party payers
        (2) Initial managed care organization was Kaiser Health Plan (California) established in 1930s
     b. Objectives
        (1) Manage use and price of healthcare delivery system

(2) Control type, level, and frequency of treatment
(3) Restrict level of reimbursement for services
c. Type of health insurance plan designed to control costs while ensuring quality care is provided
d. Obligation to manage is shared among providers, consumers, and payers
(1) Providers no longer dictate price of care delivery; must assume more financial risk for population assigned to them for care
(2) Consumers have fewer choices of coverage and providers and greater financial responsibility
(3) Payers manage healthcare dollars through benefit design, selective contracting, and shifting financial risk to providers (Hickey et al., 2000)
e. Types of managed care plans
(1) Health maintenance organizations (HMOs)
(a) Most common type
(b) By 2009, enrollment at 64.5 million
(c) Offer preestablished benefit package—including preventive, inpatient, and outpatient care
(d) HMO contracts with providers to provide care to enrollees
(e) Providers at financial risk, resulting in incentive to provide high-quality, cost-effective care
(f) Enrollees select a PCP who manages total care by authorizing specialty visits, hospitalization, and other services
(g) PCP may be MD, APRN, or PA providers; serving as "gatekeepers"
(2) Preferred provider organizations (PPOs)
(a) Compromised managed care option that is alternative between indemnity and HMO insurance
(b) Uses financial incentives to influence consumer and provider behaviors
(c) Refers to variety of arrangements between insurers, providers, and third-party payers rather than standard plan
(d) Often owned by large insurance companies such as Prudential, Travelers, and Aetna
(e) Available primarily to employed commercial population
(3) Point of service (POS) plans
(a) Consumers decide whether to use a provider network or seek care outside the network
(b) If variation of HMO plan, PCP coordinates care for enrollees; if variation of PPO plan, enrollees may choose lower-cost options outside of provider network
(c) Most rapidly growing type of managed care
(4) Integrated delivery systems
(a) Vertical integration of services across levels of care into seamless system with improved access for enrollees
(b) Capitated payment—financial risk shifts from payer to provider; unit of value is cost per member per month (PMPM); providers receive age- and sex-adjusted budget to cover services to maintain wellness of specific target population
(c) Emphasis on provision of appropriate, but not unlimited, care with financial benefit of keeping population healthy through systematic preventive services
f. Reimbursement under managed care
(1) Providers accept financial risk for care provided to specific population of enrollees
(2) Capitated payment
(a) Provider receives payment in advance
(b) Payment level reflects expected utilization by enrolled population for which provider is responsible
(3) Provider must control volume and cost
(4) Efficiency usually rewarded through bonus payments for operating within budget and meeting goals for quality and efficiency
g. Monitoring, evaluation, and accreditation in managed care
(1) Healthcare Effectiveness Data and Information Set (HEDIS)—provides quality measures and compares with benchmark standards and goals
(2) National Committee for Quality Assurance (NCQA)
(a) Major accreditation body for managed care organizations
(b) Standards in six critical areas are evaluated—quality management,

utilization management, credentialing, preventive health services, medical records, members rights/responsibilities
- h. Challenges and opportunities of managed care for APRN
  - (1) Need for balance between quality of care and costs inherent in diagnosis/management per patient visit
    - (a) Educational programs must incorporate managed-care content into curriculum
    - (b) APRN must combine strong clinical and financial skills to determine cost of providing care to target population
    - (c) Success in managed care environment requires systems-thinking skill to complement primary care skills; blended NP/CNS models may provide this necessary linkage with added focus on case management, utilization/resource management, quality improvement, and patient education/advocacy within systems of care
  - (2) APRN strategies for success within evolving managed care environment
    - (a) Determine strategies to increase efficiency without sacrificing quality of patient–provider interactions; e.g., group well-child visits
    - (b) Lobby for APN inclusion on provider panels
    - (c) Maintain partnerships with APRN educational programs for collaborative study and documentation of APRN effectiveness

# HEALTH INSURANCE PORTABILITY AND ACCOUNTABILITY ACT OF 1996 (HIPAA): PUBLIC LAW 104-191

- Purpose of HIPAA Provisions—improve efficiency and effectiveness of healthcare system by standardizing the electronic exchange of administrative and financial data

- Mandated Standards
  1. Specific transaction standards (claims, enrollment, etc.) including code sets
  2. Security and electronic signatures
  3. Privacy
  4. Unique identifiers, including allowed uses—for employers, health plans, and healthcare providers

- Privacy Rule—the privacy regulations control the use and disclosure of a patient's protected health information (PHI) where the information could potentially reveal the identity of the patient. HIPAA regulates PHI use by healthcare providers, health plans, and healthcare clearinghouses, i.e., entities that process or facilitate the processing of non-standard data elements of health information into standard elements or vice versa.

- Goals of Privacy Rule
  1. Provide strong federal protections for privacy rights
  2. Preserve quality health care

- Protected Health Information—all information
  1. Individually identifiable health information—health and demographic information; includes physical or mental health, the provision of or payment for health care; identifies the individual (includes deceased)
  2. Transmitted or maintained in any form or medium by a covered entity or its business associate

- Key Elements of Privacy Rule
  1. Covered entity—healthcare providers who transmit any health information electronically in connection with claims, billing, or payment transactions; health plans; healthcare clearinghouses
  2. Uses and disclosures of information
     a. Required
       (1) To individual when requested; to DHHS
       (2) To investigate or determine compliance with Privacy Rule
     b. Permitted
       (1) Individual
       (2) Treatment, Payment, and Health Care Operations (TPO)
       (3) Opportunity to agree or object
       (4) Public policy
       (5) "Incident to"
       (6) Limited data set
       (7) Authorized

- Individual Rights
  1. Notice of privacy practices—must contain language in Privacy Rule describing uses and disclosures of PHI
  2. Individual rights and how to exercise them; provide information as follows
     a. Covered entity duties and contact name, title, or phone number to receive complaints with effective date

- b. Access—right to inspect and obtain a copy of PHI in a designated record set (DRS) in a timely manner
- c. Amendment—individual has right to have covered entity amend PHI; request may be denied by covered entity if record is accurate and complete
- d. Accounting—individual has right to receive an accounting of disclosures of PHI made in the 6 years or less prior to date requested
- e. Request restrictions—individual may request restrictions on uses and disclosures of PHI, but covered entity may disagree
- f. Confidential communication—provider must permit and accommodate reasonable requests to receive communications of PHI by alternative means and at alternative locations
- g. Complaints to covered entity—a process must be established to document complaints and their disposition
- h. Complaints to secretary (DHHS/Office for Civil Rights [OCR])—any person may file a written complaint if he or she believes a covered entity is not complying with the Privacy Rule

- Deidentification of PHI
  1. Removal of certain identifiers so that the individual may no longer be identified
  2. Application of statistical method
  3. Stripping of listed identifiers such as names, geographic subdivisions, dates, Social Security numbers (SSNs)

- Administrative requirements
  1. Implement policies and procedures regarding PHI that are designed to comply with the Privacy Rule
  2. Implement appropriate administrative, technical, and physical safeguards to protect the privacy of PHI
  3. Provide privacy training to entire workforce and develop and apply a system of sanctions for those who violate the Privacy Rule
  4. Designate a privacy official responsible for policies and procedures and for receiving complaints
  5. Compliance and enforcement—effective April 14, 2003
  6. Office for Civil Rights (OCR) enforces the Privacy Rule

- Complaint Process
  1. Informal review may resolve issue fully without formal investigation; if not, begin investigation
  2. Technical assistance

- Civil Monetary Penalties (CMPs)
  1. $100 per violation
  2. Capped at $25,000 for each calendar year for each identical requirement or prohibition that is violated
  3. Criminal penalties for wrongful disclosures
     a. Up to $50,000 and 1 year imprisonment
     b. Up to $100,000 and 5 years imprisonment if done under false pretenses
     c. Up to $250,000 and 10 years imprisonment if intent to sell, transfer, or use for commercial advantage, personal gain, or malicious harm
     d. Enforced by Department of Justice (DOJ)

- Employment Retirement Income Security Act (ERISA)
  1. Federal law that exempts self-funded health and other benefit plans (employer and union) from state jurisdiction
  2. Seven out of 10 U.S. employees are in self-insured plans
  3. Legal challenges are in process disputing the breadth of the ERISA exemptions

# EVIDENCE-BASED PRACTICE

- Definition—the conscientious, judicious, and explicit use of current best evidence in making decisions about the care of individual patients incorporating both clinical expertise and patient values

- Major Clinical Categories of Primary Research and Their Preferred Study Designs
  1. Therapy—tests the effectiveness of a treatment: randomized, double-blinded, placebo-controlled
  2. Diagnosis and screening—measures the validity and reliability of a test or evaluates the effectiveness of a test in detecting disease at a presymptomatic stage: cross-sectional survey
  3. Causation or harm—assesses whether a substance is related to the development of an illness or condition: cohort or case-control
  4. Prognosis—determines the outcome of a disease: longitudinal cohort study
  5. Systematic review—a summary of the literature that uses explicit methods to perform a thorough literature search and critical appraisal of individual studies and that uses appropriate statistical techniques to combine these valid studies
  6. Meta-analysis—a systematic review that uses quantitative methods to summarize results

- Categories of strength of reviewed evidence from individual research and other sources
  1. Level I (A–D): Meta-analysis or multiple controlled studies

2. Level II (A–D): Individual experimental study
3. Level III (A–D): Quasi-experimental study
4. Level IV (A–D): Nonexperimental study
5. Level V (A–D): Case report or systematically obtained, verifiable quality or program evaluation data
6. Level VI: Opinion of respected authorities; this level also includes regulatory or legal opinions

- Level I is the strongest rating per type of research; however, quality for any level can range from A to D and reflects basic scientific credibility of the overall study; A indicates a very well-designed study, and D indicates the study has a major flaw that raises serious questions about the believability of the findings

## QUESTIONS

■ **Select the best answer.**

1. The Doctor of Nursing Practice:
   a. Will be the only graduate nursing degree accredited by the AACN after 2015
   b. Will be the entry-level degree for specialty nursing practice
   c. Is currently offered by > 200 colleges and universities
   d. Will replace the PhD in nursing by 2015

2. Which type of Medicare plan consists of a traditional PPO, HMO, or other managed care model?
   a. Part A
   b. Part B
   c. Part C
   d. Part D

3. Preventive health guidelines include references to:
   a. Immunizations, health screening, disease prophylaxis, education, and infection control
   b. Immunizations, counseling, health screening, disease prophylaxis, and education
   c. Health screening, disease prophylaxis, counseling, and CPR
   d. Health screening, disease prophylaxis, education, immunizations, and CPR

4. Nursing's Agenda for Health Care Reform:
   a. Is supportive of equal access, cost-effective, high-quality care
   b. Is a mandate to all nurses in the United States
   c. Is a summary of nursing research related to healthcare reform
   d. Is a report of the status of nursing in the 1990s

5. The nurse practitioner role was initially established to:
   a. Improve access to care and partially solve physician shortage
   b. Reduce the nursing shortage and improve access to care
   c. Improve working conditions of nurses while improving access to care
   d. Improve nursing's image through expansion of the role

6. Early nursing research focused on:
   a. The response of policymakers to the nursing shortage
   b. The effectiveness of the NP as a primary care giver
   c. An effort to demonstrate quality and cost-effectiveness of NPs
   d. The role of the NP as a physician extender

7. Which of the following is not a major factor influencing healthcare delivery services?
   a. Providers
   b. Payers
   c. Insurers
   d. Agencies

8. All definitions of primary health care include:
   a. The concept of universal access and accountability
   b. The concept of universal access and AIDS prevention
   c. The concept of universal access and a focus on self-responsibility for health
   d. The concept of universal access and a focus on reimbursement for services rendered

9. Standards of practice are:
   a. Authoritative statements used to measure quality
   b. Used to measure outcome but are not authoritative
   c. Designed for legal purposes
   d. Not designed for legal purposes and cannot be used to measure quality

10. Quality improvement activities include:
    a. Patient satisfaction surveys only
    b. Peer review, patient satisfaction surveys, chart audits

c. Defining four practice domains
d. Systems to decrease risk of injury to patients

11. Most risk management programs are based on the assumption that:
    a. Many injuries to patients are preventable
    b. Most legal liability is a result of poor documentation
    c. Most injuries to patients are not preventable
    d. Malpractice insurance is generally unnecessary

12. If an APRN practices beyond his/her scope:
    a. Malpractice insurance will protect him/her from a charge of practicing medicine without a license
    b. Malpractice insurance will not protect him/her from a charge of practicing medicine without a license
    c. He or she is legally accountable to the certifying body
    d. The collaborating physician is legally accountable to the certifying body

13. Standards of practice may be used to:
    a. Establish minimal levels of performance
    b. Establish reimbursement schemes for APRNs
    c. Mandate nursing practice across the nation
    d. Mandate nursing practice in certain states

14. Scope of practice:
    a. Is identical across the states
    b. Is determined by the federal government
    c. Is mandated by the federal government
    d. Varies from state to state

15. Medicaid provides health insurance coverage to:
    a. Certain categories of people whose personal income falls below the federal poverty level
    b. Anyone whose personal income falls below the federal poverty level
    c. Newborns, pregnant women, and those older than 65 years whose personal income falls below the federal poverty level
    d. Those who are elderly

16. Medicaid reimbursement is available to an APRN:
    a. Practicing in federally designated areas
    b. At a rate that is between 70% and 100% of the physician rate
    c. Only if the APRN is in collaborative practice with a physician
    d. Practicing in nursing homes only

17. Medicare reimbursement for services:
    a. Is not dependent on the patient's income level
    b. Depends on the patient's income level
    c. Is not available to APRNs under any circumstances
    d. Is only available to APRNs who are in collaborative practice with a physician

18. Medicare Part A covers:
    a. Hospital, skilled nursing facility, and hospice care
    b. All medically necessary services
    c. Skilled nursing facility care only
    d. Hospice care only

19. Medicare Part B covers:
    a. All medically necessary services
    b. Inpatient hospital care
    c. Outpatient physician services only
    d. Skilled nursing facility and hospice care

20. To receive Medicare reimbursement, APRNs must:
    a. Be nationally certified and maintain prescriptive privileges
    b. Maintain a current license in the state in which they are practicing
    c. Practice in a designated medically underserved area
    d. Practice with a physician

21. The term "incident to" refers to:
    a. The occasions when an APRN practices independently but occasionally consults with a physician
    b. The notion that the physician must be present in the office suite and immediately available to provide assistance in order for the APRN to bill for services rendered
    c. The notion that a physician must examine the patient along with the APRN if Medicare is to be billed for services rendered
    d. Medicaid only and is not pertinent to Medicare billing

22. "Incident to" billing is specific to:
    a. Medicare
    b. Medicaid
    c. Medicare and Medicaid
    d. Private insurance companies

23. TRICARE (formerly the Civilian Health and Medical Program of the Uniformed Services [CHAMPUS]):
    a. Is a federal health plan that covers health care for military personnel and their families and recognizes APRNs as reimbursable providers

b. Is a federal health plan that covers health care for military personnel and recognizes APRNs as reimbursable providers
c. Is a federal health plan that covers health care for military personnel and their families but does not recognize APRNs as reimbursable providers
d. Covers only hospital expenses of military personnel and their families

24. The knowledge base of the APRN is based on:
    a. Medical content
    b. Theoretical content only
    c. Scientific content and theory
    d. Theory and research

25. What has the role of the APRN traditionally focused on?
    a. The delivery of primary health care to all people
    b. The delivery of acute health care to all people
    c. Chronic care
    d. The medical model

26. The nurse practitioner role began:
    a. With the establishment of a pediatric nurse practitioner program in an effort to expand the role of the registered nurse to meet the needs of the children of the nation
    b. As a result of the new entitlement programs, Medicare and Medicaid
    c. When it was evident that medical schools across the United States could not prepare enough family practitioners to meet the nation's need
    d. As an experimental program at Duke University Medical Center

27. Legal authority for APRN practice is granted by:
    a. Federal law
    b. Regulations from the Department of Health and Human Services
    c. State law and regulations
    d. The board of medicine in most states

28. Direct reimbursement to APRNs has resulted in:
    a. Increased access to cost-effective, quality primary care
    b. Increased malpractice claims against APRNs
    c. Decreased consumer choice of healthcare providers
    d. Proliferation of APRNs in independent practice

29. Malpractice insurance:
    a. Protects APRNs from charges of practicing medicine without a license when they are practicing outside the legal scope of practice
    b. Does not protect APRNs from charges of practicing medicine without a license when they are practicing outside the legal scope of practice
    c. Does not pay for legal defense if the APRN is practicing beyond the legal scope of practice
    d. Is important but should not be purchased if the facility in which the APRN is employed carries good coverage

30. Collaborative practice:
    a. Limits autonomy and is not reasonable in current managed care environment
    b. Will enhance quality of care and improve patient outcomes
    c. Will limit consumer choice of providers
    d. Excludes the concept of interdisciplinary teams

31. Case management:
    a. Balances quality and cost of patient care
    b. Has not been found to be cost-effective
    c. Decreases the autonomy of the APRN
    d. Is rarely used today

32. What is the major trend in health policy research today?
    a. Outcome studies
    b. Primary care studies
    c. Studies that compare practice strategies of MDs and NPs
    d. Studies that compare patient satisfaction with care delivered by MDs versus NPs

33. Current prescriptive authority for APRNs:
    a. Varies among the states
    b. Is fairly consistent among the states
    c. Provides DEA numbers for APRNs
    d. Allows APRNs to move freely from state to state

34. *Managed care* is a term that describes:
    a. An established system of healthcare delivery that is mandated by the federal government
    b. A network of providers who contract to provide services for a specific group of enrollees
    c. A system that does not recognize APRNs as primary providers
    d. A network of hospitals and nursing homes that provide care to chronically ill people

35. Certification is:
   a. A procedure through which the government appraises and grants certification to the APRN
   b. Granted by the individual states
   c. Governed by each state's board of nursing
   d. A process in which a nongovernmental agency or group verifies that an APRN has met certain predetermined standards for specialty practice

36. Licensure:
   a. Is a federal process that is used to standardize healthcare facilities
   b. Is granted by a state government agency and grants permission to engage in the practice of a given profession
   c. Cannot be used to prohibit anyone from practicing a given profession
   d. Is a federal process that is used to standardize educational programs

37. Reimbursement under managed care:
   a. Requires that the provider accept the financial risk for the care provided to a specific population of enrolled patients
   b. Requires that the managed care organization accept the financial risk for the care provided to a specific population of enrolled patients
   c. Does not reward efficient care delivery
   d. Is not available to APRNs

38. An integrated delivery system:
   a. Is one that delivers high-quality care but is often not cost-effective
   b. Delivers a vertical integration of services with capitated payment
   c. Does not include rationing of resources
   d. Does not include a capitated payment scheme

## ■ Answers

| | | |
|---|---|---|
| 1. b | 14. d | 27. c |
| 2. c | 15. a | 28. a |
| 3. b | 16. b | 29. b |
| 4. a | 17. a | 30. b |
| 5. a | 18. a | 31. a |
| 6. c | 19. a | 32. a |
| 7. d | 20. b | 33. a |
| 8. a | 21. b | 34. b |
| 9. a | 22. a | 35. d |
| 10. b | 23. a | 36. b |
| 11. a | 24. c | 37. a |
| 12. b | 25. a | 38. b |
| 13. a | 26. a | |

## BIBLIOGRAPHY

American Association of Colleges of Nursing. (1996). *The essentials of master's education for advanced practice nursing.* Washington, DC: Author.

American Association of Critical-Care Nurses. (2012). *AACN Scope and standards of acute care nurse practitioner practice.* Alisa Viejo, CA: Author. Retrieved from http://www.aacn.org/wd/practice/docs/acnp-scope-and-standards.pdf

American Nurses Association. (2003). *Nursing's social policy statement* (2nd ed.). Washington, DC: American Nurses Publishing.

American Nurses Association. (2004). Scope of nursing practice: Advanced practice registered nurses. In *Nursing: Scope and standards of practice* (pp. 14–16). Washington, DC: Nursesbooks.org

American Nurses Association. (2008). *ANA's health system reform agenda.* Retrieved from http://www.nursingworld.org/content/healthcareandpolicyissues/agenda/anashealthsystemreformagenda.pdf

Association of Faculties of Pediatric Nurse Practitioner and Associate Programs. (1996). *Philosophy, conceptual model, terminal competencies for the education of pediatric nurse practitioners.* Cherry Hill, NJ: NAPNAP.

Benner, P. (1984). *From novice to expert, excellence, and power in nursing practice.* Menlo Park, CA: Addison-Wesley.

Bodenheimer, T. S. (2002). *Understanding health policy: A clinical approach* (3rd ed). New York, NY: McGraw-Hill.

Bosna, J. (1997). Using nurse practitioner certification for state nursing regulation: An update. *Nurse Practitioner: The American Journal of Primary Health Care, 22*(6), 213–216.

Bryant-Lukosious, D., DiCenzo, A., Brown, G., & Pinelli, J. (2004). Advance practice nursing roles: Development, implementation, and evaluation. *Journal of Advanced Nursing, 48*(5), 519–529.

Buppert, C. (2012). *Nurse practitioners business practice and legal guide* (4th ed.). Burlington, MA: Jones & Bartlett Learning.

Cady, A. F. (2003). *The advanced practice nurse's legal handbook.* Philadelphia, PA: Lippincott Williams & Wilkins.

Calkin, J.D. (1984). A model for advanced nursing practice. *Journal of Nursing Administration, 14*(1), 24–30.

Case Management Society of America. (2010). *CMSA's standards of practice for case management (revised 2010).* Little Rock, AR: Author.

Centers for Medicare & Medicaid Services. (1999). Balanced Budget Act—HCFA implementation. Retrieved from http://www.thecre.com/fedlaw/legal17/release.htm

Centers for Medicare & Medicaid Services. (2012). CY 2012 physician fee schedule final rule correction notice. Retrieved from https://www.cms.gov/PhysicianFeeSched/

Cherry, B., & Jacob, S. R. (2002). *Contemporary nursing: Issues, trends, and management* (2nd ed.). St. Louis, MO: Mosby.

Hamric, A. B., Spross, J. A., & Hanson, C. M. (2000). *Advanced practice nursing: An integrative approach* (2nd ed.). Philadelphia, PA: Saunders.

Hawkins, J. W., & Thibodeau, J. A. (2002). *The advanced practice nurse: Current issues* (5th ed.). New York, NY: Tiresias Press.

Health Care Financing Administration. (1999). *Medicare+Choice part C statutory requirement and regulatory implementation.* Baltimore, MD: Author.

Hickey, J. V., Ouimette, R. M., & Venegoni, S. L. (2000). *Advanced practice nursing: Changing roles and clinical applications* (2nd ed.). Philadelphia, PA: Lippincott Williams & Wilkins.

Institute of Medicine. (1990). *Clinical practice guidelines: Directions for a new program.* Washington, DC: National Academy Press.

Institute of Medicine. (1996). *20-20 vision: Health care in the 21st century. Primary care: America's health in a new era.* Washington, DC: National Academy Press.

Juran, M. (1999). *Juran's quality handbook* (5th ed.). New York, NY: McGraw-Hill.

Mezey, M. D., & McGivern, D. O. (1998). *Nurses, nurse practitioners: Evolution to advanced practice* (3rd ed.). Philadelphia, PA: Saunders.

National Association of Pediatric Nurse Practitioners. (1987). *Standards of practice for PNP/As.* Cherry Hill, NJ: Author.

National Association of Pediatric Nurse Practitioners. (1989). *Risk management for pediatric nurse practitioners.* Cherry Hill, NJ: Author.

National Association of Pediatric Nurse Practitioners. (2000). *Scope of practice.* Cherry Hill, NJ: Author.

National Council of State Boards of Nursing. (2008). *Consensus model for APRN regulation: Licensure, accreditation, certification and education.* Retrieved from https://www.ncsbn.org/Consensus_Model_for_APRN_Regulation_July_2008.pdf

National Organization of Nurse Practitioner Faculties. (2008). *Criteria for evaluation of nurse practitioner programs: A report of the National Task Force on Quality Nurse Practitioner Education.* Washington, DC: Author.

Pearson, L. (2010). *The Pearson Report.* Retrieved from http://www.pearsonreport.com/overview

Shuler, P. A., & Davis, J. E. (1993a). The Shuler nurse practitioner model: A theoretical framework for nurse practitioner clinicians, educators, and researchers, part I. *Journal of the American Academy of Nurse Practitioners, 5*(1), 11–18.

Shuler, P. A., & Davis, J. E. (1993b). The Shuler nurse practitioner model: Clinical application, part 2. *Journal of the American Academy of Nurse Practitioners, 5*(2), 73–88.

Shuler, P. A., & Huebscher, R. (1998). Clarifying nurse practitioners' unique contributions: Application of the Shuler nurse practitioner practice model. *Journal of the American Academy of Nurse Practitioners, 10*(11), 491–499.

Snyder, M., & Mirr, M. P. (1999). *Advanced practice nursing: A guide to professional development* (2nd ed.). New York, NY: Springer.

Social Security Administration. (n.d.). Compilation of the Social Security laws: Entitlement to hospital insurance benefits. Retrieved from http://www.ssa.gov/OP_Home/ssact/title02/0226.htm

Trandel-Korenchuk, D. M., & Trandel-Korenchuk, K. M. (1998). *Nursing and the law* (5th ed.). Gaithersburg, MD: Aspen.

U.S. Department of Health and Human Services. (2000). *Healthy people 2010 and leading health indicators.* Washington, DC: Government Printing Office.

U.S. Department of Health and Human Services. (2010). Healthy people 2020. Retrieved from http://www.healthypeople.gov/2020/topicsobjectives2020/default.aspx

U.S. Preventive Services Task Force. (2014). *The guide to clinical preventive services: Recommendations of the United States Preventive Services Task Force.* Retrieved from http://www.ahrq.gov/professionals/clinicians-providers/guidelines-recommendations/guide/index.html

# APPENDIX A

# Supplement for the Primary Care Provider

*Beth M. Kelsey*

*Susan B. Moskosky*

## PREGNANCY

- Definition—the condition of having a developing embryo or fetus within the female body (usually within the uterus)

- Incidence
  1. Birth rate, or number of live births per 1,000 estimated population, in the United States for 2012 was 12.6
  2. Birth rate for teenagers during 2012 was 29.4 per 1,000 females aged 15–19 years
  3. Fertility rate, or number of live births per 1,000 females of childbearing age (15–44 years), for 2012 was 63

- Early Diagnosis of Pregnancy Is Essential
  1. Begin prenatal care; physical examination; laboratory tests; risk assessment; discontinue use of tobacco, alcohol, street drugs, and/or teratogenic medications; provide educational materials
  2. If pregnancy is unintended, make timely decision regarding pregnancy options (e.g., continuation, termination, adoption)

- Signs and Symptoms
  1. Presumptive—subjective; frequently reported with pregnancy, but not conclusive for pregnancy
     a. Nausea with or without vomiting
     b. Urinary frequency
     c. Fatigue
     d. Perception of fetal movement by mother (quickening); with pregnancy, usually occurs 16–20 weeks
     e. Amenorrhea
     f. Breast changes
     g. Vaginal mucosa discoloration (Chadwick's sign)
     h. Increased skin pigmentation and abdominal striae
  2. Probable—more objective; often noted on physical examination or with laboratory testing
     a. Enlargement of abdomen and uterus
     b. Uterine changes in size, shape, consistency; softening of lower uterine segment at 6–8 weeks gestation (Hegar's sign)
     c. Softening of cervix at 6–8 weeks gestation (Goodell's sign)
     d. Braxton-Hicks contractions—often present by 4th month
     e. Ballottement—fetus can be pushed against the mother's abdomen and felt to bounce back against an examining finger in the vagina
     f. Outlining of fetus by examiner
     g. Pregnancy tests—detect human chorionic gonadotropin (hCG) in maternal blood or urine
  3. Positive—noted with absolute confirmation of pregnancy
     a. Detection of fetal heartbeat—auscultation with fetoscope at 17–20 weeks gestation;

*Note:* This appendix was coauthored by Susan Moskosky in her private capacity. No official support or endorsement by the Department of Health and Human Services or any component thereof is intended or should be inferred.

auscultation with Doppler by 10–12 weeks gestation
  b. Palpation of fetal movement by examiner
  c. Visualization of fetus by ultrasonography

- Differential Diagnosis
  1. Myomas, hematometra, adenomyosis
  2. Ovarian tumor or extrauterine mass
  3. Amenorrhea/irregular menses of other origin
  4. Gastrointestinal problem
  5. Gestational trophoblastic disease

- Physiological Changes (Maternal)
  1. Cardiovascular/respiratory
     a. Blood volume increased by 30–50% at term
     b. Increased cardiac output
     c. Heart displaced by uterus upward and to left
     d. Pulse rate increased by 10–15 beats per minute
     e. Dependent edema of feet and hands by third trimester
     f. Exaggerated heart sounds; functional systolic murmurs common
     g. Physiological anemia common due to unequal expansion of red cell volume (30%) and plasma volume (50%)
     h. Physiological dyspnea may occur during pregnancy due to increased tidal volume that slightly lowers blood $PCO_2$
  2. Gastrointestinal
     a. Decreased smooth muscle tone and decreased motility due to progesterone resulting in
        (1) Decreased intestinal peristalsis, which may lead to constipation
        (2) Gastric reflux and heartburn
        (3) Increased risk for gallstones
     b. Hemorrhoids are common during pregnancy; caused by constipation and elevated pressure in veins below the level of the enlarged uterus
     c. Hypertrophy and bleeding of gums possibly due to estrogen
  3. Musculoskeletal
     a. Progesterone-induced relaxation of pelvic structures and joints (may cause discomfort)
     b. Center of gravity shifts, causing lordosis and posture changes; lower back pain common; waddling gait develops
     c. Diastasis recti possible (separation of rectus abdominis muscles)
  4. Integumentary
     a. Cutaneous vascular changes—spider angiomas, palmar erythema
     b. Increased pigmentation of face (chloasma), areolae, abdomen (linea nigra), and genitalia
     c. Striae gravidarum
     d. Increased sebaceous and sweat gland activity
  5. Endocrine
     a. Diffuse thyroid gland enlargement
     b. Insulin resistance increases as a result of action of human placental lactogen (hPL)
  6. Breasts
     a. Early tenderness and tingling
     b. Increase in size and nodularity; striae may develop
     c. Veins prominent
     d. Nipples erectile; areolae darken
     e. Montgomery follicles hypertrophy
     f. Colostrum after first few months
  7. Genitalia/reproductive
     a. External genitalia
        (1) Increased pigmentation
        (2) Pelvic congestion; swelling of labia majora near term
        (3) Vulvar varicosities possible
     b. Vagina
        (1) Increased vascularity causing bluish/purple color (Chadwick's sign)
        (2) Rugations of vaginal mucosa prominent
        (3) Increased secretions (leukorrhea)
     c. Cervix
        (1) Pronounced softening and cyanosis (early)
        (2) Proliferation of endocervical glands
        (3) Mucus plug blocks endocervical canal
     d. Musculature—broad ligament softening
     e. Uterus
        (1) Increases in size and weight
        (2) Softening of lower uterine segment (Hegar's sign)
        (3) Blood supply increased
     f. Ovaries
        (1) Anovulation secondary to hormonal interruption of feedback loop
        (2) Corpus luteum—continues for first 10–12 weeks of pregnancy; produces progesterone until placenta develops
     g. Urinary
        (1) Dilation of ureters and kidneys (especially on right), decreased bladder tone—increased risk for urinary stasis and infection
        (2) Urinary frequency common early and late in pregnancy
        (3) Incontinence may occur, particularly with multiparity

- Prenatal Care
  1. Initial visit
     a. Laboratory confirmation of pregnancy—urine and serum tests available, all test for hCG

b. Expected date of birth (EDB), expected date of delivery (EDD)—Naegele's rule subtract 3 months from last normal menstrual period (LNMP) and add 7 days; duration of human gestation is 266 days
c. History—emphasize factors that may affect maternal or fetal outcome
    (1) Menstrual history—extremely important for estimating gestational age
    (2) Sexual history
    (3) Contraceptive history
    (4) Maternal history—attention to acute or chronic health problems
    (5) Family history—multiple gestation, congenital anomalies, inherited diseases, maternal family history of diabetes or hypertension
    (6) Medication history—including over-the-counter (OTC) and herbal supplements
    (7) Immunizations
    (8) Substance use—tobacco; alcohol; recreational, prescription, or herbal drugs
    (9) Exposure to environmental or occupational toxins or hazards
    (10) History of or current domestic violence
    (11) Risk factors for HIV and other sexually transmitted infections (STIs), hepatitis B
    (12) Dietary habits
    (13) Ethnic background
    (14) Reproductive/obstetric history
        (a) Each previous pregnancy including outcome—e.g., **T**erm birth, **P**reterm birth, **A**bortion (spontaneous or induced), and number of **L**iving children (T-P-A-L)
        (b) Complications during previous pregnancy/delivery/postpartum—e.g., gestational diabetes, pregnancy-induced hypertension (PIH), preterm labor (PTL) and/or preterm birth, postpartum hemorrhage, postpartum depression
        (c) Previous pregnancy loss, including gestational age and related factors
        (d) Method of delivery for previous pregnancies—vaginal or cesarean
d. Physical examination
    (1) Vital signs and complete head-to-toe examination—attention to any preexisting medical conditions
    (2) Assess uterine size to confirm pregnancy and determine gestational age—most accurately assessed by bimanual examination up to 14 weeks
        (a) 8 weeks—approximately 9 cm
        (b) 10 weeks—approximately 10 cm
        (c) 12 weeks—uterine fundus at symphysis pubis
        (d) 16 weeks—fundus midway between symphysis pubis and umbilicus
        (e) 20 weeks—fundus at umbilicus
        (f) 20 weeks to term—abdominal measurement of fundal height
            (i) Measure from top of symphysis pubis to top of uterine fundus
            (ii) Between 18 and 32 weeks gestation, good correlation between gestational age in weeks and measurement of fundal height in centimeters
    (3) Evaluate pelvic dimensions (pelvimetry)
    (4) Obtain Pap smear and cervical cultures
    (5) Auscultation of fetal heart by Doppler (usually audible by 10–12 weeks with Doppler)
e. Laboratory testing (routine)
    (1) ABO blood group/Rh factor determination
    (2) Complete blood count (CBC)
    (3) Antibody screen and titer
    (4) Rubella titer—titer of > 1:10 indicates immunity
    (5) Syphilis screening—Venereal Disease Research Laboratories test (VDRL), rapid plasma reagin (RPR)
    (6) Hepatitis B surface antigen screening
    (7) Urinalysis; urine culture if indicated
    (8) Chlamydia/gonorrhea screening
    (9) Offer human immunodeficiency virus (HIV) antibody testing
    (10) Other tests indicated by individual risk status or general patient population, e.g., postprandial 50-g glucose screen, sickle cell screen, tuberculin testing
f. Risk assessment—major categories for increased risk
    (1) Preexisting medical illness
    (2) Previous pregnancy complications
    (3) Evidence of poor maternal nutrition
    (4) Exposure to possible teratogens
g. Referral for genetic counseling if indicated
    (1) Maternal age of 35 years or older by delivery
    (2) Family history of genetic anomaly—e.g., Down syndrome, other chromosomal abnormality, hemophilia, muscular dystrophy, cystic fibrosis

                (3) History of three or more spontaneous abortions
                (4) Previous unexplained pregnancy loss
                (5) Parents possible carriers of sickle cell, thalassemia, or Tay-Sachs disease
            h. Education
                (1) Nutrition
                    (a) Dietary assessment
                    (b) Ideal weight gain during pregnancy is 25–35 pounds for woman of normal weight (BMI 18.6–24.9); 15–25 pounds for overweight women (BMI 25–29.9); 11–20 pounds for obese women (BMI > 30); 28–40 pounds for underweight women (BMI < 18.5)
                        (i) First trimester—1–4.5 pounds
                        (ii) Second and third trimesters—1–2 pounds per week
                    (c) Discourage weight loss during pregnancy
                    (d) Nutritional requirements
                        (i) Calories—1,800 kilocalories daily in first trimester, 2,200 kilocalories daily in second trimester, and 2,400 kilocalories per day in third trimester recommended for women who get less than 30 minutes of exercise each week
                        (ii) Protein—60 g per day
                        (iii) Calcium—1,000 mg per day for adult; 1,600 mg per day for adolescent
                        (iv) Iron—30-mg supplement per day
                        (v) Zinc—11-mg supplement per day
                        (vi) Folic acid—0.4 mg per day, higher in first trimester if increased risk of neural tube defect
                        (vii) Other vitamin and mineral needs can usually be met from a balanced diet; encourage fiber and fluids
                (2) Encourage good hygiene; douching not recommended
                (3) Exercise
                    (a) Regular exercise recommended throughout pregnancy
                    (b) May continue with prepregnancy exercise routine but should not begin new strenuous exercise program
                    (c) Walking and swimming are ideal during pregnancy
                    (d) Avoid excessive fatigue and excessive overheating
                (4) Sexual activity
                    (a) Coitus not contraindicated during normal pregnancy
                    (b) Changes in position may be required as pregnancy progresses
                    (c) Sexual intercourse contraindicated during pregnancy with undiagnosed vaginal bleeding, rupture of membranes, preterm labor, threatened abortion
                (5) Warning signs—patient should contact provider promptly
                    (a) Signs of ectopic pregnancy or threatened abortion
                        (i) Abdominal pain
                        (ii) Vaginal bleeding
                        (iii) Passage of tissue
                        (iv) Syncope
                    (b) Hyperemesis—severe nausea and vomiting; unable to retain food or fluids
                    (c) Signs of pyelonephritis
                        (i) Fever above 100.6° F
                        (ii) Dysuria, flank pain
                    (d) Signs of PIH
                        (i) Severe headache, dizziness
                        (ii) Scotomata, blurring of vision
                        (iii) Swelling of face; severe dependent edema that does not respond to rest/elevation
                        (iv) Epigastric pain
                    (e) Signs of PTL
                        (i) Loss of fluid from vagina
                        (ii) Lower back pain or lower abdominal cramping
                        (iii) Frequent, palpable uterine contractions with or without pain
                        (iv) Heaviness or pressure
                        (v) Increased vaginal discharge, especially if blood-tinged, mucoid, or watery
                    (f) Decreased or absent fetal movement
                (6) Signs and symptoms of labor
                    (a) True labor
                        (i) Contractions—timed from beginning of one contraction to beginning of the next
                            a) Occur at regular intervals, which gradually shorten
                            b) Initially felt in back, then radiate to lower abdomen
                            c) Duration and strength of contractions increase

d) Intensity of contractions increase with walking
e) Sedation does not stop contractions
  (ii) Bloody "show"—pink or blood-tinged mucus discharge from cervix may indicate loss of mucus plug
  (iii) Cervix dilates and effaces
  (iv) Presenting part has descended into pelvis
(b) False labor
  (i) Contractions irregular in timing, duration, and intensity
  (ii) Discomfort is felt mainly in abdomen
  (iii) Intensity of contractions not affected by walking
  (iv) No changes in cervix; no bloody show, dilation, or effacement
  (v) Fetal head remains free in pelvis
  (vi) Sedation will stop contractions
(c) Rupture of membranes
  (i) Occurs spontaneously at onset of labor in 50%
  (ii) Premature rupture of membranes associated with increased risk for
    a) PTL if occurs prior to 37 weeks gestation
    b) Ascending intrauterine infection if not delivered within 24 hours
    c) Prolapse of umbilical cord
2. Interval visits
  a. For low-risk, routine monthly visits up to 28 weeks, every 2–3 weeks until 36 weeks, then weekly until delivery
  b. Components of routine visits
    (1) Measurement of maternal weight and blood pressure
    (2) Screen urine for protein and glucose; ketones and nitrites if indicated
    (3) Obtain interval history, evaluate client complaints and risk-related symptoms, answer questions, and provide anticipatory guidance
    (4) Assess fetal heart tones by fetoscope or Doppler (normal rate is 120–160 beats per minute)
    (5) Evaluate fetal growth
      (a) Determine fundal height
      (b) Leopold's maneuvers—abdominal palpation performed using four maneuvers to determine fetal presentation and position (used later in pregnancy—beginning approximately 26 weeks)
    (6) Specific needs or screening tests as indicated by gestational age or patient history
      (a) First trimester (LNMP through 13th week)
        (i) Chorionic villus sampling (CVS)—refer when indicated for genetic reasons; generally performed at 10–13 weeks
        (ii) 1-hour postprandial 50-g glucose screen (initial visit or first trimester) for women at high risk for gestational diabetes mellitus (GDM)—prior history of GDM; first-degree relative with type 2 diabetes; prior delivery of macrosomic infant; previous unexplained stillbirth or spontaneous abortions; obesity; glucosuria
        (iii) Assess physical and psychological impact of pregnancy, including support system
        (iv) Discuss warning signs and early complications
      (b) Second trimester (14th–27th week)
        (i) Maternal serum alpha-fetoprotein (MSAFP) and multiple marker (quad) screening—screen at 15–19 weeks (16–18 weeks optimal)
          a) Elevated levels of MSAFP associated with fetal congenital abnormalities—open neural tube defects, congenital nephrosis, abdominal wall defects; also elevated with multiple gestation
          b) Low levels of MSAFP associated with Down syndrome (trisomy 21)
        (ii) Amniocentesis performed at 15–18 weeks if indicated for genetic screening—mother > 35 years, history of previous child with chromosomal, congenital, or metabolic abnormality
        (iii) 1-hour post 50-g glucose test—between 24 and 28 weeks

- a) May choose universal screening of all women or selective screening based on risk factors
- b) Selective screening guidelines—perform blood glucose testing if older than 25 years, ethnic group with high prevalence of diabetes (Hispanic, African American, Native American, South or East Asian), obese, strong family history of type 2 diabetes, prior gestational diabetes, or for glucosuria or other signs of hyperglycemia
- c) 1-hour post 50-g glucose test of 130–190 mg/dL—follow with 3-hour glucose tolerance test (GTT)
- d) 1-hour post 50-g glucose test > 190 mg/dL—presumptive diagnosis of gestational diabetes
- e) Diagnosis of gestational diabetes with a 3-hour GTT if two or more values are met or exceeded—fasting blood sugar (FBS) 105 mg/dL, 1-hour 190 mg/dL, 2-hour 165 mg/dL, 3-hour 145 mg/dL
- (iv) Assess for fetal movements (quickening)—usually between 16 and 20 weeks
- (v) Discuss warning signs for complications, including PTL
- (c) Third trimester (28th week to term—usually 40 weeks)
  - (i) Repeat VDRL and hemoglobin (Hgb)
  - (ii) Reevaluate antibody screen titer
  - (iii) Rh (D) immune globulin (RhoGAM) to unsensitized Rh-negative mother—28 weeks
  - (iv) Discuss importance of monitoring fetal movement as indicator of fetal well-being
  - (v) Review signs and symptoms of labor
  - (vi) Perform group B strep screen (35–37 weeks)
  - (vii) Assess fetal lie and presentation (36–40 weeks)
  - (viii) Perform cervical assessment for position, consistency, length, and dilation near term
3. Tests for assessment of fetal well-being
   a. Ultrasound (ultrasonography)
      (1) Definition—high-frequency sound waves reflected from tissues of varying densities and converted into images
         (a) Level 1 (basic ultrasound)—establishes gestational age, location, and grade of placenta; determines fetal presentation, number of fetuses, stage of fetal growth, cardiac activity; assesses amniotic fluid volume; detects gross fetal anomalies and maternal pelvic masses
         (b) Level II (targeted ultrasound)—confirms information obtained in Level I and surveys fetal anatomy for malformations
      (2) Indications—determination of gestational age; assess fetal growth pattern; size/date discrepancy; suspected ectopic pregnancy; suspected hydatidiform mole; determine fetal presentation/lie; suspected hydramnios/oligohydramnios; suspected fetal anomaly or fetal demise; determine placental location, integrity, maturity; identify number of fetuses; aid in diagnostic procedures, e.g., amniocentesis, CVS
   b. Nonstress test (NST)
      (1) Definition—diagnostic test that monitors fetal heart rate acceleration in response to fetal movement (noninvasive); both NST and contraction stress test (CST) were developed to assess any indication of uteroplacental insufficiency and to predict ability of fetus to endure stress of labor
      (2) Indications—decreased fetal movement; post-term pregnancy; intrauterine growth restriction; hypertensive disorders
      (3) Procedure—fetal heart rate (FHR), fetal movement, and uterine contractions are assessed (using external monitoring) over a 20-minute period; may be extended to 40 minutes if no FHR accelerations occur
      (4) Interpretation
         (a) Reactive NST—two or more accelerations in FHR of 15 or more

beats per minute, lasting for 15 seconds or more; fetal well-being assured for 1 week (repeat weekly)
            (b) Nonreactive NST—absence of appropriate heart rate accelerations over a 40-minute period; consider additional testing, e.g., contraction stress test (CST) or biophysical profile
      c. Contraction stress test (CST)
         (1) Definition—diagnostic test performed to evaluate fetal response to uterine contractions; mimics labor
         (2) Procedure—baseline tracing obtained for 10–20 minutes; if fewer than three contractions occur in 10-minute period, contractions stimulated by intravenous oxytocin infusion or nipple stimulation
         (3) Interpretation
            (a) Positive CST—late decelerations following 50% or more of contractions; delivery recommended or further tests (test has 30% false-positive rate)
            (b) Negative CST—no late or variable decelerations; subsequent testing based on fetal and maternal conditions and institutional protocol
            (c) Equivocal CST—late decelerations in fewer than 50% of contractions, or significant variable decelerations; repeat in 24 hours or do biophysical profile
         (4) Contraindications—premature rupture of membranes, history of PTL during current pregnancy, incompetent cervix or cerclage, previous vertical uterine incision, third-trimester bleeding, polyhydramnios, placenta previa, multiple pregnancy
      d. Biophysical profile (BPP)
         (1) Definition—use of real-time ultrasound to assess fetal tone, breathing, body movements, and amniotic fluid volume combined with NST to evaluate FHR accelerations (total of five variables)
         (2) Indications—high-risk pregnancy, e.g., postdate pregnancy, decreased fetal movement, maternal disease, suspected oligohydramnios, intrauterine growth restriction
         (3) Interpretation—each of five variables is scored as 2 (normal) or 0 (abnormal), with total possible score of 10
            (a) 8–10—normal (in absence of oligohydramnios)
            (b) 6—equivocal (repeat according to agency protocol)
            (c) < 4—abnormal (consider delivery)
      e. Fetal movement/kick counts
         (1) Definition—fetal movement assessment by mother
         (2) Indications—generally start at 28 weeks if identifiable risks present or 34–36 weeks if low risk for uteroplacental insufficiency
         (3) Interpretation—various methods of counting are used
            (a) Optimal number of movements and ideal duration of counting has not been established
            (b) Cardiff "count to 10" method—start at approximately same time each day and chart how long it takes to count 10 movements; if fewer than 10 movements in 10 hours or amount to reach 10 movements increases, consider NST
            (c) More important than a quantitative guideline is the mother's perception of a decrease in fetal activity in relation to a previous level

- Common Complaints in Pregnancy
  1. Nausea and vomiting
     a. Etiology—high levels of hCG in first trimester, changes in carbohydrate metabolism, delayed gastric emptying
     b. Management
        (1) Rule out hyperemesis gravidarum, pyelonephritis
        (2) Small, frequent, high-carbohydrate meals; avoid high-fat or spicy meals; avoid empty or overdistended stomach
        (3) Ginger in the form of ginger ale or supplement
  2. Backache
     a. Etiology—softening and relaxation of pelvic structures and joints; increased lordosis of spine caused by shift in center of gravity
     b. Management
        (1) Rule out pyelonephritis, labor, musculoskeletal disease
        (2) Teach pelvic tilt exercise; use proper body mechanics; avoid excessive twisting, bending, and stretching

3. Varicosities
   a. Etiology—pressure of enlarged uterus causing impaired venous circulation and increased venous pressure in lower extremities; relaxation of vein walls and valves; hereditary factors; weight gain
   b. Management
      (1) Rule out thrombophlebitis
      (2) Support pantyhose; frequent leg elevation; avoid standing for long periods, crossing legs, and knee-high hose
4. Hemorrhoids
   a. Etiology—pressure of enlarging uterus; constipation; predisposition to varicosities
   b. Management
      (1) Rule out abscessed or thrombosed hemorrhoids
      (2) Topical anesthetics; prevent or treat constipation by increasing fluids and roughage in diet; warm or cool sitz baths; ice packs or cold compresses
5. Constipation
   a. Etiology—decreased intestinal motility caused by progesterone and compression of bowel by enlarging uterus; oral iron supplements
   b. Management—increase high-fiber foods and fluids; regular exercise; bulk-forming, nonnutritive laxative
6. Heartburn
   a. Etiology—decreased gastrointestinal peristalsis and relaxation of cardiac sphincter; reflux of gastric contents into lower esophagus; upward displacement and compression of the stomach by uterus
   b. Management
      (1) Rule out cardiac, gallbladder, epigastric, or pancreatic disease, PIH
      (2) Small, frequent meals; avoid fatty foods; fluids between, but not with, meals; after eating do not lie down for at least 1 hour; low-sodium antacids
7. Pica and food cravings
   a. Etiology—unknown
   b. Management—evaluate diet to determine adequacy; explain need to maintain healthy diet; problems may occur if craved substance is substituting for nutritious food or is harmful to mother or fetus
8. Ptyalism (increased salivation)
   a. Etiology—unknown
   b. Management—reassurance of resolution following pregnancy; good oral hygiene; avoid excessive starch intake; adequate fluid intake
9. Fatigue—most common in first and third trimesters
   a. Etiology
      (1) Early pregnancy—increased oxygen consumption, increased progesterone level, fetal demands
      (2) Late pregnancy—sleep deprivation from physical discomforts
   b. Management
      (1) Rule out iron-deficiency anemia, depression
      (2) Reassurance; encourage adequate sleep and rest periods
10. Headache
    a. Etiology—increased circulatory volume; vasodilation caused by high progesterone levels; vascular congestion; stress; fatigue; hypoglycemia
    b. Management
       (1) Rule out PIH, migraine headache, sinus infection
       (2) Teach symptoms of PIH; encourage adequate rest; stress reduction; massage; moist hot or cold compresses; avoid intake of foods that trigger headaches; acetaminophen
11. Vaginal discharge (leukorrhea)
    a. Etiology—estrogen-induced increase in vascularity and hypertrophy of cervical glands and vaginal cells
    b. Management
       (1) Rule out ruptured membranes, vaginitis, cervicitis, STI
       (2) Reassurance; cotton underwear and loose clothing; avoid douching or tampon use; keep vulva clean and dry
12. Urinary frequency
    a. Etiology—enlargement of uterus compresses bladder; hyperplasia and hyperemia of pelvic organs and increased kidney output
    b. Management
       (1) Rule out urinary tract infection (UTI)
       (2) Void frequently; maintain adequate fluid intake; discontinue fluids 2–3 hours prior to bedtime; avoid caffeine
13. Leg cramps
    a. Etiology—pressure of uterus on pelvic nerves and blood vessels; imbalance in phosphorus/calcium ratio caused by inadequate or excessive calcium intake (postulated)
    b. Management
       (1) Rule out thromboembolic disease, varicosities
       (2) Avoid stretching legs, pointing toes, and lying on back; dorsiflexion of foot

to relieve cramp in calf; diet evaluation to correct excessive or inadequate intake of calcium
14. Round ligament pain
    a. Etiology—growth of uterus causes round ligaments to stretch
    b. Management
        (1) Rule out PTL, ectopic pregnancy, ruptured ovarian cyst, appendicitis
        (2) Reassurance of resolution following pregnancy; avoid sudden, twisting movements; heating pad; avoid excessive exercise, standing, or walking
15. Dyspnea (breathlessness)
    a. Etiology—increased sensitivity to lower levels of $CO_2$ (progesterone effect) in early pregnancy; later in pregnancy caused by displacement of diaphragm by enlarging uterus
    b. Management
        (1) Rule out upper respiratory infection, pulmonary or cardiac problem
        (2) Sleep with head elevated; reassure improvement will occur when fetus drops into pelvis; avoid exercise if a precipitating factor
16. Edema
    a. Etiology—increased capillary permeability (hormonal); pressure of uterus impedes venous return; increased fluid in intracellular spaces
    b. Management
        (1) Assess for PIH
        (2) Instruct about symptoms of PIH; rest in left lateral recumbent position for 1–2 hours during day and at night; elevate legs several times during day; avoid constrictive clothing; avoid long periods of sitting or standing

- Immunizations and Medication Use in Pregnancy
    1. Immunizations
        a. Preconception immunization of women to prevent infections harmful to fetus is recommended
        b. Postpartum vaccination for rubella and varicella in susceptible women is encouraged
        c. The use of live attenuated vaccines during pregnancy is contraindicated—e.g., measles, mumps, rubella, varicella
        d. Women should be advised not to become pregnant for at least 4 weeks after receiving a live attenuated vaccine
        e. Influenza vaccine—indicated for women who are pregnant in the second or third trimester during the flu season and for women at high risk for pulmonary complications regardless of trimester
        f. Hepatitis A and B—indicated preexposure and postexposure for women at risk of infection
        g. Pneumococcus—indications not altered by pregnancy
        h. Tetanus-diphtheria acellular pertussis (Tdap) should be given with each pregnancy
        i. Immune globulins for hepatitis A and B, rabies, tetanus, and varicella may be used during pregnancy
        j. Refer to Centers for Disease Control and Prevention (CDC) at http://www.cdc.gov/vaccines/pubs/preg-guide.htm for the most up-to-date immunization recommendations
    2. Medication use—Food and Drug Administration (FDA) risk factor categories for prescription drugs in pregnancy
        a. Category A—adequate, well-controlled studies in pregnant women have not shown an increased risk of fetal abnormalities
        b. Category B—animal studies have revealed no evidence of harm to the fetus; however, there are no adequate and well-controlled studies in pregnant women OR animal studies have shown an adverse effect, but adequate and well-controlled studies in pregnant women have failed to demonstrate a risk to the fetus
        c. Category C—animal studies have shown an adverse effect and there are no adequate and well-controlled studies in pregnant women OR no animal studies have been conducted and there are no adequate and well-controlled studies in pregnant women
        d. Category D—adequate and well-controlled or observational studies in pregnant women have demonstrated risk to the fetus; however, the benefits of therapy may outweigh the potential risks
        e. Category X—adequate and well-controlled or observational studies in pregnant women or animals have demonstrated positive evidence of fetal abnormalities that clearly outweigh any possible benefit to the woman

- Pregnancy Complications
    1. Bleeding disorders
        a. Spontaneous abortion (SAB)
            (1) Definition—naturally occurring termination of pregnancy before 20 weeks' gestation

(2) Etiology—chromosomal abnormalities of fetus; chronic maternal disease, infection, or endocrine imbalance; faulty implantation; immune factors; advanced maternal age
(3) Signs and symptoms/physical examination findings
  (a) Threatened abortion—occurs in one of four pregnancies
    (i) Vaginal bleeding with or without cramping; may be accompanied by low backache
    (ii) No cervical changes; cervix closed
  (b) Inevitable
    (i) Vaginal bleeding with contractions; possible gush of fluid from vagina
    (ii) Cervical dilation and rupture of membranes
  (c) Missed abortion—prolonged retention of fetus after fetal death
    (i) Loss of symptoms of pregnancy; may have brownish vaginal discharge
    (ii) Gradual decrease in uterine size; cervix closed and firm
  (d) Incomplete abortion—incomplete expulsion of products of conception (POC), usually placenta retained
    (i) Bleeding (may be profuse); cramping
    (ii) May observe tissue in cervical canal
  (e) Complete abortion—complete expulsion of all POC
    (i) Bleeding; cramping
    (ii) No retained POC; cervix dilated
(4) Differential diagnosis
  (a) Vaginal/cervical infection
  (b) Cervical polyp
  (c) Ectopic pregnancy
  (d) Molar pregnancy
  (e) Implantation bleeding
(5) Diagnostic tests/findings
  (a) Ultrasound for evidence of fetal heart action and uterine size
  (b) Serial hCG levels
  (c) Pelvic exam to evaluate cervical dilation, uterine size, and bleeding
(6) Management/treatment
  (a) Pelvic rest (nothing in vagina); hydration; counsel regarding signs of infection and when to report symptoms
  (b) May require hospitalization, dilation and curettage (D&C), transfusion, IV fluids
  (c) RhoGAM for unsensitized Rh-negative women
  (d) Emotional support
b. Ectopic pregnancy
  (1) Definition—implantation of fertilized ovum outside the uterine cavity (usually in fallopian tube)
  (2) Etiology—any condition that prevents or slows passage of fertilized ovum into uterus—e.g., tubal damage from previous pelvic infection, tubal surgery, previous ectopic; progestin-only contraceptive use
  (3) Signs and symptoms/physical findings
    (a) Before rupture—early pregnancy symptoms; amenorrhea followed by spotting/bleeding; lower abdominal pain, unilateral or bilateral; uterus normal to slightly enlarged; may have unilateral, tender adnexal mass
    (b) After rupture—sharp, unilateral abdominal pain, may radiate to shoulder; syncope/fainting/shock; spotting/bleeding; adnexal tenderness, possible fullness; cervical motion tenderness; bulging of posterior cul-de-sac
  (4) Differential diagnosis
    (a) Acute appendicitis
    (b) Pelvic inflammatory disease (PID)
    (c) Ruptured corpus luteum cyst
    (d) SAB
  (5) Diagnostic tests/findings
    (a) Ultrasound—no evidence of intrauterine pregnancy; may be gestational sac with no apparent heartbeat
    (b) CBC—may indicate anemia, slight leukocytosis
    (c) Serum beta hCG—positive, but hCG level lower than expected for gestational age
    (d) Serial beta hCG levels—level rises slowly or plateaus; with intrauterine pregnancy, doubles every 2 days
  (6) Management/treatment—hospitalization; surgery for repair or removal of damaged tube; medical management

with methotrexate; fluid replacement; transfusion if needed; RhoGAM administration for Rh-negative woman
- c. Placenta previa
  - (1) Definition—abnormal implantation of placenta in lower uterine segment
  - (2) Etiology—unknown; may be associated with multiparity, multiple gestation, previous cesarean, previous uterine surgery, smoking
  - (3) Signs and symptoms/physical findings
    - (a) Painless bleeding after 20 weeks' gestation; usually in third trimester
    - (b) Uterus nontender; usually no evidence of fetal distress
  - (4) Differential diagnosis
    - (a) Abruptio placentae
    - (b) Cervical lesion or cervicitis
    - (c) Nonvaginal bleeding (rectal or urinary)
  - (5) Diagnostic tests/findings
    - (a) Ultrasound—indicates low-lying placenta
    - (b) *No* pelvic exam
  - (6) Management/treatment
    - (a) Gestation less than 36 weeks—expectant management; hospitalization and bed rest; fetal surveillance; monitor mother for increased bleeding
    - (b) Gestation 36 weeks or more—anticipate delivery; may need amniocentesis to assess fetal lung maturity
- d. Abruptio placentae
  - (1) Definition—partial or complete detachment of normally implanted placenta any time prior to delivery
  - (2) Etiology—unknown; contributing factors include maternal hypertension, cocaine use, smoking, advanced maternal age, multiparity, trauma, preterm rupture of membranes, uterine anomalies
  - (3) Signs and symptoms/physical findings
    - (a) Vaginal bleeding of varying amount with severe, unremitting abdominal pain
    - (b) Uterine tenderness, increased uterine tone, contractions, signs of fetal distress, signs of shock
  - (4) Differential diagnosis
    - (a) Placenta previa
    - (b) Appendicitis
    - (c) Labor
  - (5) Diagnostic tests/findings—ultrasound for placental location
  - (6) Management/treatment
    - (a) Immediate transport for emergency care
    - (b) Immediate delivery if massive bleeding or fetal distress
    - (c) Expectant management in emergency facility if fetus immature, no evidence of fetal distress or maternal hypovolemia or anemia
2. Pregnancy-induced hypertension (PIH)
   - a. Definitions
     - (1) Chronic hypertension (HTN)—blood pressure (BP) > 140/90 mm Hg present before pregnancy, diagnosed before 20 weeks of gestation, or not resolved in postpartum; preeclampsia may be superimposed on chronic hypertension
     - (2) Preeclampsia—pregnancy-specific syndrome of reduced organ perfusion secondary to vasospasm and activation of a coagulation cascade
       - (a) Usually occurs after 20 weeks' gestation
       - (b) Elevated blood pressure (> 140/90 mm Hg) accompanied by proteinuria and edema
       - (c) Clinical spectrum ranges from mild to severe forms
     - (3) HELLP syndrome—seen with severe preeclampsia, multiorgan system failure; **H**emolytic anemia, **E**levated **L**iver enzymes, **L**ow **P**latelets
     - (4) Eclampsia—occurrence of seizures in woman with preeclampsia that cannot be attributed to other causes
   - b. Etiology
     - (1) Cause is unknown
     - (2) Predisposing factors—primigravidas, age < 19 or > 35 years, family history of preeclampsia, multiple gestation, antiphospholipid antibody syndrome, thromboembolic disorders, diabetes mellitus, or other chronic diseases
   - c. Signs and symptoms/physical findings
     - (1) Mild preeclampsia—HTN with BP < 160/110 mm Hg, proteinuria, edema, no maternal symptoms
     - (2) Severe preeclampsia—BP > 160/100 mm Hg, proteinuria, generalized edema, oliguria, cerebral disturbances (severe headaches, disorientation), visual disturbances (scotoma, blurred vision), hyperreflexia, epigastric or right upper

quadrant pain, enlarged liver, pulmonary edema, fetal growth restriction
- d. Differential diagnosis
  - (1) Chronic hypertension
  - (2) Gestational trophoblastic disease
  - (3) Renal disease
  - (4) Liver disease
  - (5) Brain tumor
- e. Diagnostic tests/findings
  - (1) Findings dependent on severity of PIH (laboratory tests other than proteinuria normal with mild preeclampsia)
  - (2) Proteinuria—> 300 mg/24 hours or persistent > 30 mg/dL (1+ dipstick) in random urine samples
  - (3) Serum creatinine, ALT/AST, uric acid elevated
  - (4) Platelet count—< 100,000 cells/mm$^3$
  - (5) Hemoglobin/hematocrit elevated (hemoconcentration)
  - (6) Increased lactate dehydrogenase (LDH)—microangiopathic hemolysis
  - (7) Ultrasound—may indicate fetal growth restriction
- f. Management/treatment—goal is prevention of seizures and hematological, renal, and hepatic complications in mother and birth of uncompromised newborn as close to term as possible
  - (1) Antepartum
    - (a) Intermittent bed rest in left lateral position throughout day
    - (b) Adequate nutrition and hydration
    - (c) Careful monitoring of mother—BP, proteinuria, edema, weight, intake and output, deep tendon reflexes (DTR), subjective symptoms, laboratory tests
    - (d) Careful monitoring of fetus—NST, BPP, fetal movement counts, serial ultrasounds, fetal maturity tests
    - (e) Educate mother to report headaches, visual disturbances, disorientation, epigastric/abdominal pain, decreased urinary output
    - (f) Hospitalization and early delivery may be necessary
  - (2) Intrapartum
    - (a) Goal is to prevent seizures and deliver newborn
    - (b) Magnesium sulfate—used as an anticonvulsant
      - (i) Drug action—interferes with the release of acetylcholine at the synapses, decreasing neuromuscular and CNS irritability
      - (ii) Side effects/adverse reactions—drowsiness, hypotension, bradycardia, diarrhea, flushing, sweating, respiratory depression, muscular paralysis
      - (iii) Monitor for signs of toxicity—vital signs, DTR, magnesium levels, urinary output (decreased output increases chance for toxicity)
      - (iv) Overdose antidote is calcium gluconate
    - (c) Hydralazine—most commonly used antihypertensive for severe HTN
    - (d) Diuretics should not be used because they may further compromise placental perfusion
3. Preterm labor (PTL)
   - a. Definition—documented persistent uterine contractions (at least four in 20 minutes or eight in 60 minutes) and at least one of the following (documented cervical change or cervix < 1 cm dilated and/or 80% effaced when gestational age is 20 weeks or greater and less than 37 weeks)
   - b. Etiology
     - (1) Not always known—often multifactorial
     - (2) Predisposing factors—maternal chronic disease, PIH, uterine anomalies, trauma to abdomen, genitourinary infection, chorioamnionitis, systemic infections, previous history of PTL, incompetent cervix, multiple gestation, hydramnios, placenta previa or abruption, premature rupture of membranes, lower socioeconomic status
   - c. Signs and symptoms/physical findings
     - (1) Menstrual-like cramps, pelvic pressure, constant or intermittent low backache, change in vaginal discharge (increased, watery, pink-tinged)
     - (2) Contractions documented by fetal monitoring or palpation, cervical dilation and/or effacement, ruptured membranes
   - d. Differential diagnosis
     - (1) Braxton-Hicks contractions
     - (2) Urinary tract infection/pyelonephritis
     - (3) Vaginal infection
   - e. Diagnostic tests and findings
     - (1) Urinalysis—negative for infection
     - (2) Positive ferning and nitrazine tests if rupture of membranes
   - f. Management/treatment

(1) Conservative measures if cervical changes not advanced—hydration (no evidence to support but often advised), modified bed rest (up to bathroom, meals, and shower)—prolonged bed rest may increase risk for thromboembolic complications; avoid bladder distention, avoid sexual intercourse and orgasm, avoid breast stimulation, continue to monitor fetal status and status of contractions
(2) Tocolytics—useful in postponing birth to allow time for administration of corticosteroids to enhance fetal lung maturity
 (a) Use if 20–34 weeks, membranes intact, cervical dilation < 4 cm, effacement < 80%, and fetus not in distress
 (b) Contraindications—chorioamnionitis, severe preeclampsia, placenta previa, fetal distress, lethal fetal anomalies, maternal hemodynamic instability, cardiac disease, or cardiac rhythm disturbance
 (c) Beta-adrenergic agonists (ritodrine, terbutaline)
  (i) Drug action—interferes with smooth muscle contractility
  (ii) Side effects/adverse reactions—tachycardia, tremors, anxiety, hyperglycemia, hypokalemia, pulmonary edema, fetal tachycardia
 (d) Magnesium sulfate
  (i) Drug action—acts on vascular smooth muscle causing vasodilation
  (ii) Side effects/adverse reactions—drowsiness, hypotension, bradycardia, diarrhea, flushing, sweating, respiratory depression, muscular paralysis
  (iii) Monitor for signs of toxicity—vital signs, DTR, magnesium levels, urinary output (decreased output increases chance for toxicity)
  (iv) Overdose antidote is calcium gluconate
(3) Corticosteroids (betamethasone, dexamethasone)—stimulate fetal surfactant production and reduce risk for neonatal respiratory distress syndrome
 (a) May be given between 24 and 34 weeks unless there is an indication for immediate delivery
 (b) Optimal benefits begin 24 hours after starting therapy

## FERTILITY CONTROL

- Combination Oral Contraceptives (COC)
 1. Description—pill taken daily for contraception or for specific noncontraceptive benefits; combination of estrogen and progestin
  a. Monophasic pills—deliver constant amount of estrogen/progestin throughout cycle
  b. Multiphasic pills—vary amount of estrogen and/or progestin delivered throughout cycle; concept is to mimic natural menstrual cycle more closely
 2. Mechanism of action
  a. Estrogen—inhibits ovulation through suppression of follicle-stimulating hormone (FSH), alters cellular structure of the endometrium, stabilizes endometrium, potentiates progestin
   (1) Ethinyl estradiol ($E_2$)—most prevalent synthetic estrogen in COC
   (2) Mestranol—weaker estrogen; utilized in older COC formulations
  b. Progestin—inhibits ovulation through suppression of luteinizing hormone (LH); produces atrophic endometrium; thickens cervical mucus; decreases ovum transport through fallopian tube; may inhibit capacitation of sperm; numerous forms are available
 3. Effectiveness/first-year failure rate
  a. Perfect use—0.1%
  b. Typical use—5%
 4. Advantages
  a. Ease of use
  b. Reversible
  c. Effective
  d. May reduce incidence of/afford protection against
   (1) Acne
   (2) Dysmenorrhea
   (3) Pelvic inflammatory disease
   (4) Ectopic pregnancy
   (5) Endometriosis
   (6) Osteoporosis
   (7) Functional ovarian cysts
   (8) Ovarian cancer; endometrial cancer
   (9) Premenstrual syndrome
 5. Disadvantages/side effects
  a. Does not prevent transmission of STI/HIV

b. Requires user compliance/daily dosing schedule
c. Side effects may include
    (1) Estrogenic effects
        (a) Nausea
        (b) Increased breast size
        (c) Cyclic weight gain
        (d) Leukorrhea
        (e) Hypertension
        (f) Increased cholesterol concentration in gallbladder bile
        (g) Growth of leiomyomata
        (h) Telangiectasia
        (i) Chloasma
        (j) Cerebrovascular accidents
        (k) Thromboembolic complications, including pulmonary emboli
        (l) Stimulation of breast neoplasia
    (2) Progestogenic side effects (alone or in combination with estrogen)
        (a) Breast tenderness
        (b) Headaches
        (c) Hypertension
        (d) Decreased libido
    (3) Androgenic effects
        (a) Increased appetite/weight gain
        (b) Depression, fatigue
        (c) Acne, oily skin
        (d) Increased breast tenderness/size
        (e) Increased low-density lipoprotein (LDL) cholesterol
        (f) Decreased high-density lipoprotein (HDL) cholesterol
        (g) Decreased carbohydrate tolerance/increased insulin resistance
6. Contraindications (World Health Organization [WHO] category 4 use represents unacceptable risk)
    a. Refrain from providing if any of the following conditions exist
        (1) Venous thromboembolism
        (2) Cerebrovascular accident, coronary artery/ischemic heart disease
        (3) Structural heart disease
        (4) Pregnancy
        (5) Breast cancer
        (6) Lactation (less than 6 weeks' postpartum)
        (7) Benign hepatic adenoma, liver cancer, or history thereof; active viral hepatitis; severe cirrhosis
        (8) Headaches (migraine) with focal neurological symptoms
        (9) Major surgery with prolonged immobilization, any surgery on legs
        (10) Age 35 years or older smoking 15 or more cigarettes daily
        (11) Hypertension systolic > 160 or diastolic > 100
        (12) Vascular disease
        (13) Known thrombotic mutations
    b. Exercise caution WHO category 3 risks outweigh benefit
        (1) Postpartum less than 21 days
        (2) Lactation (6 weeks–6 months)
        (3) Undiagnosed, abnormal vaginal/uterine bleeding
        (4) Age 35 years or older smoking fewer than 15 cigarettes daily
        (5) Past history breast cancer with no recurrence for 5 years
        (6) Adequately controlled hypertension or BP of systolic 140–159 or diastolic 90–99 mm Hg
        (7) Untreated stage 1 hypertension
        (8) Bariatric bypass procedures (only combined oral options)
        (9) Age 35 years or older with migraine headache, but no focal neurological symptoms
        (10) Use of drugs that alter liver enzymes—rifampin, phenytoin, griseofulvin, carbamazepine, barbiturates, topiramate, primidone
        (11) Gallbladder disease/history of COC-related cholestasis
        (12) Diabetes mellitus (DM) type 1 or 2 of > 20 years duration and/or comorbid vascular disease
7. Management
    a. Health assessment prior to initiation of method
        (1) Elicit information from thorough history concerning any contraindications/risk to use of COCs
        (2) Blood pressure
        (3) Pelvic examination/Pap smear not required but recommended if patient sexually active, now or in past
        (4) Clinical breast examination not required but recommended if age > 20 years
        (5) Mammogram not required but recommended if age > 40 years
    b. Health assessment at follow-up visits
        (1) Patients may be assessed yearly if no risk factors
        (2) Patients with risk factors may be seen at 3- to 6-month intervals
    c. Special considerations
        (1) Management of breakthrough bleeding/spotting
            (a) Common side effect first 3 months of use
            (b) Reinforce to take pills daily at the same time

- (c) Change to 30–35 mcg estrogen if on 20 mcg COC and bleeding is during first half of cycle
- (d) Change to COC with different progestin
- (e) If problem persists, consider another cause for bleeding, e.g., infection, polyps
(2) Management of absence of withdrawal bleeding
- (a) Occurs in about 5% of women after several years of COC use
- (b) Rule out pregnancy
- (c) No intervention required if woman is okay with no menses
- (d) Change to 30–35 mcg estrogen if on 20 mcg COC
- (e) Add supplemental estrogen to regimen for first 3 weeks of one cycle
8. Instructions for use
   a. General instructions
      (1) Backup method used (e.g., condoms) for first 7 days of first pack
         (a) Necessary only if patient is on Sunday start pack or begins pills after day 5 of menstrual cycle
         (b) Initiation on first day of cycle ensures protection
      (2) Pill taken at approximately same time each day
      (3) If nausea occurs, pill taken with meals or at bedtime
      (4) Backup method (condoms) used if efficacy/absorbency compromised by severe vomiting/diarrhea
      (5) Condom use considered for prevention of STI/HIV
   b. Missed pills
      (1) If 1 pill missed, take as soon as remembered and take next pill at normal time; use backup method for 7 days if pill missed in week 1
      (2) If 2 pills missed in week 1 or 2, 2 pills taken on day remembered and 2 pills the next day; pack finished as usual; backup method used for 7 days
      (3) If 2 pills missed in week 3
         (a) Sunday start—1 pill taken each day until Sunday; remainder of pack discarded; new pack started; backup method used for 7 days
         (b) First day menses start—remainder of pack discarded and new pack started immediately; backup method used for 7 days
      (4) Emergency contraception considered if unprotected intercourse occurred during days when backup method should have been used
   c. Warning signs (ACHES)
      (1) **A**bdominal pain (severe)
      (2) **C**hest pain (sharp, severe, shortness of breath)
      (3) **H**eadache (severe, dizziness, unilateral)
      (4) **E**ye problems (scotoma, blurred vision, blind spots)
      (5) **S**evere leg pain (calf or thigh)

- Progestin-Only Pills (POP)
  1. Description—pill taken daily for purposes of contraception; comprised of synthetic progestins in lower doses than those used in combination oral contraceptive pills
  2. Mechanism of action
     a. Inhibits ovulation through suppression of FSH and LH
     b. Produces atrophic endometrium
     c. Thickens cervical mucus
     d. Slows ovum transport through fallopian tube
     e. May inhibit sperm capacitation
  3. Effectiveness/first-year failure rate
     a. Perfect use—0.5%
     b. Typical use—5%
  4. Advantages
     a. Ease of use
     b. Reversible
     c. Effective
     d. Contains no estrogen for women in whom it is contraindicated or who cannot tolerate estrogenic side effects
     e. Can be used during lactation
  5. Disadvantages and side effects
     a. Decreased availability/increased expense compared to COC
     b. Strict daily dosing schedule
     c. No protection against STI/HIV
  6. Contraindications (WHO recommendations)
     a. Refrain from providing if any of the following conditions exist
        (1) Pregnancy
        (2) Breast cancer
     b. Exercise caution if any of the following conditions exist
        (1) Use of drugs that alter liver enzymes (same as with COC)
        (2) Lactation (less than 6 weeks' postpartum)
        (3) History of breast cancer with 5-year disease-free interval
        (4) Current deep vein thrombosis or pulmonary emboli
        (5) Liver conditions such as cirrhosis, adenoma, cancer, active viral hepatitis

(6) Current/history of ischemic heart disease or cerebrovascular accident
(7) Development of migraine headaches with focal neurological symptoms while using the method
7. Management
   a. Health assessment prior to initiation of method—refer to COC section earlier in this appendix
   b. Health assessment at follow-up visits—refer to COC section earlier in this appendix
   c. Special considerations—ectopic pregnancy more likely if pregnancy occurs
8. Instructions for using the method
   a. General instruction
      (1) Pills started on cycle day 1 (first day of menses)
      (2) Pill taken at same time each day every day; no placebo/off week
         (a) If more than 3 hours late taking pill, backup method should be used for 48 hours
         (b) If more than 1 pill is missed, 2 pills should be taken for 2 days, backup method should be used for rest of cycle, clinician should be notified if no bleeding occurs in 4–6 weeks
   b. Warning signs
      (1) Severe low abdominal pain
      (2) No bleeding after series of regular cycles
      (3) Severe headache

- Transdermal Contraceptive System
  1. Description—patch applied to skin; delivers continuous daily systemic dose of progestin (norelgestromin) and estrogen (ethinyl estradiol), new patch applied each week for 3 weeks followed by 1 week without patch to induce withdrawal bleeding
  2. Mechanism of action—same as COC
  3. Effectiveness/first-year failure rate
     a. Perfect use—0.99%
     b. Typical use—1.24%
  4. Advantages
     a. Ease of use—no daily dosing regimen
     b. Reversible
     c. Effective
     d. Good menstrual cycle control
  5. Disadvantages and side effects
     a. Does not prevent transmission of STI/HIV
     b. Skin irritation at application site
     c. Other side effects similar to those of COC
  6. Contraindications (WHO recommendations)
     a. Refrain from providing if any of the following conditions exist—same as with COC
     b. Exercise caution if any of the following conditions exist—same as with COC
  7. Management
     a. Health assessment prior to initiation—same as with COC
     b. Health assessment at follow-up visits—same as with COC
     c. Special considerations
        (1) May be less effective in women who weigh > 90 kg (198 pounds)
        (2) Probably same drug interactions as with COC
  8. Instructions for using the method
     a. First patch applied on first Sunday after menstrual period starts; backup method used for first 7 days
     b. Patch applied first day of menses; no backup method needed
     c. Patch applied to buttocks, abdomen, upper torso front or back (excluding breasts), upper outer arm
     d. New patch applied on same day each week for total of 3 weeks
     e. Patch not worn on week 4; withdrawal bleeding will occur
     f. Use of condoms considered for STI/HIV prevention
     g. New patch applied if current patch partially or completely pulls away from skin
     h. Healthcare provider contacted if warning signs occur—same as COC warning signs

- Contraceptive Vaginal Ring (NuvaRing)
  1. Description—soft, malleable, clear plastic ring; delivers continuous, systemic dose of estrogen (ethinyl estradiol) and progestin (etonogestrel); worn in vagina for 3 weeks followed by 1 week without ring to induce withdrawal bleeding
  2. Mechanism of action—same as COC
  3. Effectiveness/first-year failure rate
     a. Perfect use—data not available
     b. Typical use—2%
  4. Advantages
     a. Ease of use—no daily dosing regimen
     b. Reversible
     c. Effective
     d. Good menstrual cycle control
  5. Disadvantages and side effects
     a. Does not prevent transmission of STI/HIV
     b. Side effects similar to those of COC
     c. Vaginal discharge/vaginal irritation
  6. Contraindications (WHO recommendations)
     a. Refrain from providing if any of the following conditions exist—same as with COC
     b. Exercise caution if any of the following conditions exist—same as with COC

7. Management
   a. Health assessment prior to initiation—same as with COC
   b. Health assessment at follow-up visits—same as with COC
   c. Special considerations—probably same drug interactions as with COC
8. Instructions for using the method
   a. First vaginal ring inserted within 5 days of start of menstrual period
   b. Ring folded and gently inserted into vagina
   c. Exact position of ring in vagina is not important
   d. Ring left in vagina for 3 weeks, then removed
   e. New ring inserted in 7 days
   f. If ring is expelled or removed for 3 hours or more, backup method used for next 7 days after ring is reinserted in vagina
   g. If ring is left in vagina for more than 3 weeks but less than 4 weeks, it should be removed; new ring inserted after 1-week ring-free period
   h. If ring is left in vagina more than 4 weeks, it may not protect from pregnancy; backup method used until new ring in vagina for 7 days
   i. Healthcare provider contacted if warning signs occur—same as COC warning signs

- Progestin-Only Injectable Contraception (Depo-Provera [DMPA])
  1. Description—intramuscular, injectable progestin administered in 3-month intervals for contraception
  2. Mechanism of action
     a. Inhibits ovulation through suppression of FSH and LH
     b. Produces atrophic endometrium
     c. Thickens cervical mucus
     d. Slows ovum transport through fallopian tube
     e. May inhibit sperm capacitation
  3. Effectiveness/first-year failure rate
     a. Perfect use—0.3%
     b. Typical use—0.3%
  4. Advantages
     a. Ease of use
     b. Effective
     c. Long-term contraceptive option
     d. Does not require compliance with daily/event regimen
     e. Does not have drug interaction profile
     f. Results in absence of menstrual bleeding in up to 50% of women by end of first year of use (4 injections); by end of second year 70% are amenorrheic
     g. Can be used during lactation
  5. Disadvantages/side effects
     a. Menstrual cycle irregularities
     b. Mastalgia
     c. Depression
     d. No protection against STI/HIV
     e. Not immediately reversible—requires 3 months to be eliminated
     f. Requires routine 3-month injection schedule
     g. Weight gain
        (1) Average 5.4 pounds first year
        (2) 13.8 pounds after 4 years
     h. 6- to 12-month delay in return to fertility in some women
     i. Decreased bone density in long-term (greater than 5 years) user—returned to normal following discontinuance
     j. May decrease HDL cholesterol
  6. Contraindications (WHO recommendations)
     a. Refrain from providing if any of the following conditions exist
        (1) Pregnancy
        (2) Breast cancer
     b. Exercise caution if any of the following conditions exist
        (1) Lactation (less than 6 weeks' postpartum)
        (2) History of breast cancer with 5-year disease-free interval
        (3) Current deep vein thrombosis or pulmonary emboli
        (4) Liver conditions such as cirrhosis, adenoma, cancer, or active viral hepatitis
        (5) Current/history of ischemic heart disease or cerebrovascular disease
        (6) Hypertension—systolic > 160 or diastolic > 100 mm Hg or vascular disease
        (7) Multiple risk factors for arterial cardiovascular disease
        (8) Unexplained vaginal bleeding before evaluation
        (9) Development of migraine headaches with neurological symptoms while using the method
  7. Management
     a. Health assessment prior to initiation of method
        (1) Refer to COC section earlier in this appendix
        (2) Include relevant health history
        (3) Baseline weight assessment
     b. Health assessment at follow-up visits
        (1) Return every 3 months for injection
        (2) Determine bleeding pattern—hematocrit/hemoglobin if excessive

(3) Assess for side effects/problems
(4) Weight
c. Special considerations
(1) Consider DMPA as contraceptive of choice for women with
(a) Seizure disorder
(b) Sickle cell disease
(2) DMPA may be administered within 7 days postpartum with no adverse effects on breastfeeding
8. Instructions for using the method
a. Explain importance of adherence to 3-month injection schedule—contraceptive efficacy maintained for 14 weeks after injection
b. Administer first injection within first 5 days of menstrual period
c. Rule out pregnancy prior to first injection if administered other than within first 5 days of menstrual period
d. Counsel patients regarding possibility of irregular bleeding; use of backup contraception if more than 3 months between injections; use of condoms for STI/HIV prevention
e. Warning signs
(1) Frequent intense headache
(2) Heavy, irregular bleeding
(3) Depression
(4) Abdominal pain (severe)
(5) Signs of infection at injection site (prolonged redness, bleeding, pain, discharge)

- Progestin-Only Implants
1. Description—long-term contraceptive system of rod-shaped implant placed subdermally that provides low-dose sustained release of progestin; Nexplanon is the only one currently available in the United States
   a. One rod containing etonogestrel
   b. Effective for 3 years
2. Mechanism of action
   a. Suppresses LH—ovulation inhibited
   b. Produces atrophic endometrium
   c. Thickens cervical mucus
   d. Decreases ovum transport through fallopian tubes
   e. May inhibit sperm capacitation
3. Effectiveness/first-year failure rate
   a. Perfect use—0.05%
   b. Typical use—0.05%
4. Advantages
   a. Ease of use
   b. Effective
   c. Reversible—fertility returns immediately upon removal
   d. Contains no estrogen for women with contradictions to estrogen or who cannot tolerate estrogenic side effects
   e. Can be used during lactation
   f. Affords long-term contraception
   g. High continuation rate
5. Disadvantages and side effects
   a. Requires surgical procedure for insertion and removal; insertion/removal fees expensive
   b. Irregular bleeding
   c. No protection against STI/HIV
6. Contraindications (WHO recommendations)
   a. Refrain from providing if any of the following conditions exist
      (1) Pregnancy
      (2) Breast cancer
   b. Exercise caution if any of the following conditions exist
      (1) Use of drugs that alter liver enzymes (same as with COC)
      (2) Lactation (less than 6 weeks' postpartum)
      (3) History of breast cancer with 5-year disease-free interval
      (4) Current deep vein thrombosis or pulmonary emboli
      (5) Liver conditions such as cirrhosis, adenoma, cancer, active viral hepatitis
      (6) Current/history of ischemic heart disease or cerebrovascular accident
      (7) Development of migraine headaches with focal neurological symptoms while using method
      (8) Unexplained vaginal bleeding before evaluation
7. Management
   a. Health assessment prior to initiation of method
      (1) Refer to COC section earlier in this appendix
      (2) Include relevant health history
   b. Health assessment at follow-up visits
      (1) Return 1 month after insertion to assess site
      (2) Routine annual visits
   c. Special considerations
      (1) Drug interaction—same as with COC
      (2) Good option for diabetic women—no impact on carbohydrate metabolism
8. Instructions for using the method
   a. Use backup contraception for 3–7 days following insertion
   b. Insert within 7 days of start of menstrual period
   c. Rule out pregnancy if inserted other than within 7 days of start of menstrual period

d. Inform patient of replacement date for implants
- Emergency Contraception
  1. Definition—method used to prevent conception after unprotected coitus; involves use of either progestin-only pills (POP) or a copper-containing IUD
  2. Mechanism of action
     a. POP
        (1) Inhibits ovulation (refer to POP mechanism of action section)
        (2) Alters sperm/ova transport
        (3) Will not disrupt an established pregnancy—minimal endometrial effect
     b. Copper-containing IUD
        (1) Prevents fertilization (regular use)
        (2) Interferes with implantation
  3. Effectiveness
     a. POP
        (1) Depends on preexisting fertility
        (2) Reduces risk of pregnancy by at least 75%
        (3) Effective up to 5 days after unprotected intercourse; the sooner taken, the greater the efficacy
     b. IUD—reduces risk of pregnancy by more than 99%
  4. Advantages
     a. Provides means of emergency contraception in event of
        (1) Unplanned intercourse
        (2) Method failure—condom breaks/leaks; IUD expelled; cap/diaphragm dislodged/improperly placed
        (3) Missed COC pills at beginning of pack
        (4) Late for contraceptive injection
        (5) POP may be provided with instructions for use for women using any contraceptive method
     b. Can provide continuous contraception (IUD)
  5. Disadvantages and side effects
     a. POP
        (1) Nausea/vomiting—23% and 6%, respectively
        (2) Change in next menses
     b. Copper-containing IUD
        (1) Irregular, heavy bleeding
        (2) Uterine cramping/abdominal pain
        (3) Refer to following section on intrauterine devices/systems
  6. Precautions and risks
     a. POP
        (1) Contraindication—pregnancy
        (2) Consider actual risk of pregnancy vs. theoretical risk
     b. Copper-containing IUD
        (1) Contraindications
           (a) Pregnancy
           (b) Pelvic inflammatory disease
        (2) See following section on intrauterine devices/systems for details
  7. Management
     a. Health assessment prior to initiation of method
        (1) Urine hCG as needed to determine preexisting pregnancy
        (2) If using IUD
           (a) Speculum examination; wet prep/cervical cultures to assess for STI
           (b) Bimanual examination; determine size/position/consistency of uterus
        (3) Discuss/provide ongoing contraception
     b. Health assessment at follow-up visits
        (1) Follow-up visit if no menses within 1 month or if pregnancy symptoms
        (2) Check placement of IUD (visible string) after first menses
        (3) Perform pregnancy test as needed to determine efficacy
        (4) Discuss/provide ongoing contraception
        (5) Discourage use of emergency contraception as contraceptive method
  8. Instructions for using the method
     a. Progestin-only pills (Plan B)
        (1) Begin first dose within 120 hours after coitus (most effective if initiated within 72 hours)
        (2) Two-dose and single-dose options available
     b. Progesterone receptor modulator (Ella)
        (1) Available as a single pill regimen
        (2) Effective up to 5 days after an act of unprotected intercourse; best efficacy when taken as soon as possible
     c. IUD—can be inserted up to 5 days after intercourse

## INTRAUTERINE DEVICES/SYSTEMS

1. Description—device placed in uterus for purpose of long-acting contraception
2. Mechanism of action
   a. Copper T 380A
      (1) Copper may inhibit sperm capacitation
      (2) Alters tubal/uterine transport of ovum
      (3) Enzymatic influence on endometrium
   b. Progesterone T and levonorgestrel-releasing intrauterine system (LNG IUS)—progestin influence

(1) Thickens cervical mucus
(2) Produces atrophic endometrium
(3) Slows ovum transport through tube
(4) Inhibits sperm motility and function
3. Effectiveness/first-year failure rate
   a. Perfect use
      (1) Copper T—0.6%
      (2) Progesterone T—1.5%
      (3) LNG IUS—0.71%
   b. Typical use
      (1) Copper T—0.8%
      (2) Progesterone T—2.0%
      (3) LNG IUS—0.71%
4. Advantages
   a. Ease of use
   b. Not coitally dependent
   c. Effective
   d. Reversible
   e. No systemic side effects
   f. Cost effective (if used longer than 1 year)
   g. Progestin IUD/IUS can decrease blood loss during menses
   h. Effective choice for women who cannot use other hormonal methods
   i. Can be used during lactation
5. Disadvantages and side effects
   a. Altered menstrual bleeding patterns
      (1) Increased amount and length of menstrual bleeding—Copper T; first few months of LNG IUS
      (2) Increased dysmenorrhea—Copper T
      (3) Absence of bleeding—LNG IUS
   b. Risk of PID
      (1) Increased risk first few weeks following insertion
      (2) Poor choice for women exposed to STI
         (a) Recent history of STI
         (b) Multiple sexual partners
   c. Risk of spontaneous expulsion
      (1) May go undetected by the woman
      (2) More likely at time of menses
6. Contraindications (WHO category 4)
   a. Refrain from providing if any of the following conditions exist
      (1) Known/suspected pregnancy
      (2) PID current or within past 3 months
      (3) Severely distorted uterine cavity
         (a) Leiomyomata
         (b) Endometrial polyps
         (c) Cervical stenosis
         (d) Bicornuate uterus
         (e) Small uterus
      (4) Unexplained vaginal bleeding before evaluation
      (5) Cervical cancer awaiting treatment
      (6) Breast cancer
      (7) Endometrial cancer
   b. Exercise caution WHO category 3 theoretical risks outweigh benefit
      (1) Increased risk for STI—multiple partners, partner with multiple partners
      (2) AIDS-defining illness
      (3) Active hepatitis, severe cirrhosis, benign/malignant liver tumor—LNG IUS only
7. Management
   a. Health assessment prior to initiation of method
      (1) History to include
         (a) STI/PID—current, history of, or symptoms
         (b) Risk factors for STI
         (c) Vaginitis symptoms
         (d) Contraceptive history (e.g., condom use)
         (e) HIV status/exposure
         (f) Pap smear—abnormal results
         (g) Heavy menses/anemia
         (h) Menstrual history
      (2) Physical examination to include
         (a) Speculum examination with wet prep to assess for possible vaginal/cervical infection
            (i) Cervicitis/cervical discharge
            (ii) Suspect infection if numerous white blood cells (WBCs)
         (b) Pap smear (if none within past year)
         (c) Cervical cultures (if history/physical examination indicates)
         (d) Bimanual examination—contour; size; consistency; mobility; position of uterus
         (e) Hemoglobin (Hgb)/hematocrit (Hct) if history of anemia
   b. Health assessment at follow-up visits
      (1) Speculum examination at first menses after insertion—check for IUD strings
      (2) Assessment for any signs/symptoms of pelvic infection
      (3) Hgb/Hct if increased bleeding
   c. Special considerations
      (1) Prophylactic antibiotics at time of insertion
         (a) No consensus regarding risk reduction for postinsertion infection
         (b) May use doxycycline 1-time dose at time of insertion
      (2) Timing of insertion
         (a) Not necessary to wait for menses if evidence patient is not pregnant
         (b) May be inserted at any time if patient not pregnant
            (i) May be inserted immediately after childbirth
            (ii) May be inserted when breast-feeding
            (iii) May be inserted immediately after spontaneous or induced abortion

(3) Menstrual abnormalities (spotting, bleeding)
    (a) Hgb/Hct
        (i) Ferrous sulfate for 2 months if Hgb less than 11.5 g—repeat Hgb/Hct 3 months
        (ii) Remove IUD if Hgb less than 9 g—repeat Hgb/Hct 1 month
    (b) Assess for endometritis/PID if associated with pain
        (i) Cervical cultures
        (ii) Uterine tenderness
        (iii) Treat with antibiotics if suspicious
    (c) If more than 40 years old and prolonged heavy bleeding, remove IUD
(4) Cramping and pain
    (a) If severe—rule out perforation
    (b) If mild—nonsteroidal anti-inflammatory drug (NSAID)/other analgesic or remove IUD
    (c) May indicate infection, pregnancy
(5) Expulsion
    (a) Symptoms—cramping, spotting, dyspareunia, lengthening of string
    (b) Partial expulsion
        (i) Remove IUD
        (ii) Rule out pregnancy/infection
        (iii) Replace IUD if patient desires
        (iv) Doxycycline for 5–7 days
    (c) Complete expulsion
        (i) Pregnancy test
        (ii) Replace IUD if patient desires
(6) Pregnancy
    (a) SAB
        (i) Remove IUD
        (ii) Doxycycline/ampicillin for 7 days
        (iii) Ferrous sulfate if anemic/heavy bleeding
    (b) Patient requests abortion—refer
    (c) Patient wants to continue pregnancy—visible strings
        (i) Advise concerning risk for spontaneous abortion—decreased risk with IUD removal early in pregnancy
        (ii) Gently remove IUD
        (iii) Warning about possible ectopic
    (d) Patient wants to continue pregnancy—no visible strings
        (i) Advise concerning risk for spontaneous abortion
        (ii) Ultrasound to determine if IUD present
        (iii) Monitor for intrauterine infection throughout pregnancy and retrieve IUD at delivery
        (iv) If intrauterine infection occurs, refer for evacuation of uterus
(7) Perforation, embedding
    (a) Perforation occurs 1 in 1,000 insertions
        (i) Ultrasound to determine location—refer for treatment
        (ii) If protrusion through cervix, can be removed in office with local anesthetic
        (iii) May/may not be associated with severe pain
    (b) Embedding
        (i) Can remove IUD from uterus with forceps if visualized
        (ii) May need to be removed with D&C
(8) PID
    (a) Most IUD-related PID occurs within the first 20 days after insertion
    (b) If symptomatic PID occurs, antibiotic therapy should be initiated and the IUD removed
(9) Actinomycosis on Pap smear
    (a) Asymptomatic
        (i) Repeat Pap smear in 1 year
        (ii) If actinomycosis present on repeat Pap smear
            a) Remove IUD; replace after one menstrual cycle
            b) Keep IUD and treat with doxycycline for 14 days; repeat Pap smear
            c) Keep IUD and do not treat; advise to notify healthcare provider if PID symptoms develop
    (b) Symptoms of PID
        (i) Preload with antibiotic
        (ii) Remove IUD
        (iii) Treat PID
8. Instructions for using the method
    a. Check IUD strings
        (1) After each menses
        (2) If increased cramping
        (3) If absent—use backup birth control and notify healthcare provider
        (4) If longer
            (a) May be in process of expulsion
            (b) Use backup birth control and notify healthcare provider
    b. Signs of infection—notify healthcare provider if
        (1) Pelvic pain
        (2) Vaginal discharge
        (3) Unexplained vaginal bleeding
    c. Monitor menses—notify provider if
        (1) Heavy, irregular bleeding
        (2) Missed menses
        (3) Increased cramping

d. Warning signs (PAINS)
   (1) **P**eriod late/missed; abnormal spotting or bleeding
   (2) **A**bdominal pain
   (3) **I**nfection—vaginal discharge
   (4) **N**ot feeling well—fever, aches, chills
   (5) **S**tring missing, shorter or longer

- Vaginal Spermicides
  1. Description—cream, foam, suppository, tablet, film, gel, or other preparation that destroys sperm when placed in vagina
  2. Mechanism of action
     a. Nonoxynol-9 or octoxynol-9 is active ingredient
     b. Destroys sperm cell membrane
  3. Effectiveness/first-year failure rate
     a. Perfect use—6%
     b. Typical use—21–28%
  4. Advantages
     a. Accessible
     b. Inexpensive
     c. Readily available backup method
     d. No systemic effects
  5. Disadvantages and side effects
     a. Coitally dependent
     b. Does not protect against STI/HIV
     c. Potential for allergy/sensitivity/irritation
     d. Must follow instructions for effective use
  6. Precautions and risks
     a. Individuals with skin sensitivities may want to test/avoid use
     b. Individual must be capable of following instructions for use
     c. Vaginal abnormalities (septa, prolapse) may preclude use
  7. Management
     a. No health assessment needed prior to initiation of method
     b. Special considerations—encourage use of spermicide with condom for increased effectiveness
  8. Instructions for using method
     a. Spermicide used with each act of intercourse
     b. All instructions read carefully
     c. Spermicide left in place (no douching) for 6 hours following last intercourse
     d. Instructions should be followed regarding how long prior to intercourse the spermicide may be inserted—if too much time has lapsed, pregnancy may occur
     e. Spermicide placed deep within vagina
     f. Adequate time should be allowed for spermicide to dissolve (if film, tablets, or suppositories)
     g. With foam use—canister should be shaken well, as directed, prior to filling applicator

- Male Condoms
  1. Description—latex/polyurethane/natural membranous sleeve placed over erect penis prior to intercourse to prevent transmission of semen/sperm into vaginal vault
  2. Mechanism of action—barrier; prevents transmission of semen/sperm into vagina
  3. Effectiveness/first-year failure rate
     a. Perfect use—3%
     b. Typical use—14%
  4. Advantages
     a. Accessible
     b. Cost effective
     c. Prevents transmission of STI (except membrane condoms)
     d. Active involvement of male partner
     e. Prevents allergic reaction to semen
     f. Arrests development of antisperm antibodies in infertility patients
     g. May help prevent premature ejaculation
     h. Does not require visit to healthcare provider
  5. Disadvantages and side effects
     a. Decreased penile sensitivity
     b. Interrupts act of sex
     c. Not appropriate for men with erectile dysfunction
     d. Requires active involvement of male partner
     e. Possibility of condom rupture
  6. Contraindications
     a. Latex allergy (male or female partner)—use polyurethane
     b. Spermicide allergy (if condoms lubricated with spermicide)
  7. Management
     a. No health assessment needed prior to initiation of method
     b. Special considerations
        (1) Membrane condoms may not protect against STI/HIV
        (2) Petroleum/oil-based lubricants may decrease effectiveness of latex condoms (okay for polyurethane condom)
  8. Instructions for using method
     a. New condom used with each act of intercourse
     b. Use only water-soluble lubricants—K-Y jelly, Astroglide, Replens, Lubrin
     c. Condom unrolled over penis completely (to the base)
     d. Penis withdrawn from vagina soon after ejaculation—condom secured at base of penis to prevent spillage
     e. If condom slips/breaks
        (1) Before ejaculation—apply new condom

(2) After ejaculation—consider emergency contraception
- Female Condom
  1. Description—polyurethane sheath placed in the vagina that acts as a barrier to prevent direct contact with seminal fluid during intercourse
  2. Mechanism of action—barrier, protects vagina/vulva from direct contact with penis/seminal fluid
  3. Effectiveness/first-year failure rate
     a. Perfect use—5%
     b. Typical use—21%
  4. Advantages
     a. Prevents transmission of STI
        (1) Decreases risk of cervical dysplasia/neoplasia related to HPV
        (2) Decreases risk of PID and sequelae as a result of decreased transmission of gonococcal (GC) infection and chlamydia
     b. Does not require use of spermicide
     c. Accessible
     d. Controlled by the woman
     e. Does not require visit to healthcare provider
  5. Disadvantages and side effects
     a. Coitally dependent
     b. Noisy
     c. May be aesthetically unappealing
     d. Expensive
  6. Precautions and risks
     a. Must be properly inserted/positioned
     b. Polyurethane allergy
  7. Management
     a. No health assessment needed prior to initiation of method
     b. Special considerations—women with vaginal abnormalities should not use this method
  8. Instructions for using the method
     a. Pouch held with open end down—inner ring should be at bottom of pouch
     b. Inner ring squeezed together and inner ring and pouch inserted into vagina
     c. Inner ring pushed deep into vagina
     d. Outer ring should rest outside vulva
     e. Condom removed immediately after intercourse
     f. Outer ring squeezed together and twisted to prevent spillage
     g. Discard
     h. New condom used with each act of intercourse
     i. Male condom should not be used when using female condom—may adhere together, causing dislodgement

- Diaphragm
  1. Description—reusable latex dome that covers anterior vaginal wall, including cervix; spermicide placed in dome covers cervix, affording increased contraceptive protection; types include
     a. Flat spring
        (1) Good for women with firm vaginal tone
        (2) Gentle spring strength
     b. Coil spring
        (1) Good for women with average vaginal tone
        (2) Firm spring strength
     c. Arcing spring
        (1) Good for women with lax vaginal tone
        (2) Firm spring strength
     d. Wide seal
        (1) Good for women with average/lax vaginal tone
        (2) Available as arcing or coil spring
  2. Mechanism of action
     a. Barrier—prevents direct cervical contact with seminal fluid
     b. Spermicide—nonoxynol-9/octoxynol-9 destroys sperm cell membrane
  3. Effectiveness/first-year failure rate
     a. Perfect use—6%
     b. Typical use—20%
  4. Advantages
     a. Cost effective—may be used for 1–2 years
     b. Affords some protection against STI—possible decreased incidence of PID
     c. No systemic effects
  5. Disadvantages and side effects
     a. Requires sizing by trained clinician and instructions in use
     b. May have sensitivity to latex/spermicide
     c. Increased risk of bacterial vaginosis and UTI
        (1) Due to increased colonization with *E. coli*
        (2) Related to use of spermicide
        (3) Mechanical irritation/compression against urethra
     d. Does not afford absolute protection from STI/HIV
     e. Risk of toxic shock—2–3/100,000 per year
     f. Inability to learn correct insertion technique
  6. Contraindications
     a. Known allergy to latex or spermicide
     b. Inability to follow directions for insertion
     c. Significant vaginal relaxation—prolapse/cystocele/rectocele
     d. Frequent/recurrent UTI
     e. History of toxic shock
  7. Management

a. Health assessment prior to initiation of method
   (1) Routine annual Pap smear
   (2) Proper fit by trained professional—determine appropriate size and type for woman's anatomy
b. Health assessment at follow-up visits—recheck fit following childbirth or if patient gains/loses 15 pounds or more

8. Instructions for using the method
   a. General instructions (patient)
      (1) Insert just prior to intercourse or up to 6 hours before
      (2) Coat inner dome with 1 tablespoon of spermicide
      (3) Pinch sides of diaphragm and insert fully into vagina
         (a) Tuck anterior rim behind symphysis
         (b) Be certain that dome covers cervix
      (4) If repeated intercourse, insert another application of spermicide in vagina; do not remove diaphragm
      (5) Leave diaphragm in place for at least 6 hours following last intercourse
      (6) Do not leave in place for more than 24 hours
      (7) After each use wash and store diaphragm in clean, cool, dark environment
      (8) Do not use with oil-based lubricants or vaginal medications
      (9) Replace diaphragm yearly
      (10) Assess for holes/tears periodically by filling with water and inspecting for leaks
   b. Warning signs (toxic shock)
      (1) High fever
      (2) Nausea, vomiting, diarrhea
      (3) Syncope, weakness
      (4) Joint/muscle aches
      (5) Rash resembling sunburn

- Fertility Awareness Methods
  1. Description—method of contraception using abstinence during estimated fertile period based on all or some of the following methods:
     a. Menstrual cycle pattern (calendar method)
     b. Basal body temperature (BBT)—determines ovulation
     c. Evaluation of cervical mucus (ovulation/Billings method)—determines ovulation
     d. Sympto-thermal method—combines BBT with evaluation of cervical mucus and cervical position/consistency
  2. Mechanism of action—intercourse is avoided during fertile period
     a. Ovum remains fertile for 24 hours
     b. Sperm viability approximately 72 hours
     c. Most pregnancies occur when intercourse occurs before ovulation
  3. Effectiveness/first-year failure rate
     a. Perfect use
        (1) Calendar method—9%
        (2) BBT—2%
        (3) Ovulation method—3%
        (4) Sympto-thermal—2%
     b. Typical use for all methods—25%
  4. Advantages
     a. Minimal cost
     b. Natural
        (1) No systemic effects
        (2) No localized side effects, e.g., latex allergy
     c. Can be utilized for contraception and conception planning
  5. Disadvantages and side effects
     a. Requires motivation from both partners
     b. Requires periodic abstinence
     c. No protection against STI/HIV
  6. Precautions and risks
     a. Not reliable for women
        (1) With irregular menses (consider sympto-thermal and ovulation methods)
        (2) Who are perimenopausal
        (3) Who are recently postpartum
        (4) Who have had recent menarche
     b. Not a suitable method for
        (1) Women who cannot accurately evaluate their fertile period
           (a) Inability to use/read thermometer
           (b) Inability to understand cervical mucus/changes
           (c) Inability to time intercourse based on calendar evaluation
        (2) Couples unwilling to abstain during fertile time period
        (3) If nonconsensual coitus is likely to occur
  7. Management
     a. Health assessment prior to initiation of method
        (1) History to reflect pattern of menses
        (2) Evaluation of client's willingness/ability to check cervical mucus/consistency/position
     b. Health assessment at follow-up visits—BBT/sympto-thermal chart evaluation
     c. Special considerations—combination of fertility awareness methods more effective than single method
  8. Instructions for using the method
     a. Calendar method
        (1) Keep record of menstrual cycle intervals for several months

(2) From the shortest cycle length, subtract 18 days—this determines first fertile day
(3) From the longest cycle length, subtract 11 days—this determines last fertile day
(4) Use these numbers to determine days of abstinence for every cycle
  b. BBT method
    (1) Take temperature each morning before rising
      (a) BBT thermometer
      (b) Temperature can be oral, vaginal, or rectal (maintain same route)
    (2) Record on BBT chart
    (3) Temperature increase of 0.4° F or higher at ovulation—remains elevated for at least 3 days
    (4) Abstain from intercourse until 3-day temperature increase occurs
  c. Ovulation method
    (1) Inspect cervical mucus/secretions on underwear, toilet tissue, with fingers beginning day after menses
    (2) Determine consistency—elastic, slippery, wet by touch indicates preovulatory
      (a) Amount increases; becomes thinner and more elastic around time of ovulation
      (b) After ovulation, mucus becomes thick, tacky, and cloudy
    (3) Abstain from intercourse during "wet days" at onset of increased, slippery, thin mucus discharge until 4 days past the peak day (last day of clear, stretchy, slippery secretions)
    (4) Abstain from intercourse during menses because of inability to assess mucus
  d. Sympto-thermal method—combines ovulation, BBT, and assessment of consistency/position of cervix in vagina
    (1) Uses cervical assessment method and BBT
    (2) Ovulatory pain "mittelschmerz" may be indicator
    (3) Abstain until latter of two methods indicates "safe" time

- Female Sterilization
  1. Description—permanent contraception for woman achieved through surgical means; commonly performed on outpatient basis or postpartum prior to discharge using laparoscopy
  2. Mechanism of action
    a. Fallopian tubes are obstructed to prevent union of sperm and ovum
    (1) Surgical ligation—Pomeroy procedure
    (2) Surgical ligation and attachment to uterine body—Irving procedure
    (3) Electrocauterization
    (4) Section of tube excised—Pritchard procedure, fimbriectomy
    (5) Occluded—compressed with falope ring
    (6) Transcervical method—micro insert device inserted into fallopian tubes with catheter; expands and occludes tubes
  3. Effectiveness/first-year failure rate
    a. Perfect use—0.5%
    b. Typical use—0.5%
  4. Advantages
    a. Affords permanent contraception
    b. Highly effective
    c. Cost effective over long term
    d. Not coitally dependent
  5. Disadvantages and side effects
    a. Invasive surgical procedure requiring anesthesia
    b. Reversal is difficult, expensive, and often unsuccessful
    c. No protection against STI/HIV
    d. Initially expensive
  6. Precautions and risks
    a. Surgical procedure
      (1) Operative complications—bladder/uterine/intestinal injury may occur
      (2) Anesthetic complications—death (rare)
    b. Wound infection
    c. If pregnancy occurs following procedure, increased risk of ectopic
  7. Management
    a. Health assessment prior to initiation of method
      (1) Is patient candidate for surgery
      (2) Assess psychological readiness for permanent contraceptive method
    b. Health assessment at follow-up visits—assess for signs/symptoms of infection
      (1) Fever
      (2) Wound tenderness
      (3) Wound drainage
      (4) Abdominal pain
    c. Special considerations
      (1) Consent form signed in advance
      (2) Patient should be advised procedure is irreversible
  8. Instructions for using the method
    a. Nothing by mouth at least 8 hours prior to procedure
    b. Need transportation assistance from hospital/clinic to home

              c. Rest for at least 24 hours recommended following procedure
              d. Light lifting only for 1 week
              e. No coitus for 1 week
              f. Warning signs (notify healthcare provider)
                 (1) Fever greater than 100° F
                 (2) Severe pain
                 (3) Drainage from incision
                 (4) Dizziness/fainting/vertigo

- Male Sterilization
     1. Description—permanent contraception involving occlusion of vas deferens, preventing transmission of sperm through semen
          a. Surgical resection—surgical incision made in scrotum; vas deferens is resected
          b. Occlusion—surgical incision made in scrotum; vas deferens is divided and fulgurated/tied/cauterized
          c. No scalpel—ring forceps secures vas deferens; dissecting forceps punctures skin of scrotum; vas deferens lifted out and occluded
     2. Mechanism of action—sperm not present in ejaculate
     3. Effectiveness/first-year failure rate
          a. Perfect use—0.10%
          b. Typical use—0.15%
     4. Advantages
          a. Cost effective
          b. Highly effective
          c. Affords permanent contraception
          d. Not coitally dependent
          e. No systemic effects/artificial devices
     5. Disadvantages and side effects
          a. Initial expense
          b. Should be considered irreversible
          c. Invasive surgical procedure
          d. No protection against STI/HIV
     6. Precautions and risks
          a. Surgical procedure
          b. Wound infection
     7. Management
          a. Health assessment prior to initiation of procedure—assess psychological readiness for permanent contraceptive method
          b. Health assessment at follow-up visits—assess for signs/symptoms infection
               (1) Fever
               (2) Wound tenderness
               (3) Wound drainage
               (4) Swelling
          c. Special considerations
               (1) Relationship between vasectomy and prostate cancer unclear
                    (a) Study data conflicting
                    (b) Prostate screening postvasectomy is same as for men in general population
               (2) Procedure does not confer immediate sterility—up to 20 ejaculations will contain sperm
     8. Instructions for using the method
          a. Rest recommended for approximately 48 hours following procedure
          b. Apply ice pack to scrotum for minimum of 4 hours after procedure
          c. Avoid lifting/exercise for minimum of 1 week
          d. Keep area dry for 48 hours
          e. Abstain from intercourse for 48 hours
          f. Continue using other contraception until minimum of 20 ejaculations; obtain semen analysis to confirm azoospermia
          g. Warning signs
               (1) Fever greater than 100° F
               (2) Increasing pain
               (3) Increasing swelling/tension on stitches
               (4) Bleeding/drainage from incision

- Abortion
     1. Medical methods
          a. Mifepristone plus misoprostol
               (1) Most effective at 7 weeks' gestation or earlier
                    (a) 95% effective at 7 weeks LMP or earlier
                    (b) 80% effective in the 9th week LMP
               (2) Mifepristone
                    (a) 19-nor steroid
                    (b) Progesterone antagonist
               (3) Misoprostol—prostaglandin analogue
               (4) Avoid use of nonsteroidal anti-inflammatory medications during procedure; may inhibit action of misoprostol
               (5) Method requires three clinic visits
                    (a) Mifepristone orally at initial visit
                    (b) Misoprostol 48 hours later if expulsion not complete—observe for 4 hours
                    (c) 1- to 2-week follow-up appointment to assess for complete abortion
          b. Methotrexate plus misoprostol
               (1) 95% effective in early pregnancy
               (2) Methotrexate
                    (a) Destroys trophoblastic tissue
                    (b) Blocks folic acid, preventing cell division
               (3) Two clinic visits
                    (a) Methotrexate IM at initial visit

(b) Misoprostol vaginally 3–7 days later
(4) Avoid use of folic acid during procedure; may inhibit action of methotrexate
c. Hypertonic saline (2nd trimester)—instilled intra-amniotically
d. Hypertonic urea (2nd trimester)—instilled intra-amniotically
e. Misoprostol (2nd trimester)
f. Dinoprostone—prostaglandin vaginal suppository
2. Surgical methods
a. Vacuum aspiration (1st trimester)
(1) Suction curettage
(2) Local anesthetic
b. Dilation and evacuation (D&E)—can be performed up to 20 weeks' gestation
3. Pre-abortion health assessment and counseling
a. History
(1) LMP and menstrual history
(2) Surgical history, including gynecological surgeries
(3) Contraceptive history
(4) Medical history
(5) Current medications/history of allergic responses
b. Physical examination
(1) Size of uterus
(2) Note uterine/cervical position
(3) Presence of uterine/cervical/adnexal abnormalities
(a) Fibroids
(b) Adnexal masses (rule out ectopic)
(4) Laboratory tests
(a) Pregnancy test—urine/serum
(b) Hgb/Hct
(c) Blood type and Rh
(d) STI evaluation if warranted, e.g., sexual assault/patient concern
c. Counseling
(1) Discuss all pregnancy options
(2) Discuss options for termination—medical, surgical

## MENOPAUSE

1. Definitions
a. Menopause—cessation of menses; average age in United States is 51 years; genetically predetermined; confirmed after 12 consecutive months without a period
b. Climacteric—term used to describe the physiological changes associated with the change from reproductive to nonreproductive status; 2–8 years before menopause until 1 year after last period
c. Perimenopause—another term for climacteric
d. Postmenopause—phase of life following menopause
e. Premature menopause (premature ovarian failure)—cessation of menses before age 40
2. Physiology
a. As climacteric begins, the rhythmic ovarian and endometrial responses of the menstrual cycle decline and eventually stop
b. Number of responsive follicles decreases with resultant decreased production of estradiol throughout climacteric
c. With decreasing estradiol, FSH levels increase
d. At the end of the climacteric, ovary contains no follicles and endometrium atrophies so that reproductive capability is terminated
e. After menopause, estrone becomes principal estrogen
f. Estrone produced through aromatization of androstenedione; androstenedione is an androgen produced by adrenal cortex and ovarian stroma; converted to estrone in peripheral fat cells
g. After menopause, both FSH and LH levels are elevated
h. Generally rely on cessation of menses, hypoestrogenic symptoms, age, and consistently elevated FSH for diagnosis of menopause
3. Laboratory findings
a. FSH—> 40 mIU/mL
b. LH—threefold elevation after menopause (20–100 mIU/mL)
c. Estradiol—< 20 pg/mL
4. Possible menstrual changes in climacteric
a. No change
b. Oligomenorrhea/polymenorrhea—cycles shorter or longer than usual
c. Hypomenorrhea/hypermenorrhea—bleeding lighter/shorter or heavier/longer than usual
d. Metrorrhagia—irregular intervals, amount variable
5. Physical changes
a. Reproductive organs
(1) Labia—decrease in subcutaneous fat and tissue elasticity
(2) Vagina
(a) Thinning of epithelium; decreased rugae, increase in pH (> 5)
(b) May have pruritus, leukorrhea, friability, increased susceptibility to infection
(c) May have dyspareunia
(3) Cervix—decrease in size, or may become flush with vaginal walls, may become stenotic
(4) Uterus and ovaries—decrease in size and weight; ovaries usually not palpable

b. Urinary tract
   (1) Decreased muscle tone—urethra and trigone area of bladder
   (2) Atrophic changes in urethra and periurethral tissue—stress incontinence may occur
   (3) Hypoestrogenic effects in trigone area; lowered sensory threshold to void—sensory urge incontinence may occur
   (4) Urinary urgency, frequency, and dysuria due to atrophic changes in urethra and periurethral tissue
c. Breasts—reduction in size and flattened appearance; decrease in glandular tissue
d. Skin
   (1) Thinning/decreased activity of sebaceous and sweat glands
   (2) Hyperpigmentation/hypopigmentation
   (3) Scalp, pubic, and axillary hair becomes thinner and drier
e. Bone integrity—increased bone loss associated with decrease in estrogen

6. Vasomotor symptoms—hot flashes
   a. Observed in 75% of women during climacteric
   b. Mechanism responsible not known; gonadotropin-related effect on the central thermoregulatory function of the hypothalamus (measurable increase in body surface heat and decrease in core temperature)
   c. Sudden feeling of warmth followed by visible redness of upper body and face
   d. May be associated with profuse sweating and palpitations
   e. May awaken during the night, leading to insomnia, sleep disturbance, cognitive (memory) and affective (anxiety) disorders with loss of REM sleep
   f. Generally cease within 2–3 years after menopause

7. Cardiovascular system effects
   a. Lipid levels—increase in low-density lipoproteins (LDL), very-low-density lipoproteins (VLDL), and triglycerides; possible decrease in high-density lipoproteins (HDL)
   b. Regulation of clotting processes—increase in certain fibrinolytic and procoagulation factors
   c. Vasoactive substances—increase in endothelin and decrease in angiotensin-converting enzyme (vasoconstrictors), increase in nitric oxide and decrease in prostacyclin (vasodilators)
   d. Extent of impact of decreased estrogen levels on cardiovascular disease not definitively established

8. Alterations in mood
   a. Majority of women do not have psychological problems attributable to menopause
   b. Depression in menopause often related to history of previous depression
   c. Depression/irritability may be related to sleep disturbances caused by hot flashes
   d. Perceived health shown to be a major factor related to depression in perimenopausal women; individual characteristics and self-perception appear to be important determinants of each woman's experience of the climacteric
   e. More research is needed to establish hormonal influences on mood changes that occur during perimenopause

9. Cognitive function
   a. Memory impairment may be indirectly related to decreased estrogen secondary to hot flashes and sleep disturbance
   b. Women's Health Initiative Memory Study (Shumaker et al., 2002)—use of estrogen plus progestin does not prevent dementia or mild cognitive impairment

10. Sexuality
    a. Diminished genital sensation, less vaginal expansion, and decreased vasocongestion may cause some changes in orgasm experience—increased time to reach orgasm, shorter duration of orgasm, decreased strength of orgasmic contractions
    b. Freedom from fear of pregnancy, freedom from contraceptives, and increased privacy as children leave home may increase sexual enjoyment
    c. Dyspareunia, loss of partner, medications, and chronic illness may affect sexual desire and activity

11. Health assessment/health promotion
    a. Health history
       (1) Family and personal history—focus on risks for cancer, heart disease, osteoporosis
       (2) High-risk behavior evaluation—smoking, alcohol, drugs, STI/HIV risks
       (3) Menstrual history—focus on irregular bleeding problems
       (4) Nutrition and exercise assessment
       (5) Psychosocial assessment—sexuality, stressors, support system, domestic violence
    b. Physical assessment
       (1) Blood pressure
       (2) Height and weight
       (3) Complete physical examination
    c. Screening tests
       (1) Pap smear every 3 years to age 70
       (2) Colorectal cancer screening beginning age 50—fecal occult blood test annually; colonoscopy every 10 years, or

double-contrast barium enema every 5 years
(3) Mammography every year starting at age 40
(4) Cholesterol with HDL every 5 years beginning at age 20, more frequent and additional lipid tests as needed (National Cholesterol Education Program [NCEP] of the National Heart, Lung, and Blood Institute, 2004)
(5) Plasma glucose every 3 years age 45 years or older and for younger women with risk factors
(6) Bone mass density screening—age 65 and older, earlier in postmenopausal women with risk factors (National Osteoporosis Foundation, 2013)
(7) Screening for visual acuity and glaucoma by ophthalmologist every 2–4 years from age 40–64 and every 1–2 years beginning at age 65, earlier and more frequent screening if risk factors are present (USPSTF, 2014)
(8) Other as determined by risk factors
d. Immunizations (CDC, 2014)
(1) Tetanus-diphtheria (Td) vaccine every 10 years; should have tetanus-diphtheria acellular pertussis (Tdap) once in place of Td one time
(2) Annual influenza vaccine
(3) Pneumoccocal vaccine once
(4) Varicella zoster vaccine once after age 60
e. Contraception for women over 40
(1) Continue contraception until FSH level indicates no longer fertile or no menses for 1 year
(2) Nonsmokers with no cardiovascular disease (CVD) risk factors may continue combination hormonal methods until age 53–55, then assume menopause and discontinue contraception
(3) A single elevated FSH during hormone-free week is not a reliable indicator of menopause
(4) Options
(a) Low-dose combination oral contraception (COC)—noncontraceptive benefits of COC may be especially attractive to the perimenopausal woman
(i) Decreased incidence of endometrial and ovarian cancer
(ii) Relief of vasomotor symptoms
(iii) Increased menstrual regularity and decreased dysmenorrhea
(iv) Possible increased bone density
(b) Other hormonal contraception methods are also options if there are no contraindications
(c) IUD/IUS
(i) Long-lasting, effective contraceptive option
(ii) LNG IUS may also be therapeutic for perimenopausal women with heavy bleeding
(d) Barrier methods are acceptable options
(e) Sterilization—most prevalent contraceptive method among married women in the United States
(f) Fertility awareness methods less effective during perimenopause with irregular menstrual cycles
12. Hormone therapy (HT)
a. Indications
(1) Relief of moderate to severe menopausal symptoms related to estrogen deficiency—vasomotor instability, vulvar/vaginal atrophy
(2) Prevention of osteoporosis—consider nonestrogen medications if not also treating for vasomotor and/or vulvovaginal symptoms
b. Other potential benefits—reduction in risk for colon cancer
c. Contraindications
(1) Active or recent arterial thromboembolic disease (myocardial infarction, angina)
(2) Untreated hypertension
(3) Venous thromboembolic disorders or thrombophlebitis
(4) Known or suspected breast cancer
(5) Endometrial hyperplasia
(6) Estrogen-dependent cancer
(7) Liver dysfunction or disease
(8) Undiagnosed abnormal uterine bleeding
(9) Known or suspected pregnancy
(10) Porphyria cutanea tarda
d. Potential risks
(1) Endometrial hyperplasia/cancer
(2) Breast cancer
(a) Relationship with HT inconclusive
(b) Possible small but significant increase of breast cancer with long-term HT
(3) Gallbladder disease
(4) Thromboembolic disorders
e. Assessment prior to initiation of HT
(1) Health history with attention to specific contraindications and precautions
(2) General physical examination, gynecological examination with Pap smear, breast examination, mammogram
(3) Base decisions concerning HT use on woman's symptoms, treatment goals, benefit-risk analysis
f. Routine follow-up after HT initiation

(1) Reevaluate in 3 months—assess therapeutic effectiveness and any problems
(2) Annual follow-up thereafter if no problems
    (a) Evaluate continuing need for HT—limit use to shortest duration consistent with treatment goals and risks for individual woman
    (b) Consider nonhormonal drugs for osteoporosis prevention if long-term therapy needed
g. Regimen options
    (1) Consider use of lowest dose of estrogen needed for symptom relief—0.3–0.625 mg conjugated estrogen or equivalent
    (2) 10–14 days each month of 5–10 mg of medroxyprogesterone acetate (MPA) or equivalent or daily doses of 1.5–5 mg recommended for prevention of endometrial hyperplasia
    (3) Continuous-combined regimen
        (a) Estrogen and progestin every day
        (b) Lower cumulative dose of progestin than with cyclic regimens
        (c) May have unpredictable bleeding
        (d) After several months endometrium atrophies and amenorrhea usually results
        (e) No estrogen-free period during which vasomotor symptoms can occur
    (4) Continuous-cyclic regimen
        (a) Estrogen every day
        (b) Progestin added 10–14 days each month
        (c) No estrogen-free period during which vasomotor symptoms can occur
        (d) Withdrawal bleeding when progestin withdrawn each month
    (5) Cyclic regimen
        (a) Estrogen days 1–25
        (b) Progestin added last 10–14 days
        (c) Followed by 3–6 days of no therapy
        (d) Withdrawal bleeding when progestin withdrawn each month
    (6) Continuous unopposed estrogen—for woman without uterus
h. Progestin only may be used if estrogen is contraindicated
    (1) Effective in relieving vasomotor symptoms; may have a positive impact on calcium balance
    (2) Not effective in relief of vulvovaginal symptoms; may have adverse effect on lipid metabolism
i. Testosterone may be added if extreme vasomotor symptoms not relieved by estrogen alone; oral, transdermal, injections, subcutaneous implants
    (1) May be especially useful after surgical menopause
    (2) May increase energy level, feeling of well-being, libido
    (3) Side effects—acne, hirsutism, clitoromegaly
    (4) Long-term effects of low-dose testosterone treatment in women are not known
j. Side effects of HT
    (1) Breast tenderness—estrogen or progestin (usually subsides after first few weeks)
    (2) Nausea—estrogen (relieved if taken at mealtime or at bedtime)
    (3) Skin irritation with transdermal patches
    (4) Fluid retention and bloating—estrogen or progestin
    (5) Alterations in mood—estrogen or progestin
k. Management of bleeding during HT
    (1) Continuous-cyclic regimen—usually experience some uterine bleeding; starts last few days of progestin administration or during hormone-free days; earlier bleeding, heavy or persistent bleeding may indicate endometrial hyperplasia and warrants endometrial evaluation
    (2) Continuous-combined regimen—erratic spotting and light bleeding of 1–5 days' duration in first year; endometrial biopsy if bleeding heavier or longer than usual

13. Nonhormonal management of vasomotor symptoms
    a. Drugs FDA approved for other indications that have shown some effectiveness in relieving hot flashes—clonidine, gabapentin, selective serotonin reuptake inhibitors (SSRIs)
    b. Avoiding caffeine, alcohol, cigarettes, spicy foods, and big meals
    c. Regular, moderate exercise—may also help alleviate insomnia
    d. Wearing layers and natural fibers
    e. Sleeping in a cool room
    f. Keeping a thermos of ice water available
    g. Stress management and relaxation techniques
    h. Vitamin E—anecdotal reports of relief, placebo controlled studies not supportive
    i. Soy foods and isoflavone supplements
14. Nonhormonal management of vulvovaginal symptoms
    a. Water-soluble lubricants
    b. Regular sexual activity
    c. Noncoital methods of sexual expression—massage, mutual masturbation if penetration is painful

## QUESTIONS

**Select the best answer.**

1. Which of the following is a positive sign of pregnancy?
   a. Goodell's sign
   b. Urinary frequency/urgency
   c. Braxton-Hicks contractions
   d. Fetal movement felt by examiner

2. Which of the following statements is correct regarding maternal physiological changes in pregnancy?
   a. Pulse rate decreases
   b. Insulin requirements decrease
   c. Sweat gland activity increases
   d. Intestinal peristalsis increases

3. Examination of the breasts in pregnancy may normally show:
   a. Increased nodularity
   b. Linea nigra
   c. Retractions in skin
   d. Loss of nipple pigmentation

4. Examination of a woman in the 30th week of pregnancy would normally reveal:
   a. Cervical dilation of 2 cm
   b. Diastolic heart murmur
   c. Fundal height of 29 cm
   d. Thyroid nodularity

5. Examination of a woman in her 14th week of pregnancy would normally reveal:
   a. Fundal height of 14 cm
   b. Fetal heart tones audible with fetoscope
   c. Milk expressed from breasts
   d. Cyanosis of the cervix

6. Chadwick's sign is described as:
   a. Softening of the uterine isthmus
   b. A bluish discoloration of the cervix
   c. Palpable uterine softening to palpation
   d. Manipulation of the uterus displaces fetus to examiner's finger in the vagina

7. Which of the following complications is most likely to occur in the first trimester?
   a. Pregnancy-induced hypertension
   b. Bleeding
   c. Placenta previa
   d. Gestational diabetes

8. What is the recommended weight gain in pregnancy for a woman beginning pregnancy with a BMI of 27?
   a. Less than 20 pounds
   b. 20 pounds
   c. 25 pounds
   d. More than 30 pounds

9. How is the EDD determined using Naegele's rule?
   a. Subtract 3 months from LNMP and add 7 days
   b. Subtract 7 days and add 9 months from the start of the LNMP
   c. Add 9 months from start of the LNMP
   d. Subtract 7 from last day of LNMP and count back 3 months

10. During pregnancy, sexual intercourse is contraindicated when:
    a. Increased whitish vaginal discharge is present
    b. 36 weeks' gestation has been reached
    c. Rupture of membranes is suspected
    d. Weight gain is inadequate

11. Which of the following statements is true regarding diagnostic testing during pregnancy?
    a. Chorionic villus sampling is performed between weeks 14 and 24 when indicated for genetic reasons
    b. Alpha-fetoprotein in maternal blood is assessed between weeks 16 and 18
    c. Gestational diabetes screening is performed between weeks 15 and 18
    d. Amniocentesis is performed between weeks 22 and 26 when indicated for advanced maternal age

12. Laboratory testing ordered in the first trimester of pregnancy should include all of the following *except*:
    a. HbsAg screening
    b. VDRL screening
    c. HIV test
    d. Quad screening

13. True labor is characterized by:
    a. Contractions initially felt in back and that radiate to lower abdomen
    b. Decrease of intensity of contractions with walking
    c. Discomfort of contractions felt mainly in abdomen
    d. Contractions relieved with sedation

14. A predisposing factor for preterm labor is:
    a. Hypothyroidism
    b. Gestational diabetes
    c. Pyelonephritis
    d. Oligohydramnios

15. Which of the following is a risk factor for the development of gestational diabetes?
    a. Multiple gestation
    b. Prior macrosomic infant
    c. Oligohydramnios in prior pregnancy
    d. Maternal age younger than 19

16. A 19-year-old female patient reports that she has not had a normal period in 6 weeks, but she has had bleeding for several days and bilateral lower abdominal/groin pain. A urine hCG is positive. Further evaluation must include:
    a. A serum hCG
    b. A pelvic examination
    c. A transvaginal ultrasound
    d. Serial quantitative hCGs

17. Which of the following increases a woman's chances of having an ectopic pregnancy?
    a. Use of combination oral contraceptives
    b. Uterine myoma
    c. Maternal age older than 30
    d. Previous ectopic pregnancy

18. *Inevitable abortion* refers to:
    a. Death of embryo or fetus without expulsion
    b. Gross rupture of membranes in the presence of cervical dilation
    c. Expulsion of products of conception without medical intervention
    d. Presence of bleeding and uterine cramping without cervical dilation

19. Which of the following is a sign of increasingly severe preeclampsia?
    a. Hemoconcentration with decreased platelets
    b. Increased urinary output
    c. Patellar hyporeflexia
    d. Elevated serum glucose

20. Presentation with placenta previa is differentiated from abruptio placentae by:
    a. Abruptio placentae occurs earlier in gestation
    b. Amount of bleeding is more with placenta previa
    c. Severe abdominal pain with abruptio placentae
    d. PIH usually accompanies placenta previa

21. Which of the following patterns in laboratory values would be expected in menopause?
    a. Decreased FSH, increased LH, decreased estradiol
    b. Decreased LH, increased FSH, increased estradiol
    c. Increased FSH, increased LH, decreased estradiol
    d. Increased LH, decreased FSH, increased estradiol

22. All of the following are contraindications to hormone therapy (HT) in menopause *except*:
    a. A history of angina chest pain currently managed with beta-adrenergic blockade
    b. Hypothyroidism currently managed with 100 mcg/day of synthetic thyroxine
    c. Endometrial hyperplasia
    d. Breast cancer treated 6 years ago

23. What is the most prevalent contraceptive method among married women in the United States?
    a. Combination oral contraceptives
    b. Condoms
    c. Sterilization
    d. Withdrawal

24. A 54-year-old female with vaginal dryness causing irritation and dyspareunia has no problem with hot flashes. Bone densitometry reveals a T score of 1. What is the best treatment?
    a. Continuous-combined regimen HT
    b. Cyclic HT with added testosterone
    c. Estrogen vaginal ring
    d. Progestin-only therapy

25. Which of the following women should have an endometrial biopsy/evaluation?
    a. Woman on continuous-cyclic HT regimen with amenorrhea
    b. Woman on continuous-cyclic HT regimen with bleeding starting last few days of progestin administration each month
    c. Woman on continuous-combined HT regimen with irregular bleeding in the first year of use
    d. Woman on continuous-combined HT regimen with spotting that occurs after several months of amenorrhea

26. A 53-year-old female who had a hysterectomy 10 years ago for dysfunctional uterine bleeding presents with complaints of severe hot flashes and night sweats for the past few months. Her lipid profile is significant for cholesterol of 220 mg/dL and triglycerides of 350 mg/dL. What is the most appropriate therapy for her vasomotor symptoms at this time?

    a. Continuous-combined oral HT
    b. Selective estrogen receptor modulator (raloxifene)
    c. Transdermal estrogen patch
    d. Vaginal estrogen cream

27. A 24-year-old female presents to your office with a request for combination oral contraceptives. Her current medications include a bronchodilator for asthma. Management for this client should include advising her that:

    a. Combination oral contraceptives are not recommended for women with asthma
    b. Combination oral contraceptives may potentiate the action of her bronchodilator
    c. She should use a backup method if using the bronchodilator several days in a row
    d. Use of progestin-only contraceptive injections may reduce her asthma attacks

28. Which of the following contraceptive methods would be best for a woman with a seizure disorder who is taking phenytoin?

    a. Combination oral contraceptives
    b. Combination contraceptive injections
    c. Progestin-only oral contraceptives
    d. Progestin-only contraceptive injections

29. A 22-year-old female calls the clinic on Monday morning stating that the condom broke when she and her partner had sex on Saturday night at about 11:00 p.m. She is interested in emergency contraception. In discussing options with this client, it is important to explain that the latest she should wait before initiating emergency contraception is:

    a. Monday at 11:00 a.m.
    b. Monday at 11:00 p.m.
    c. Tuesday at 11:00 a.m.
    d. Thursday at 11:00 p.m.

30. The second dose of emergency contraceptive pills should be taken how many hours after the first dose?

    a. 4
    b. 6
    c. 12
    d. 24

31. When counseling a woman about the use of POP emergency contraception, it is appropriate to tell her:

    a. There is an increased risk of birth defect if pregnancy does occur
    b. It is not safe to use if she has a history of arterial or venous thromboembolic disease
    c. There is a 25% chance she will experience nausea as a side effect
    d. The same contraindications apply as for any hormonal contraception

32. What is an advantage of progestin-only hormonal contraception?

    a. It is significantly less expensive than combined forms are
    b. It has a lesser side effect profile
    c. It provides an option for women who have contraindications to estrogen
    d. It can be taken within 4 weeks of giving birth

33. Following a vasectomy, a man should use another method of contraception until he has had a minimum of how many ejaculations?

    a. 5
    b. 10
    c. 15
    d. 20

34. A woman who is undergoing a medically induced abortion using mifepristone and misoprostol should be advised to avoid which of the following during the procedure?

    a. Acetaminophen
    b. Folic acid supplements
    c. Nonsteroidal anti-inflammatory drugs
    d. Vitamin $B_6$ supplements

35. Which of the following abortion methods may be used in the second trimester?

    a. Hypertonic saline instillation
    b. Methotrexate and misoprostol
    c. Mifepristone and misoprostol
    d. Vacuum aspiration

36. Studies have indicated that HT, although not an approved indication, may have the benefit of decreasing the risk for:

    a. Colon cancer
    b. Rheumatoid arthritis

c. Osteoarthritis
d. Cognitive dysfunction

37. A woman who is requesting contraception and who also wants to get pregnant in 1 year should avoid using:

   a. Combination oral contraceptives
   b. Fertility awareness methods
   c. Progestin-only oral contraceptives
   d. Progestin-only contraceptive injections

38. Which of the following statements by a client indicates that she needs additional information about use of the contraceptive vaginal ring?

   a. I should insert a new ring every 7 days
   b. I should expect to have regular periods while using the ring
   c. My partner can use a male condom while I am wearing the ring
   d. The exact position of the ring in the vagina is not important

39. Your patient is on combination oral contraceptives and calls to tell you that she has missed her pills for 2 days in a row. It is the second week of her cycle. You advise her to:

   a. Double her pills for the next 2 days; no backup is required
   b. Take 1 pill daily until Sunday; discard the pack and start a new one at that time
   c. Take 2 pills a day for the next 2 days, using backup contraception for 7 days
   d. Begin a new pack immediately; use a backup method for 7 days

40. A 3-week postpartum woman who is breast-feeding presents in your office to discuss her contraceptive options. Currently, she is breastfeeding on demand and is not providing any supplements. She plans to continue breastfeeding for at least 6 months. The woman asks if she can restart birth control pills now because she wants to be sure that she does not become pregnant. The best response would be:

   a. Combination oral contraceptives are contraindicated during the duration of breastfeeding
   b. All hormonal methods of contraception should be avoided while she is breastfeeding
   c. She should wait until she is having regular periods before restarting her birth control pills
   d. Progestin-only pills may be a better option for her to start at 6 weeks' postpartum

41. A woman using a diaphragm for contraception has sexual intercourse at 8:00 a.m. on Friday, at 2:00 a.m. on Saturday, and again at 8:00 a.m. on Saturday. When can she safely remove her diaphragm for effective contraception while minimizing problems related to leaving the diaphragm in for extended periods of time?

   a. 10:00 a.m. on Saturday
   b. 2:00 p.m. on Saturday
   c. 10:00 p.m. on Saturday
   d. 8:00 a.m. on Sunday

42. When counseling patients about emergency contraception, in the interest of full disclosure it is important to advise that:

   a. Depending on the timing in the cycle, it may interrupt an established pregnancy
   b. There is a possibility of teratogenicity if a pregnancy does occur
   c. An increased risk of embolic disease occurs as a result of the relatively large dose
   d. Although it may be taken up to 5 days later, it is most effective when used earliest

43. Which of the following is an advantage of the female condom?

   a. It can be used with a male condom for added protection
   b. It can be used for repeated acts of intercourse
   c. It may be used by individuals with latex allergy
   d. It has a lower failure rate than the male condom does

44. Noncontraceptive benefits of combination oral contraceptives include all of the following except:

   a. Decrease in risk for benign breast disease
   b. Decrease in risk for cervical cancer
   c. Decrease in risk for endometrial cancer
   d. Decrease in risk for ovarian cancer

45. For which of the contraceptive methods is there the least difference between the perfect use and typical use failure rates?

   a. Combination oral contraceptives
   b. Diaphragm
   c. Intrauterine device
   d. Male condom

46. A woman who weighs 200 pounds or more may have decreased effectiveness with which of the following contraceptive methods?

a. Combination injectable contraception
b. Contraceptive vaginal ring
c. Levonorgestrel intrauterine system
d. Transdermal contraceptive system

47. When performing a routine assessment of a woman who is 18 weeks' gestation, what would you expect her to report?

    a. Worsening nausea and heartburn
    b. Round ligament discomfort
    c. Having just recently felt fetal movement
    d. Increased leukorrhea

48. A 20-year-old female who is 30% overweight presents for her first Depo-Provera injection. Concerns in administering Depo-Provera to this woman include:

    a. She may need a larger dose than the usual 150 mg
    b. She should return for repeat injections every 2 months
    c. You should massage the injection site well to ensure absorption
    d. You should choose a site that ensures deep IM injection

49. Instructions for progestin-only oral contraceptive users should include:

    a. If you are more than 3 hours late taking a pill, use a backup method for 48 hours
    b. If 2 pills are missed in the third week of the pack, throw away the pack and start a new one
    c. If you miss pills in the fourth week of the pack, you do not have to use a backup method
    d. If you miss 2 pills in the first week of the pack, make them up and use a backup method for 7 days

50. The menopausal woman may experience some changes in sensation or the orgasmic experience during sexual activity related to:

    a. Decreased vasocongestion and decreased vaginal expansion
    b. Decreased vasocongestion and increased vaginal expansion
    c. Increased vasocongestion and decreased vaginal expansion
    d. Increased vasocongestion and increased vaginal expansion

51. Which of the following contraceptive choices should not be recommended for the perimenopausal woman who is having irregular menses?

    a. Combination oral contraceptives
    b. Diaphragm
    c. Fertility awareness methods
    d. LNG intrauterine system

52. The mechanism of action of mifepristone in inducing abortion is:

    a. Antiprogesterone effect on the endometrium
    b. Cervical dilation effect
    c. Stimulatory effect on the myometrium
    d. Toxic effect on the fertilized egg

53. When a patient on combination oral contraceptives has persistent breakthrough bleeding during the first half of the cycle, the appropriate intervention is to:

    a. Advise that this may occur for up to 1 year
    b. Consider progestin-only options
    c. Counsel regarding the need to switch to non-hormonal methods
    d. Increase the estrogen component of the method

54. What is considered to be the main mechanism of action of oral contraceptives when used for emergency contraception?

    a. Disruption of implanted fertilized ovum
    b. Inhibition of ovulation
    c. Prevention of implantation of fertilized ovum
    d. Toxic effect on the fertilized ovum

55. According to WHO recommendations, which of the following is considered to be a condition that represents an unacceptable health risk (refrain from providing) for the use of the indicated contraceptive method?

    a. Initiation of progestin-only oral contraceptives by a woman with a history of deep vein thrombosis
    b. Initiation of progestin-only injectable contraception for a woman with hypertension
    c. Initiation of combination injectable contraception in a lactating woman who is less than 6 weeks' postpartum
    d. Insertion of an IUD in a woman who is at risk for HIV infection

## Answers

| | | | |
|---|---|---|---|
| 1. | d | 31. | c |
| 2. | c | 32. | c |
| 3. | a | 33. | d |
| 4. | c | 34. | c |
| 5. | d | 35. | a |
| 6. | b | 36. | a |
| 7. | b | 37. | d |
| 8. | c | 38. | a |
| 9. | a | 39. | c |
| 10. | c | 40. | d |
| 11. | b | 41. | b |
| 12. | d | 42. | d |
| 13. | a | 43. | c |
| 14. | c | 44. | b |
| 15. | b | 45. | c |
| 16. | c | 46. | d |
| 17. | d | 47. | b |
| 18. | b | 48. | d |
| 19. | a | 49. | a |
| 20. | c | 50. | a |
| 21. | c | 51. | c |
| 22. | b | 52. | a |
| 23. | c | 53. | d |
| 24. | c | 54. | b |
| 25. | d | 55. | c |
| 26. | c | | |
| 27. | b | | |
| 28. | d | | |
| 29. | d | | |
| 30. | c | | |

## BIBLIOGRAPHY

American Association of Clinical Endocrinologists. (2011). Medical guidelines for clinical practice for the diagnosis and treatment of menopause. *Endocrine Practice, 17*(Suppl. 6), 1–26.

American Cancer Society. (2013). *Breast cancer early detection.* Retrieved from http://www.cancer.org/acs/groups/cid/documents/webcontent/003165-pdf.pdf

American College of Obstetricians and Gynecologists. (2007). *Guidelines for women's health care* (3rd ed.). Washington, DC: Author.

American College of Obstetricians and Gynecologists & American Academy of Pediatrics. (2012). *Guidelines for perinatal care* (7th ed.). Washington, DC: Author.

Centers for Disease Control and Prevention. (2012). National Vital Statistics System: Birth data. Retrieved from http://www.cdc.gov/nchs/births.htm

Centers for Disease Control and Prevention. (2014). Adult immunization schedules. Retrieved from http://www.cdc.gov/vaccines/schedules/hcp/adult.html

Hatcher, R. (2011). *Contraceptive technology* (20th ed.). New York, NY: Thomas Reuters.

Leveno, K., Cunningham, F., & Bloom, S. (2012). *Williams manual of pregnancy complications* (23rd ed.). New York, NY: McGraw-Hill.

Lucidi, R. S. (2013). Polycystic ovarian syndrome. Retrieved from http://www.emedicine.com/med/TOPIC2173.htm

Massad, L. S., Einstein, M. H., Huh, W. K., Katki, H. A., Kinney, W. K., Schiffman, M., ... Lawson, H. L. (2013). 2012 updated consensus guidelines for the management of abnormal cervical cancer screening test and cancer precursors. *Journal of Lower Genital Tract Disease, 17*(5), S1–S27. Retrieved from http://www.omniaeducation.com/images/hpv_resource2.pdf

National Cholesterol Education Program. (2004). Third Report of the Expert Panel on Detection, Evaluation, and Treatment of High Blood Cholesterol in Adults (Adult Treatment Panel III) 2004 update. Retrieved from http://www.nhlbi.nih.gov/guidelines/cholesterol/index.htm

National Institutes of Health. (2000). *Working group report on high blood pressure in pregnancy.* Washington, DC: Author.

National Osteoporosis Foundation. (2013). *Clinician's guide to prevention and treatment of osteoporosis.* Retrieved from http://nof.org/files/nof/public/content/file/950/upload/523.pdf

North American Menopause Society. (2004). Treatment of menopause associated vasomotor symptoms: Position statement of the North American Menopause Society. *Menopause: The Journal of NAMS, 11*(1), 11–33.

Shumaker, S. A., Reboussin, B. A., Espeland, M. A., Rapp, S. R., McBee, W. L., Dailey, M., & Jones, B. N. (2002). The women's health initiative memory study (WHIMS): A trial of the effect of estrogen therapy in preventing and slowing the progression of dementia. *Controlled Clinical Trials, 19*(6), 604–621.

U.S. Preventive Services Task Force (USPSTF). (2014). The guide to clinical preventive services: Recommendations of the United States Preventive Services Task Force. Retrieved from http://www.uspreventiveservicestaskforce.org/adultrec.htm

Youngkin, E. Q., Davis, M. S., Schadewald D., & Juve, C. (2012). *Women's health: A primary care clinical guide* (4th ed.). Upper Saddle River, NJ: Prentice Hall.

# APPENDIX B

# Supplement for the Acute Care Provider

*Sally K. Miller*

## MANAGEMENT OF THE PREOPERATIVE PATIENT

- Definition—includes the *preoperative evaluation*, which is an assessment of overall health and serves primarily to identify risk factors for complicated recovery, the *diagnostic evaluation*, which focuses on the assessment of information (history, physical examination, and diagnostic evaluation) of those factors relative to the surgical problem, and *preoperative preparation*, which includes any interventions indicated by the preoperative and diagnostic evaluation and prepares the patient and any caregivers physiologically and psychologically for the postoperative experience (Doherty, 2009)

- History and Physical Examination—emphasis on identification of undiagnosed cardiopulmonary disease, risk factors for bleeding, risk for infection
    1. Past medical history
    2. Past surgical history
    3. Family history
    4. Psychosocial history
    5. Allergies
    6. Review of systems
    7. Current medications
    8. Head-to-toe physical examination

- Laboratory and Diagnostic Screening—evidence-based guidelines recommend against a battery of routine tests for patients without clear indication or risk; current evidence-based recommendations include focused assessment based on the preoperative evaluation
    1. Complete blood count (CBC)
        a. Underlying disease increases risk of anemia
        b. Significant blood loss is anticipated
        c. Infection or immune compromise is suspected
    2. Urinalysis
        a. Patients undergoing urologic surgery
        b. Procedure involves implantation of foreign material
    3. Chest radiography
        a. Patients with new or unstable cardiopulmonary signs or symptoms
        b. Procedure is thoracic
    4. Electrolyte studies and measure of renal function
        a. Underlying endocrine, metabolic, or vascular disease
        b. Current pharmacological management that may affect electrolyte concentration or renal function
        c. Other risk for renal dysfunction exists
    5. Random glucose or HgbA1c
        a. Underlying diabetes mellitus (DM)
        b. Result would affect postoperative management
    6. Coagulation studies
        a. Patients on anticoagulant therapy

b. History of abnormal bleeding
c. Underlying disease that increases risk of coagulopathy, e.g., liver or renal disease
7. Cardiac testing
   a. Patients with signs or symptoms of active cardiac disease and those having cardiac surgery should have appropriate cardiac testing under the supervision of a cardiologist
   b. Patients undergoing noncardiac surgery with no signs and symptoms of active disease
      (1) Electrocardiography is indicated in all patients having high-risk surgery (aortic and major or peripheral vascular surgery)
      (2) Electrocardiography is indicated in patients having intermediate-risk surgery (intraperitoneal, intrathoracic, carotid endarterectomy, head or neck, orthopedic, or prostate surgery) who have other cardiac risk factors
      (3) Electrocardiography is not indicated for patients having low-risk surgery (ambulatory surgery, breast surgery, endoscopic or superficial procedures, cataract surgery)
8. Pulmonary function testing
   a. Not routinely obtained
   b. Consider for
      (1) Patients with asthma requiring daily medication
      (2) Patients with chronic obstructive pulmonary disease (COPD)
      (3) Patients having lung surgery
      (4) Patients having coronary artery bypass grafting (CABG) and upper or lower abdominal surgery with a history of smoking longer than 10 pack years
9. Cardiac consultation and clearance for patients undergoing noncardiac surgery
   a. Myocardial infarction < 6 weeks ago
   b. Unstable angina
   c. Decompensated congestive heart failure (CHF)
   d. Significant dysrhythmia
   e. Severe valvular disease

- Assessment of Surgical Risk
  1. Nutritional status
     a. Dietary history
     b. Poor dentition
     c. Serum albumin < 3 g/dL and serum transferrin < 150 mg/dL correlate with prolonged recovery and increased mortality
     d. Preoperative weight loss of > 20% caused by illness correlates with prolonged recovery, risk of infection 3 × greater than the general population, and increased mortality
     e. Obesity is correlated with an increased risk of poor surgical outcomes in some procedures, but not all (obesity paradox); in terms of general health, controlled weight reduction is recommended prior to elective procedures when possible
  2. Immune competence
     a. Total leukocyte (white blood cell [WBC] count) with differential
        (1) Leukocytes—reference range 5,000 to 12,000 cells/mm$^3$
        (2) Leukocytes comprised of five cell types
           (a) Neutrophils—fight bacterial infection; comprise 50–70% of the total count (average 60%)
           (b) Lymphocytes—fight viral infection; comprise 25–35% of the total count (average 30%)
           (c) Monocytes—clear noninfectious cellular debris; comprise 4–8% of the total differential (average 6%)
           (d) Eosinophils—respond to allergic events and parasitic infection; comprise 1–4% of the total differential (average 3%)
           (e) Basophils—role less clear; respond to many types of inflammatory events—prevalent in the allergic response; comprise up to 3% of the total differential (average 1%)
        (3) A "left shift" is said to occur when the differential suggests bacterial infection, e.g., when the presence of neutrophils increases; this may present as
           (a) Leukocytosis—total number of WBCs increases; because the majority of the total WBC count is neutrophils, an increase in neutrophils often increases the total WBC count above upper limits of normal
           (b) Neutrophil fraction > 70%
           (c) Absolute neutrophil count (ANC) exceeds 7,000 cells/mm$^3$ (ANC = WBC × neutrophil percentage)
           (d) Bands (immature WBCs) exceed 4% of the total differential (immature WBCs typically not found in circulation, but up to 4% is consistent with normal variability; > 4% suggests systemic response consistent with bacterial infection)

(e) Absolute band count (ABC) exceeds 400 cells/mm³ (ABC = WBC × band percentage)
   b. Cell-mediated immunity measured by serology
   c. Known immunodeficiency such as human immunodeficiency virus (HIV) with a CD4⁺ count < 350 cells/mm³
   d. Corticosteroid use
   e. Immunosuppressive agents, e.g., those used in the transplant patient, monoclonal antibody preparations used in autoimmune disease
   f. Cytotoxic drugs
   g. Chemotherapy
   h. Prolonged antibiotic therapy
   i. Renal failure
   j. Irradiation
3. Bleeding risk factors
   a. Patient history
      (1) Prolonged bleeding after procedure or injury
      (2) Bleeding one day after tooth extraction
      (3) Spontaneous bruising
      (4) Liver or kidney disease
      (5) Menorrhagia with iron deficiency
      (6) Unprovoked bruising > 5 cm
      (7) Recent thrombolytics, anticoagulants, nonsteroidal anti-inflammatory drugs (NSAIDs), or other drugs that prolong bleeding
      (8) Herbal medications
      (9) Personal (moral, ethical, religious) contraindication to transfusion
   b. Physical examination
      (1) Hepatosplenomegaly
      (2) Petechiae
      (3) Ecchymoses
      (4) Findings consistent with anemia
   c. Diagnostic findings
      (1) Anemia
      (2) Prolonged prothrombin time (PT), partial thromboplastin time (PTT), or international normalized ratio (INR)
      (3) Thrombocytopenia
      (4) Abnormal liver function tests (LFT)
      (5) Prolonged bleeding time (normal range 1–9 minutes)
4. Thromboembolism risk factors
   a. Cancer
   b. Obesity
   c. Age > 45 years
   d. Myocardial dysfunction
   e. History of thrombosis
   f. Use of hormonal contraception
   g. Anticipated decrease in postoperative mobility
5. Delayed wound healing
   a. Protein deficiency or depletion
   b. Volume contraction
   c. Vitamin C deficiency
   d. Smoking
   e. Poorly controlled vascular disease
      (1) Hypertension
      (2) Diabetes mellitus
      (3) Dyslipidemia
   f. Polycythemia

- Control of Chronic Illness
   1. Diabetes mellitus—no strong consensus on one single management strategy; general principles include
      a. Discontinue any oral agents on the day of surgery
      b. Patients on maintenance insulin should decrease p.m. dose the evening prior to surgery to avoid hypoglycemia when n.p.o.
      c. Goals of perioperative glycemic control
         (1) General surgical patient: fasting 90–126 mg/dL, random < 200 mg/dL
         (2) Cardiac surgery and critically ill patients: < 150 mg/dL
         (3) Acute neurological disorders: 80–140 mg/dL
      d. A variety of protocols and computer-based programs are available to calculate perioperative insulin dosing; most guidelines include a separate piggyback insulin infusion of regular insulin 100 units per 100 mL of normal saline solution (NSS) with rate calculated at insulin in units/hour = serum glucose mg/dL/150
   2. Coronary artery disease
      a. Continue antiplatelet therapy unless concerns about hemostasis are overriding; all things being equal, the risk of rebound clotting is higher when antiplatelet therapy is stopped than is the risk of bleeding when continued
      b. Medical management of existing coronary artery disease in the perioperative period typically managed by cardiology consultation
      c. Preoperative regimens of beta-adrenergic antagonists, calcium channel antagonists, and nitrates generally continued through the perioperative period
   3. Congestive heart failure
      a. Surgery should be postponed in decompensated CHF if possible
      b. Assess fluid status
      c. Inotropes as indicated throughout the perioperative period

d. Optimize preoperative management to minimize postoperative decompensation
e. Continue preoperative regimen in the stable patient
4. Hypertension
   a. Continue preoperative beta blockers and centrally acting agents on the day of surgery to avoid withdrawal syndromes
   b. Consider withholding drugs that affect the renin–angiotensin system the morning of surgery to avoid hypovolemic syndromes intraoperatively; resume only when euvolemic
   c. 75% of surgical patients will have some form of perioperative hypertension 2–6 hours postoperatively—use short-acting agents so that effect does not persist past physiological normalization
5. Anemia
   a. Hgb < 8 mg/dL is associated with increased complications
   b. Transfuse preoperatively as indicated by low hemoglobin (Hgb), presence of cardiopulmonary disease, type of surgery, and anticipated blood loss
6. Renal disease
   a. Patients with chronic kidney disease not requiring maintenance therapy (CKD stages 1–4)
      (1) Ensure adequate preoperative hydration—preoperative blood urea nitrogen (BUN) and creatinine should be at patient's best baseline
      (2) Ensure renal dosing of medications in patients with glomerular filtration rates < 30 mL/min
   b. Patients with dialysis-dependent chronic kidney disease
      (1) Admit morning prior to surgery to ensure dialysis occurs either the day before or morning of surgery
      (2) Transfuse to hematocrit of 24% if indicated
   c. In all patients with CKD
      (1) Optimize any electrolyte abnormalities
      (2) Optimize any risk of bleeding due to renal dysfunction—increases risk of anemia and thrombocytopenia

- Ensure Physical and Emotional Readiness
  1. Nutritional status
     a. Preoperative supplementation if indicated by the physical or laboratory evaluation
     b. Preoperative supplementation if prolonged n.p.o. status indicated postoperatively is anticipated
  2. Fluid and electrolyte status
     a. Fluid supplementation/diuresis preoperatively as indicated by the preoperative and diagnostic evaluations
     b. Correction of $Na^+$, $K^+$, $Ca^{++}$, $Mg^{++}$, and phosphorus to normal limits as possible
  3. Acid-base balance
     a. Correction of acid-base imbalance as indicated by preoperative condition
     b. Correction of abnormal anion gap to < 20; $Na^+ - (Cl^- + HCO_3^-)$
  4. Anxiety
     a. Will accelerate physiological stress responses
     b. Keep patient well informed—answer questions
     c. Nonpharmacological and pharmacological anxiety reduction measures as indicated
        (1) Guided imagery
        (2) Relaxation exercises
        (3) Medium-length-acting benzodiazepine to promote sleeping the night prior to surgery
  5. Prepare patient for the postoperative period, including anticipation of
     a. Ventilator support
     b. Pulmonary artery monitoring
     c. Nasogastric tube
     d. Chest tubes and/or drains
     e. Foley catheter
     f. Other drains/monitoring equipment
     g. Mobility restraints
     h. Pain
  6. Morning of surgery
     a. Answer patient and family questions
     b. Ensure patient has remained n.p.o.
     c. Document informed consent
     d. Ensure all preoperative medications have been administered
        (1) Antibiotics
        (2) Analgesics, anxiolytics
        (3) Fluids and blood products

## MANAGEMENT OF THE POSTOPERATIVE PATIENT

- Definition—the body exists in a dynamic state of equilibrium, with a complex series of compensatory mechanisms that are employed in response to any physiological stressor to achieve and maintain equilibrium. In the immediate postoperative period, these compensatory mechanisms are responsible for most physiological occurrences; the body is trying to recover from a major insult and restore homeostasis

- Events That Trigger Compensatory Mechanisms
  1. Tissue damage
  2. Volume loss
  3. Tissue hypoperfusion
  4. Pain
  5. Fear
  6. Consideration that infection and starvation will perpetuate the compensatory responses

- Responses to Volume Loss and Tissue Hypoperfusion
  1. Pressure detectors sense volume loss and signal the brain
  2. Brain stimulates catecholamine release, releases antidiuretic hormone (ADH)
  3. Aldosterone release stimulated by adrenocorticotropic hormone (ACTH) and renal mechanisms (ACE)
  4. Peripheral arteriolar smooth muscle constricts

- Responses to Tissue Damage
  1. Hypermetabolism
  2. Fever
  3. Increased mobilization and utilization of glucose, protein, fat

- Responses to Pain and Fear
  1. Varied pain responses linked to anxiety—helplessness, fear, and uncertainty will increase pain perception
  2. Physiology of postoperative pain
     a. Pain impulses transmitted to the central nervous system (CNS) from splanchnic afferent fibers, causing spinal, brain stem, and cortical responses
        (1) Spinal responses may include muscle spasm, vasospasm, and ileus
        (2) Brain stem responses include changes in ventilation, blood pressure, and endocrine function
        (3) Cortical responses include fear and apprehension, which in turn lower the threshold for pain perception and perpetuate pain sensation

- Considerations for Maintaining Homeostasis (see **Figure B-1**)
  1. The patient should be as emotionally prepared as possible for the postoperative experience
  2. Nutritional status should be as close as possible to optimal; postoperative nutritional needs should be anticipated and supplementation begun without delay
  3. Underlying chronicities should be controlled, e.g., hypertension, angina, asthma, DM, thyroid disorders, anemias, coagulopathies
  4. Pain should be managed liberally with adequate doses of appropriate medications

- Postoperative Documentation
  1. Postoperative orders
     a. Admit to (surgical) service
     b. Diagnosis—list surgical diagnosis and any medical diagnosis to be managed until transfer
     c. Condition—critical, serious, stable, etc.
     d. Activity—bed rest, out-of-bed (OOB) to chair, ambulate ad lib
     e. Diet—n.p.o., clear liquids, diabetic or caloric restrictions, advance as tolerated
     f. Intravenous fluids (IVF)—solution, rate, volume
     g. Oxygen—amount and delivery mechanism, pulse oximetry or arterial blood gas parameters for titration
     h. Monitor—telemetry, cardiopulmonary pressures, end-tidal $CO_2$, EEG, etc.
     i. Incision observation or care as indicated
     j. Vital signs (VS) and intake/output (I/O) monitoring with parameters for notification if indicated
     k. Drains or tubes—gravity, suction, parameters for fluid replacement or provider notification
     l. Pulmonary toilet
     m. Medications—name, dose, frequency, route, and parameters to administer, hold, or notify
     n. Deep vein thrombosis (DVT) prophylaxis
     o. Laboratory and other diagnostic orders
     p. Consultations
  2. Postoperative progress note
     a. Summarize the events of the procedure to include estimated blood loss (EBL), any significant deviations in patient response, and patient tolerance
     b. Outline plan for postoperative management and follow-up
     c. Be specific about the plan for ongoing monitoring

- Postoperative Complications
  1. Bleeding
     a. The best way to reduce risk is to ensure a thorough preoperative evaluation
     b. All patients should be monitored for subtle signs of bleeding
        (1) Unexplained elevation of pulse or drop in blood pressure
        (2) Unanticipated blood in urine, stool, or drainage
        (3) Unexplained ecchymoses

**FIGURE B-1** Systemic Responses to Physiological Stress

- Hypothalamus
  - Elaboration of ACTH, ADH, GH
- Efferent neural pathways
- Afferent neural pathways
- Pancreatic response
  - ↑ glucagon
  - ↓ insulin
- Heart (baroreceptors)
- Trauma (injured tissue)
- Cardiac responses
  - ↑ stroke volume
  - ↑ heart rate
- Pancreas
- Local inflammatory mediators
  - Cytokines
  - Prostaglandins
  - Platelet-activating factor
- Adrenal responses
  - ↑ cortisol release
  - ↑ catecholamine release
- Renal volume conserving mechanisms
  - Aldosterone
  - ADH
- Humoral cascades
  - Complement
  - Kinins
- Mobilization of amino acids from skeletal muscle
- Peripheral vasoconstriction (redistributes blood to more vital organs)

    (4) Increased or change in character of pain
    (5) Decrease in Hgb/hematocrit (Hct) not explained by documented blood loss or fluid replacement
  c. If bleeding occurs
    (1) Laboratory assessment to quantify blood loss and identify cause
      (a) CBC
      (b) PT/INR, PTT
    (2) Specific measures as indicated to stop bleeding if site identified
    (3) Ensure hemodynamic stability with crystalloids; transfuse as necessary

2. Atelectasis
  a. Affects 25% of postoperative patients
  b. Has obstructive and nonobstructive features
  c. Obstruction may come from COPD, intubation, anesthesia, blood clots, malposition of the endotracheal tube
  d. Often caused by closed bronchioles when the lung reaches closing volume (closing volume higher in older people and smokers as a result of the loss of elasticity)—immediate effect is hypoxemia; later result is infection of the atelectatic segment with clinical indicators to include:

- (1) Tachycardia
- (2) Fever
- (3) Tachypnea
- (4) Elevated diaphragm
- (5) Rales
  e. Treatment
   - (1) Chest percussion
   - (2) Cough
   - (3) Airway expansion
   - (4) Nasotracheal suction
   - (5) Bronchodilators
   - (6) Mucolytic agents
   - (7) Fiber-optic bronchoscopy
   - (8) Place patient with the uninvolved side in dependent position
3. Pulmonary aspiration
   a. Nasogastric (NG) and endotracheal (ET) tubes depress protective sphincters
   b. Esophageal reflux, food in the stomach, and patient position increase risk
   c. Two-thirds of cases of aspiration follow thoracic or abdominal surgery
   d. 50% cases of aspiration result in pneumonia
   e. Death rate for aspiration pneumonia is 50%
   f. Aspiration of highly acidic contents causes chemical pneumonitis
   g. Aspiration occurs in 80% of patients with tracheostomies
   h. Prevention is the best approach—if aspiration occurs, treat for hospital-acquired pneumonia as indicated by clinical diagnosis and chest radiography
4. Fat embolism
   a. Very common postoperatively—rarely causes symptoms
   b. Fat embolism syndrome—most often related to bone surgery or liposuction but does occur in other circumstances
      (1) Neurological dysfunction
      (2) Respiratory insufficiency
      (3) Petechiae of axilla, chest, and proximal arms
      (4) Onset 12–72 hours after procedure
      (5) Diagnosis is clinical—a variety of clinical criteria have been proposed, including Gurd's criteria, Lindeque's criteria, and Schonfeld's criteria
      (6) Decreased hematocrit, platelets, and other coagulopathies common
      (7) Treatment is supportive until symptoms subside—mortality estimated at 5–15%
5. Deep vein thrombosis (DVT)
   a. Typical risk factors include bed rest, immobility, obesity, old age
   b. Edema is the most specific symptom; up to 50% of patients may be asymptomatic
   c. Diagnostic evaluation should include
      (1) Validated clinical prediction rules
      (2) High-sensitivity D-dimer assay
      (3) Venous ultrasound
      (4) Coagulation studies if hypercoagulable state suspected
   d. Management
      (1) Anticoagulation with heparin, low-molecular-weight heparins, factor Xa inhibitors, or warfarin as indicated; duration of therapy depends on clinical circumstances and location of thrombus
      (2) Ambulation as tolerated after initial stabilization
      (3) Thrombus removal in severe iliofemoral cases with limb ischemia
      (4) Inferior vena cava filters when:
         (a) Confirmed thrombus in patients with contraindication to anticoagulation
         (b) Recurrent thromboembolism while on anticoagulants
6. Renal failure
   a. Most commonly due to volume contraction/renal hypoperfusion (prerenal failure)
      (1) Renal failure is due to glomerular hypoperfusion
      (2) Any urine formed is characterized by normal urinalysis
      (3) Unlike other forms of renal failure, BUN/Cr ratio typically wide at > 20:1
      (4) Restoration of volume/renal perfusion typically corrects the problem
   b. Intrarenal failure
      (1) Occurs as a consequence of nephron damage
      (2) May occur postoperatively following renal ischemia
      (3) Acute oliguria is characteristic of early phase
      (4) BUN/Cr ratio < 10:1
      (5) Urine sediment shows tubular cells and casts
      (6) Urine sodium concentration > 40 mEq/L
      (7) Treatment is supportive until resolution—patient may require renal replacement therapy (RRT)

- Postoperative Fluid Management
  1. Short-term replacement
     a. Not necessary to measure serum electrolytes

b. Typically replace 2,000–2,500 mL 5% dextrose in normal saline solution (D5NSS) or lactated Ringer's (LR) per 24-hour period
   c. No potassium in the first 24-hour period
   d. Losses from fluid sequestration at the operative site usually replaced intraoperatively
   e. Sensible and insensible losses can be approximated by multiplying weight in kilograms (wt in kg) by 30 cc
2. Following complex operation—fluid and electrolyte replacement should be calculated based on
   a. Maintenance requirements
   b. Extra needs (fever, burns)
   c. Losses from drains
   d. Third space losses
3. Fluid maintenance requirements
   a. As noted above, fluid maintenance calculated by 30 cc × wt in kg
   b. Fluid replacement must be isotonic
   c. Most body fluids are isosmolar—replacing extensive body fluid losses with isotonic saline only will result in electrolyte abnormalities
4. Electrolyte maintenance requirements
   a. Most common electrolyte abnormalities—hyponatremia, hypochloremia, hypokalemia
   b. Hypochloremia often results in compensatory renal retention of $HCO_3^-$, resulting in metabolic alkalosis—most common postoperative acid-base disorder
   c. Hyponatremia and hypochloremia may occur as a result of excess D5W
   d. Hypernatremia is less common but can result from excess postoperative losses, e.g., diarrhea, tube drainage without adequate replacement of free water
   e. Although mechanisms exist for calculating sodium deficits, both hyponatremia and hypernatremia will be corrected with the infusion of normal saline unless sodium < 110 or > 150 mEq
   f. Potassium must be corrected to normal pH
5. Extra needs
   a. Febrile patients (temp > 101.0° F) are at twice the normal metabolic rate
   b. Burn patients require 3–4 mL/kg body weight/% burn in the first 24 hours; at least half should be given in the first 8 hours
   c. Losses from drains
      (1) Most gastrointestinal (GI) losses of < 500 cc can be replaced with isotonic fluid
      (2) Add 20 mEq of potassium for every liter of fluid loss
      (3) Losses of > 1,500 cc from any single site require electrolyte measurement every 4–6 hours

## COMMON PROBLEMS IN ACUTE CARE

### ■ Fever

- Definition—an elevation in body temperature that usually occurs as a protective or compensatory mechanism to protect the body from an infectious organism or to augment the inflammatory response by facilitating vasodilation and the migration of inflammatory mediators to a site of injury; management of fever should include a risk–benefit analysis and antipyretics instituted only when the metabolic costs of fever pose a threat to the patient that are not outweighed by the benefits

- Physiological Benefits of Fever
  1. Fever is both a diagnostic and prognostic indicator
  2. Fever augments several aspects of the inflammatory response
  3. Fever complements antibiotic activity
  4. Fever enhances survival in animal studies

- Metabolic Costs of Fever
  1. Oxygen consumption increases by 13% for each centigrade degree of temperature elevation
     a. Easily tolerated by a patient with no cardiopulmonary disease
     b. May produce dangerous hypoxia in a patient with clinically significant disease
  2. Relatively minor decreases in temperature elevation double caloric requirements
     a. Tolerable in a patient with normal weight or in whom calorie supplement is easily administered
     b. May rapidly lead to malnutrition in a patient who is already underweight or a poor candidate for effective nutritional supplementation, e.g., an elderly patient who is not tolerating tube feedings
  3. Fever reduces mental acuity and may cause delirium—risk does not outweigh benefit in elderly adults and those otherwise at risk for mental status changes
  4. Fever above 102° F commonly causes patient discomfort, which can lead to decreased activity and ambulation and contribute to complications associated with immobility

- Key Points in Fever Assessment
  1. An immunocompetent body develops fever when challenged with an infectious microorganism

2. Invading organisms usually infect the host because the host's environment is compatible with the organism's physiological needs, e.g., temperature of 98.6° F
3. Elevation of body temperature usually inactivates the infecting organism
4. Not all fevers are of infectious origin (see **Table B-1**)—noninfectious tissue damage triggers an inflammatory response that includes the liberation of pyrogens; heat facilitates healing (see **Figure B-2**)

**TABLE B-1   Noninfectious Causes of Fever**

| | | |
|---|---|---|
| ARDS | Autoimmune disease | Cirrhosis |
| CVA/MI | Decubitus ulcer | Drug reactions |
| ETOH/drug withdrawal | Fat emboli | Gout |
| Hematoma | Inflammatory disease | Ischemic bowel |
| Neoplastic fever | Neuroleptic malignant syndrome | Pancreatitis |
| Post-transfusion | Serotonin syndrome | Thrombophlebitis |

**FIGURE B-2   Inflammation as a Cause of Fever**

Infectious agents/toxins/mediators of inflammation (Pyrogens)
↓
Monocytes/macrophages/endothelial cells/other cell types release
↓
Pyrogenic cytokines – IL-1, TNF, IL-6 stimulate
↓
Anterior hypothalamus (mediated by $PGE_2$) (*Antipyretics/NSAIDs act here*) results
↓
Elevated thermoregulatory set point leads to
↓
Increased heat conservation (Vasoconstriction/behavior changes)
Increased heat production (involuntary muscular contractions) result in
↓
FEVER

5. Other indicators of infection are usually present when fever is of infectious origin
   a. Erythema, edema, heat, and pus at insertion point of tubes and lines or infected soft tissue
   b. Foul-smelling and purulent urine if urinary tract infection present
   c. Consolidation on radiograph if pneumonia present
   d. Sinus opacities on maxillofacial CT scan if sinusitis present
   e. Positive blood cultures
   f. Appropriate white blood cell shift to support bacterial or viral infection
6. Diagnostic cues
   a. Fever due to common infection usually demonstrates diurnal variation
      (1) In common viral and bacterial infection, temperature peaks late in the day; drops to normal or near normal levels in the morning hours
      (2) Use caution when fever is a criterion for transfer to lower level of care or discharge
   b. Absent normal diurnal variation, consider other causes of fever
      (1) Central nervous system damage
      (2) Fictitious fever (manipulated by the patient to prolong hospital stay)
      (3) Gram-negative pneumonia
   c. Fever that does not return to normal in a 24-hour period suggests drug fever
   d. Noninfectious fever rarely exceeds 102° F; infection, drug fever, or transfusion reaction are leading differentials if > 102° F
   e. Fever that occurs > 5 days postoperatively suggests abscess formation
   f. Fever that occurs after at least 10 days on inpatient antibiotics requires assessment for fungal infection
7. Prognostic cues
   a. Pattern of fever suggestive of response of treatment
   b. Presence of fever suggestive of anticipated outcome depending on the underlying condition
      (1) Pancreatitis characterized by fever suggests a more serious hospital course
      (2) Sepsis characterized by fever is associated with better patient outcomes

- Postoperative Fever
1. Postoperative fever may also be infectious or noninfectious
2. Most fever in postoperative patients is noninfectious and is likely due to

a. Increased basal metabolic rate as a response to physiological stress
b. Volume contraction due to operative loss
c. Postoperative atelectasis—greater risk in those with prolonged intubation
d. Drug reaction
3. Like fever in any febrile patient, postoperative fever typically is accompanied by other indices of infection

- Fever of Unknown Origin (FUO)
    1. A variety of criteria exist to categorize fever as FUO
        a. Fever of > 101° F on several occasions with no obvious cause AND
        b. More than 3 weeks duration AND
        c. No cause is identified despite 1 week of inpatient evaluation AND
        d. Fictitious fever is ruled out
    2. FUO statistical disposition—ultimately an origin is determined in at least 85% of cases
        a. 30–40% are infectious
        b. 20–30% are neoplasms
        c. 10–20% are collagen vascular disease
        d. 15–20% are miscellaneous causes
        e. 5–15% are truly unknown—usually ultimately characterized by a benign course if no other substantial disease present

- Management of Fever—depends on the underlying cause; antipyretics are symptom management and should be administered only when they do not hinder diagnosis, when curative treatment is targeted to the underlying problem, and when the metabolic risks of fever outweigh the benefits
    1. Postoperative fever
        a. In the absence of clear indicators of infection—and in the first 3 days post-operatively—presume atelectasis and/or volume contraction
            (1) Encourage spirometry use
            (2) Ambulation
            (3) Cough and deep breathe
            (4) Use of sigh setting on ventilated patients
            (5) Increase isotonic fluid administration
        b. Consider all other noninfectious causes of fever that may occur in nonoperative patients, especially those associated with immobility such as DVT
        c. In the presence of indicators of infection—such as a white blood cell shift—discontinue any suspect invasive device and institute diagnostic evaluation
            (1) Discontinue any lines or drains that appear purulent
            (2) Culture urine, blood, and sputum
            (3) Diagnostic imaging of the lungs, abdomen, sinuses, and operative site if appropriate
            (4) Begin broad spectrum antibiotics targeted to likely organisms pending culture
    2. The medical patient
        a. Determine underlying source as able—antibiotics indicated only in the setting of bacterial infection
            (1) Local signs and symptoms
            (2) Constitutional signs and symptoms
            (3) Leukocytosis with neutrophilia +/− bandemia
            (4) Fever likely > 102° F
        b. Antipyretics only when the metabolic costs of fever outweigh the diagnostic and prognostic benefits
            (1) Should not be given routinely
            (2) Clear indications to treat
                (a) Acute brain insult
                (b) Limited cardiopulmonary reserve
                (c) Body mass index (BMI) < 18
                (d) Temperature > 104° F
                (e) Delirium
        c. External therapies
            (1) Cooling blankets
                (a) No more effective than antipyretics are
                (b) Associated with large fluctuations in temperature; produce peripheral vasoconstriction that ultimately shunts hot blood to the deeper tissues and organs, increasing risk of adverse outcomes
            (2) Ice packing—used in emergent situations
            (3) Cool sponge bathing—more efficacious as a comfort measure than a temperature-reduction technique
    3. Fever of unknown origin
        a. "Treatment" really centers around a systematic approach to identifying cause
        b. Must first exclude the possibility of fictitious fever
        c. Daily questioning about symptoms from all major organ systems, including generalized complaints
        d. Record all complaints even if no longer present
        e. Review all previous illnesses, including psychiatric history
        f. Detailed history
            (1) Family history
            (2) Immunization status

(3) Occupational history
(4) Travel history
(5) Nutrition
(6) Drug history (prescribed, over-the-counter [OTC], recreational)
(7) Sexual history
(8) Recreational habits
(9) Animal contacts, including vector

g. Document fever pattern
   (1) 24-hour diurnal variation with nadir in a.m. and peaks in p.m. suggests infection
   (2) No 24-hour variability suggests drug fever, gram-negative pneumonia, or CNS thermoregulatory disease
   (3) Peaks < 102° F increase likelihood of noninfectious cause (see Table B-1)

h. Physical examination daily—special notice to
   (1) Rashes
   (2) New/changing cardiac murmur
   (3) Joint pain
   (4) Abdominal pain, tenderness/rigidity
   (5) Lymph node enlargement
   (6) Neurological deficits
   (7) Edema

i. Diagnostic evaluation—at a minimum must include
   (1) CBC with differential and microscopic
   (2) Urinalysis
   (3) Liver function tests
   (4) Bacteria, fungal, stool, cerebrospinal fluid, urine, pleural fluid, peritoneal fluid, and mycobacterial cultures
   (5) Serology for Epstein-Barr virus, HIV, amebiasis, toxoplasmosis, sexually transmitted infections
   (6) Serum protein electrophoresis
   (7) Antinuclear antibodies (ANA), rheumatoid factor (RF, thyroid-stimulating hormone (TSH), erythrocyte sedimentation rate (ESR)
   (8) CT scan of the chest, abdomen, pelvis
   (9) MRI if osteomyelitis or vasculitides a possibility
   (10) Upper and lower endoscopy and retrograde cholangiography
   (11) Biopsies (lymph node) when all other explorations negative

j. Disposition
   (1) No evidence to support continued inpatient care when all evaluation is negative
   (2) Transfer to another facility only if all testing is not available or the patient experiences clinical deterioration

# Nutritional Support

- Definition—nutritional considerations in the acutely ill patient are not unlike those in patients who are well, but there are some important differences; although nurse practitioners may not be ordering the specifics of parenteral therapy, the primary service is always responsible for the general hospital course and care of the patient. Poor nutrition can precede a wide variety of complications that may prolong hospital stay and lead to complications and poor outcomes
    1. Nutritional considerations for all patients
        a. Nutrition should come from the three physiological fuel sources; carbohydrates, proteins, and fats
        b. The patient's primary service assumes responsibility for ensuring that the patient's nutritional needs are met—this may involve the utilization of consulting services, but the responsibility remains with the primary service
    2. Nutritional considerations for the acutely ill patient
        a. In times of physiological stress a patient's caloric need is double its baseline requirement as a result of the hypercatabolic state; a patient who normally requires 1,500 kcal/day now requires 3,000 kcal/day to sustain existing weight
        b. In times of physiological stress, the goal of nutritional therapy is to sustain the patient's existing weight, *even if the patient is obese*—this may require the administration of a large number of calories
        c. Typical caloric requirement to sustain existing weight is 30–35 kcal/kg of body weight daily; consequently most hospitalized patients will require 60–70 kcal/kg daily.
    3. Patients requiring nutritional support include those
        a. Who are unable to ingest adequate amounts
            (1) Obtunded or comatose
            (2) Impaired swallow, e.g., new cerebrovascular accident (CVA) or other cerebral event
            (3) Mouth or gut surgery
        b. With severe, prolonged hypercatabolic states
        c. Requiring prolonged, therapeutic bowel rest
        d. With severe, protein-calorie malnutrition with a treatable disease who have lost 25% of body weight

4. Principles of nutritional support
    a. Determine the patient's daily caloric requirement
    b. Always use the gut if able
    c. Use the least invasive method of administration (see **Figure B-3**)
    d. Determine whether support will be short or long term
        (1) Enteral support—long term defined as > 6 weeks
        (2) Parenteral support—long term defined as > 2 weeks
    e. Enteral support
        (1) Use nasogastric access (nasoduodenal if increased risk of aspiration) if short term
        (2) Use direct gastric access, e.g., percutaneous endoscopic gastrostomy (PEG) tube if long term
    f. Parenteral support
        (1) Use peripheral parenteral nutrition (PPN) if short term
        (2) Use total parenteral nutrition (TPN) if long term
5. Complications of nutritional support
    a. Enteral
        (1) Usually the result of the feeding solution itself
            (a) Feeding solution is very hyperosmolar and draws water into the gut
            (b) Diarrhea is the most common complication
            (c) Treatment includes slowing/withdrawing the feeding and gradually reintroducing with slowly escalating amounts
        (2) Emesis
        (3) Dehydration
        (4) Hypernatremia
        (5) Mechanical obstruction of the tube
        (6) Aspiration
    b. Parenteral
        (1) Most PPN/TPN ordered by specialty services; problems with solution not usually a problem
        (2) Complications typically related to the delivery mechanism
            (a) Catheter sepsis
            (b) Pneumothorax
            (c) Arterial laceration
            (d) Air emboli
            (e) Catheter thrombosis
        (3) Parenteral nutrition not properly calculated can cause serious metabolic abnormalities (see **Table B-2**)
            (a) Hyperglycemia
            (b) Hyperosmolar hyperglycemic state (HHS)
            (c) Hyperchloremic metabolic acidosis
            (d) Azotemia

**FIGURE B-3** Decision Tree—Methods of Nutritional Supplementation

## Electrolyte Abnormalities

- Definition—electrolyte deficiencies and excesses can occur in a variety of diagnoses, are consistent with many disease states, and are presented throughout this text. However, in the acute care setting three electrolytes—sodium, potassium, and calcium—frequently present with abnormalities that have immediate clinical implications. Because imbalances of these electrolytes often need to be managed immediately in the acute care setting, independent of the underlying disease state, they are presented here
    1. Hyponatremia (serum $Na^+$ < 135 mEq/L)
        a. The most common electrolyte abnormality in the acute care setting
        b. Clinical relevance is that $Na^+$ is the most abundant extracellular solute
            (1) Hyponatremia may result in hypo-osmolality
            (2) Hypo-osmolality may result in intracellular fluid shift
            (3) Intracellular fluid shift may result in intracellular edema
            (4) Intracellular edema will decrease intracellular function
            (5) Neurological changes that occur in hyponatremic patients are a consequence of intracellular edema of the neuron

### TABLE B-2  Calculating Parenteral Nutrition

**Determining nutritional requirements: A complete nutritional support solution should include water, energy, protein, electrolytes, vitamins, minerals, and essential fatty acids.**

| | |
|---|---|
| Water | 1,500 cc for first 20 kg body wt + 20 cc for every kg > 20<br>Additional losses replaced as they occur |
| Energy | Indirect calorimetry is preferred—can estimate energy requirements by wt × 30–35 kcal |
| Protein | If adequate calories are provided, give 0.8–1.2 g/kg/day of protein<br>If client is in moderate to severe distress, 1.5 g/kg/day |
| Electrolytes/vitamins/minerals | Requirements for electrolytes are greatly varied, by range 45–145 mEq/d. Actual requirements depend on patient's CV, renal, GI, and endocrine function.<br>Clients on enteral support should receive vitamins and minerals according to RDA<br>Clients on parenteral support should get daily vitamins, smaller amounts of minerals, and trace elements (zinc, copper)<br>** Parenteral iron should not be given routinely ** |
| Essential fatty acids | Clients on enteral support should get EFA as 2–4% of total calories as linoleic acid<br>Clients on parenteral nutrition should get 250 cc of 20% IV fat 2–3 times per week |

   c. When a patient is hyponatremic, the next assessment must be of serum osmolality; hyponatremia is characterized by one of three osmolar states (see **Table B-3**)
      (1) Isotonic hyponatremia ($Na^+ < 135$ mEq/L with normal serum osmolality [270–290 mOsm/L])
      (2) Hypotonic hyponatremia ($Na^+ < 135$ mEq/L with low serum osmolality [< 270 mOsm/L])
      (3) Hypertonic hyponatremia ($Na^+ < 135$ mEq/L with high osmolality [> 290 mOsm/L])
   d. Treating hyponatremia depends on underlying cause
      (1) Isotonic hyponatremia—no treatment required because hyponatremia not clinically significant
      (2) Hypotonic hyponatremia
         (a) Hypervolemic—treat cause of free water excess; infuse isotonic saline or hypertonic saline depending on the presence/absence of neurological symptoms
         (b) Hypovolemic—treat cause of fluid and sodium loss and infuse isotonic saline
         (c) Isotonic—treat cause and infuse isotonic saline
2. Hypernatremia (serum $Na^+ > 145$ mEq/L)
   a. Virtually always a result of free water loss; excess $Na^+$ intake to the point of serum hypernatremia does not occur
   b. Clinical concern is that hypernatremia may produce extracellular hyperosmolality with resultant extracellular fluid shift
      (1) Fluid shifts out of the cell
      (2) Intracellular volume contraction occurs
      (3) Cell morphology changes and function declines
   c. Primary assessment includes clinical volume state, patient history, and urine osmolality—need to determine where patient is losing free water
      (1) Urine osmolality < 250 mOsm/L is characteristic of central and nephrogenic diabetes insipidus (DI)—patient is unable to conserve water at the nephron
      (2) Urine osmolality > 400 mOsm/L is characteristic of water-conserving ability; water loss is occurring at some site other than the nephron
         (a) Gastrointestinal losses—evaluate for vomiting and/or diarrhea
         (b) Normal GI function—evaluate for excess diaphoresis
   d. Treatment
      (1) Severe hypernatremia with hypovolemia should be treated with NSS followed by ½ NSS
      (2) Hypernatremia with euvolemia should be treated with free water (D5W)
      (3) Hypernatremia with hypervolemia should be treated with free water and loop diuretics—may need dialysis
3. Hypokalemia (serum $K^+ < 3.5$ mEq/L)
   a. Primary consequence is cardiac myocyte irritability as a consequence of an inability to maintain membrane resting potential

## TABLE B-3  Types of Hyponatremia

| Isotonic | Hypotonic | Hypertonic |
|---|---|---|
| – Amount of plasma water decreased as a result of increase in indissolvable solute (hyperlipidemia most common)<br>– Each liter of serum typically comprised of 900 mL plasma water and 100 mL indissolvable solute—serum sodium reported in the metabolic panel is actually a representation of the amount of sodium dissolved in the 900 mL plasma water<br>• Reported serum sodium of 140 mEq/L (140 mmol/L) actually 140 mEq/900 mL plasma water, or 0.15 mEq/mL<br>• When indisolvable solute elevated, may only have 800 mL plasma water and 200 mL of solute—sodium dissolves only in the plasma water; therefore, a serum sodium of 120 mEq/L (120 mmol/L) in this patient would be 120 mEq/800 mL plasma water, or 0.15 mEq/mL, rendering the patient isotonic<br>– Treatment involves reducing the indissolvable solute; as plasma water per L increases, sodium will rise | – Assess clinical volume state and urine sodium<br>• Clinically wet (volume overload)<br>• Patient is retaining free water<br>• Serum sodium is diluted<br>• Common causes include cardiac, hepatic, or renal failure<br>• Treatment will include free water restriction ± diuresis<br>• Clinically dry (volume contracted)<br>• Patient is losing sodium and water<br>• Sodium loss exceeds water loss; net result is hyponatremia<br>• Need to assess urine sodium to determine site of loss<br>• Urine sodium < 10 mEq/L (10 mmol/L), renal function is intact, investigate GI or diaphoretic losses<br>• Urine sodium normal or > 20 mEq/L (20 mmol/L), renal loss is apparent, diuretic excess is likely<br>• In either case treatment is to replace sodium, water, and treat underlying cause<br>• Clinically normal (euvolemic)<br>• Mild free water retention<br>• Hypothyroidism is most common cause. | – Increase in some other solute raises osmolality (hyperglycemia is most common)<br>– In an effort to maintain an isotonic state, the kidney begins dumping solute<br>– Sodium is the most abundant extracellular solute and is frequently excreted<br>– When hyperglycemia (or other solute excess) normalizes, the hyponatremia resolves |

    b. Clinically, patients are at risk for dysrhythmias such as premature ventricular beats, ventricular tachycardia, and ventricular fibrillation; it is difficult to correct ventricular dysrhythmia in a hypokalemic patient
    c. Causes
       (1) Chronic diuretic use
       (2) Gastrointestinal fluid loss
       (3) Excess renal loss
          (a) Transtubular potassium concentration gradient (TTKG) distinguishes renal from nonrenal losses
          (b) TTKG > 4 suggests renal loss with increased distal secretion

$$TTKG = \frac{Urine\ K^+ / Plasma\ K^+}{Urine\ Osm / Plasma\ Osm}$$

       (4) Alkalosis
          (a) Serum $K^+$ drops 0.3 mEq for each 0.1 increase in pH due to metabolic alkalosis
          (b) Serum $K^+$ drops 0.2 mEq for each 0.1 increase in pH due to respiratory alkalosis
       (5) Elevated serum epinephrine, e.g., trauma
    d. Clinical signs and symptoms
       (1) Muscle weakness
       (2) Fatigue
       (3) Cramping
       (4) Constipation
       (5) Ileus
       (6) Palpitations
       (7) If $K^+$ < 2.5 mEq/L
          (a) Flaccid paralysis
          (b) Tetany
          (c) Hyporeflexia
          (d) Rhabdomyolysis
    e. Cardiac rhythm strip
       (1) Decreased amplitude on ECG
       (2) Broad T waves
       (3) Prominent U waves
       (4) Ventricular tachycardia or fibrillation

- f. Treatment
  - (1) Oral replacement if > 2.5 mEq and no ECG abnormalities
  - (2) IV replacement at 10 mEq/hour if cannot take oral replacement
  - (3) If < 2.5 mEq or severe signs or symptoms
    - (a) Give 40 mEq/L/hour IV
    - (b) Monitor at least q.3.h.
    - (c) Continuous ECG monitoring
  - (4) Ensure normal $Mg^{++}$; deficit may impair $K^+$ correction
4. Hyperkalemia (serum $K^+$ > 5.5 mEq/L)
  - a. Primary consequence is a decreased ability to depolarize myocardium; eventually, cardiac myocytes will not contract, and if untreated, patient becomes bradycardic and asystolic
  - b. Causes
    - (1) Acidosis—$K^+$ increases 0.7 mEq/L with each 0.1 drop in pH
    - (2) Excess exogenous replacement
    - (3) Renal failure
    - (4) Medications that contain $K^+$ or promote retention
      - (a) NSAIDs
      - (b) Heparin
      - (c) Angiotensin-converting enzyme (ACE) inhibitors
      - (d) Renin inhibitors
      - (e) Angiotensin receptor antagonists
      - (f) $K^+$-sparing diuretics
    - (5) Hemolysis
  - c. Signs and symptoms
    - (1) Muscle weakness
    - (2) Flaccid paralysis
    - (3) Ileus
  - d. Cardiac rhythm strip (may not occur until very late)
    - (1) Peaked T waves
    - (2) Wide QRS complex
    - (3) Bundle branch blocks
    - (4) Atrioventricular blocks
    - (5) Bradycardia
  - e. Treatment
    - (1) Exchange resins
    - (2) If > 6.5 mEq/L or cardiac toxicity or muscle paralysis is present
      - (a) Insulin 10 U with 1 amp D50
      - (b) Calcium gluconate as antagonist
      - (c) Beta-adrenergic agonists reduce serum $K^+$ 0.5–1 mEq/L in 30 minutes
      - (d) $NaHCO_3^-$ in emergency
5. Hypocalcemia (serum $Ca^{++}$ < 8.5 mEq/L)
  - a. Primary consequence is a decreased ability to achieve and maintain muscle contraction; severe hypocalcemia may also produce bleeding abnormalities
  - b. Causes
    - (1) Hypoparathyroidism
    - (2) Hypomagnesemia
    - (3) Chronic kidney disease
    - (4) Pancreatitis
    - (5) Severe trauma
    - (6) Multiple transfusion
    - (7) Decreased serum albumin
  - c. Signs and symptoms
    - (1) Increased deep tendon reflexes (DTR)
    - (2) Muscle/abdominal cramps
    - (3) Carpopedal spasm
    - (4) Convulsions
    - (5) Trousseau's sign—carpal spasm with occlusion of brachial artery
    - (6) Chvostek's sign—tapping the facial nerve produces contraction of facial muscle
  - d. Cardiac rhythm strip
    - (1) Prolonged QT interval
    - (2) Dysmorphic QRS complex
  - e. Treatment
    - (1) Oral replacement for chronic or asymptomatic patients
    - (2) If paralysis, seizure, or dysrhythmia present
      - (a) Continuous calcium gluconate infusion
      - (b) 10–15 mg/kg to 1 L D5W infused over 4–6 hours; monitor $Ca^{++}$ every 4–6 hours and titrate drip to serum level > 7 mg/dL
6. Hypercalcemia (serum $Ca^{++}$ > 10 mEq/L)
  - a. Primary consequence is a progressive decline in mental status that may lead to coma and death if untreated; otherwise, symptoms and signs are vague and ill defined
  - b. Causes
    - (1) Hyperparathyroidism
    - (2) Vitamin D excess
    - (3) Acromegaly
    - (4) Adrenal insufficiency
    - (5) Thyrotoxicosis
    - (6) Thiazide diuretics
    - (7) Lithium
    - (8) Immobility
  - c. Signs and symptoms
    - (1) Nausea/vomiting
    - (2) Muscle weakness
    - (3) Depression
    - (4) Anorexia
    - (5) Constipation
    - (6) Renal colic

(7) Neurological decline
    (a) Drowsiness and confusion
    (b) Stupor
    (c) Obtundation
    (d) Coma
d. Treatment
    (1) Stop calcium-containing medications
    (2) Loop diuretics with isotonic saline replacement
    (3) Calcitonin if impaired cardiac or renal function
    (4) Dialysis in extreme cases
    (5) Investigate underlying cause—malignancy should be considered

# Acid-Base Disorders

- Definition—an imbalance in pH that is either below lower limits of normal (< 7.35) or above upper limits of normal (> 7.45); may be a consequence of metabolic imbalance, respiratory imbalance, or both
  1. Key concepts in acid-base disorders
     a. Assessment requires measurement of arterial blood gas (ABG) for pH, $pCO_2$, and $HCO_3^-$; total venous $CO_2$ is a more direct determination of arterial bicarbonate
     b. Venous blood gases are also useful because arteriovenous differences are constant with the exception of cardiopulmonary arrest
     c. Two types of acid-base disorders are acidosis (pH < 7.35) and alkalosis (pH > 7.45)
     d. Acidosis and alkalosis may be either respiratory or metabolic
        (1) Respiratory disorders are a consequence of $pCO_2$
            (a) Increased $pCO_2$ produces respiratory acidosis
            (b) Decreased $pCO_2$ produces respiratory alkalosis
        (2) Metabolic disorders are a consequence of $HCO_3^-$
            (a) Increased $HCO_3^-$ produces metabolic alkalosis
            (b) Decreased $HCO_3^-$ produces metabolic acidosis
     e. The unaffected system will compensate
        (1) Primary respiratory acidosis
            (a) Primary problem is respiratory $CO_2$ retention (e.g., COPD)
            (b) Metabolic compensatory mechanisms promote renal $HCO_3^-$ retention to compensate
            (c) Compensatory mechanisms will not exceed a minimum threshold; compensated respiratory acidosis will result in an arterial pH between 7.35 and 7.39
        (2) Primary respiratory alkalosis
            (a) Primary problem is increased respiratory $CO_2$ exhalation
            (b) Metabolic compensatory mechanisms promote renal $HCO_3^-$ excretion to compensate
            (c) Compensatory mechanisms will not exceed minimum threshold; compensated respiratory alkalosis will result in an arterial pH between 7.41 and 7.45
        (3) Primary metabolic acidosis
            (a) Primary problem is accelerated renal excretion of $HCO_3^-$
            (b) Respiratory compensatory mechanisms promote respiratory $CO_2$ exhalation to compensate
            (c) Compensatory mechanisms will not exceed minimum threshold; compensated metabolic acidosis will result in an arterial pH between 7.35 and 7.39
        (4) Primary metabolic alkalosis
            (a) Primary problem is renal retention of $HCO_3^-$
            (b) Respiratory compensatory mechanisms promote respiratory $CO_2$ retention to compensate
            (c) Compensatory mechanisms will not exceed minimum threshold; compensated metabolic alkalosis will result in an arterial pH between 7.41 and 7.45
     f. Disorders may present as mixed acid-base disorders; the primary problem should be determined by analysis of the ABG (see **Table B-4**)
     g. Anion gap should always be calculated
        (1) Anion gap represents the difference between positive and negative ions
        (2) An anion gap > 20 mEq/L indicates a primary metabolic disturbance regardless of ABG analysis
        (3) Corrected bicarbonate should be calculated in high-gap metabolic acidosis
  2. Metabolic acidosis
     a. Characterized by decreased pH and decreased $HCO_3^-$
     b. Classified as either normal gap or high-gap acidosis
     c. Increased anion gap acidosis—typically indicates an acute, unstable patient
        (1) Lactic acidosis—lactate levels exceed 5 mEq/L—often much higher
            (a) Decreased tissue perfusion (shock states)
            (b) Carbon monoxide poisoning
            (c) Hepatic disease

| **TABLE B-4** Assessment of Compensated Acid-Base States ||||
|---|---|---|---|
| **Respiratory Acidosis** | **Respiratory Alkalosis** | **Metabolic Acidosis** | **Metabolic Alkalosis** |
| pH 7.36 | pH 7.43 | pH 7.36 | pH 7.44 |
| pCO$_2$ 55 mm Hg | pCO$_2$ 30 mm Hg | pCO$_2$ 31 mm Hg | pCO$_2$ 50 mm Hg |
| HCO$_3^-$ 32 mm Hg | HCO$_3^-$ 19 mm Hg | HCO$_3^-$ 19 mm Hg | HCO$_3^-$ 32 mm Hg |
| Pt is exhibiting compensated respiratory acidosis | Pt is exhibiting compensated respiratory alkalosis | Pt is exhibiting compensated metabolic acidosis | Pt is exhibiting compensated metabolic alkalosis |
| Elevated pCO$_2$ indicates CO$_2$ retention, which produces an acidotic state | Decreased pCO$_2$ indicates CO$_2$ loss, which produces an alkalotic state | Decreased HCO$_3^-$ indicates renal bicarb excretion, which produces an acidotic state | Increased HCO$_3^-$ indicates renal bicarb retention, which produces an alkalotic state |
| HCO$_3^-$ is elevated, which would produce an alkalotic state | HCO$_3^-$ is decreased, which would produce an acidotic state | pCO$_2$ is decreased, which would produce an alkalotic state | pCO$_2$ is increased, which would produce an acidotic state |
| This patient has a respiratory acidosis with metabolic compensation as evidenced by the fact that the pH is just above lower limits of normal | This patient has a respiratory alkalosis with metabolic compensation as evidenced by the fact that the pH is just below upper limits of normal | This patient has a metabolic acidosis with respiratory compensation as evidenced by the fact that the pH is just above lower limits of normal | This patient has a metabolic alkalosis with respiratory compensation as evidenced by the fact that the pH is just below upper limits of normal |
| Clinical examples include COPD and respiratory failure | Clinical examples include anxiety with hyperventilation and pulmonary embolus with tachypnea | Clinical examples include diabetic ketoacidosis and renal failure | Clinical examples include volume contraction and hyperaldosteronism |

      (d) Renal tubular acidosis
      (e) Propylene glycol
   (2) Diabetic ketoacidosis—characterized by elevated glucose, metabolic acidosis, and high anion gap
   (3) Alcoholic ketoacidosis—exaggerated by coincident thiamine deficiency; patients often hypoglycemic
   (4) Uremic acidosis—occurs as a consequence of decreased renal H$^+$ secretion; typically accompanied by hyperchloremia
   (5) Salicylate poisoning
 d. Normal-gap acidosis
   (1) Gastrointestinal HCO$_3^-$ loss
   (2) Renal tubular acidosis—abnormalities in renal H$^+$ excretion
 e. Treatment
   (1) Centers on identification and treatment of underlying disorder
   (2) HCO$_3^-$ administration for hyperkalemia or pH < 7.1
   (3) Normal-gap acidosis more likely to require chronic alkali administration
   (4) Chelation or dialysis in some poisoned states
3. Metabolic alkalosis
 a. Characterized by increased pH and HCO$_3^-$
 b. Classified as saline-responsive and saline-unresponsive
 c. Saline-responsive metabolic alkalosis
   (1) Comprises majority of cases
   (2) Occurs as a response to extracellular volume contraction
      (a) Diarrhea, vomiting
      (b) Diuretic excess
      (c) Postoperative volume loss
      (d) Decreased Cl$^-$ promotes renal HCO$_3^-$ retention
      (e) Frequently results in hypokalemia as a consequence of bicarb-mediated renal excretion of potassium
      (f) Compensatory increase in aldosterone promotes sodium retention with resultant potassium excretion
   (3) Treatment
      (a) Treat cause of Cl$^-$ loss—stop diuretics, treat diarrhea
      (b) Replace volume with NaCl
      (c) Replace K$^+$ as necessary
 d. Saline-unresponsive
   (1) Relatively uncommon—when it occurs, it is usually a consequence of hyperaldosteronism (aldosterone-secreting tumor) or excess bicarbonate administration in renal disease
   (2) Hyperaldosteronism
      (a) Excess aldosterone produces increased Na$^+$ retention
      (b) Excess serum Na$^+$ retention results in increased K$^+$ and H$^+$ excretion
   (3) Alkali administration

(a) Chronic kidney disease decreases renal excretion of $HCO_3^-$
(b) Increased $HCO_3^-$ administration/ingestion (antacids) will produce metabolic alkalosis
　(4) Treatment
　　(a) Hyperaldosteronism requires treatment of underlying problem; consider $K^+$ repletion
　　(b) Excess administration often responds to correction of the excess; pH of > 7.6 is an emergent state
4. Respiratory acidosis
　a. Characterized by decreased pH and increased $CO_2$
　b. Causes may be pulmonary or extrapulmonary
　　(1) Alveolar hypoventilation
　　(2) COPD or asthma
　　(3) Central nervous system respiratory depression
　　(4) Obesity-hypoventilation syndrome
　　(5) Drug-induced respiratory suppression (e.g., opiates)
　　(6) Neuromuscular disease with diaphragmatic impairment
　　(7) Myasthenia gravis
　　(8) Amyotrophic lateral sclerosis
　　(9) Guillain-Barré syndrome
　　(10) Decreased responsiveness of chemoreceptors
　　(11) Obstructive sleep apnea
　　(12) Acute respiratory distress syndrome
　　(13) Hypothyroidism
　c. Diagnostic evaluation
　　(1) Centers around identification of underlying condition
　　　(a) Drug screenings as indicated by history and physical examination
　　　(b) Pulmonary function testing may demonstrate obstructive dysfunction
　　　(c) Other studies as indicated by history and physical examination, e.g., brain imaging, chest imaging, diaphragmatic assessment
　　(2) Primary respiratory acid-base disorders are typically uncompensated in the acute state—metabolic compensation may lag by days
　　(3) Chronic respiratory acidosis
　　　(a) Elevated serum bicarbonate as compensatory mechanism
　　　(b) Renal excretion of acid as $NH^4Cl$ produces hypochloremia
　　　(c) Serum hypokalemia may occur as a response to chronic acidosis
　　　(d) Patients who are chronically hypoxic may develop polycythemia
　d. Treatment
　　(1) Rapid correction of respiratory acidosis may result in metabolic alkalosis; caution with ventilator-assisted expiration of $CO_2$
　　(2) Opiate or benzodiazepine reversal agents as indicated
　　(3) Primary efforts at treating underlying cause
　　(4) Oxygen therapy should be considered with caution against suppressing hypoxic drive; when indicated for hypoxemia, titrate to $saO_2$ low 90% range or $paO_2$ 60–65 mm Hg
5. Respiratory alkalosis
　a. Characterized by increased pH and decreased $CO_2$
　b. Most common causes are hyperventilation
　　(1) Anxiety-related hyperventilation
　　(2) Neurological disease
　　(3) Infection and fever
　　(4) Heat exposure
　　(5) Pulmonary embolism
　　(6) Pulmonary edema
　　(7) Mechanical overventilation
　　(8) Drug stimulation
　　(9) Acetylsalicylic acid (ASA)
　　(10) Nicotine
　　(11) Theophylline
　　(12) Decreased responsiveness of chemoreceptors
　　(13) Obstructive sleep apnea
　　(14) Acute respiratory distress syndrome
　　(15) Pain
　　(16) Psychiatric disease
　c. Clinical findings
　　(1) Stocking-glove paresthesia
　　(2) Chest tightness
　　(3) Perioral numbness
　　(4) Vertigo, lightheadedness, confusion due to cerebral vasoconstriction
　　(5) Tetany in severe cases due to increased ionized calcium
　d. Diagnostic evaluation
　　(1) Centers around identification of underlying condition
　　(2) Mild hyponatremia and hypokalemia may occur
　　(3) Increased ionized calcium
　　(4) Drug screens as appropriate
　　(5) TSH (rule out hyperthyroidism)

(6) WBC differential and cultures if sepsis suspected
(7) Chest and brain imaging as appropriate to rule out underlying pulmonary etiology (e.g., pulmonary embolism, CNS tumor)
e. Treatment
(1) Primary efforts directed toward identification and treatment of underlying cause
(2) Emergent treatment not indicated unless pH > 7.5
(3) Rebreathing into a paper bag is controversial but still advocated in some cases
(4) Sedatives only in cases that do not respond to more conservative reassurance
(5) Reduce tidal volume and respiratory rate in ventilated patients
(6) Ensure adequate pain control

# Poisoning and Toxicity

- Definition—*poisoning* refers to the administration of a toxic substance; *overdose* refers to the administration of a benign or therapeutic substance that produces dangerous effects when serum levels exceed the therapeutic window; best management of poisonings and toxicities
  1. General concepts for all poisonings and toxicities
     a. Call poison control for guidance 1-800-222-1222
     b. Initial approach involves four steps
        (1) Assess potential danger
            (a) Substance and amount ingested or absorbed
            (b) Time since exposure
            (c) Underlying metabolic disease that may affect metabolism or excretion
        (2) Consider gut decontamination
        (3) Treat symptoms and complications
        (4) Observe asymptomatic patient for an appropriate time frame
            (a) All asymptomatic patients should be observed for a 6-hour minimum
            (b) Longer observation indicated for ingestion of delayed-release substances or those that slow GI motility
     c. Identify the substance
        (1) When a reliable historian is available, the substance is easily identified
        (2) When patient cannot/will not give history, a physical exam may direct initial care
            (a) Stimulants (cocaine, amphetamine, Ecstasy)
                (i) Tachycardia
                (ii) Hypertension
                (iii) Pupil dilation
                (iv) Agitation
                (v) Dry membranes; thirsty
                (vi) Psychosis
            (b) Depressants (benzodiazepines, opiates, ethanol, sedative-hypnotics)
                (i) Hypotension
                (ii) Bradycardia
                (iii) Hypothermia
                (iv) Pupil constriction
                (v) Obtundation or coma
            (c) Cholinergics (organophosphates [pesticides], cholinesterase-inhibiting drugs [edrophium, donazepil])
                (i) Bradycardia
                (ii) Hypotension
                (iii) Excess salivation
                (iv) Lacrimation
                (v) Vomiting and diarrhea
                (vi) Urinary incontinence
                (vii) Wheezing
            (d) Anticholinergics (atropine, tricyclic antidepressants, first-generation antihistamines)
                (i) Warm skin
                (ii) Tachycardia
                (iii) Pupil dilation
                (iv) Constipation
                (v) Urine retention
                (vi) Delirium
        (3) Elevated anion gap
            (a) Carbon monoxide
            (b) Ethylene glycol
            (c) Salicylates
            (d) Ibuprofen
            (e) Metformin
        (4) Urine screen for drugs of abuse if indicated by history
        (5) Radiographic assessment of the abdomen if suspicion exists for drug muling (rupture of drug-filled, swallowed condoms)
     d. Decontaminate as indicated
        (1) Anesthetize eyes and flush with copious amounts of saline (water if saline unavailable)
            (a) Flush from nasal bridge laterally

(b) Use at least 1 L of saline
(c) Flush to pH of 6–8
(2) Flush skin with lukewarm water or saline; special attention to skin folds and subungal regions
    (a) Add soap or shampoo if substance is oily
    (b) Diluted bleach may be indicated for some toxins (discuss with poison control)
(3) Gastrointestinal decontamination
    (a) Gastric emptying (emesis or diarrhea) not generally indicated; exceptions may include
      (i) Ingestions of large amounts of toxins that delay gastric emptying (anticholinergics, salicylates)
      (ii) Sustained-release substances
      (iii) Use lavage when gastric emptying indicated; emesis is no longer advocated
    (b) Activated charcoal
      (i) Data are conflicting
      (ii) Absorbs most drugs if given rapidly
      (iii) Always consult poison control
    (c) Cathartics
      (i) No clear data to support use
      (ii) Contraindicated in suspected obstruction
(4) Hemodialysis—indicated in some toxicities when symptoms are life-threatening
  e. Treat immediate symptoms
    (1) Airway
    (2) Breathing
    (3) Circulation
    (4) Drugs—when agent is unknown in a comatose patient
      (a) Dextrose 50% IV
      (b) Thiamine 100 mg parenterally
      (c) Nalaxone 0.4 to 2 mg or nalmefene 0.5 to 1 mg IV
    (5) Treat any other apparent immediate consequences pending identification of agent and specific antidote
      (a) Extremes of blood pressure or pulse
      (b) Dysrhythmia
      (c) Seizure
      (d) Hyperthermia
2. Acetaminophen
  a. 7,000 mg/24-hour period is a lethal dose—presentation has four phases
  b. Phase 1 (0–24 hours)
    (1) Asymptomatic, anorexia, nausea or vomiting, malaise
    (2) Subclinical rise in serum transaminase levels begins at about 12 hours post-ingestion
  c. Phase 2 (18–72 hours)
    (1) Right-upper-quadrant abdominal pain, anorexia, nausea, vomiting
    (2) Continued rise in serum transaminase levels
  d. Phase 3 (72–96 hours)
    (1) Centrilobular hepatic necrosis with continued abdominal pain
    (2) Jaundice
    (3) Coagulopathy
    (4) Hepatic encephalopathy
    (5) Nausea and vomiting
    (6) Renal failure
    (7) Fatality
  e. Phase 4 (4 days to 3 weeks)
    (1) Complete resolution of symptoms
    (2) Complete resolution of organ failure
  f. Treatment
    (1) IV fluids
    (2) Activated charcoal if patient presents < 2 hours from ingestion
    (3) N-acetylcysteine 150 mg/kg over 60 minutes followed by 50 mg/kg over 4 hours, and then 100 mg/kg over 16 hours
3. Salicylate
  a. Present in a variety of OTC medications including ASA
  b. Single ingestion of 200 mg/kg is toxic
  c. Symptoms include
    (1) Nausea and vomiting
    (2) Tinnitus
    (3) Diaphoresis
    (4) Hyperventilation
    (5) Confusion and lethargy
    (6) Convulsions and coma
    (7) Cardiovascular failure
  d. Laboratory assessment
    (1) Elevated salicylate level—symptomatic > 60 mg/dL
    (2) Metabolic acidosis
  e. Treatment
    (1) Activated charcoal at a 10:1 ratio of aspirin ingested
    (2) Urinary alkalinization to facilitate renal excretion—100 mEq of $NaHCO_3$ to 1 L of fluid at 150–200 mL/hour—add $K^+$ unless patient is hyperkalemic
    (3) May need hemodialysis if levels very high (> 700 mg/dL)
    (4) Monitor pH closely on intubated patients; do not allow fall in pH

4. Carbon monoxide
   a. Colorless, odorless gas resulting from combustion of carbon-containing materials
   b. Poisonings include accidental exposure and suicide attempts
   c. Binds to Hgb with an affinity 250× greater than oxygen, leading to tissue hypoxia
   d. Causes
      (1) Suicide attempt typically via car exhaust
      (2) Smoke inhalation from fire
      (3) Poorly ventilated gas heater
      (4) By-product from generator
   e. Clinical signs and symptoms
      (1) Low-level exposure (carboxyhemoglobin saturation < 20%)
         (a) Severe headache
         (b) Nausea
         (c) Abdominal discomfort
         (d) Vertigo
      (2) High-level exposure (carboxyhemoglobin saturation > 50%)
         (a) Hypotension
         (b) Mental status changes
         (c) Seizure
         (d) Coma
   f. Laboratory assessment
      (1) Document carboxyhemoglobin level
      (2) Evaluate cardiac rhythm strip for hypoxia-related dysrhythmia
      (3) Traditional pulse oximetry and ABGs not useful and will give false normal oxygen assessments
      (4) Oximetry devices available that differentiate oxyhemoglobin (normal) from carboxyhemoglobin (carbon monoxide)
   g. Treatment
      (1) Remove patient immediately from exposure
      (2) High-flow 100% oxygen administration
      (3) Manage consequences as indicated, e.g., hypotension, seizures
      (4) Encourage CO detectors in the home
5. Stimulants—amphetamine, cocaine, MDMA (Ecstasy)
   a. Often abused because of resultant euphoria
   b. A variety of forms available for oral, inhalant, or parenteral administration
   c. Symptoms and signs include
      (1) Anxiety
      (2) Agitation
      (3) Psychosis
      (4) Hypertension
      (5) Tachycardia, palpitations
      (6) Muscle hyperactivity—may lead to rhabdomyolysis
      (7) Hyperthermia
      (8) Seizure
      (9) Excessive thirst and water ingestion—may lead to hyponatremia
      (10) Extreme states may produce myocardial infarction (MI), cerebrovascular accident (CVA)
   d. Laboratory assessment
      (1) Elevated salicylate level—symptomatic > 60 mg/dL
      (2) Metabolic acidosis
   e. Treatment
      (1) ABCs as with any emergency
      (2) Benzodiazepines for seizure, agitation, psychosis
      (3) Vasodilators for hypertension
         (a) Alpha-beta combination, e.g., labetalol 10–20 mg IV
         (b) Do *not* use pure beta blockade because of risk of unopposed alpha stimulation
      (4) Treat hyperthermia as indicated
      (5) Monitor for electrolyte abnormalities, e.g., hyponatremia
6. Cholinergics—pesticides, cholinesterase inhibitor drugs (edrophium, donazepil)
   a. Cholinergics often used in home gardening
   b. Cholinesterase-inhibiting drugs are used to treat disease such as myasthenia gravis and Alzheimer's dementia
   c. Toxicity results in cholinergic excess (increased parasympathetic activity)
      (1) SLUD symptoms—salivation, lacrimation, urination, defecation
      (2) Cholinergic-mediated bradycardia
   d. Symptoms and signs include
      (1) Nausea and vomiting
      (2) Diarrhea
      (3) "Watery" mouth
      (4) "Leaking" eyes
      (5) Cholinergic-mediated bronchoconstriction
         (a) Wheeze
         (b) Excess sputum production
   e. Laboratory assessment
      (1) Serology not especially helpful unless specific agent known
      (2) Cardiac rhythm strip to assess for bradycardia
   f. Treatment
      (1) Atropine 2 mg IV

            (2) Activated charcoal for oral poisonings
            (3) Vasodilators for hypertension
                (a) Alpha-beta combination, e.g., labetalol 10–20 mg IV
                (b) Do *not* use pure beta blockade because of risk of unopposed alpha stimulation
            (4) Treat hyperthermia as indicated
            (5) Monitor for electrolyte abnormalities, e.g., hyponatremia
    7. Ethylene glycol and methanol
        a. Methanol (wood alcohol) used as a substitute for ethanol in alcoholic patients
        b. Ethylene glycol is major component of antifreeze
        c. Both compounds metabolize to dangerous toxic organic acids
        d. Symptoms and signs include
            (1) Methanol
                (a) Visual disturbances
                (b) Nausea and vomiting
                (c) Abdominal pain
                (d) Lethargy, confusion
                (e) Seizures, coma
            (2) Ethylene glycol
                (a) Stage I
                    (i) Intoxication
                    (ii) Slurred speech
                    (iii) Ataxia
                    (iv) Stupor
                    (v) Hallucinations
                    (vi) Seizures, coma
                (b) Stage II
                    (i) Hypertension
                    (ii) Tachycardia
                    (iii) High-output renal failure
                    (iv) Myositis
                (c) Stage III
                    (i) Costovertebral angle tenderness
                    (ii) Oliguria or anuria
        e. Laboratory assessment
            (1) Evaluate levels of suspected toxin
            (2) Increased anion gap
            (3) Urine microsopy
        f. Treatment
            (1) Empty stomach by nasogastric aspiration if patient presents within 1 hour
            (2) Consider dialysis
            (3) Ethanol as antidote
            (4) Fomepizole may be primary treatment; contact poison control
            (5) Folic acid, thiamine, and pyridoxine to promote breakdown of toxic metabolites

# THE TRANSPLANT PATIENT

- Definition—organ transplantation includes a wide variety of topics, including donor, recipient, living and nonliving donors, general indications and contraindications, and management of the patient both in the immediate postoperative period as well as long term. A variety of organs are transplanted each year, and a number of these issues are addressed individually based on the specific organs

- General Considerations
    1. Criteria for inclusion on transplant list are organ-dependent
    2. Patients are referred to transplant evaluation by primary care or specialty provider
    3. Extensive evaluation by the transplant team
        a. Thorough history and physical examination
        b. Laboratory evaluation—organ-specific
        c. Determination is made for eligibility
        d. Waiting times are prioritized and the following are considered:
            (1) Medical urgency
            (2) Transplanted organ
            (3) Time on list
            (4) Distance between donor and potential organ
            (5) Number of donors in a local area
            (6) Blood and tissue types
    4. 246 transplant centers exist in the United States; there are 58 organ procurement organizations
    5. Five steps of organ matching
        a. An organ is donated
        b. United Network for Organ Sharing (UNOS) generates a list of potential recipients
        c. Transplant center is notified of available organ
        d. Transplant team considers the organ for the patient
        e. Organ is accepted or declined
    6. Types of donors
        a. Living donors (partial donation)
            (1) Lung
            (2) Liver
            (3) Intestine
            (4) Pancreas
        b. Deceased—brain death
            (1) Age criteria—organ-specific
            (2) Expanded donor criteria
                (a) Age > 50 years with hypertension (HTN), CVA, creatinine > 1.5 mg/dL
                (b) Age > 60 years
                (c) HTN at time of death
                (d) CVA as cause of death

c. Donation after cardiac death (DCD)
   (1) The potential DCD donor:
       (a) Has suffered a devastating neurological injury, such as head trauma, anoxic injury, or intracranial bleeding
       (b) Is maintained on a ventilator
       (c) Does not meet brain death criteria
       (d) Family wants withdrawal of support
       (e) Is likely to die from cessation of cardiopulmonary function within 60 minutes
7. Donor disqualifiers
   a. HIV
   b. Actively spreading cancer
   c. Severe infection
8. Contraindications—organ-specific
   a. Heart
      (1) Age > 70 years
      (2) Fixed pulmonary hypertension
      (3) HIV/AIDS
      (4) Sarcoidosis or systemic lupus erythematosus (SLE)
      (5) Irreversible renal or hepatic dysfunction
      (6) Nondermal neoplasm
      (7) A variety of relative contraindications are considered case by case
          (a) Substance abuse
          (b) COPD
          (c) Psychiatric illness
          (d) Gastric disease
   b. Lung
      (1) Age > 70 years
      (2) HIV/AIDS
      (3) Hepatitis B or C
      (4) Malignancy
      (5) Active smoker
      (6) Psychiatric disease
      (7) Irreversible deconditioning
   c. Liver
      (1) Uncontrolled bacterial or fungal infection outside hepatobiliary system
      (2) Active nonhepatobiliary malignancy
      (3) Advanced cardiopulmonary disease
      (4) Active drug or alcohol use
      (5) Relative contraindications
          (a) Age > 70 years
          (b) Portal vein thrombosis
          (c) Pulmonary hypertension
          (d) Congenital cardiac anomalies
          (e) Psychiatric disease
          (f) HIV
          (g) Cholangiocarcinoma
   d. Kidney
      (1) Few absolute contraindications
          (a) Untreated infection
          (b) Metastatic disease
          (c) Chronic illness
          (d) Uncontrolled psychiatric disease
          (e) Substance abuse
      (2) Several relative contraindications
          (a) Active hepatitis
          (b) Coronary artery disease
          (c) Cerebrovascular disease
          (d) Active peptic ulcer disease
          (e) HIV/AIDS
          (f) Noncompliance
          (g) Obesity
9. Types of rejection
   a. Hyperacute
      (1) Immediate rejection when graft is perfused
      (2) Is a consequence of antigens/antibodies to the graft
      (3) When circulation returned, antibodies bind to the graft and inhibit perfusion
      (4) Uncommon as a result of good pre-transplant management
   b. Acute
      (1) Character and timing are organ-specific
      (2) May occur within the first month to first year
      (3) Management includes
          (a) High-dose corticosteroids
          (b) Optimize immunosuppressants
          (c) Humanized antilymphocytic monoclonal antibody
   c. Chronic rejection
      (1) Increased risk in patient with
          (a) Atherosclerosis
          (b) History of acute rejection
      (2) Occurs as a consequence of increased immune activation
      (3) Best management is prevention
10. Survival statistics
    a. Heart—1 year 82%; 5 year 70%
    b. Lung—1 year 78%; 5 year 50%
    c. Liver—1 year 86%; 5 year 72%
    d. Kidney—1 year 90%; 5 year 80%

## SHOCK STATES

- Definition—shock is a state in which cardiac output is inadequate to achieve tissue perfusion, characterized by a systolic blood pressure (SBP) < 90 mm Hg. The immediate risk is of decreased perfusion to the vital organs; immediate management strategies are centered on maintaining an adequate blood pressure while identifying and treating the underlying problem

- Four general shock states, each characterized by predictable abnormalities in cardiac pressures (see **Table B-5**).
  1. In all types of shock, general patient assessment is consistent with tissue hypoperfusion and hypoxia
  2. Hypovolemic
     a. Cause—occurs in any circumstance that produces intravascular hypovolemia
        (1) Acute blood loss
        (2) Dehydration
        (3) Extravascular third-spacing
     b. Cardiac pressures consistent with intravascular hypovolemia and compensatory peripheral arterial constriction and increased tissue extraction of oxygen
        (1) Pulmonary capillary wedge pressure (PCWP) decreased
        (2) Cardiac index (CI) and cardiac output (CO) decreased
        (3) Systemic vascular resistance (SVR) increased
        (4) Central venous pressure (CVP) decreased
        (5) $SvO_2$ decreased
        (6) Pulmonary artery pressure (PAP) decreased
     c. Treatment—increasing intravascular volume is the mainstay of therapy
        (1) Isotonic fluids if appropriate
        (2) Colloid fluids if third-spacing present
        (3) Blood products as necessary
  3. Cardiogenic shock
     a. Cause—any condition that decreases cardiac systolic function
        (1) Congestive heart failure
        (2) Acute myocardial infarction
        (3) Cardiomyopathy
        (4) Dysrhythmia

**TABLE B-5** Normal Range of Cardiac Pressures and Indices

| | |
|---|---|
| Right atrial (RA) | 0 to 7 mm Hg |
| Right ventricular (RV) | 20 to 30 mm Hg (systolic) |
| | 0 to 5 mm Hg (diastolic) |
| Pulmonary artery (PA) | 20 to 30 mm Hg (systolic) |
| | 8 to 12 mm Hg (diastolic) |
| | < 20 mm Hg (mean) |
| Pulmonary artery occlusion pressure (PAOP) | 6 to 12 mm Hg |
| Saturation of mixed venous oxygen ($SvO_2$) | 75% |
| Systemic vascular resistance (SVR) | 900–1,300 (dyn.s/cm$^5$) |
| Cardiac output (CO) | 4.8 to 6.4 L/min |
| Cardiac index (CI) | CO / body surface area (BSA) |

  b. Cardiac pressures consistent with cardiac congestion, decreased cardiac output, compensatory peripheral arterial constriction, and increased tissue oxygen extraction
     (1) PCWP increased
     (2) SVR increased
     (3) $SvO_2$ decreased
     (4) CVP increased
     (5) CI/CO decreased
     (6) CVP increased
  c. Treatment—correct cause of systolic dysfunction, support blood pressure
     (1) Acute coronary syndrome (ACS) protocol
     (2) Isotonic fluids as tolerated—caution against fluid overload; intravascular volume is not the primary problem, but controlled fluid support is necessary to maintain blood pressure while acute
     (3) Inotropic agents as indicated
        (a) Dobutamine
        (b) Phosphodiesterase inhibitors
  4. Obstructive shock
     a. Causes—any circumstance that obstructs ventricular filling
        (1) Pulmonary embolus
        (2) Cardiac tamponade
        (3) Pneumothorax
     b. Cardiac pressures consistent with decreased ventricular volume and impaired forward flow (decreased fluid in ventricles and arterial tree), increased fluid in atria and venous system due to impaired ventricular filling, compensatory peripheral and pulmonary artery constriction and increased tissue oxygen extraction
        (1) CI/CO decreased
        (2) SVR and pulmonary vascular resistance (PVR) increased
        (3) PCWP decreased
        (4) CVP increased
        (5) $SvO_2$ decreased
     c. Treatment—support blood pressure while relieving cause of obstructed filling
        (1) Isotonic fluids
        (2) Decompress pneumothorax
        (3) Relieve cardiac tamponade
        (4) Consider embolectomy when pulmonary embolus produces shock
  5. Distribute shock
     a. Causes—any circumstance that produces a maldistribution of vascular volume with disproportionate flow in arteries and veins resulting in impaired cardiac return
        (1) Neurogenic—spinal cord injury may produce paradoxical vasodilation above level of the injury

(2) Anaphylaxis—IgE-mediated vasodilation promotes volume distribution into arterial and venous circulation
            (3) Sepsis—sepsis produces maladaptive vasodilation that promotes volume distribution into arterial and venous circulation
    b. Cardiac pressures consistent with relative hypovolemia in arterial and venous circulation, decreased intracardiac volume and output, and an inability to maintain peripheral arterial resistance; in septic shock, tissue extraction of oxygen is impaired
        (1) CI/CO initially increased as the healthy heart tries to compensate; eventually both measures decrease as a result of decreased ventricular filling
        (2) PCWP decreased
        (3) SVR decreased
        (4) CVP decreased
        (5) SvO$_2$ increased in septic shock; decreased in neurogenic and anaphylaxis
    c. Treatment—support blood pressure while treating underlying cause
        (1) Isotonic fluids
        (2) Consider vasopressors
        (3) Epinephrine for anaphylaxis
        (4) Antibiotic therapy for septic shock
        (5) Monitor septic shock for disseminated intravascular coagulation

## QUESTIONS

1. A 54-year-old man is postoperative day 1 following an uncomplicated open cholecystectomy. Nursing staff pages to report that he has a temperature of 100.5° F. The best response for the ACNP would be to:

    a. Order acetaminophen 650 mg p.o. now and q.i.d. prn temp > 100.5° F
    b. Do nothing at this time because this low-grade temperature is likely a normal physiological response to surgery
    c. Increase intravenous fluids to 125 cc/hour and reassess in 8 hours
    d. Begin a third-generation cephalosporin antibiotic to cover gram-negative organisms

2. In the febrile postoperative patient, which of the following signs or symptoms is most consistent with infection?

    a. Pain at the incision site
    b. Azotemia
    c. Anorexia
    d. Neutrophilia

3. Which of the following types of hyponatremia is likely to respond best to diuretic therapy with normal saline infusion?

    a. Hypotonic, hypovolemic
    b. Hypertonic
    c. Hypotonic, hypervolemic
    d. Isotonic

4. An 80-year-old female is admitted to your service with dehydration and a change in mental status. Fully expecting that she will be hypernatremic as a result of extracellular concentration of sodium, you are surprised to find that she has a serum sodium of 116 mEq/dL. Your next action should be to:

    a. Order 3% NaCl solution for 1 L; and then change to NSS
    b. Order a urine sodium
    c. Order a serum osmolality
    d. Order NSS at 150 cc/hour

5. What is the most likely cause of hyponatremia in a patient with a urine sodium of 50 mEq/dL?

    a. Chronic diarrhea
    b. Hyperglycemia
    c. Diuretic excess
    d. Diabetes insipidus

6. What is the appropriate intervention for a patient with a serum calcium of 14 mEq/dL?

    a. 10 U of humulin R, 1 amp of D50W, 1 amp of NaHCO$_3$ intravenously
    b. Consult nephrology for dialysis—this is a medical emergency
    c. Lasix 60 mg intravenously with NSS at 125 cc/hour
    d. 1 amp of intravenous calcium carbonate

7. A 42-year-old female presents for preadmission testing for a uterine ablation scheduled for the following Monday. She denies any significant medical or surgical history, and the only medication she takes is the occasional acetaminophen tablet for headache. Which of the following diagnostic studies is least appropriate:

    a. A complete blood count
    b. A urinalysis
    c. An ECG
    d. A urine hCG

8. An 81-year-old woman with a permanent tracheostomy is admitted for treatment of pneumonia. Her baseline mental status is confused, and with the infectious process she has become almost obtunded. She will need nutritional support as

her p.o. intake has decreased to almost nothing since she has become ill. What is the most appropriate choice for nutritional support?

a. A nasoduodenal tube
b. A PEG tube
c. Peripheral parenteral nutrition
d. A nasogastric tube

9. Which acid-base disorder is most common in the postoperative period?

a. Metabolic acidosis
b. Metabolic alkalosis
c. Respiratory acidosis
d. Respiratory alkalosis

10. In which of the following scenarios is it appropriate to give intravenous $NaHCO_3$?

a. In a patient with respiratory acidosis due to drug overdose
b. In a patient with diabetic ketoacidosis and a pH of 7.1
c. A patient with hyperkalemia and ECG changes
d. A patient with chronic acidosis secondary to chronic kidney disease

11. Many electrolyte abnormalities are fairly easy to recognize because they produce specific clinical findings. Which of the following electrolyte abnormalities is particularly dangerous because its only findings are fatigue, anorexia, and maybe depression?

a. Hyponatremia
b. Hyperkalemia
c. Hypercalcemia
d. Hypokalemia

12. What is the most common cause of hypertonic hyponatremia?

a. Diuretic use
b. Renal salt wasting
c. Diarrhea
d. Hyperglycemia

13. A high anion gap represents a large difference between:

a. The positive and negative extracellular ions
b. The charged and uncharged extracellular solutes
c. The positive extracellular and intracellular ions
d. The charged and uncharged intracellular solutes

14. A normal gap acidosis is typically treated with:

a. Fluid resuscitation
b. Oral bicitra with meals
c. Calcium gluconate
d. Dialysis

15. Which of the following metabolic states will decrease ionized calcium?

a. Hypo-osmolality
b. Normal-gap acidosis
c. Alkalosis
d. Hyperglycemia

16. Which of the following is not a cause of volume-contraction alkalosis?

a. Diuretics
b. NG suctioning
c. Posthypercapnia states
d. Hyperaldosteronism

17. A patient with a long history of congestive heart failure has been on loop diuretics for 6 years. He recently experienced 3 days of nausea and vomiting that he attributed to food poisoning. Today he presents with weakness, hypotension, and decreased skin turgor. ABG reveals a pH of 7.47 and an elevated serum bicarbonate. Therapy should include an infusion of:

a. $HCO_3^-$
b. D5W
c. Colloids
d. Normal saline

18. A patient with chronic respiratory acidosis secondary to COPD is admitted in acute respiratory failure. Mechanical ventilation is initiated. During the period in which his kidneys are compensating, you would expect to see:

a. Increased pH and increased bicarbonate
b. Increased pH and decreased bicarbonate
c. Decreased pH and increased bicarbonate
d. Decreased pH and decreased bicarbonate

19. A 65-year-old alcoholic male is found to have a serum $Ca^{++}$ of 7.5 mEq/dL. He is carefully questioned regarding symptoms of the disorder and reports generalized muscle cramps and paresthesias around his lips. Which additional laboratory would you need to rule out a calcium abnormality?

a. Hemoglobin
b. Glucose
c. Albumin
d. Potassium

20. A 63-year-old patient is admitted with a recent onset of nausea, vomiting, diarrhea, and new onset confusion. Past medical history is positive for seizures. Physical findings include a heart rate of 110 bpm, supine BP of 110/80 mm Hg, upright BP of 90/58 mm Hg, and poor skin turgor. Serum electrolytes reveal a serum Na+ of 128 mEq/L. Which laboratory examination should be the next step in evaluating the cause of the sodium imbalance?

   a. Serum osmolality
   b. Serum chloride
   c. Urine catecholamines
   d. Urine sodium

21. An important complication of inadequately treated acute hyponatremia is:

   a. Atrioventricular block
   b. Paralytic ileus
   c. Cerebral edema
   d. Tetany

22. With respect to the management of congestive heart failure in the preoperative period, what is the appropriate procedure in terms of medication management?

   a. No medication should be administered after 10:00 p.m. the night prior to surgery
   b. Patients should be diuresed intravenously as needed the morning of surgery
   c. Routine medications should be administered the morning of surgery
   d. Congestive heart failure should be controlled before surgery is performed

23. Harold is 5'6", 269 lbs, and 59 years old. He is scheduled for a bowel resection of a malignant obstructing tumor in the ascending colon. He has a complex medical history including type 2 DM controlled on glyburide, CAD with an MI 3 years ago, hypertension, and seizure disorder. His multiple medical conditions are relatively stable, and he is having surgery today. What is the appropriate intraoperative management of Harold's DM?

   a. Administer his morning dose of glyburide and monitor intraoperative sugars q.2.h.
   b. Infuse 0.1u/kg/hour of insulin and maintain sugars at about 250 mg/dL via separate glucose infusion
   c. Hold his glyburide preoperatively and follow sugars intraoperatively; administer short-acting insulin per protocol (IV or SQ) to maintain glucose < 250 mg/dL
   d. Hold oral agents preoperatively and infuse 5% dextrose at 100 cc/hour intraoperatively

24. Bleeding and infection are the two most common causes of postoperative complication. Which of the following is not an indicator of increased risk for infection?

   a. Corticosteroid use
   b. Prolonged antibiotic therapy
   c. Renal failure
   d. A leukocyte count of 5,500

25. What is the most accurate indicator of general preoperative nutritional status?

   a. Serum albumin
   b. Serum transferrin
   c. Dietary history
   d. Height-to-weight ratio

26. Renal failure patients:

   a. Should be dialyzed the morning of surgery to optimize their metabolic status preoperatively
   b. Should be dialyzed immediately after surgery to correct fluid loss/excesses created intraoperatively
   c. Should not be dialyzed the day of surgery because the traumatic induction of cellular fluid shifts can predispose to hypotension
   d. Should be dialyzed in accordance with their typical schedule without regard to surgery

27. One of the primary emphases of the preoperative history and physical examination is the:

   a. Detection of risk factors for intraoperative renal failure
   b. Identification of undiagnosed cardiopulmonary disease
   c. Prevention of complications related to nutritional deficits
   d. Documentation of existing chronic illnesses

28. During a preoperative evaluation, a patient is found to have several large bruises on the arms and legs. The remainder of the physical examination is benign. The nurse practitioner orders additional testing with results as follows:

   | Hgb | 13.5 |
   | --- | --- |
   | Hct | 40% |
   | INR | 1.2 |
   | WBC | 9.5 |
   | PT | 12 seconds |
   | PTT | 28 seconds |
   | Plt | 300 K |

   The next appropriate action would be to:

a. Cancel the surgery pending more extensive evaluation
b. Notify the surgeon
c. Call social services
d. Repeat the laboratory assessment

29. A 72-year-old woman presents with complaints of nausea, polyuria, and constipation. Her muscles are weak upon examination, and she exhibits depressed deep tendon reflexes. She has been supplementing her diet with calcium antacids in an effort to prevent osteoporosis. Her serum calcium is 13 mEq/L. Serum albumin is normal. In an effort to correct the calcium, you would begin treatment with:

a. Hypotonic saline and thiazide diuretics
b. Normal saline and loop diuretics
c. Colloids and magnesium
d. Normal saline and insulin

30. Enteral feedings often produce diarrhea when first begun. The best intervention is to:

a. Decrease the amount of feeding and reintroduce gradually
b. Begin *C. difficile* prophylaxis
c. Order a mild antidiarrheal
d. Supplement with parenteral nutrition

31. What is the best intervention for fever of unknown origin?

a. Acetaminophen if the fever is > 101° F
b. Nothing until the diagnosis is confirmed
c. Broad spectrum IV antibiotics
d. Broad spectrum p.o. antibiotics

32. Who is at greatest risk for developing a deep vein thrombosis?

a. A 32-year-old male with cirrhosis of the liver
b. An 18-year-old female on oral contraceptives
c. A 22-year-old female paraplegic
d. A 41-year-old-male with atrial fibrillation

33. Before instituting anticoagulant therapy in the treatment of deep vein thrombosis, the diagnosis must be supported with which of the following diagnostic studies?

a. A venogram
b. No diagnostic testing is required—a clinical diagnosis is adequate
c. A prothrombin time
d. A Doppler ultrasound

34. When assessing a patient for potential surgical risk factors, the AGACNP knows that patients who report using herbal medications should be evaluated closely for:

a. Infection
b. Depression
c. Bleeding
d. Fluid retention

35. A patient on your service is scheduled for a right lower lobectomy. Preoperative PFTs are as follows:

FVC 80% of predicted
$FEV_1$ 65% of predicted
$FEV_{25-75}$ 65% of predicted
RV 100% of predicted

These results are consistent with:

a. Mild obstructive disease
b. Mild restrictive disease
c. Moderate obstructive disease
d. Moderate restrictive disease

36. You have placed a patient with ARDS on an $FIO_2$ of 100% and PEEP of 10 cm. The ABGs are as follows: pH 7.36, $paCO_2$ 37, $paO_2$ 60, $HCO_3^-$ 23. Which of the following indicators of improvement do you anticipate?

a. pH of 7.4
b. $paCO_2$ of 40
c. $paO_2$ of 70
d. $HCO_3^-$ of 25

37. Which of the following factors will likely have the greatest impact on a patient's ability to wean from mechanical ventilation?

a. COPD
b. Anemia
c. Diabetes
d. Azotemia

38. A 28-year-old-male is brought into the emergency department with a methamphetamine overdose. The patient reported "body packing," or ingesting a bag full of methamphetamine, when the police pulled him over for speeding. The AGACNP determines the most important risk reduction intervention should be directed toward:

a. Hyperthermia
b. Paranoia
c. Acute coronary syndrome
d. Pain

39. You are discussing organ donation with a patient who is interested in registering for organ

donation. The patient has a history for traumatic brain injury 10 years ago, CVA 2 years ago, and breast cancer 5 years ago now in remission. The patient is currently being treated for gram-negative sepsis for *E. coli*. In your discussion, you relay that the patient does not qualify for organ donation because of:

   a. *E. coli* infection
   b. Traumatic brain injury
   c. CVA
   d. Breast cancer

40. Post-transplant patients are at high risk for infection due to immunosuppression and steroid use to decrease rejection. In the first postoperative month, which of the following infections are of greatest concern?

   a. Community-acquired
   b. Bacterial
   c. Fungal
   d. All of the above

41. In evaluating a patient for a liver transplant, the nurse practitioner recognizes the following as a contraindication for transplantation:

   a. Alcoholic cirrhosis
   b. Biliary cirrhosis
   c. Encephalopathy
   d. Spontaneous bacterial peritonitis

42. In a plan of care for the post-transplant patient in the first 3 months, the focus will be prevention and monitoring of:

   a. Infection
   b. Nephrotoxicity
   c. Rejection
   d. Cancer

43. You are the first practitioner to arrive to a rapid response call for a patient who is postoperative day 2 following a heart transplant. The patient is unresponsive with a heart rate of 28 beats per minute. The AGACNP knows that all of the following are appropriate choices in treating bradyarrhythmias in a postoperative heart transplant *except*:

   a. Isoproterenol 0.2–0.6 mg IV bolus
   b. Atropine 0.5 mg IV bolus
   c. Transcutaneous pacing at a rate of 95
   d. Epinephrine 1 mg IV bolus

44. A 59-year-old male comes to the clinic for his routine examination. He has a history of a liver transplant, and the nurse practitioner notes no corticosteroids on the medication list he provides. The nurse practitioner knows:

   a. The main drug for immunosuppression in liver transplant patients is a corticosteroid
   b. The patient must be on a regimen of three medications
   c. A referral should be made to see the transplant physician
   d. Liver transplantation often requires less immunosuppression than transplantation of other organs does, and corticosteroids can often be discontinued

45. While on call you are asked to evaluate a deteriorating patient. This patient was admitted for pneumonia and exacerbation of CHF. The systolic blood pressure is < 90 mm Hg, and urine output is < 10 mL/hour. ECG reveals no acute processes but reveals previously noted changes consistent with bilateral atrial and ventricular enlargement and a marked left axis deviation. You insert a PA line and anticipate which of the following pressures?

   a. Cardiac index of 1.3 L/min, PAOP of 27 mm Hg; RA of 18 mm Hg
   b. Cardiac index of 1.9 L/min, PAOP of 12 mm Hg; RA of 6 mm Hg
   c. Cardiac index of 2.4 L/min, PAOP of 18 mm Hg; RA of 8 mm Hg
   d. Cardiac index of 1.4 L/min, PAOP of 7 mm Hg; RA of 4 mm Hg

46. The $svO_2$ is increased in which shock state?

   a. Cardiogenic
   b. Hypovolemic
   c. Septic
   d. Obstructive

47. The ACNP knows that patients in _____ shock initially exhibit an increased cardiac output followed by a decreased cardiac output.

   a. Cardiogenic
   b. Hypovolemic
   c. Distributive
   d. Neurogenic

48. Which type of shock places the patient at highest risk for disseminated intravascular coagulation?

   a. Septic
   b. Hypovolemic
   c. Obstructive
   d. Neurogenic

49. All of the following have indications for gut decontamination of ingested poisons *except*:

a. Induced emesis
b. Gastric lavage
c. Activated charcoal
d. Catharsis

50. A comatose patient is being seen in the emergency department for suspected poisoning. There is no one to provide a history, and no empty containers or medication bottles were found at the scene. Physical examination reveals a pulse of 129 bpm, blood pressure of 190/110 mm Hg, temperature of 101.9° F, and dry mucous membranes. The pupils are dilated bilaterally. Bowel sounds are hyperacute, and there appears to be some dried vomit around the patient's mouth. The AGACNP suspects what kind of poisoning?

a. Depressant
b. Stimulant
c. Cholinergic
d. Anticholinergic

## Answers

| | | | |
|---|---|---|---|
| 1. | c | 26. | a |
| 2. | d | 27. | b |
| 3. | c | 28. | d |
| 4. | c | 29. | b |
| 5. | c | 30. | a |
| 6. | c | 31. | b |
| 7. | c | 32. | c |
| 8. | a | 33. | d |
| 9. | b | 34. | c |
| 10. | c | 35. | a |
| 11. | c | 36. | c |
| 12. | d | 37. | b |
| 13. | a | 38. | c |
| 14. | b | 39. | a |
| 15. | c | 40. | b |
| 16. | d | 41. | d |
| 17. | d | 42. | c |
| 18. | c | 43. | b |
| 19. | c | 44. | d |
| 20. | a | 45. | a |
| 21. | c | 46. | c |
| 22. | b | 47. | c |
| 23. | c | 48. | a |
| 24. | d | 49. | a |
| 25. | a | 50. | b |

## BIBLIOGRAPHY

Bongard, F., Sue, D., & Vintch, J. (2008). *Current diagnosis & treatment in critical care* (3rd ed.). New York, NY: McGraw-Hill Medical.

Bronfenbrener, R. (2013). Acid–base interpretation. Retrieved from http://emedicine.medscape.com/article/2058760-overview#aw2aab6b3

Brown, L. K. (2010). Hypoventilation syndromes. *Clinics in Chest Medicine, 31*(2), 249–270.

Chan-Tack, K. M. (2014). Fever of unknown origin. Retrieved from http://emedicine.medscape.com/article/217675-overview

Chassot, P. G., Marcucci, C., Spahn, D. R., & Delabays, A. (2010). Perioperative antiplatelet therapy. *American Family Physician, 82*(12), 1444–1489.

Doherty, G. M. (2009). *Current surgical diagnosis and treatment* (13th ed.). New York, NY: McGraw-Hill.

Feeley, M. A., Collins, S. C., Daniels, P. R., Kebede, E. B., Jatoi, A., & Mauck, K. F. (2013). Preoperative testing before noncardiac surgery: Guidelines and recommendations. *American Family Physician, 87*(6), 414–418.

Fleisher, L. A., Beckman, J. A., Brown, K. A., Calkins, H., Chaikof, E. L., Fleischmann, K. E., . . . Yancy, C. W. (2007). ACC/AHA 2007 guidelines on the perioperative cardiovascular evaluation and care for noncardiac surgery. *Journal of the American College of Cardiology, 50*(17), 1707–1732. Retrieved from http://circ.ahajournals.org/content/116/17/e418.full

Gupta, A., & Reilly, C. S. (2007). Fat embolism. *Continuing Education in Anaesthesia, Critical Care & Pain, 7*(5), 148–151.

Laffey, J. G. (2002). Hypocapnia. *New England Journal of Medicine, 347*(1), 43–53.

Lo-Trivedi, M. (2013). Perioperative management of the diabetic patient. Retrieved from http://emedicine.medscape.com/article/284451-overview#aw2aab6b8

Madappa, T. (2014). Atelectasis. Retrieved from http://emedicine.medscape.com/article/296468-overview

Marino, P. L. (2013). *The ICU book* (4th ed.). Philadelphia, PA: Wolters Kluwer Health/Lippincott Williams & Wilkins.

McPhee, S. J., & Papadakis, M. A. (2012). *Current medical diagnosis and treatment* (51st ed.). New York, NY: McGraw-Hill.

Mullen, J. T., Moorman, D. W., & Davenport, D. L. (2009). The obesity paradox: Body mass index and outcomes in patients undergoing nonbariatric general surgery. *Annals of Surgery, 250*(1), 166–172.

Washington University School of Medicine. (2010). *The Washington manual of medical therapeutics* (33rd ed.). Philadelphia: Wolters Kluwer Health/Lippincott Williams & Wilkins.

# Index

**Note:** Page numbers followed by *f* or *t* indicate material in figures or tables respectively.

## A

abortion, 314–315
abruptio placentae, 299
abstinence, 312
acarbose, 162–163
ACE inhibitors. *See* angiotensin-converting enzyme inhibitors
acetaminophen, 346
acid-base balance, preoperative patient management, 330
acid-base disorders
    assessment of, 342, 343*t*
    definition of, 342
    metabolic acidosis, 342–343
    metabolic alkalosis, 343–344
    respiratory acidosis, 344
    respiratory alkalosis, 344–345
acne vulgaris, 47–48
acquired immunodeficiency syndrome (AIDS), 181–184
acronyms, in developing memory, 5
acrostics technique, for memory development, 5
actinic keratosis, 37
acute bacterial prostatitis, 196
acute care, problems in
    acid-base disorders, 342–345
    electrolyte abnormalities, 338–342
    fever, 334–337
    nutritional support, 337–338, 338*f*, 339*t*
    poisoning and toxicity, 345–348

acute gastroenteritis, 145–148, 147*t*
acute iodiopathic polyneuropathy, 240
acute lymphocytic leukemia (ALL), 126*t*
acute myelogenous leukemia (AML), 126*t*
acute otitis media (AOM), 70–71
acyclovir, 189
Addison's disease, 171–172
adolescents
    anticipatory guidance for health, 25–27
    health monitoring, 23–25
    immunization schedule, 28
    interviewing guidelines for, 22–23
adult hypothyroidism, 168–170, 169*t*
adults
    health
        anticipatory guidance for, 26–27
        immunization schedule, 28
        monitoring, screenings for, 25
    older. *See* elderly
advanced practice nursing, 267–281
    conceptual models for, 269
    definition of, 267–268
    under managed care, 277–279
    practice issues, 269–276
    professional organizations, 276
    regulations/credentialing, 270–271
    reimbursement, 273–276
    research, 276
    role development, 268–269
    scope/standards, 269–270

Advanced Practice Registered Nurse (APRN). *See* advanced practice nursing
AFPNP/AP. *See* Association of Faculties of Pediatric Nurse Practitioner and Associate Programs
African Americans, cultural beliefs, 17
aging theories, 32–34
AIDS. *See* acquired immunodeficiency syndrome
alcoholism
    definition, 255
    diagnosis, 256
    etiology/incidence, 255
    management/treatment, 256–257
    signs and symptoms, 255–256, 255*t*
ALL. *See* acute lymphocytic leukemia
allergic rhinitis, 78–79
alopecia, 48–49
alpha-glucosidase inhibitor, 162–163
alphabet technique, for memory development, 5
Alzheimer's disease (AD), 238–239
amantadine, 237
amenorrhea, 205–206
AML. *See* acute myelogenous leukemia
amniocentesis, 293
amylin analogs, 163
analysis, definition of, 4
anemias, 330
    of chronic disease, 120*t*, 124
    definition of, 117

357

anemias (Continued)
  diagnostic tests for, 119t
  folic acid-deficiency, 122–124
  iron-deficiency, 117–120, 120t
  macrocytic, 120t, 121
  microcytic, 117, 120t
  normocytic, 120t, 124
  pernicious, 121–122
  sickle cell, 124–125
  thalassemia, 120–121, 120t
angina, 103–106, 105f
angiotensin-converting enzyme inhibitors (ACE inhibitors), 103, 108
ankle sprain, 224
antacids, 137
anterior drawer test, 223
anticholinergics, 237
antidepressants, 251
antiretroviral therapy (ART), 183
antisecretory agents, 137
antiseizure medications, 236
antithyroid drugs, 167–168
anxiety, 330
  categories, 253
  diagnosis, 254
  etiology/incidence, 253
  management/treatment, 254–255
  signs and symptoms, 253–254
AOM. See acute otitis media
Apley's grind test, 223
appendicitis, 140–141
application/analysis, developing as thinking skill, 4–6
APRN. See advanced practice nursing
ART. See antiretroviral therapy
aseptic meningitis, purulent vs., 241t
Asian Americans, cultural beliefs, 17
aspiration, pulmonary, 333
Association of Faculties of Pediatric Nurse Practitioner and Associate Programs (AFPNP/AP), 268
asthma, 88–90, 95t–96t
atelectasis, postoperative complications, 332–333
atopic dermatitis, 51, 52
attitude, for test taking, 11
autonomic dysreflexia, 242t

## B

$B_{12}$ deficiency, 120t
backaches
  low, 298
  during pregnancy, 295
bacterial infections, of skin, 49–51
bacterial prostatitis, 196
bacterial vaginosis (BV), 192–193
barium radiographs, 136
basal cell carcinoma (BCC), 37, 56–58
benign prostatic hyperplasia (BPH), 198–199
beta blockade, 347–348
beta blockers, 55, 69, 88–89, 105
beta cell stimulants (secretagogues), 162
biguanide (metformin), 162
bilirubin, 119t
biophysical profile (BPP), 295
bipolar disorder, 248
bleeding
  dysfunctional uterine, 201–203
  nosebleed, 74–75
  postoperative complications, 331–332
  during pregnancy, 297
  risk factors, preoperative patient management, 329
blepharitis, 67
blood pressure, cardiovascular disorders and, 101
blood sugar testing, 161
body mass index (BMI), 19
bone marrow smear, 119t
Botulism gastroenteritis, 145, 147t
BPH. See benign prostatic hyperplasia
BPP. See biophysical profile
breasts
  cancer, 200–201
  fibrocystic changes of, 200
  physical assessment, 38
bronchitis
  acute, 86
  chronic, 90–91
Brown–Sequard syndrome, 242t
bursitis, 221–222
BV. See bacterial vaginosis

## C

CAD. See coronary artery disease
calcium channel blockers, 105
calcium, recommended dietary intakes, 18, 18t
Campylobacter gastroenteritis, 145, 147t
cancer
  breast, 200–201
  cervical, screening for, 203
  colorectal, 150–151
  lung, 93
  prostate, 199
  skin, 56–58
candidiasis of skin, 53–54
capitation model, 276
carbon monoxide, 347

carbuncle, 49, 50
cardiac risk factors, 23
cardiac testing, preoperative patient management, 328
cardiogenic shock, 350
cardiovascular disorders
  chronic venous insufficiency, 109–110
  congestive heart failure, 107–108
  coronary artery disease, 103–106, 105f
  dyslipidemia, 106
  endocarditis, 110
  hypertension, 101–103
  pericarditis, 110
  peripheral arterial disease, 108–109
  thrombophlebitis, 109
cardiovascular system, 38
carpal tunnel syndrome, 222–223
case management, 271–272
cataracts, 70
catechol-o-methyltransferase (COMT), 237
CBC. See complete blood count
cellulitis, 49–51
Centers for Medicare and Medicaid Services (CMS), 275
central cord syndrome, 242t
cervarix, 190
cervical cancer screening, 203
CGL. See chronic granulocytic leukemia
Change Theory, 16
chest radiography, preoperative patient management, 327
CHF. See congestive heart failure
chlamydial infection, genital, 185–186
cholecystitis, 139–140
cholesterol-lowering diet, 106
cholinergics, 347–348
chorionic villus sampling (CVS), 293
chronic bacterial prostatitis, 196–197
chronic bronchitis, 90
chronic disease. See also specific chronic diseases
  anemias of, 120t, 124
chronic granulocytic leukemia (CGL), 126t
chronic illness control, preoperative patient management, 329–330
chronic lymphocytic leukemia (CLL), 126t
chronic myelogenous leukemia (CML), 126t
chronic obstructive pulmonary disease (COPD), 90–91
chronic venous insufficiency, 109–110
cimetidine, 137

Civil Monetary Penalties (CMPs), 280
CK-MB. *See* creatine kinase muscle-brain
CLL. *See* chronic lymphocytic leukemia
cluster headaches, 232
CML. *See* chronic myelogenous leukemia
CMPs. *See* Civil Monetary Penalties
CMS. *See* Centers for Medicare and Medicaid Services
COC. *See* combination oral contraceptives
colorectal cancer, 150–151
combination oral contraceptives (COC), 301–303
common cold. *See* nasopharyngitis
complete blood count (CBC), 136
   preoperative patient management, 327
comprehension, 4
COMT. *See* catechol-o-methyltransferase
concentration peaks, 7
condoms
   female, 311
   male, 310
condylomata acuminata (genital warts), 189–191
confusion. *See* delirium
congestive heart failure (CHF), 107–108, 329–330
conjunctivitis, 65–67, 66*t*
constipation, during pregnancy, 296
contact dermatitis, 51, 52
content
   assessment, for test taking, 6, 6*t*–7*t*
   knowledge, in test taking, 6–9, 6*t*–8*t*
contraception methods
   abortion, 314–315
   abstinence, 312
   diaphragms, 311–312
   female sterilization, 313–314
   fertility awareness methods, 312–313
   male sterilization, 314
   pharmacological contraceptives
      combination oral, 301–303
      emergency, 307
      progestin-only, 303–304
      progestin-only implants, 306–307
      transdermal, 304
      vaginal rings, 304–305
   for women over, 317
contraceptive vaginal ring (NuvaRing), 304–305

contraction stress test (CST), 295
Cooley's anemia, 120
COPD. *See* chronic obstructive pulmonary disease
corneal abrasion, 68
coronary angiography, 104
coronary artery disease (CAD), 103–106, 105*f*, 329
coronary revascularization, 105–106
corticosteroids, for preterm labor, 301
counseling, exercise, 20
cramming, for tests, 8
creatine kinase muscle-brain (CK-MB), 111
CST. *See* contraction stress test
cultural beliefs, in healthcare encounters, 16–17
CURB-65 criteria, 88
Cushing's syndrome, 170–171
CVS. *See* chorionic villus sampling
cystitis, 194–195

# D

dawn phenomenon, 165
deep vein thrombosis (DVT), postoperative complications, 333
delirium
   definition, 259
   diagnosis, 260
   etiology/incidence, 259
   management/treatment, 260–261
   signs and symptoms, 259–260
dementia, 238–239
Depo-Provera (progestin-only injectable contraception), 305–306
depression
   definition, 247
   diagnosis, 249
   etiology/incidence, 248–249
   management/treatment, 250–251
   signs and symptoms, 249
   suicide and, 251–253
   types of, 247–248
dermatitis, 51–53
dermatological disorders, 47
   acne vulgaris, 47–48
   alopecia, 48–49
   dermatitis, 51–53
   fungal/yeast infections, 53–54
   papulosquamous disorders, 54–56
   pyodermas, 49–51
   scabies, 56
   skin cancer, 56–58
   viral dermatoses, 58–60

diabetes mellitus (DM), 329
   diagnosis, 160
   etiology/incidence, 159–160
   exercise for, 162
   management/treatment, 161–166, 161*t*, 163*t*, 165*t*
   signs/symptoms, 160
diabetic ketoacidosis (DKA), 172–173
diagnostic evaluation, 327
diaphragms, 311–312
diet therapy. *See under specific disorders*
dipeptidyl peptidase-4 (DPP-4) inhibitors, 163
distribute shock, 350–351
diuretics, 102, 103, 108
diverticulitis, 141–142
DKA. *See* diabetic ketoacidosis
DM. *See* diabetes mellitus
donors, types of, 348–349
dopamine agonists, 236–237
drug abuse, psychoactive, 257–259
Drugs. *See* medications; *specific medications*
DUB. *See* dysfunctional uterine bleeding
duodenal ulcer, 135
DVT. *See* deep vein thrombosis
dysfunctional uterine bleeding (DUB), 201–203
dyslipidemia, 106
dysmenorrhea, 206
dysplasia, 203–205
dyspnea, during pregnancy, 297
dysthymia, 247

# E

*E. coli* gastroenteritis, 145, 147*t*
ear disorders
   acute otitis media, 70–71
   hearing loss, 72–73
   otitis externa, 71–72
   otitis media, 70–71
   serous otitis media, 71
   vertigo, 73–74
echocardiography, 112
ECT. *See* electroconvulsive therapy
ectopic pregnancy, 298–299
edema, during pregnancy, 297
elderly
   anticipatory guidance for health, 26–27
   biological aging theories, 32–33
   demographics of, 31–32
   functional assessment, 36–37
   health monitoring, 25
   interview and health history, 34–36

elderly (Continued)
    interviewing guidelines for, 23
    living situations/income status, 36
    nutritional risk factors, 19
    pharmacotherapy and, 40–41
    physical assessment, 37–40
    psychosocial aging theories, 33–34
    safety for, 21
electrocardiography, 104
    preoperative patient management, 328
electroconvulsive therapy (ECT), 251
electrolyte abnormalities
    definition, 338
    hypercalcemia, 341–342
    hyperkalemia, 341
    hypernatremia, 339
    hypocalcemia, 341
    hypokalemia, 339–341
    hyponatremia, 338–339, 340t
emergency contraceptives, 307
emphysema, 90–91
Employment Retirement Income Security Act (ERISA), 280
endocarditis, 110
endocrine disorders
    Addison's disease, 171–172
    adult hypothyroidism, 168–170, 169t
    Cushing's syndrome, 170–171
    diabetes mellitus. See diabetes mellitus (DM)
    physical assessment, 39
    thyroid nodule, 170
    thyrotoxicosis, 166–168, 167t
endoscopy, 136
enteral nutritional support, 338
environment, health and, 21–22
epicondylitis, 222
epididymitis, 197–198
episodic model, 276
epistaxis, 74–75
Erikson's Stages of Psychosocial Development, 15
ERISA. See Employment Retirement Income Security Act
ERV. See expiratory reserve volume
ethylene glycol, 348
evidence-based practice, 280–281
exam day, preparation for, 11
exentide, 163
exercise
    benefits of, 20
    counseling, 20
    for diabetes mellitus, 162
    electrocardiography (stress testing), 104
    plan, 20
    prescription components, 20–21
    tension-relaxation, 17
exercise thallium imaging, 104
expiratory reserve volume (ERV), 85
eye disorders
    blepharitis, 67
    cataracts, 70
    conjunctivitis, 65–67, 66t
    corneal abrasion, 68
    foreign bodies, 67–68
    glaucoma, 66t, 68–70
    iritis, 66t
eyelid margins, inflammation of, 67

# F

failure, dealing with, 11
famciclovir, 189
family history, 22
famotidine, 137
fat embolism, postoperative complications, 333
fatigue, during pregnancy, 296
Federal Employee Health Benefits Program (FEHBP), 276
fee-for-service model, 276
$FEF_{25-75}$. See forced expiratory flow 25–75
FEHBP. See Federal Employee Health Benefits Program
female condoms, 311
ferritin, serum, 118, 119t
fertility awareness methods, 312–313
fetal movements, 295
$FEV_1$. See forced expiratory volume
fever
    assessment of, 334–335, 335f
    definition of, 334
    FUO, 336
    management of, 336–337
    metabolic costs of, 334
    noninfectious causes of, 335t
    physiological benefits of, 334
    postoperative, 335–336
fever blister (herpes simplex I), 58–60
fever of unknown origin (FUO), 336
    management of, 336–337
fibrocystic breast changes, 200
fluid management, postoperative patient management, 333–334
folic acid-deficiency anemias, 120t, 122–124
folliculitis, 49, 50
food cravings, during pregnancy, 296
forced expiratory flow 25–75 ($FEF_{25-75}$), 85
forced expiratory volume ($FEV_1$), 85, 90
forced vital capacity (FVC), 85
foreign body, in eye, 67–68
FRC. See functional residual capacity
functional bowel syndrome, 148–149
functional residual capacity (FRC), 85
fungal infections, of skin, 53–54
furunculosis, 49, 50
FVC. See forced vital capacity

# G

gallbladder inflammation, 139–140
Gardasil, 190
gastric ulcer, 135
gastroenteritis, acute, 145–148, 147t
gastroesophageal reflux disease, 138–139, 138t
gastrointestinal decontamination, 346
gastrointestinal disorders
    acute gastroenteritis, 145–148, 147t
    appendicitis, 140–141
    cholecystitis, 139–140
    colorectal cancer, 150–151
    diverticulitis, 141–142
    gastroesophageal reflux disease, 138–139, 138t
    inflammatory bowel disease, 149–150
    irritable bowel syndrome, 148–149
    peptic ulcer disease, 135–138
    physical assessment, 38
    viral hepatitis, 142–145, 144t, 146t
General Adaptation Syndrome, 17
General Systems Theory, 16
genetic cellular theories, 33
genital chlamydial infection, 185–186
genital warts, 189–191
genitourinary/gynecological disorders
    acquired immunodeficiency syndrome, 181–184
    acute bacterial prostatitis, 196
    acute pyelonephritis, 195–196
    amenorrhea, 205–206
    benign prostatic hyperplasia, 198–199
    breast cancer, 200–201
    chronic bacterial prostatitis, 196–197
    dysfunctional uterine bleeding, 201–203
    dysmenorrhea, 206
    dysplasia, 203–205
    epididymitis, 197–198
    fibrocystic breast changes, 200
    genital chlamydial infection, 185–186
    genital warts, 189–191
    gonorrhea, 184–185
    herpes genitalis, 188–189

lower urinary tract infection, 194–195
pelvic inflammatory disease, 191–192
physical assessment, 39
premenstrual syndrome, 206–207
prostate cancer, 199
syphilis, 186–188
upper urinary tract infections, 195
vulvovaginitis, 192–194
giant cell arteritis, 217
*Giardia lamblia* gastroenteritis, 145, 147t
glaucoma, 66t, 68–70
Goeckerman regimen, 55
gonorrhea, 184–185
gout, 217–218
Graves' disease, 166
Guillain-Barré syndrome, 240

## H

$H_2$ receptor antagonists, 137
hair loss (alopecia), 48–49
hallucinogenic abuse, 259
HAV. *See* hepatitis A vaccine
HBV. *See* hepatitis B vaccine
headaches, 229–232
    cluster, 232
    evaluation, 229–230
    migraine, 230–232
    during pregnancy, 296
    tension, 230
Health Behavior Change Models, 16
Health Belief Model, 15
health history, 22, 34–36
Health Insurance Portability and Accountability Act of 1996 (HIPAA; Public Law 104-191), 279–280
Health maintenance organizations (HMOs), 278
health policy, 276–279
health promotion/evaluation, 15
    age-related monitoring, 23–25, 24t
    cultural beliefs and, 16–17
    environment and, 21–22
    evaluation, across lifespan, 22–28
    lifestyle factors and, 17–22, 18t
    prevention levels and, 16
    safety and, 21–22
    theories/models of, 15–16
Health Promotion Model, 15
healthcare delivery systems, 277–279
Healthcare Effectiveness Data and Information Set (HEDIS), 278
*Healthy People 2020*, 276–277
hearing loss, 34, 72–73
    physical assessment, 39
heartburn, during pregnancy, 296

HEDIS. *See* Healthcare Effectiveness Data and Information Set
*Helicobacter pylori*, 136
hematocrit, 118, 119t
hematological and oncological disorders
    anemias. *See* anemias
    Hodgkin's disease, 127–128
    leukemia, 125–126, 126t
    non-Hodgkin's lymphoma, 126–127
hemoglobin, 118, 119t
hemoglobin H disease, 121
hemorrhoids, during pregnancy, 296
hepatitis A vaccine (HAV), 27
hepatitis B vaccine (HBV), 27
hepatitis, viral, 142–145, 144t, 146t
herpes genitalis, 188–189
herpes simplex I (fever blister), 58–60
herpes zoster (shingles), 58–60
hidradentitis suppurativa, 49, 50
Hierarchy of Needs, Maslow, 15
Hispanic Americans, cultural beliefs, 16
HIV infection. *See* human immunodeficiency virus infection
HMG CoA reductase inhibitors, 106
HMOs. *See* Health maintenance organizations
Hodgkin's disease, 127–128
homeostasis, postoperative patient management, 331, 332f
hormone therapy (HT), 317–318
HPV. *See* human papillomavirus
HT. *See* hormone therapy
human immunodeficiency virus (HIV) infection, 181–184
human papillomavirus (HPV), 27, 58–60, 190
hyperaldosteronism, 343
hypercalcemia, 341–342
hypercortisolism, 170–171
hyperkalemia, 341
hypernatremia, 339
hypertension, 101–103, 330
hypocalcemia, 341
hypoglycemia, 164–165
hypokalemia, 339–341
hyponatremia, 338–339, 340t
hypoperfusion, tissue, 331
hypothyroidism, adult, 168–170, 169t
hypovolemic shock, 350

## I

IBD. *See* inflammatory bowel disease
IBS. *See* irritable bowel syndrome
ideal body weight (IBW), calculation of, 162

imaging technique, in developing memory, 5
immune competence, preoperative patient management, 328–329
immunizations, 27–28, 297
impetigo, 49, 50
incretin mimetics, 163
indirect Coombs test, 119t
infectious mononucleosis, 77–78
inflammatory bowel disease (IBD), 149–150
influenza, 75–76
influenza vaccine, 27
Ingram regimen, 55
insulin allergy, 165
insulin resistance, 165
insulins, 163–164, 163t
    metabolism/action, 165t
integrated delivery systems, 278
integumentary system, 37–38
intrauterine devices (IUDs), 307–315
iritis, 66t
iron-deficiency anemias, 117–120, 120t
iron replacement therapy, 118
iron, serum, 119t
irritable bowel syndrome (IBS), 148–149
ischemic cerebrovascular accident, 240–241
IUDs. *See* intrauterine devices

## K

Kaposi's sarcoma (KS), 56–58
knee pain, 223–224
knowledge, test taking and, 4
KS. *See* Kaposi's sarcoma

## L

labor
    preterm, 300–301
    signs/symptoms of, 292–293
Lachman test, 223
lactic dehydrogenase (LDH), 111
LBP. *See* low back pain
leg cramps, during pregnancy, 296–297
Leopold's maneuvers, 293
leukemia, 125–126, 126t
leukorrhea, during pregnancy, 296
levodopa/carbidopa, 236, 237
links technique, in developing memory, 5
lipids, serum, 104
lipodystrophy, 165
liraglutide, 163
low back pain (LBP), 220–221
lower urinary tract infection (LUTI), 194–195

# Index

lung cancer, 93
LUTI. *See* lower urinary tract infection
lyme disease, 27

## M

macrocytic anemias, 120*t*, 121
major depression (MD), 247
male condoms, 310
male sterilization, 314
malignant melanoma (MM), 38, 56–58
malpractice, 272
managed care, 277–279
Maslow's Hierarchy of Needs, 15
maternal serum alpha-fetoprotein (MSAFP), 293
maximum voluntary ventilation (MVV), 85
MCH. *See* mean corpuscular Hgb
MCHC. *See* mean corpuscular Hgb concentration
McMurray's test, 223
MCV. *See* mean corpuscular volume
mean corpuscular Hgb (MCH), 119*t*
mean corpuscular Hgb concentration (MCHC), 119*t*
mean corpuscular volume (MCV), 119*t*
measles-mumps-rubella vaccine (MMR), 27
Medicaid, 273
medical history, past, 22, 35
Medicare, 273–274
medications. *See also specific medications*
   problems with use of, 41
   use during pregnancy, 297
meglitinides, 162
memory, 4–5, 8
meningococcal vaccine, 27
menopause, 315–318
metabolic acidosis, 342–343
metabolic alkalosis, 343–344
metformin (biguanide), 162
methanol, 348
methimazole, 168
microcytic anemias, 117, 120*t*
miglitol, 162–163
migraine headache, 230–232
Mini-Mental State Exam (MMSE), 37
MM. *See* malignant melanoma
MMR. *See* measles-mumps-rubella vaccine
motivation, for test taking, 12
MSAFP. *See* maternal serum alpha-fetoprotein
multiple choice questions (MCQs), 9
multiple sclerosis (MS), 237–238

muscle strain, 224–225
musculoskeletal disorders
   ankle sprain, 224
   bursitis, 221–222
   carpal tunnel syndrome, 222–223
   epicondylitis, 222
   giant cell arteritis, 217
   gout, 217–218
   knee pain, 223–224
   low back pain, 220–221
   muscle strain, 224–225
   osteoarthritis, 213–214
   osteoporosis, 218–220
   physical assessment, 39
   rheumatoid arthritis, 214–216
   systemic lupus erythematosus, 216–217
music technique, for memory development, 5
MVV. *See* maximum voluntary ventilation
*Mycobacterium avium* complex, 183
*Mycobacterium tuberculosis*, 183
myocardial infarction, 42

## N

nasopharyngitis, 75
National Committee for Quality Assurance (NCQA), 278–279
National Council of State Boards of Nursing (NCSBN), 267–268
National Organization of Nurse Practitioner Faculties (NONPF), 268
Native Americans, cultural beliefs, 16
nausea/vomiting, during pregnancy, 295
NCQA. *See* National Committee for Quality Assurance
NCSBN. *See* National Council of State Boards of Nursing
neck disorders, physical assessment, 39–40
negligence, 273
*Neisseria gonorrhoeae*, 184
Neuman's Systems Model, 16
neurological disorders, 229–242
   dementia, 238–239
   headaches, 229–232
   MS, 237–238
   Parkinson's disease, 236–237, 239
   seizure disorder, 234–236
   TIA, 232–234
neurological system, 40
neurosyphilis, 186–188
nizatidine, 137
non-Hodgkin's lymphoma, 126–127

nongenetic cellular theories, 33
nonhormonal management
   vasomotor symptoms, 318
   vulvovaginal symptoms, 318
NONPF. *See* National Organization of Nurse Practitioner Faculties
nonstress test (NST), 294–295
normal-gap acidosis, 343
normocytic anemias, 120*t*, 124
nose disorders
   allergic rhinitis, 78–79
   epistaxis, 74–75
   infectious mononucleosis, 77–78
   influenza, 75–76
   nasopharyngitis, 75
   pharyngitis, 76–77
   physical assessment, 39–40
   sinusitis, 79–80
nosebleed, 74–75
NSAID-induced ulcers, 137
NST. *See* nonstress test
nurse practice acts, 269–270
nurse practitioners (NPs), role development, 268–269
Nursing's Agenda for Health Care Reform, 277
*Nursing's Social Policy Statement*, 271
nutrition
   assessment for weight loss, 18–19
   for athletic performance, 21
   dietary guidelines, 18
   evaluation, 35
   prenatal, 292
   risk factors for elderly, 19
nutritional status, preoperative patient management, 328
nutritional support, 337–338, 338*f*, 339*t*
NuvaRing (vaginal contraceptive rings), 304–305

## O

OA. *See* osteoarthritis
obesity, as risk factor, 23
OBRA. *See* Omnibus Budget Reconciliation Act
obsessive-compulsive disorder (OCD), 253
obstructive shock, 350
occupational and environmental history, 22
OCD. *See* obsessive-compulsive disorder
OGTT. *See* oral glucose tolerance test
older adults. *See* elderly
Omnibus Budget Reconciliation Act (OBRA), 274

oncological disorders. *See* hematological and oncological disorders
OPQRST symptom analysis, 22
oral glucose tolerance test (OGTT), 161
organ transplantation, 348–349
organic mood syndrome, 248
organization, for study preparation, 6–7, 6t–8t
osteoarthritis (OA), 213–214
osteoporosis, 218–220
otitis externa, 71–72
otitis media, 70–71
overpreparation, for tests, 12

**P**
PAD. *See* peripheral arterial disease
pap smear, abnormal, 203–205
papulosquamous disorders, 54–56
parenteral nutritional support, 338, 339t
Parkinson's disease, 236–237, 239
past medical history, 35
pathogens. *See under specific disorder*
Patient Self-Determination Act (1990), 36
peak expiratory flow rate (PEFR), 85
PEFR. *See* peak expiratory flow rate
pelvic inflammatory disease (PID), 191–192, 309
peptic ulcer disease (PUD), 135–138
pericarditis, 110
peripheral arterial disease (PAD), 108–109
peripheral blood smear, 119t
pernicious anemias, 121–122
persistent generalized lymphadenopathy (PGL), 182
personal habits, in health history, 22
PFTs. *See* pulmonary function tests
PGL. *See* persistent generalized lymphadenopathy
pharmacotherapy. *See also under specific disorder*
  and elderly, 40–41
pharyngitis, 76–77
PHI. *See* protected health information
physical activity, health and, 19–21
physical fitness
  evaluation of, 21
  health benefits and, 20
physiological systems theories, 33
pica, during pregnancy, 296
PID. *See* pelvic inflammatory disease
PIH. *See* pregnancy induced hypertension

pink puffer (emphysema), 5
pityriasis rosea, 54–56
placenta previa, 299
plantar warts, 59
PMS. *See* premenstrual syndrome
pneumococcal vaccine, 27
*Pneumocystis jiroveci* pneumonia, 183
pneumonia, 87–88
point of service plans (POS), 278
poisoning and toxicity
  acetaminophen, 346
  carbon monoxide, 347
  cholinergics, 347–348
  concepts for, 345–346
  definition, 345
  ethylene glycol and methanol, 348
  salicylate, 346
  stimulants, 347
polio, 27
POP. *See* progestin-only pills
POS. *See* point of service plans
positive attitude, for test taking, 11
post-traumatic stress disorder (PTSD), 253
postoperative fever, 335–336
postoperative patient management
  complications, 331–333
  definition, 330
  documentation, 331
  fluid management, 333–334
  homeostasis, 331, 332f
  pain and fear response, 331
  tissue damage response, 331
  volume loss and tissue hypoperfusion, 331
postzoster neuralgia, 60
PPD. *See* purified protein derivative
PPI. *See* proton pump inhibitors
practice tests, 11
pramlintide, 163
PRECEDE Model, 16
pregnancy, 289–301
  backaches, 295
  bleeding, 297
  complaints, common, 295–297
  complications, 297–301
  constipation, 296
  diagnosis, 289, 290
  ectopic, 298–299
  edema, 297
  fatigue, 296
  food cravings, 296
  headaches, 296
  heartburn, 296
  hemorrhoids, 296
  immunizations, 297
  leg cramps, 296–297

  leukorrhea, 296
  medication use, 297
  physiological changes, 290
  prenatal care, 290–295
  round ligament pain, 297
  urinary frequency, 296
  vaginal discharge (leukorrhea), 296
  varicosities, 296
pregnancy-induced hypertension (PIH), 291, 299–300
premenstrual syndrome (PMS), 206–207
prenatal nutrition, 292
preoperative evaluation, 327
preoperative patient management
  chronic illness, control of, 329–330
  definition, 327
  history and physical examination, 327
  laboratory and diagnostic screening, 327–328
  physical and emotional readiness, 330
  surgical risk assessment, 328–329
preoperative preparation, 327
preterm labor (PTL), 291, 300–301
prevention, levels of, 16
primary adrenocortical insufficiency, 171–172
primary health care, 277
primary prevention, 16
Prinzmetal's angina, 103
procrastination, 7
professional organizations, 276
progestin-only implants, 306–307
progestin-only injectable contraception (Depo-Provera), 305–306
progestin-only pills (POP), 303–304
propylthiouracil (PTU), 168
prostate cancer, 199
protected health information (PHI), 279
  deidentification of, 280
proton pump inhibitors (PPI), 136–137
psoriasis vulgaris, 54–56
psychoactive substance abuse
  definition, 257
  diagnosis, 258
  etiology/incidence, 257
  management/treatment, 258–259
  signs and symptoms, 257–258
psychosocial development, stages of, 15
psychosocial disorders, 247–261
  alcoholism, 255–257, 255t
  anxiety, 253–255

psychosocial disorders (*Continued*)
  delirium, 259–261
  depression. *See* depression
  psychoactive substance abuse, 257–259
  suicide, 251–253
psychosocial history, 22
PTL. *See* preterm labor
PTSD. *See* post-traumatic stress disorder
ptyalism, during pregnancy, 296
Public Law 104-191 (Health Insurance Portability and Accountability Act of 1996), 279–280
PUD. *See* peptic ulcer disease
pulmonary aspiration, postoperative complications, 333
pulmonary disease. *See* respiratory disorders
pulmonary function tests (PFTs), 85–86
  preoperative patient management, 328
purified protein derivative (PPD), 86, 91–92
purulent meningitis *vs*. aseptic, 241*t*
pyelonephritis, 292
  acute, 195–196
pyodermas, 49–51

## Q
quality improvement (QI), 272

## R
RA. *See* rheumatoid arthritis
radioactive iodine ($^{131}$I), 167
radioactive iodine uptake (RAIU), 167*t*
radionuclide ventriculography, 104
ranitidine, 137
RBC. *See* red blood cell count
RDW. *See* red cell distribution width
reciprocal determinism, 15
recombinant tissue plasminogen activator (rtPA), characteristics of, 241*t*
red blood cell count (RBC), 119*t*
red cell distribution width (RDW), 119*t*
reimbursement issues for advance nursing practice, 273–276
reimbursement, under managed care, 278
renal disease, 330
renal failure, postoperative complications, 333
residual volume (RV), 85
respiratory acidosis, 344
respiratory alkalosis, 344–345

respiratory disorders
  acute bronchitis, 86
  asthma, 88–90, 95*t*–96*t*
  chronic obstructive pulmonary disease, 90–91
  lung cancer, 93
  pneumonia, 87–88
  pulmonary function tests and, 85–86
  tuberculosis, 91–92
  VAP prevention strategies, 97*f*
respiratory system, 38
retrieval of information, memory skills, 5
rheumatoid arthritis (RA), 214–216
rhymes technique, in developing memory, 5
Rinne test, 73
risk factors, identification of, 23
risk management, 272
round ligament pain, during pregnancy, 297
rtPA. *See* recombinant tissue plasminogen activator
RV. *See* residual volume

## S
safety
  assessment, 35–36
  health and, 21–22
salicylate, 346
scabies, 56
SCC. *See* squamous cell carcinoma
screening guidelines, age-related, 23–25, 24*t*
seborrheic dermatitis, 51, 52
secondary prevention, 16
secretagogues (beta cell stimulants), 162
seizure disorder, 234–236
selegiline, 237
Self-Efficacy Theory, 15
self-fulfilling prophecy, 11
self-worth, positive, 11
serological tests, 136
serous otitis media (SOM), 71
*Shigella/Salmonella* gastroenteritis, 145, 147*t*
shingles (herpes zoster), 58–60
shock
  cardiac pressures, 350, 350*t*
  definition, 349
  types of, 350–351
Short Portable Mental Status Questionnaire (SPMSQ), 36
sickle cell anemias, 124–125
sinusitis, 79–80

skin
  bacterial infections of, 49–51
  cancer, 56–58
  candidiasis of, 53–54
  disorders. *See* dermatological disorders
  fungal infections of, 53–54
  yeast infections of, 53–54
SLE. *See* systemic lupus erythematosus
slow vital capacity (SVC), 85
SMI. *See* Supplementary Medical Insurance
social support, health and, 18
SOM. *See* serous otitis media
somogyi phenomenon, 165
spermicides, vaginal, 310
spinal cord syndromes, 242*t*
spirometry, 85
spontaneous abortion, 297
squamous cell carcinoma (SCC), 37, 56–58
*Staphylococcus* gastroenteritis, 145, 147*t*
starvation, 19
stasis dermatitis, 51, 52
sterilization
  female, 313–314
  male, 314
stimulants, 347
stress
  management, 17–18
  reduction technique, 17
  theoretical basis of, 17
stress testing (exercise electrocardiography), 104
stressors, types of, 17
study aids, 9
study plan development, 7, 8*t*
studying
  active participation in, 9
  areas of concentration for, 9
  breaks in, 8
  creating space for, 6
  preparation for, 6–7, 6*t*–7*t*
  stopping, 9
  time considerations, 8
substance abuse
  alcoholism, 255*t*
  psychoactive drug, 257–259
sucralfate, 137
suicide
  definition, 251
  diagnosis, 252
  elderly and, 252
  etiology/incidence, 251–252
  management/treatment, 252–253
  risk factors for, 23
  signs and symptoms, 252

sulfonylureas, 162
Supplementary Medical Insurance (SMI), 274
SVC. *See* slow vital capacity
swimmer's ear. *See* otitis externa
syphilis, 186–188
systemic lupus erythematosus (SLE), 216–217
Systems Theories, 16

## T

Tanner staging, 24
taste, physical assessment, 40
TB. *See* tuberculosis
tennis elbow (epicondylitis), 222
tension headaches, 230
tertiary prevention, 16
tests
    content assessment, 6, 6*t*–7*t*
    questions, components of, 9–11, 10*t*
    taking, strategies/techniques for, 1
        become test-wise, 9–11, 10*t*
        develop your thinking skills, 4–6
        know the content, 6–9, 6*t*–8*t*
        know yourself, 3
        psych yourself up, 11–12
        rules, 10, 12
    types, study methods for, 6
tetanus-diphtheria vaccine (Td), 27
thalassemia, 120–121, 120*t*
thiazolidinediones, 162
thinking
    levels of, 4
    skills, development of, 4–6
throat disorders
    allergic rhinitis, 78–79
    infectious mononucleosis, 77–78
    influenza, 75–76
    pharyngitis, 76–77
    physical assessment, 39–40
thromboembolism risk factors, preoperative patient management, 329
thrombophlebitis, 109
thyroid assessment tests, 167, 167*t*
thyroid nodule, 170
thyrotoxicosis, 166–168, 167*t*
TIA. *See* transient ischemic attack
TIBC. *See* total iron binding capacity
tinea, 53–54
tissue
    damage response, 331
    hypoperfusion, 331
TLC. *See* total lung capacity
tocolytics, 301
total iron binding capacity (TIBC), 118, 119*t*
total lung capacity (TLC), 85
touch, physical assessment, 40
transdermal contraceptive system, 304
transferrin saturation percentage, 119*t*
transient ischemic attack (TIA), 232–234
transplant patient, 348–349
Transtheoretical Model, 16
*Trichomonas vaginalis*, 192–194
troponin T, 111
tuberculosis (TB), 91–92
Tzanck stain, 188

## U

ultrasonography, 294
upper urinary tract infection, 195–196
urea breath test, 136
urinalysis, preoperative patient management, 327
urinary frequency, during pregnancy, 296
urinary tract infection
    lower, 194–195
    upper, 195–196

## V

vaginal contraceptive rings (NuvaRing), 304–305
vaginal discharge (leukorrhea), during pregnancy, 296
vaginal spermicides, 310
valacyclovir, 189
varicella vaccine, 27
varicosities, during pregnancy, 296
vascular dementia (VaD), 239
vasomotor symptoms, nonhormonal management of, 318
verruca plantaris, 59
verruca vulgaris, 59
vertigo, 73–74
viral dermatoses, 58–60
viral hepatitis, 142–145
    adult prophylaxis for, 146*t*
    serology tests for, 144*t*
vision impairments, 39
vulvovaginal candidiasis (VVC), 192–194
vulvovaginal symptoms, nonhormonal management of, 318
vulvovaginitis, 192–194
VVC. *See* vulvovaginal candidiasis

## W

warts
    common, 59
    genital, 189–191
wasting syndrome, 182
Weber test, 73
weight loss
    body mass index and, 19
    guidelines for healthy, 19
    nutrition assessment for, 18–19
    prognostic factors, 19
    strategies, 19

## Y

yeast infections, of skin, 53–54

## Z

zostavax vaccine, 27